LEFT VENTRICULAR DIASTOLIC DYSFUNCTION AND HEART FAILURE

LEFT VENTRICULAR DIASTOLIC DYSFUNCTION AND HEART FAILURE

William H. Gaasch, M.D.

Professor of Medicine
University of Massachusetts Medical School
Chief of Cardiology
The Medical Center of Central Massachusetts
Worcester, Massachusetts

Martin M. LeWinter, M.D.

Professor of Medicine
University of Vermont
Director, Cardiology Unit
Medical Center Hospital of Vermont
Burlington, Vermont

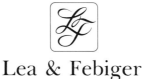

Lea & Febiger

PHILADELPHIA • BALTIMORE • HONG KONG
LONDON • MUNICH • SYDNEY • TOKYO
A WAVERLY COMPANY
1994

Lea & Febiger
Box 3024
200 Chester Field Parkway
Malvern, Pennsylvania 19355-9725
U.S.A.
(215) 251-2230

Executive Editor—R. Kenneth Bussy
Development Editor—Tanya Lazar
Manuscript Editor—Jessica Howie Martin
Production Manager—Michael DeNardo

Library of Congress Cataloging-in-Publication Data

Left ventricular diastolic dysfunction and heart failure / [edited by]
    William H. Gaasch, Martin M. LeWinter.
        p.   cm.
    Includes bibliographical references and index.
    ISBN 0-8121-1509-0
    1. Congestive heart failure—Pathophysiology.   2. Heart—Left
ventricle—Pathophysiology.   3. Diastole (Cardiac cycle)
I. Gaasch, William H.   II. LeWinter, Martin M.
    [DNLM: 1. Ventricular Function, Left—physiology.   2. Diastole—
physiology.   3. Heart Diseases—therapy.   4. Heart Diseases—
physiopathology.   5. Heart Diseases—diagnosis.   WG 200 L495 1993]
RC685.C53L44   1993
616.1'29071—dc20
DNLM/DLC
for Library of Congress   93-9991
                                                                    CIP

NOTE: Although the author(s) and the publisher have taken reasonable steps to ensure the accuracy of the drug information included in this text before publication, drug information may change without notice and readers are advised to consult the manufacturer's packaging inserts before prescribing medications.

Reprints of chapters may be purchased from Lea & Febiger in quantities of 100 or more. Contact Sally Grande in the Sales Department.

PRINTED IN THE UNITED STATES OF AMERICA

Print Number: 5   4   3   2   1

Dedication

*To our wives
Rita Gaasch and Barbara LeWinter*

Preface

The clinical syndrome of congestive heart failure has long been recognized to be caused by disorders of left ventricular systolic contraction, but only in the past two decades have physiologists and clinicians recognized the importance of the diastolic properties of the heart in the genesis of this disorder. During the 1970s, investigators studied the pathophysiology of diastole and the mechanisms causing left ventricular diastolic dysfunction. These studies emphasized the physical properties of the fully relaxed ventricle (i.e., chamber and myocardial stiffness) and the dynamic factors that are intrinsic to the myocardium (i.e., myocardial relaxation) as well as those extrinsic to the ventricle (i.e., pericardium and right ventricle). During the 1980s, numerous articles reflecting the clinical importance of diastolic dysfunction appeared in the medical literature. These studies documented the frequency of congestive failure in the presence of normal left ventricular systolic function. Myocardial ischemia, hypertrophy, and infiltrative processes were found to be the leading disorders causing diastolic dysfunction of the left ventricle. This large body of evidence indicates that pathophysiology, therapy, and prognosis are distinctly different in heart failure caused by systolic and diastolic dysfunction.

In this text, we review our current knowledge of diastolic dysfunction with special emphasis on its relation to heart failure. Our goals are to review the normal and abnormal physiology of diastole and to provide a basis for the clinical diagnosis of left ventricular diastolic dysfunction. The major emphasis is on diseases causing diastolic dysfunction and their treatment. This book will be of interest to clinical investigators, to those interested in cardiac function, and especially to those who care for patients with heart failure caused by myocardial hypertrophy and ischemia.

Worcester, Massachusetts   William H. Gaasch, M.D.
Burlington, Vermont   Martin M. LeWinter, M.D.

Contributors

Norman R. Alpert, Ph.D.
Professor and Chair
Department of Physiology and Biophysics
University of Vermont College of Medicine
Burlington, Vermont

Carl S. Apstein, M.D.
Professor of Medicine and Physiology
Boston University School of Medicine
Chief of Cardiology
Boston City Hospital
Boston, Massachusetts

Edward M. Blanchard, Ph.D.
Research Assistant Professor
Department of Physiology and Biophysics
University of Vermont College of Medicine
Burlington, Vermont

Alvin S. Blaustein, M.D.
Associate Professor of Medicine
University of Cincinnati School of Medicine
Director, Cardiology Noninvasive Laboratory
Veterans Administration Medical Center
Cincinnati, Ohio

Robert O. Bonow, M.D.
Goldberg Professor of Medicine
Northwestern University Medical School
Chief, Division of Cardiology
Northwestern Memorial Hospital
Chicago, Illinois

Jean G. F. Bronzwaer, M.D.
Department of Cardiology
Free University Hospital
Amsterdam, The Netherlands

Carolyn A. Burns, M.D.
Research Fellow, Cardiology
Medical College of Virginia
Richmond, Virginia

Eugenia P. Carroll, M.D.
Assistant Professor of Medicine
Northwestern University Medical School
Chicago, Illinois

John D. Carroll, M.D.
Associate Professor of Medicine
Pritzker School of Medicine
University of Chicago
Director, Hans Hecht Cardiac Catheterization
   Laboratory
University of Chicago Hospitals
Chicago, Illinois

Michael Courtois, M.A.
Research Assistant Professor of Medicine
Washington University School of Medicine
St. Louis, Missouri

Bernard de Bruyne, M.D.
Cardiovascular Center
O.L.V. Ziekenhuis
Aalst, Belgium

William H. Gaasch, M.D.
Professor of Medicine
University of Massachusetts Medical School
Chief of Cardiology
The Medical Center of Central Massachusetts
Worcester, Massachusetts

Derek G. Gibson, M.D.
Consultant Cardiologist
Royal Brompton Hospital
London, England

Thierry C. Gillebert, M.D., Ph.D.
Associate Professor of Medicine
University of Antwerp
Antwerp, Belgium

Stanton A. Glantz, Ph.D.
Professor of Medicine
University of California
San Francisco, California

William Grossman, M.D.
Herman Dana Professor of Medicine
Harvard Medical School
Chief, Cardiovascular Division
Beth Israel Hospital
Boston, Massachusetts

Gerd Hasenfuss, M.D.
Assistant Professor
Department of Medicine, Cardiology
University of Freiburg
Freiburg, Germany

Liv Hatle, M.D.
Professor of Medicine
University of Trondheim, Norway
Head, Section of Adult Cardiology
King Faisal Specialist Hospital
Saudi Arabia

Otto M. Hess, M.D.
Professor of Medicine
University Hospital
Zurich, Switzerland

Brian D. Hoit, M.D.
Associate Professor of Medicine
University of Cincinnati Medical School
Director, Echocardiographic Laboratory
University Hospital
Cincinnati, Ohio

Christian Holubarsch, M.D.
Assistant Professor
Department of Medicine, Cardiology
University of Freiburg
Freiburg, Germany

Joseph S. Janicki, Ph.D.
Professor of Medicine and Physiology
Department of Internal Medicine
University of Missouri
Columbia, Missouri

Hans P. Krayenbuehl, M.D.
Professor of Medicine
University Hospital
Zurich, Switzerland

Herbert J. Levine, M.D.
Professor of Medicine
Tufts University School of Medicine
Senior Physician
New England Medical Center
Boston, Massachusetts

Wilbur Y. W. Lew, M.D.
Associate Professor of Medicine
Director, Cardiovascular Training Program
University of California
San Diego, California

Martin M. LeWinter, M.D.
Professor of Medicine
University of Vermont College of Medicine
Director, Cardiology Unit
Medical Center Hospital of Vermont
Burlington, Vermont

Beverly H. Lorell, M.D.
Associate Professor of Medicine
Harvard Medical School
Director, Hemodynamic Research Laboratory
Beth Israel Hospital
Boston, Massachusetts

Philip A. Ludbrook, M.B., B.S., F.R.A.C.P.
Professor of Medicine and Radiology
Director, Cardiac Catheterization Laboratory
Washington University School of Medicine
St. Louis, Missouri

Beatriz B. Matsubara, M.D.
Research Associate
Department of Internal Medicine
University of Missouri
Columbia, Missouri

Jon N. Meliones, M.D.
Assistant Professor of Pediatrics and
    Communicable Diseases
University of Michigan Medical Center
Ann Arbor, Michigan

L. LuAnn Minich, M.D.
Fellow, Pediatric Cardiology
University of Michigan Medical Center
Ann Arbor, Michigan

James P. Morgan, M.D., Ph.D.
Associate Professor of Medicine
Harvard Medical School
Associate Physician
Beth Israel Hospital
Boston, Massachusetts

Louis A. Mulieri, Ph.D.
Research Associate Professor
Department of Physiology and Biophysics
University of Vermont College of Medicine
Burlington, Vermont

Eivind E. S. P. Myhre, M.D., Ph.D.
Visiting Scientist
Section of Cardiology
University of Vermont College of Medicine
Burlington, Vermont

Yasuyuki Nakamura, M.D.
Assistant Professor of Medicine
Shiga University of Medical Science
Shiga, Japan

Srdjan D. Nikolic, Ph.D.
Associate Staff Scientist
Research Institute, Palo Alto Medical
  Foundation
Consulting Assistant Professor
Department of Cardiothoracic Surgery
Stanford University Medical School
Stanford, California

Rick A. Nishimura, M.D.
Associate Professor of Internal Medicine
Mayo Medical School
Rochester, Minnesota

J. V. Nixon, M.D.
Professor of Medicine
Director, Echocardiography Laboratories
Associate Director, Heart Station
Medical College of Virginia
Richmond, Virginia

Walter J. Paulus, M.D., Ph.D.
Director, Cardiac Catheterization Laboratory
Cardiovascular Center
O.L.V. Ziekenhuis
Aalst, Belgium

Howard A. Rockman, M.D.
Assistant Professor of Medicine
University of California, San Diego
San Diego, California

Shigetake Sasayama, M.D.
Professor of Medicine
Kyoto University
Kyoto, Japan

Hideo Shintani, M.D.
Visiting Scientist
Cardiovascular Research Institute
University of California
San Francisco, California

Bryan K. Slinker, Ph.D., D.V.M.
Associate Professor
Veterinary and Cooperative Anatomy,
  Pharmacology, and Physiology Department
Washington State University
Pullman, Washington

A. Rebecca Snider, M.D.
Professor of Pediatrics and Communicable
  Diseases
University of Michigan Medical Center
Ann Arbor, Michigan

Stanislas U. Sys, M.D., Ph.D.
Associate Professor of Physiology
University of Antwerp
Antwerp, Belgium

James D. Thomas, M.D.
Director of Cardiovascular Imaging
Department of Cardiology
The Cleveland Clinic Foundation
Cleveland, Ohio

James E. Udelson, M.D.
Assistant Professor of Medicine
Tufts University School of Medicine
Director, Nuclear Cardiology Laboratory
Tufts-New England Medical Center Hospitals
Boston, Massachusetts

Richard A. Walsh, M.D.
Professor of Medicine, Pharmacology and Cell
  Biophysics
Director, Division of Cardiology
University of Cincinnati College of Medicine
Cincinnati, Ohio

E. Douglas Wigle, M.D.
Professor of Medicine
University of Toronto
Senior Physician
Toronto General Hospital
Toronto, Ontario, Canada

Edward L. Yellin, Ph.D.
Professor of Cardiothoracic Surgery
Professor of Physiology and Biophysics
Albert Einstein College of Medicine
Bronx, New York

Michael R. Zile, M.D.
Professor of Medicine
Medical University of South Carolina
Charleston, South Carolina

Contents

Part One

THE PHYSIOLOGY OF LEFT VENTRICULAR RELAXATION AND FILLING

Chapter 1

CELLULAR MECHANISMS UNDERLYING LEFT VENTRICULAR DIASTOLIC DYSFUNCTION

Carl S. Apstein and James P. Morgan

Approximately one third of patients with symptomatic congestive heart failure have a normal ejection fraction and symptoms that are entirely or in large measure a result of diastolic dysfunction. In many cases, such diastolic dysfunction is caused by one or more abnormalities of cardiac structure, e.g., hypertrophy, fibrosis, infiltrative diseases, or pericardial constraint; however, many patients appear to have diastolic dysfunction resulting from abnormalities of cellular mechanisms of myocyte relaxation, usually because of ischemia and/or hypoxia. The occurrence of ischemia or hypoxia in a hypertrophied heart causes exaggerated diastolic dysfunction. Also, metabolic processes such as alkalosis, many cardiovascular drugs, and the hypertrophy process itself can alter cellular mechanisms of myocardial relaxation and may predispose to diastolic dysfunction.

This chapter will focus on cellular mechanisms of myocardial relaxation. The calcium and sodium movements that reverse the processes of excitation-contraction coupling, can be thought of as processes of *repolarization-relaxation coupling*. Just as drugs, metabolic processes, or pathologic conditions may exert a positive or negative inotropic effect by influencing the movement and sensitivity to calcium as part of the excitation-contraction coupling process, a positive or negative lusitropic (relaxation-enhancing) effect can result from alteration of the processes of repolarization-relaxation coupling. Much pharmacologic research has been directed toward enhancing contractile function by developing drugs that alter excitation-contraction coupling events to produce a positive inotropic response. A similar approach to re-polarization-relaxation coupling has the potential to bring about therapies with positive lusitropic effects.

EXCITATION-CONTRACTION AND REPOLARIZATION-RELAXATION COUPLING

Central Role of Calcium

Rapid changes in intracellular levels of free-ionized calcium (Ca_i^{2+}) regulate the contraction and relaxation of cardiac muscle. The modulation of Ca_i^{2+} levels during systole and diastole occurs at several sites within the cell, which are outlined in Figure 1–1. Synchronous function of each of these steps allows the heart to sustain normal function and to maintain a 10,000-fold concentration gradient for calcium across the sarcolemma. Abnormal function at any one of these multiple sites can lead to cardiac dysfunction, heart failure, and both systolic and diastolic dysfunction (1-4).

Excitation-contraction coupling in the mammalian heart is modulated by at least one important second messenger other than Ca^{2+}, i.e., cyclic AMP. This nucleotide activates a series of protein kinases, which in turn phosphorylate proteins at several subcellular sites, including the sarcolemma, the sarcoplasmic reticulum (SR), and the troponin-tropomyosin regulatory complex on the myofilaments (Figs. 1–1 and 1–2). Phosphorylation of the Ca^{2+} channels in the sarcolemma increases Ca^{2+} entry and force generation; phosphorylation of phospholamban on the SR, and Troponin I on the regulatory complex of the contractile elements, enhances $[Ca^{2+}]_i$ resequestration and diastolic relaxation. This important pathway is initiated in vivo

3

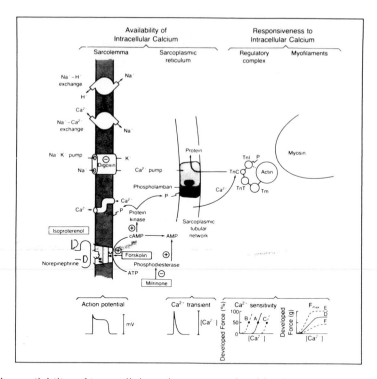

Figure 1–1. The availability of intracellular calcium is regulated by the sarcolemma and sarcoplasmic reticulum, and calcium responsiveness is controlled by the myofilaments and the regulatory troponin-tropomyosin complex. The figure shows four major cellular sites for the regulation of excitation-contraction and repolarization-relaxation coupling in the mammalian heart: sarcolemma, sarcoplasmic reticulum, regulatory complex, and myofilaments. Cardiac contractility and lusitropy may be altered by changing either the availability of intracellular calcium for activation or the responsiveness of the myofilaments to intracellular calcium. Calcium availability is regulated predominantly by sites in the sarcolemma and sarcoplasmic reticulum that can be functionally monitored by means of the action potential and calcium transient, respectively. Responsiveness to intracellular calcium is regulated predominantly by the troponin-tropomyosin complex, attached to actin, and the myofilaments, actin and myosin. These components can be functionally assessed by the calcium sensitivity and maximal calcium-activated force (F_{max}) of fibers rendered hyperpermeable to calcium. The Ca^{2+} transient is the depolarization-induced release and decrease in the intracellular calcium concentration ($[Ca^{2+}]$); Ca^{2+} sensitivity is the relation between the intracellular calcium concentration and cardiac activation, expressed as a percentage of peak developed force. Curves A and D are baseline values of the sensitivity of myofilaments to calcium and F_{max}, respectively. Ca^{2+} sensitivity and F_{max} can change independently of each other. Curves B and E show enhancement, and curves C and F depression, of sensitivity and F_{max}, respectively. TnI = troponin I, TnC = troponin C, TnT = troponin T, Tm = tropomyosin, bR = beta-adrenergic receptor, ATP = adenosine triphosphate, cAMP = cyclic AMP, and P = phosphorylation. Reproduced with permission from Morgan JP: Mechanisms of disease. Abnormal intracellular modulation of calcium as a major cause of cardiac contractile dysfunction. N Engl J Med *325*:625, 1991.

by activation of the beta-adrenergic receptors. Other second messengers in the heart may modulate excitation-contraction coupling, including inositol triphosphate (which has been reported to induce the release of calcium from the sarcoplasmic reticulum) and diacylglycerol (which has been reported to activate various enzymatic processes, including myosin light chain phosphorylation and sodium-hydrogen exchange): however, the role of these other second messengers in the heart remains controversial (4).

It is useful to view the regulation of the cardiac contractile state from the vantage point of troponin C, the Ca^{2+} receptor protein of the contractile apparatus (Fig. 1–2) (5). Inotropic and lusitropic mecha-

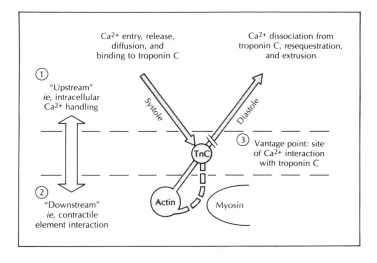

Figure 1–2. Diagram of three major mechanisms (1, 2, 3) regulating the contractile state. TnC = troponin C. Dashed line connecting TnC to actin depicts the inhibitory action of troponin-tropomyosin complex on actin-myosin interaction. This inhibition is removed and cross-bridges allowed to attach when Ca^{2+} binds to TnC.

nisms can then be divided into those that are "upstream" from troponin C and modulate the availability of free-ionized Ca^{2+} ions for activation of the contractile apparatus, in contrast to "downstream" mechanisms affecting the ability of the myofilaments to respond to any given level of occupancy of the Ca^{2+}-receptor sites on troponin C. Myocardial contraction and relaxation can also be affected by changing the affinity of troponin C for Ca^{2+}. Many of the steps involved in contraction and relaxation of the heart require the expenditure of energy in the form of ATP, which provides a fourth way by which the contractile state may be altered, i.e., by a change in the rate of energy use or supply to the myocytes (6).

Abnormal Calcium Modulation in Hypertrophy and Failure

Abnormal modulation of intracellular calcium has been proposed as a major mechanism underlying the systolic and diastolic dysfunction that develops with cardiac hypertrophy and failure (1, 2, 4). (See Chap. 20.) Systolic force generation is depressed in most models of heart failure, but this change does not always correlate with decreased availability of activator calcium (7, 8). For example, in right ventricular pressure-overload hypertrophy with failure in the ferret, systolic force generation is depressed, but intracellular calcium levels are normal. The major abnormality appears to be in the cardiac interstitium in

this model, where significant changes occur in connective tissue content, which, in turn, impairs systolic force generation (9). Conversely, an excellent correlation exists between systolic dysfunction and decreased availability of activator calcium in cardiac muscle from Syrian hamsters with end-stage dilated cardiomyopathy (10, 11), from diabetic rats with failure (12), and from rats after myocardial infarction (13).

In contrast to this somewhat variable relationship between systolic function and intracellular calcium, there appears to be a highly positive correlation between end-diastolic calcium levels and diastolic relaxation abnormalities. The duration of diastole is prolonged in most models of failure, and this correlates with a prolongation of the intracellular calcium transient measured with the calcium indicator acquorin (7). In some cases, such as digitalis toxicity and hypoxia, elevated end-diastolic calcium levels are associated with increased end-diastolic tension or pressure. On the other hand, marked increases in systolic and diastolic calcium occur in myocardial ischemia, and appear to be uncoupled from force production, which, in contrast, falls to very low levels (14–20). Therefore, in ischemia, decreased myofilament calcium responsiveness may affect both systolic force generation and diastolic relaxation.

In comparison to the models just discussed, in hypertrophic cardiomyopathy, systolic function is normal or hyperdynamic, but diastolic relaxation may become so abnormally slow as to prevent complete relaxation between contractions. (See Chap. 22.) At rapid heart rates, this can produce elevated end-diastolic calcium, and mechanical dysfunction caused by fusion of the prolonged Ca_i^{2+} transients and contractions (21, 22). Because systolic function is normal or hyperdynamic in hypertrophic cardiomyopathy, this raises the possibility that the abnormalities in excitation-contraction coupling may more closely correlate with the presence of significant hypertrophy rather than heart failure, per se. In support of this point, cardiac muscle from patients with end-stage chronic heart failure characteristically shows a significant degree of compensatory hypertrophy, and the degree of hypertrophy that is present (i.e., moderate to severe) positively correlates with the abnormalities in excitation-contraction coupling that are present (23).

Human Heart Failure

Three characteristic signatures of failure have been consistently noted in physiologic studies of human heart muscle loaded with the Ca^{2+} indicator aequorin over the past decade (24): (1) an abnormal second component in the Ca_i^{2+} signal recorded with aequorin (Fig. 1–3) (21); (2) reversal of the normal positive staircase of the force-frequency relationship caused by abnormal Ca_i^{2+} restitution processes (25); and (3) a depressed response to most inotropic agonists that depend on cyclic AMP generation to produce their cellular response (26). Pharmacologic studies have indicated that cyclic AMP levels are depressed in failing human myocardium, may contribute to the alterations in Ca_i^{2+} modulation shown in Figure 1–3, and may be largely responsible for the diastolic relaxation abnormalities that are present (26–28). This hypothesis may also explain why, in cardiac tissue from heart failure patients, positive inotropic agents that act by means of phosphodiesterase inhibition show decreased effectiveness. Moreover, interventions that increase intracellular cyclic AMP concentrations in myopathic human myocardium

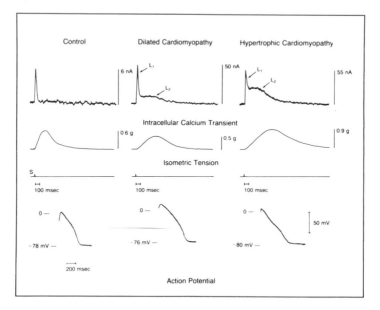

Figure 1–3. Recordings representing intracellular calcium transient (recorded with the bioluminescent indicator aequorin), isometric tension, and stimulus artifact (S) from control and myopathic human trabecular carneae, maintained in vitro, and action potentials in different muscles from the same hearts. L_1 and L_2 denote two temporally distinct components of the calcium transients that are typical of failing human muscle. L_2 appears to reflect abnormal Ca^{2+} handling by the sarcoplasmic reticulum and sarcolemma. Note the correlation of L_2 with prolonged action potential duration and delayed relaxation of the isometric contraction. Reproduced with permission from Gwathmey JK, et al.: Abnormal intracellular calcium handling in myocardium from patients with end-stage heart failure. Circ Res 61:70, 1987.

reverse or significantly ameliorate the diastolic dysfunction that is present (23). Of interest, agents that increase $[Ca^{2+}]_i$, such as digitalis, exacerbate; whereas those that lower $[Ca^{2+}]_i$, such as verapamil, ameliorate the functional abnormalities that are present. Depressed cyclic AMP generation may be caused by a heart failure-related increase in the proportion of inhibitory to stimulatory G proteins that regulate adenylate cyclase activity (29, 30). This ratio may vary with the etiology of heart failure (31, 32). The fact that abnormalities of cyclic AMP generation contribute importantly to the altered systolic and diastolic physiology of heart failure does not exclude other mechanisms from also being contributory, e.g., sarcoplasmic reticulum Ca^{2+}-ATPase gene expression (33).

Sarcolemmal Receptors and Mechanisms

The cardiac sarcolemma is a complex structure that contains multiple channels, exchangers and pumps that are necessary for maintaining cellular Ca^{2+} homeostasis (see Fig. 1–1). The structure and regulation of the adrenergic and related receptors has been the topic of recent reviews (34, 35). Significant progress has been made in understanding the genetic regulation of the beta-adrenergic receptor. Several members of this receptor family coupled with the G proteins have been found in recent years. Both beta$_1$ and beta$_2$-adrenoceptors are present in human atrial and ventricular myocardium, and both appear to increase tissue levels of cyclic AMP. Of interest, the relative proportions of beta$_2$-receptors increase in heart failure as the beta$_1$-receptors are "downregulated" (36, 37). Beta$_1$-receptors are decreased by 60 to 70%, with beta$_2$-receptors exhibiting a small, nonsignificant increase. Alpha$_1$-receptor density does not change significantly. In the nonfailing ventricle, beta$_1$-receptor density dominates, with the beta$_2$ and alpha$_1$-receptors constituting less than 30% of the total. In contrast, in the failing heart, the beta$_1$ fraction is less than 50% of the total, with the alpha$_1$ and beta$_2$-receptors constituting more than 50% of the total. These changes in receptor populations may vary with the etiology of heart failure (38) and may have therapeutic importance with regard to delivering inotropic and lusitropic support and in the use of beta-blocking agents. Partial agonists may transform a smaller proportion of the receptor pool into the activated form that serves as a substrate for beta-adrenergic receptor kinase (39). In contrast to the downregulation of beta$_1$-adrenergic receptors that occurs with heart failure, the calcium antagonist binding sites are not significantly altered in failing human left ventricular tissue from patients with idiopathic dilated cardiomyopathy (40).

In recent years, there has been an increasing appreciation that the level of intracellular Na, acting by means of Na^+/Ca^{2+} exchange, is an important determinant of $[Ca^{2+}]_i$. Cardiac disease states may be associated with increased intracellular Na levels which, taken to an extreme, may result in $[Ca^{2+}]_i$ overload and diastolic dysfunction (see reference 41 for review). The sodium-calcium and sodium-hydrogen exchange sites play important roles in governing calcium homeostasis in the mammalian heart. For example, a decrease in intracellular pH, i.e., an increase in H_i^+, has the effect of increasing Na_i by means of Na^+/H^+ exchange and secondarily increasing Ca_i^{2+} by means of Na^+/Ca^{2+} exchange. Alterations of these exchanges may contribute to the prolongation of the action potential in failing human myocardium and secondarily influence myocyte relaxation, as suggested by the work of Schouten et al. (42). Gwathmey et al. (43) demonstrated the potentially important role of intracellular sodium and sodium-calcium exchange in regulating the contractility of ventricular muscle isolated from control patients and patients with end-stage heart failure and showed the marked delay in diastolic relaxation that these mechanisms can produce. Of interest, the sensitivity of Na^+-K^+ ATPase to ouabain inhibition may shift in heart failure because of isoform conversion of the catalytic subunit indicating that changes in the function of this pump may disturb Na_i^+ homeostasis (44).

The Ca^{2+} ATPase of the cardiac sarcolemma appears to play the role of "fine tuning" Ca^{2+} homeostasis (45). To date, specific abnormalities associated with dysfunction of this relatively low-capacity pump have not been identified.

Sarcoplasmic Reticulum

The sarcoplasmic reticulum (SR) is the most important intracellular store of calcium in the mammalian heart and plays a primary part in regulating both contraction and relaxation. It is therefore not surprising that drugs affecting Ca^{2+} release and reuptake by the SR have profound effects on diastolic relaxation. For example, in most mammalian species, ryanodine, which selectively inhibits the SR Ca^{2+} release channels, markedly prolongs diastolic relaxation while producing a negative inotropic effect (46). Similarly, caffeine, a complex drug with additional effects on phosphodiesterase and myofilament Ca^{2+} responsiveness, appears to act predominantly in most mammalian species to block the ATP-dependent Ca^{2+} pump of the SR that functions to resequester $[Ca^{2+}]_i$. Caffeine's effect is also associated with a marked prolongation of contraction and delayed relaxation. Molecular genetic techniques have enhanced our understanding of Ca^{2+} release and reuptake by this organelle, as recently reviewed by MacClellan (47). Mercardier et al. (33) reported altered sarcoplasmic reticular Ca^{2+}-ATPase gene expression in the human ventricle during end-stage heart failure. Lompre et al. (48) reported similar changes in Ca^{2+}-ATPase and calsequestrin genes in rat hearts during development and aging. De la Bastie et al. (49) reported a relative diminution in density of SR Ca^{2+} pumps in pressure-overload-induced cardiac hypertrophy, an abnormality that could explain the slow velocity of relaxation of severely hypertrophied hearts. These abnormalities could also contribute to the prolonged calcium transients and slowed velocity of relaxation that occur with cardiac hypertrophy and failure. Feldman et al. (50) have found that the expression of mRNA for phospholamban, the regulatory protein of the calcium pump of the sarcoplasmic reticulum, is depressed in myocardium from patients with heart failure, whereas the mRNA for two other cellular proteins is unchanged or increased, indicating selective alterations of gene expression in heart failure. Movsesian

et al. (51) have also reported data supporting this hypothesis. The functional significance of these findings at present remains somewhat speculative, but they could contribute to the occurrence of diastolic dysfunction in these conditions.

Some, but not all, studies have shown decreased calcium uptake rates by the sarcoplasmic reticulum in myopathic human myocardium (52). Abnormal calcium modulation by the sarcoplasmic reticulum may contribute to the abnormal frequency-response relationship that is one of the characteristics of failing human myocardium (25, 53). As already discussed, interventions that prevent Ca^{2+} overload of the sarcoplasmic reticular vesicles (i.e., Ca^{2+} channel blockers) or that enhance the ability of the SR to resequester Ca^{2+} from the cytoplasm (i.e., cyclic AMP generators) can ameliorate or reverse these changes in some experimental conditions and may be able to do the same in vivo in humans.

Altered Myofilament Ca^{2+} Responsiveness

In addition to changes in Ca^{2+} availability, cardiac contractility can be regulated by changing the myofilament responsiveness to Ca^{2+}. As shown in Figure 1–1, for fibers rendered hyperpermeable to Ca^{2+}, a change in responsiveness may manifest itself as a change in (1) sensitivity (i.e., ED_{50} or potency) or (2) maximal Ca^{2+}-activated force (F_{max} or efficacy). With regard to diastolic relaxation, sensitivity changes are probably more important. Such an effect could occur through altering the affinity of Ca^{2+} binding to its receptor protein, troponin C, or by some other action on the myofilaments themselves, such as phosphorylation of the myosin light chains or the C proteins of the myosin thick filaments (54, 55). Some of the agents and interventions that have been shown to affect myofilament calcium sensitivity in animal models are shown in Figure 1–4; not all of these have been tested in human myocardium. Of interest, in recent years, it has been learned that some endogenous substances such as endothelin, alpha agonists, and opioid agonists may exert their inotropic activity largely by producing an intracellular alkalosis, which results in increased force production but delayed relaxation because

EFFECTS OF INTERVENTIONS ON Ca^{2+} SENSITIVITY
OF THE CONTRACTILE APPARATUS

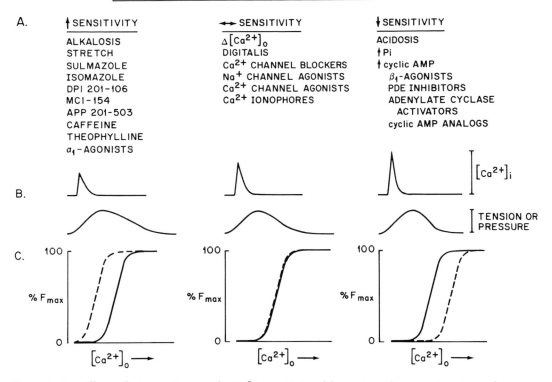

A.

↑SENSITIVITY	↔ SENSITIVITY	↓SENSITIVITY
ALKALOSIS	$\Delta[Ca^{2+}]_o$	ACIDOSIS
STRETCH	DIGITALIS	↑Pi
SULMAZOLE	Ca^{2+} CHANNEL BLOCKERS	↑ cyclic AMP
ISOMAZOLE	Na^+ CHANNEL AGONISTS	β_1-AGONISTS
DPI 201-106	Ca^{2+} CHANNEL AGONISTS	PDE INHIBITORS
MCI-154	Ca^{2+} IONOPHORES	ADENYLATE CYCLASE
APP 201-503		ACTIVATORS
CAFFEINE		cyclic AMP ANALOGS
THEOPHYLLINE		
a_1-AGONISTS		

B.

$[Ca^{2+}]_i$

TENSION OR PRESSURE

C. 100   100   100

% F_{max} % F_{max} % F_{max}

0   0   0

$[Ca^{2+}]_o \longrightarrow$ $[Ca^{2+}]_o \longrightarrow$ $[Ca^{2+}]_o \longrightarrow$

Figure 1–4. Effects of interventions on the Ca^{2+} sensitivity of the contractile apparatus. A panels summarize the effects of interventions on myofilament calcium sensitivity. B panels show the effects of equiinotropic concentrations of the agonists listed in A on the intracellular calcium transient. Note that drugs that decrease myofilament calcium sensitivity increase the amplitude of the calcium transient relative to drugs that do not change myofilament calcium sensitivity. C panels show the effects of these agents on the force versus pCa relationship of skinned or hyperpermeabilized fibers. The interventions that increase myofilament sensitivity to calcium have the potential to cause or exacerbate diastolic dysfunction; conversely agents which decrease myofilament sensitivity to calcium have a potential lusitropic effect.

of enhanced myofilament responsiveness to Ca^{2+} (48, 56–59). Several laboratories have reported that the development of end-stage heart failure in humans is not associated with changes in basal, myofibrillar Ca^{2+} sensitivity (60–62). However, although the experimental inotropic agent DPI 201-106 had no effect on the Ca^{2+} sensitivity of normal human heart muscle, it significantly increased the Ca^{2+} sensitivity of muscle from patients with end-stage failure, raising the possibility that the effects of pharmacologic agents on myofibrillar Ca^{2+} sensitivity can be altered by the development of cardiac disease states (60).

A significant theoretical problem with using Ca^{2+} sensitizers therapeutically arises as a consequence of their mechanism of action. By enhancing actin-myosin interaction, they should prolong relaxation, an effect that has been demonstrated in vivo and in vitro in animals and in humans (63). The significance of this effect in a given patient would depend on the degree of diastolic dysfunction that is present; the agents may be a treatment of choice in patients with predominant systolic dysfunction or in combination with an agent that prevents or ameliorates the diastolic slowing. On the other hand, it may be possible to develop drugs that selectively influence the F_{max} component of Ca^{2+} responsiveness (see Fig. 1–1) without adversely affecting diastolic relaxation. For example, MCI

154, a phosphodiesterase inhibitor, has been shown to produce a slight but significant increase in F_{max} of animal trabeculae made hyperpermeable to Ca^{2+} in doses that enhance or do not affect the rate of diastolic relaxation (64). Force development and shortening of cardiac muscle occur as a result of the interaction between actin and myosin within the myofibrillar lattice. Pagani et al. (65) compared the myofibrillar content and myofibrillar ATPase activity of normal human ventricular muscle with that of ventricular muscle from patients with end-stage heart failure. The amount of myofibrillar protein in hearts with end-stage heart failure was significantly lower than myofibril from patients with less severe degrees of heart failure. However, regardless of the severity, muscle from both groups of patients with heart failure had lower myofibrillar protein content than muscle from normal hearts. These data suggest that a reduction in the amount of myofibrillar protein in ventricular tissue may be a pivotal event responsible for the progression of heart disease to end-stage failure, and may also be related to the development of diastolic dysfunction.

ALTERATION OF EXCITATION-CONTRACTION AND REPOLARIZATION-RELAXATION COUPLING: EFFECTS ON DIASTOLIC FUNCTION

The analysis of the excitation-contraction and repolarization-relaxation coupling pathways predicts that alterations with the potential to increase diastolic cytosolic calcium levels may cause diastolic dysfunction by means of persistent calcium-activated tension throughout diastole. Conversely, interventions that reduce diastolic cytosolic calcium levels should have a positive lusitropic effect and the potential to ameliorate diastolic dysfunction. These predictions are borne out by several experimental studies.

Exacerbation of Ischemic and Hypoxic Diastolic Dysfunction by Sarcolemmal Sodium Pump Inhibition with Ouabain

Several studies have demonstrated that the presence of ouabain exacerbates the diastolic dysfunction caused by hypoxia or ischemia (66–68). Digitalis glycosides such as ouabain inhibit the sarcolemmal sodium-potassium ATPase (sarcolemmal sodium pump), causing an increase in intracellular sodium with a resultant increase in intracellular calcium secondary to increased sodium-calcium exchange. This increase in intracellular calcium is generally believed to be responsible for the positive inotropic effect of the digitalis glycosides, but such an increase in myocyte calcium content has the potential to cause diastolic dysfunction by a mechanism of diastolic cytosolic calcium overload, particularly under circumstances where diastolic calcium removal is impaired, (e.g., hypoxia or ischemia), or where the myocyte is put under an additional cation load, such a during tachycardia. Experimental evidence supporting these concepts comes from studies by Cunningham and associated (66). Isolated buffer perfused rabbit hearts were subjected to 15 minutes of hypoxia and diastolic function assessed. The presence of a modest, nontoxic dose of ouabain markedly increased the extent of hypoxic diastolic dysfunction (as assessed by both an increase in isovolumic left ventricular diastolic pressure and the time constant of relaxation, T) without any significant effect on coronary vasomotion or myocardial lactate production. Similar results were obtained by Lorell et al. (68) during low-flow ischemia in isolated blood perfused rabbit hearts. After 6 minutes of low-flow ischemia, left ventricular diastolic chamber distensibility did not change in the control group, but was markedly reduced in the presence of ouabain. Exposure of hearts to an equi-inotropic level of isoproterenol did not cause diastolic dysfunction during low-flow ischemia, and there was no difference between ouabain and isoproterenol groups with regard to myocardial perfusion rates, determinants of myocardial oxygen demand, myocardial oxygen consumption, lactate production, ATP, or creatine phosphate content. Thus, the greater increase in ischemic LV diastolic chamber stiffness in the ouabain group was not caused by a greater metabolic severity of ischemia. A mechanism of cytosolic calcium overload, induced by ouabain and resulting in persistent active myofilament tension development throughout diastole, was the likely cause of the observed decrease in diastolic chamber distensibility. Similar results have been obtained during sustained low-flow ischemia when low-dose ouabain was compared to low-dose isoproterenol (67). During 60 minutes of low-flow ischemia, the presence of ouabain caused a marked increase in ischemic diastolic dysfunction whereas the control and isoproterenol groups exhibited no ischemic diastolic dysfunction. Thus, these studies demonstrate the potential of a pharmacologically induced increase in myocyte sodium and calcium content to cause or exacerbate diastolic dysfunction during ischemia and/or hypoxia in an isolated heart model at physiologic coronary perfusion and work load levels.

Amelioration of Diastolic Dysfunction by Manipulation of Diastolic Calcium Level with Combined β-Adrenergic Stimulation and Calcium Channel Blockade

Weinberg et al. (69) have shown that appropriate manipulation of excitation-contraction and repolarization-relaxation coupling can significantly improve hypoxic diastolic function. Well-oxygenated and hypoxic hypertrophied and nonhypertrophied rat hearts were studied using a pharmacologic strategy designed specifically to accelerate sarcoplasmic reticular calcium reuptake. The beta-adrenergic agonist, isoproterenol, was used to exploit its dual inotropic and lusitropic actions. Its inotropic effect occurs by increasing systolic calcium availability by increasing calcium entry by way of the sarcolemmal calcium channel; its lusitropic action is caused by increasing the rate of SR calcium re-uptake by a phospholamban-mediated mechanism as well as decreasing troponin sensitivity to calcium. The calcium channel blocker diltiazem was given simultaneously with isoproterenol, and the dose of diltiazem was "titrated" so that the inotropic effect of isoproterenol was precisely negated. At this dose, the lusitropic actions of isoproterenol were not inhibited, and this combination drug therapy resulted in a net lusitropic effect, increasing both the rate and extent of LV relaxation, both under well-oxygenated conditions and during hypoxia, partially eliminating the exagger-

ated hypoxic diastolic dysfunction associated with hypertrophy (69). Thus these experiments indicate that excitation-contraction and repolarization-relaxation coupling processes can be successfully manipulated to enhance myocardial relaxation and ameliorate hypoxic diastolic dysfunction.

ROLE OF ATP IN MYOCARDIAL RELAXATION

Adenosine triphosphate (ATP) availability can influence the rate and extent of myocardial relaxation in several ways. ATP is required to fuel the ion pumps that directly remove calcium from the cytosol during diastole: the sarcoplasmic reticular calcium ATPase, and the sarcolemmal calcium extrusion pump (sarcolemmal Ca^{2+}-ATPase). Furthermore, ATP is necessary to provide energy to the sarcolemmal sodium pump (sodium-potassium ATPase). An active sodium pump is critical for achieving myocyte relaxation because the intracellular sodium concentration regulates intracellular calcium levels by means of sarcolemmal sodium-calcium exchange.

ATP also influences myocardial relaxation directly at the level of the myofilaments by interacting with actomyosin to cause its dissociation to actin and myosin, a step critical to relaxation (see Fig. 1–5). The interaction of ATP with the contractile proteins is complex because ATP has a dual role, being required for both contraction and relaxation. Low (micromolar) amounts of ATP are adequate to saturate the high-affinity ATP binding site on myosin. The myosin head then becomes energized, causing formation of an active actin-myosin complex, i.e., creating actomyosin from actin and myosin, and a "rigor complex" forms, which is responsible for the mechanical motion of the myofilaments. Dissociation of the rigor complex requires binding of ATP to the high-affinity myosin head. It is also facilitated by relatively high ATP concentrations (in the millimolar range) for actomyosin to dissociate to actin and myosin, i.e., for myofilament relaxation to occur. This relaxing effect of a millimolar ATP concentration is caused by an allosteric effect of the anionic polyphosphate chain of ATP and is referred to as a

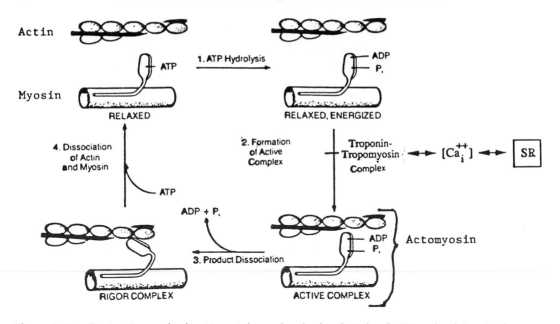

Figure 1–5. Contraction and relaxation at the molecular level: Role of ATP and calcium in the cross-bridge cycle. This diagram illustrates the cross-bridge cycle, i.e., contraction and relaxation at the molecular level. The sequence begins at the upper left, where ATP binding to myosin has dissociated the thick and thin filaments (i.e., the myosin and actin filaments), causing the muscle to relax. Hydrolysis of myosin bound ATP (Step 1) transfers the energy of the ATP molecule to the cross-bridge, which remains in a relaxed, unattached, but energized state (upper right). The affinity for ATP of the myosin head is very high, requiring only micromolar concentrations of ATP for this step in the molecular cardiac cycle. Interaction of the energized myosin cross-bridge with actin in the thin filament (Step 2) leads to the formation of the actomyosin active complex (lower right) in which the energy derived from ATP is still associated with the cross-bridge, which has yet to move. This step is regulated by the troponin-tropomyosin regulatory protein complex whose interaction with actin is regulated by the binding of troponin-C to calcium; such binding is regulated by the cytosolic calcium concentration. When the cytosolic calcium concentration is low, as in normal diastole, troponin-C has minimal or no calcium bound to it, the troponin-tropomyosin complex inhibits the formation of the actomyosin complex, and the myofilaments remain in a relaxed, but energized state. Systolic contraction is initiated by the release of calcium from the sarcoplasmic reticulum. The calcium binds to troponin C, the configuration of the troponin-tropomyosin complex changes such that the inhibition of the actin-myosin interaction is removed, and formation of the active complex of actomyosin at Step 2 occurs. Step 2 is also referred to as the step of "calcium-activated tension" because of the central role of calcium in regulating this reaction by means of the troponin-tropomyosin complex. Failure to lower cytosolic calcium adequately during diastole results in the continuous formation of active actomyosin complexes throughout the cardiac cycle because a persistently elevated calcium level prevents the troponin-tropomyosin complex from completely inhibiting Step 2 as is required for normal diastolic relaxation. At Step 3, dissociation of ADP and P_i, the products of ATP hydrolysis, leads to formation of a rigor complex in which the chemical energy of the energized cross-bridge has been expended to perform mechanical work, the motion of the cross-bridge. This rigor bond complex represents a low energy state of actomyosin. It is the state of the actomyosin complex at "end-systole" of the cross-bridge cycle. For relaxation to occur, the actomyosin rigor complex must be dissociated by ATP (Step 4). At Step 4, a rapid binding of ATP to the high-affinity myosin head of the rigor complex occurs, causing the rigor complex to dissociate to actin and myosin and the muscle to relax. This dissociation is facilitated by millimolar concentrations of ATP. This action of ATP has been called its "plasticizing effect," and is caused by an allosteric action of ATP. The ATP concentrations needed for the "plasticizing effect" are much higher than those needed to saturate the high affinity substrate site of myosin. Thus, if ATP depletion occurs, rigor complexes can still form because of the high affinity of the myosin head for ATP, but the dissociation of actin and myosin caused by the plasticizing effect of ATP is reduced. Thus, the initial net effect of ATP depletion is to cause inadequate relaxation or diastolic dysfunction. This figure indicates that diastolic dysfunction and impaired relaxation can occur by two distinct mechanisms. An inadequate lowering of cytosolic calcium during diastole can lead to

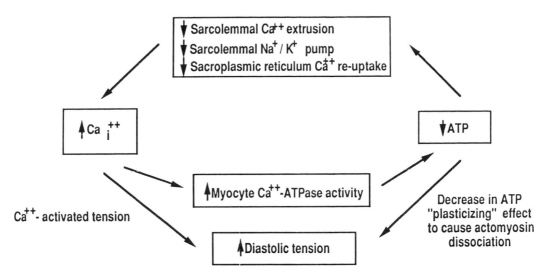

Figure 1–6. Synergistic interactions between an increase in cytosolic calcium and a decrease in ATP availability to decrease diastolic tension. This figure illustrates how an increased cytosolic calcium level or a decrease in ATP availability can increase diastolic myofilament tension and cause or exacerbate diastolic dysfunction. A decrease in ATP availability can directly increase diastolic tension by decreasing the rate or amount of actomyosin dissociation from the rigor complex state by means of the "plasticizing effect" of ATP (see Fig. 1–5). A decrease in ATP availability can also impair calcium removal from the cytosol by the sarcolemmal and sarcoplasmic reticular calcium ATPases. A decrease in ATP can also decrease the sarcolemmal sodium-potassium ATPase (sodium pump) activity resulting in an increase in intracellular sodium, which increases intracellular calcium by means of sodium-calcium exchange. Such an increase in cytosolic calcium, if it persists throughout diastole, can augment diastolic tension directly by binding to troponin C, causing persistent formation of active actomyosin complexes throughout diastole, as illustrated in Step 2 of Figure 1–5. An increase in intracellular calcium can also accelerate a decrease in ATP levels by activating a number of myocyte calcium ATPases. Thus, either cytosolic calcium overload or a decrease in ATP availability can initiate a "vicious cycle" of calcium-ATP interactions, which are synergistic in causing or exacerbating diastolic dysfunction. Therapeutic interventions designed to decrease intracellular calcium, increase ATP availability, or both, are likely to be beneficial in preventing or reversing diastolic dysfunction caused by abnormalities of cellular relaxation.

"plasticizing" effect of ATP which decreases the interaction between the thick and thin filaments. Thus, small decreases in ATP availability have the potential to significantly impair myocardial relaxation by decreasing the rate and/or extent of actomyosin dissociation to actin and myosin (see Fig. 1–5 and reference 70).

The interaction between calcium and ATP in regulating myocardial relaxation is complex (Fig. 1–6). Decreases in ATP levels are potentially synergistic, with increases in myocyte calcium content in causing diastolic dysfunction. Normally, intracellular levels of ATP are high enough (i.e., in the micromolar range) to saturate the head of myosin, except in very severe long-standing ischemia which is probably lethal. Thus, in viable myocytes it is reasonable to assume that ATP levels are ade-

persistent formation of active complexes of actomyosin throughout diastole because of failure of adequate inhibition of Step 2 by the troponin-tropomyosin complex caused by persistent binding of calcium to troponin C. A second mechanism that can cause diastolic dysfunction occurs when ATP levels are diminished such that the plasticizing effect of ATP to dissociate actomyosin at Step 4 is reduced. Both of these mechanisms can occur simultaneously and may be synergistic as illustrated in Figure 1–6. Adapted with permission from Katz AM: Physiology of the Heart. New York, Raven Press, 1992, pp. 151–177.

quate to keep the myosin head energized. Formation of the active actomyosin complex (Step Two of Fig. 1–5) is regulated by the regulatory proteins, troponin and tropomyosin. These regulatory proteins block formation of the active actomyosin complex when they are in their inhibitory state as determined by a low level of cytosolic calcium. Thus, failure to achieve a low level of cytosolic calcium during diastole will cause incomplete inhibition of Step Two of the crossbridge cycle as illustrated in Fig. 1–5, so that active actomyosin complexes will form abnormally during diastole, leading to generation of persistent diastolic myofilament tension. In other words, diastolic cytosolic calcium excess causes a fraction of the myofilaments to behave as if they are in continuous systole, never achieving diastolic relaxation. Consequently, with diastolic calcium excess, because of continuous cross-bridge cycling, ATP hydrolysis is also increased above normal values during diastole. If ATP synthesis is limited because of ischemia, hypoxia, or inadequate metabolic substrate levels, ATP levels may decrease, impairing Step Four of the crossbridge cycle, the dissociation of actin and myosin, which is required for myofilament relaxation and tension dissipation. Conversely, lower levels of intracellular ATP can increase intracellular calcium content by reducing sodium and calcium clearance from the cytosol by ATP-requiring ion pump mechanisms as discussed previously. The potential synergistic actions of an increase in cell calcium and decrease in ATP to impair relaxation are illustrated in Figure 1–6 (also see reference 66).

Decreased ATP as a Cause of Diastolic Dysfunction

Because of the central role of ATP in myocardial relaxation, the diastolic dysfunction associated with hypoxia and ischemia has been thought by many investigators to be caused by a decrease in ATP availability. Such a decrease in ATP could result in increased diastolic sodium and/or calcium levels, and/or cause direct impairment of myofilament diastolic tension dissipation, because of some degree of rigor bond formation and loss of the "plasticiz-

ing" effect of ATP. Evidence in support of decreased ATP availability as the cause of hypoxic or ischemic diastolic dysfunction comes from several sources. Hypoxia and ischemia are known to decrease the rate of ATP synthesis and decrease myocardial ATP content. Although relatively severe degrees of ischemia or hypoxia are required to reduce ATP content substantially, mild degrees can markedly decrease ATP turnover rates (71, 72). Thus, ATP availability for repolarization-relaxation coupling processes may be restricted because of a decrease in ATP turnover rate, with only a modest decrease in myocardial ATP content.

A second line of evidence supporting a causative role for ATP depletion in hypoxic and ischemic diastolic dysfunction comes from experiments in which the provision of additional glycolytic substrate improved hypoxic or ischemic relaxation, and glycolytic inhibition greatly accelerated ischemic diastolic dysfunction. For example, when rat left ventricular trabecular and papillary muscles were subjected to severe hypoxia in the presence of a normal (100 mg%) glucose level, significant diastolic dysfunction occurred within 15 minutes of hypoxia (manifested as a significant rise in resting or diastolic tension), and a severe increase in resting tension (contracture) was present after 60 minutes of hypoxia. Increasing the bath glucose level to 400 mg% completely prevented any increase in diastolic tension for as long as 120 minutes of severe hypoxia. Furthermore, the hypoxia-induced increase in diastolic tension could be reversed by increasing the bath glucose concentration after 30 minutes of hypoxia had elapsed; normal muscle relaxation was re-established despite the continued presence of hypoxia (73). The provision of a high-glucose substrate was thought to increase ATP availability by increasing glycolytic flux relative to the normal glucose condition. Thus, these studies are consistent with the concept that a decrease in ATP availability contributes importantly to the impaired myocardial relaxation associated with hypoxia.

Studies of hearts subjected to sustained low-flow ischemia have yielded results similar to the hypoxia studies (74, 75). In both buffer and blood-perfused isolated rabbit hearts, significant diastolic dysfunction occurred within 15 to 30 minutes of low-flow ischemia when the hearts were exposed to normal levels of glucose and insulin. Exposure to high levels of glucose and insulin completely prevented any increase in LV diastolic chamber stiffness for $2\frac{1}{2}$ hours of low-flow ischemia. Regardless of exogenous glucose and insulin levels, all hearts had a maximal rate of glycolytic flux as assessed by myocardial lactate production during the first 15 minutes of low-flow ischemia. However, with more sustained ischemia, the hearts provided with a normal glucose and insulin level had a progressive decrease in ischemic lactate production, consistent with depletion of myocardial glycogen stores, and this decrease in glycolytic flux was accompanied by a simultaneous increase in LV diastolic chamber stiffness. The provision of the high glucose and insulin substrate completely prevented a decrease in ischemic glycolytic flux, and maintenance of a maximal level of ischemic lactate production was accompanied by the complete absence of diastolic dysfunction (i.e., there was no increase in LV diastolic chamber stiffness) for $2\frac{1}{2}$ hours of low-flow ischemia. The high glucose and insulin substrate maintained ischemic myocardial ATP levels approximately 50% higher than the normal glucose group (74). Thus, these results also support the hypothesis that a limitation of ATP availability is directly responsible for the increase in diastolic chamber stiffness which occurs during low-flow ischemia. An increase in glycolytic ATP availability may protect against diastolic dysfunction either by fueling ion pumps and preventing cytosolic calcium overload, by a direct effect on the myofilaments, or by both mechanisms.

Is the Source of ATP (Glycolytic vs. Oxidative) Important in Preventing Ischemic or Hypoxic Diastolic Dysfunction?

During low-flow ischemia or hypoxia (in contrast to zero flow ischemia or anoxia), ATP synthesis results from both the glycolytic pathway and the reduced level of oxidative phosphorylation, which persists under conditions of partial oxygen deprivation. In hearts in which a high glucose

and insulin substrate prevented diastolic dysfunction during prolonged low-flow ischemia, *total* ATP synthesis was increased by only 18% by the presence of the increased glycolytic substrate relative to the normal glucose substrate, but the potential ATP yield from *glycolysis* increased by 340%. This observation suggested that the glycolytically produced ATP may have specifically prevented the increase in ischemic diastolic chamber stiffness, either by facilitating sodium and calcium homeostasis or by direct myofilament effects. A similar conclusion was reached by Owen et al. (76). These investigators studied the relationship between ischemic contracture (i.e., the increase in ischemic diastolic chamber stiffness) and the source and rate of ATP production in isolated rat hearts subjected to global underperfusion. The rate of glycolytic flux from glucose was the metabolic parameter that correlated best with prevention or delay of ischemic contracture during 45 minutes of global low-flow ischemia.

Such results are consistent with the hypothesis that the glycolytic pathway may provide a small but critically localized pool of ATP, which may have a high turnover rate relative to pool size (77, 78). Glycolytic ATP may play an important role in membrane ion transport and other membrane-related processes. Weiss and co-workers have demonstrated a preferential role of glycolytically synthesized ATP in inhibiting ATP-sensitive potassium channels in cardiac myocytes (79). Paul and coworkers have demonstrated that an endogenous glycolytic cascade preferentially supports calcium uptake in plasma membrane vesicles from smooth muscle cells (80). Recently Han and associates (81) have demonstrated that isolated skeletal muscle triads (i.e., membrane fragments consisting of transverse tubules connected to adjacent terminal cisternae of the sarcoplasmic reticulum) contain a compartmentalized glycolytic reaction. The ATP synthesized by this membrane "compartment" is not in equilibrium with bulk cell ATP stores; the ATP synthesized by these triads appears to be utilized by associated protein kinases and phosphatases, which are structurally associated with the triad membranes. Similarly, Entman and associated (82) reported that enzymes responsible for glycogen breakdown are associated with cardiac sarcoplasmic reticulum membrane fractions, consistent with a specific role of the glycolytic pathway in supporting intracellular calcium homeostasis. These results provide "microanatomic" evidence supporting the hypothesis of a glycolytic compartment whose ATP synthesis is preferentially utilized by membrane-associated processes such as ion transport.

Also consistent with a critical role of glycolytic ATP in maintaining normal relaxation during hypoxia and ischemia are results from experiments in which the glycolytic pathway was inhibited. Isolated perfused rat hearts with an intact glycolytic pathway tolerated 5 to 10 minutes of zeroflow ischemia without developing an increase in diastolic chamber stiffness. However, when the glycolytic pathway was specifically blocked by iodoacetic acid, ischemic diastolic chamber stiffness occurred rapidly so that severe contracture was present within 1 minute of ischemia (83). Even under well oxygenated conditions, the glycolytic pathway appears to provide a source of ATP, which is important in supporting the processes of repolarization-relaxation coupling. Gordon et al. (84) assessed the effects of glycolytic inhibition on myocardial relaxation under well oxygenated conditions in isolated rabbit hearts. Under baseline workload conditions, glycolytic inhibition did not impair myocardial relaxation. However, when the hearts were stressed by tachycardia, glycolytic inhibition was associated with significant diastolic dysfunction.

Tachycardia stresses repolarization-relaxation processes in several ways. Tachycardia shortens diastole, thereby requiring a more rapid rate of diastolic calcium and sodium clearance from the cytosol to restore a normal end-diastolic milieu and avoid incomplete relaxation. Secondly, the increased frequency of depolarization requires greater diastolic sodium and calcium sarcolemmal extrusion and sarcoplasmic reticular calcium reuptake per unit time to maintain intracellular ionic homeostasis. Lastly, the higher frequency of contractions increases ATP utilization, which is required for more frequent myofilament active tension generating cross-bridge cycles.

The results of Gordon et al. (84) suggest that glycolytic ATP may play a specific and important role in relaxation during tachycardia when the rates of repolarization-relaxation coupling processes are increased, even though the amount of glycolytic ATP synthesis relative to mitochondrial ATP synthesis is relatively small.

Additional evidence implicating an important role for glycolysis in myocardial relaxation comes from studies of hearts with certain types of hypertrophy which exhibit both a decrease in hypoxic glycolytic reserve and exaggerated hypoxic diastolic dysfunction (85). In rat hearts with hypertrophy secondary to the deoxycorticosterone-sodium overload model of hypertension, hypoxia caused much greater diastolic dysfunction than in age-matched control rats. This exaggerated diastolic dysfunction was associated with less myocardial hypoxic lactate production, suggesting a restricted ability of the hypertrophied myocardium to recruit the glycolytic pathway during hypoxia. Perfusion of the hypertrophied hearts with high glucose and insulin completely eliminated both the deficient hypoxic lactate production and the exaggerated hypoxic diastolic dysfunction of the hypertrophied hearts relative to controls (85). Similarly, after a period of ischemia, hypertrophied failing dog hearts manifested greater diastolic dysfunction than nonhypertrophied controls or hypertrophied nonfailing hearts, and this exaggerated diastolic dysfunction was associated with less ischemic myocardial lactate production (86).

ROLE OF ANGIOTENSIN AND ACE INHIBITION IN DIASTOLIC DYSFUNCTION

Angiotensin II levels are increased in patients with congestive heart failure and inhibition of angiotensin II synthesis by means of angiotensin-converting enzyme (ACE) inhibitors is associated with improvement of CHF symptoms such as pulmonary congestion. The beneficial effect of such ACE inhibition has been largely attributed to the effects of decreasing the action of angiotensin in the peripheral circulation, thereby decreasing systemic vascular (arteriolar) resistance and increasing systemic venous capacitance. However, several studies have suggested that angiotensin II may directly impair myocardial relaxation, especially in the setting of hypertrophy and/or ischemia. (See Chap. 20.) Thus, inhibition of angiotensin II synthesis may directly improve myocardial diastolic function and may be an important component of the action of ACE inhibitors in relieving heart failure symptoms.

There is now substantial evidence demonstrating the presence of an endogenous renin-angiotensin system in the heart (87–90). Schunkert and associates (90) have shown that pressure overload hypertrophy (aortic banded rat heart model) is associated with a three-to-fourfold increase in steady state levels of cardiac mRNA for the ACE gene and for cardiac tissue ACE activity. Exposure of such hypertrophied hearts under oxygenated conditions to an infusion of angiotensin I resulted in an immediate impairment of diastolic relaxation, whereas no such effect was seen in nonhypertrophied hearts (90). Eberli et al. (91) showed that, relative to nonhypertrophied controls, this hypertrophied rat heart model had exaggerated diastolic dysfunction during low-flow ischemia. In addition to having a greater capacity to convert angiotensin I to angiotensin II, these hypertrophied hearts also had an increased sensitivity to angiotensin II, exhibiting a greater degree of ischemic diastolic dysfunction in response to angiotensin II than nonhypertrophied hearts (92). The ACE inhibitor, enalaprilat, significantly ameliorated the ischemia-induced exaggerated diastolic dysfunction of the hypertrophied hearts, but had no effect on the nonhypertrophied hearts (91). Thus, these studies indicate a close association between an increased expression and activity of ACE and a marked sensitivity of myocardial relaxation to angiotensin I in pressure overload cardiac hypertrophy. Furthermore, the exaggerated ischemic diastolic dysfunction in such hypertrophied hearts was significantly reduced by treatment with ACE inhibition.

In the absence of hypertrophy, angiotensin II also had a deleterious effect on ischemic diastolic function. In nonhypertrophied rabbit hearts, Mochizuki et al. (93) demonstrated that exposure to angiotensin II markedly worsened diastolic dysfunction during low-flow ischemia, greatly augmenting the rise of isovolumic LVEDP. This impairment of ischemic myocardial relaxation was independent of any effect on myocardial ATP levels, glycolytic rate (as assessed by lactate production), or ischemic coronary flow.

The mechanisms by which angiotensin II impairs myocardial relaxation are not completely defined, but appear to involve the protein kinase C system, sodium-hydrogen exchange, and the production of intracellular alkalosis, which increases myofilament sensitivity to calcium. Angiotensin II can activate phosphoinositide "second messengers," thereby increasing both cytosolic calcium and myofilament calcium sensitivity (94–99). Angiotensin II may cause intracellular alkalization by enhanced sodium-hydrogen exchange secondary to protein kinase C activation (94, 100–102). Recent studies using isolated rabbit hearts and isolated rabbit myocytes showed that angiotensin II increased contractility in this species by increasing intracellular pH and myofilament sensitivity to calcium, rather than by increasing intracellular calcium levels (103). Such an increased myofilament sensitivity to calcium could contribute to the exaggerated ischemic diastolic dysfunction caused by angiotensin II, by increasing myofilament diastolic tension levels.

Evidence to support the hypothesis that angiotensin II impairs relaxation in hypertrophied hearts by activating the protein kinase C system comes from recent studies by Mochizuki et al. (104). The adverse effects of angiotensin II on diastolic function in hypertrophied hearts were simulated by active phorbol esters which are known to directly activate protein kinase C. Similarly, the impairment of diastolic relaxation by angiotensin II in hypertrophied hearts was prevented by coadministration of staurosporine, an inhibitor of protein kinase C. Mochizuki et al. have also provided evidence for activation of sodium-hydrogen exchange by angiotensin II in hypertrophied hearts (105). In these studies, pretreatment of hypertrophied rat hearts with amiloride, an inhibitor of sodium-hydrogen exchange, prevented the marked ischemic diastolic dysfunction caused by exposure to angiotensin II.

SUMMARY AND THERAPEUTIC IMPLICATIONS

This chapter has reviewed the major cellular mechanisms known to be involved in the regulation of myocardial relaxation and the occurrence of diastolic dysfunction. Consideration of these mechanisms leads naturally to the construction of therapeutic strategies designed to enhance myocardial relaxation, and to prevent or alleviate diastolic dysfunction. The central role of calcium in regulating myofilament tension generation, and the mechanisms regulating intracellular calcium levels and myofilament sensitivity to calcium have been presented in detail. Numerous interventions and drugs have the potential to alter diastolic cytosolic calcium levels and myofilament sensitivity to calcium, thereby exerting positive or negative inotropic and lusitropic effects. These interventions and agents are summarized in Table 1–1 and Figure 1–4. In patients with heart failure, who often have both systolic and diastolic dysfunction, a major challenge will be the manipulation of calcium regulatory mechanisms so that diastolic calcium levels and myofilament sensitivity are decreased to enhance relaxation without similarly affecting systolic tension generation and worsening systolic dysfunction. The preliminary studies of Weinberg et al. (69) are encouraging in this regard, demonstrating that a combination of a β-adrenergic agonist and a calcium channel blocker can selectively augment relaxation without altering indices of contractility.

The importance of ATP in regulating myocardial relaxation and the evidence implicating an important role for glycolytic ATP has been reviewed. The critical role of ATP availability in supporting the repolarization-relaxation process, and the specific role that glycolytically synthesized ATP appears to play in maintaining normal myocardial relaxation, have potentially significant clinical implications. First of all, maintenance of the myocyte ATP level is obviously important for normal diastolic function. In practical terms, the standard approach of avoiding myocardial ischemia

and minimizing any oxygen supply/demand imbalance are important principles, particularly in hypertrophied hearts. In addition, the clinician should consider that alterations of glycolytic substrate can have a significant influence on diastolic function particularly during stress (e.g., tachycardia), ischemia, or hypoxia. Thus, hypoglycemia is to be avoided. A high glucose and insulin substrate has been shown to be beneficial in animal studies and should be considered a potential therapy for patients with hypoxic or ischemic diastolic dysfunction. The observed beneficial hemodynamic effects when high glucose and insulin therapy was used in post-MI and postoperative patients with depressed cardiac output (106, 107) may have resulted partly from improvement of diastolic function. Other metabolic approaches to increase glycolytic ATP synthesis as a mechanism of improving cardiac lusitropy should be considered as potential future therapy for diastolic dysfunction.

Evidence implicating the renin angiotensin system as a significant culprit in contributing to ischemic diastolic dysfunction, especially in hearts with hypertrophy, has also been presented. The experimental data reviewed in this chapter summarize results obtained in rats with global concentric hypertrophy secondary to aortic banding, but the clinical implications may not be limited to patients with concentric LVH. Patients with coronary artery disease often have regional, heterogeneous hypertrophy as nonischemic regions hypertrophy to compensate for the loss of function in ischemic or infarcted regions. Therefore, it is possible that ACE inhibition and angiotensin receptor blocking agents may be beneficial in treating the diastolic dysfunction that occurs in patients with chronic coronary artery disease who exhibit impaired myocardial relaxation in the setting of recurrent ischemia. Because angiotensin II may impair relaxation by activating protein kinase C and sodium-hydrogen exchange, therapy directed towards protein kinase C inhibition or inhibition of sodium-hydrogen exchange and intracellular alkalosis may also prove beneficial in relieving ischemic diastolic dysfunction.

The processes of repolarization and relaxation have a complexity equal to that of

Table 1–1. Interventions that Theoretically Alter Diastolic Cytosolic Calcium Levels

Intervention	Theoretical Effect on Diastolic Ca_i^{2+}	Mechanisms/Comments
Ischemia or hypoxia	Increase	Decreased SR reuptake and SL extrusion
Digitalis	Increase	Increases Na_i^+ by Na^+/K^+ pump inhibition; Ca_i^{2+} increased secondary to increased Na^+-Ca^{2+} exchange. Combination of ischemia or hypoxia + digitalis causes exaggerated diastolic dysfunction (Isoyama et al.; Cunningham et al).
Ca^{2+} channel blocker	Decrease	Decreased Ca^{2+} entry by way of sarcolemma. Associated bradycardia prolongs diastole, allowing for greater calcium removal via SR and SL
β-adrenergic blocker	±	Decreased c-AMP levels decrease Ca^{2+} entry via Ca^{2+}-channel, but also decrease Ca^{2+} reuptake by SR. Associated bradycardia prolongs diastole as with Ca^{2+} channel blocker
β-adrenergic agonist	±	Increased c-AMP levels increase Ca^{2+} entry, but also increase SR calcium reuptake by phospholamban regulation.
Phosphodiesterase inhibitors	±	Same mechanisms as β-adrenergic agonist
Ca^{2+} agonist (BAYK8644)	Increase	Increased Ca^{2+} influx via L-type channels can produce Ca^{2+} overload
Ca^{2+} ionophore (A23187)	Increase	Increased transarcolemmal Ca^{2+} influx
Na^{2+} agonist (Veratridine)	Increase	$[Ca^{2+}]_i$ loading by Na/Ca^{2+} exchange
Na^{2+} ionophore (Monensin)	Increase	$[Ca^{2+}]_i$ loading by Na/Ca^{2+} exchange
Antagonist of Na/Ca^{2+} exchanger (dichlorobenzamil)	±	Potential to affect $[Na^+]_i$
Antagonist of Na^+/H^+ exchanger (Amiloride)	±	Potential to affect $[Na^+]_i$
Inhibitor of SR Ca^{2+} uptake (caffeine)	±	Multiple effects but blocks Ca^{2+} uptake after inducing Ca^{2+} release
SR Ca^{2+} ATPase inhibitor (thapsigargin)	±	Blocks Ca^{2+} uptake by inhibiting pump
Inhibitor SR Ca^{2+} release (ryanodine)	±	Blocks Ca^{2+} release channel of SR leading to Ca^{2+} overload of vesicles and decreased uptake
Phospholamban antibodies	±	May enhance SR Ca^{2+} uptake by modifying function of phospholamban
Mitochondrial inhibitors (FCCP)	±	Decreased Ca^{2+} storage capacity of mitochondria in overload state

excitation-contraction. It is likely that future therapy of diastolic dysfunction will be based on an understanding and pharmacologic exploitation of the subcellular mechanisms summarized in this chapter, as well as others yet to be elucidated, in an effort to increase cardiac lusitropy.

REFERENCES

1. Katz AM: Cardiomyopathy of overload: A major determinant of prognosis in congestive heart failure. N Engl J Med 322:100, 1990.
2. Morgan JP: Mechanisms of disease. Abnormal intracellular modulation of cal-

cium as a major cause of cardiac contractile dysfunction. N Engl J Med 325:625, 1991.

3. Katz AM: Interplay between inotropic and lusitropic effects of cyclic adenosine monophosphate on the myocardial cell. Circulation 82:I7, 1990.

4. Rasmussen H: The calcium messenger system. N Engl J Med 314:1094, 1164, 1986.

5. Blinks JR, Endoh M: Modification of myofibrillar responsiveness to Ca++ as an inotropic mechanism. Circulation 73:III-85, 1986.

6. Katz AM: Requirements of contraction and relaxation: implications for inotropic stimulation of the failing heart. Basic Res Cardiol 84:47, 1989.

7. Perreault CL, et al: Differential effects of hypertrophy and failure on right versus left ventricular calcium activation. Circ Res 67:707, 1990.

8. Perreault CL, Hague NL, Ransil BJ, Morgan JP: The effects of cocaine on intracellular Ca{+2+} handling and myofilament Ca{+2+} responsiveness of ferret ventricular myocardium. Br J Pharmac 101: 679, 1990.

9. Gwathmey JK, Morgan JP: Altered calcium handling in experimental pressure-overload hypertrophy in the ferret. Circ Res 57:836, 1985.

10. Bentivegna LA, Ablin LW, Kihara Y, Morgan JP: Altered calcium handling in left ventricular pressure overload hypertrophy as detected with aequorin in the isolated, perfused ferret heart. Circ Res 69: 1538, 1545, 1991.

11. Wikman-Coffelt J, et al.: [Ca{+2+}]{−i} transients in the cardiomyopathic hamster heart. Circ Res 68:45, 1991.

12. Maher KA, et al.: Abnormalities in excitation-contraction coupling in diabetic cardiomyopathic rats. Circulation 84 (Suppl)II:446, 1991.

13. Litwin SE, Morgan JP: Intracellular Ca2+ handling and Ā-adrenergic responsiveness in surviving myocardium from rats with large infarctions. Circulation 84 (Suppl II):II10, 1991.

14. Kihara Y, Grossman W, Morgan JP: Direct measurement of changes in intracellular calcium transients during hypoxia, ischemia, and reperfusion of the intact mammalian heart. Circ Res 65:1029, 1989.

15. Kihara Y, Gwathmey JK, Grossman W, Morgan JP: Mechanisms of positive inotropic effects and delayed relaxation produced by DPI 201–206 in mammalian working myocardium: effects on intracellular calcium handling. Br J Pharmac 96: 927, 1989.

16. Levine MJ, et al.: Excitation-contraction uncoupling during ischemia in the blood perfused dog heart. Biochem Biophys Res Commun 179:502, 1991.

17. MacKinnon R, Gwathmey JK, Morgan JP: Differential effects of reoxygenation on intracellular calcium and isometric tension. Pflugers Arch 409:448, 1987.

18. Marban E, et al.: Intracellular free calcium concentration measured with 19F NMR spectroscopy in intact ferret hearts. Proc Natl Acad Sci USA 84:6005, 1987.

19. Steenbergen C, Murphy E, Levy L, London RE: Elevation in cytosolic free calcium concentration early in myocardial ischemia in perfused rat heart. Circ Res 60: 700, 1987.

20. Mohabir R, Lee HC, Kurz RW, Clusin WT: Effects of ischemia and hypercarbia acidosis on myocyte calcium transients, contraction, and pH{−i} in perfused rabbit hearts. Circ Res 69:1525, 1991.

21. Gwathmey JK, et al.: Abnormal intracellular calcium handling in myocardium from patients with end-stage heart failure. Circ Res 61:70, 1987.

22. Morgan JP, MacKinnon R, Briggs M, Gwathmey JK: Calcium and cardiac relaxation. In Diastolic Relaxation of the Heart. Edited by W Grossman and BH Lorell. Boston: Martinus Nijhoff, 1988, pp. 17–26.

23. Gwathmey JK, et al.: Diastolic dysfunction in hypertrophic cardiomyopathy: Effect on active force generation during systole. J Clin Invest 87:1023, 1991.

24. Morgan JP, et al.: Abnormal intracellular calcium handling: a major cause of systolic and diastolic dysfunction in ventricular myocardium from patients with heart failure. Circulation 81:21, 1990.

25. Phillips PJ, et al.: Post extrasystolic potentiation and the force-frequency relationship: differential augmentation of myocardial contractility in working myocardium from patients with end-stage heart failure. J Mol Cell Cardiol 22:99, 1990.

26. Feldman MD, et al.: Deficient production of cyclic AMP: Pharmacologic evidence of an important cause of contractile dysfunction in patients with end-stage heart failure. Circulation 75:331, 1987.

27. Erdmann E: The effectiveness of inotropic agents in isolated cardiac preparations from the human heart. Klin Wochenschr 66:1, 1988.

28. Nabauer M, et al.: Positive inotropic effects in isolated ventricular myocardium from non-failing and terminally failing human hearts. Eur J Clin Invest 18:600, 1988.
29. Feldman AM, Cates AE, Veazey, et al.: Increase of the 40,000 mol wt. pertussis toxin substrate (G-protein) in the failing human heart. J Clin Invest 82:189, 1988.
30. Neumann J, et al.: Increase in myocardial Gi-proteins in heart failure. Lancet 8617:936, 1988.
31. Bhm M, Gierchik P, Jakobs KH, et al.: Increase in Gi alpha in human hearts with dilated but not ischemic cardiomyopathy. Circulation 82:1249, 1990.
32. Fleming JW, Wisler PL, Watanabe AM: Surgical transduction by G proteins in cardiac tissues. Circulation 85:420, 1992.
33. Mercadier JJ, Lompre AM, Duc P, et al.: Altered sarcoplasmic reticulum Ca{2+} ATPase gene expression in the human ventricle during end-stage heart failure. J Clin Invest 85:305, 1990.
34. Lefkowitz RJ, Caron MG: Role of phosphorylation in desensitization of the beta adrenoceptor. Trends Pharmacol Sci 11:190, 1990.
35. Collins S, Bolanowski MA, Caron MG, Lefkowitz RJ: Genetic regulation of beta-adrenergic receptors. Annu Rev Physiol 51:203, 1989.
36. Brodde OE: Ā1 and Ā2-adrenoceptors in the human heart: properties, function and alterations in chronic heart failure. Pharmacol Rev 43:203, 1991.
37. Bristow MR, Hershenberger RE, Port JD, et al.: Beta-adrenergic pathways in non-failing human ventricular myocardium. Circulation 82:I12, 1990.
38. Bristow MR, Anderson FL, Poat JD, et al.: Differences in beta-adrenergic neuro effector mechanisms in ischemic versus idiopathic dilated cardiomyopathy. Circulation 84:1024, 1991.
39. Benovic JL, et al.: Ā-adrenergic receptor kinase. Activity of partial agonists for stimulation of adenylate cyclase correlates with ability to promote receptor phosphorylation. J Bio Chem 263:3893, 1988.
40. Rasmussen RP, Minobe W, Bristow MR: Calcium antagonist binding sites in failing and non-failing human ventricular myocardium. Biochem Pharmacol 39:691, 1990.
41. Kaczorowski GJ, Slaughter RS, King VF, Garcia ML: Inhibitors of sodium-calcium exchange: identification and development of probes of transport activity. Biochem Biophys Acta 988:287, 1989.
42. Schouten VJA, Ter Keurs HEDL, Quaegebeur JM: Influence of electrogenic Na/Ca exchange on the action potential in human heart failure. Cardiovasc Res 24:758, 1990.
43. Gwathmey JK, Slawsky MT, Briggs GM, Morgan JP: The role of intracellular sodium in the regulation of intracellular calcium and contractility. Effects of DPI 201–206 on excitation-contraction coupling in human ventricular myocardium. J Clin Invest 82:1592, 1988.
44. Grupp G, Grupp IL, Melvin DB, Schwartz A: Functional evidence in diseased human heart fibers for multiple sensitivities of the inotropic ouabain receptor Na+, K+-ATPase. Prog Clin Biol Res 258:215, 1988.
45. Caroni P, Carafoli E: An ATP-dependent pumping system in dog heart sarcolemma. Nature 283:765, 1980.
46. Sutko JL, Ito K, Kenyon JL: Ryanodine: A modifier of sarcoplasmic reticulum calcium release in striated muscle. Fed Proc 44:2984, 1985.
47. MacLennan DH: Molecular tools to elucidate problems in excitation-contraction coupling. Biophys J 58:1355, 1990.
48. Lompre AM, Lambert F, Lakatta EG, Schwartz K: Expression of sarcoplasmic reticulum Ca2+-ATPase and calsequestrin genes in rat heart during ontogenic development and aging. Circ Res 69:1380, 1991.
49. De La Bastie D, et al.: Function of the sarcoplasmic reticulum and expression of its Ca2+-ATPase gene in pressure overload-induced cardiac hypertrophy in the rat. Circ Res 66:552, 1990.
50. Feldman AM, et al.: Selective gene expression in failing human heart. Quantification of steady state levels of messenger RNA in endomyocardial biopsies using the polymerase chain reaction. Circulation 33:1866, 1991.
51. Movsesian MA, et al.: Identification and characterization of proteins in sarcoplasmic reticulum from normal and failing human left ventricles. J Mol Cell Cardiol 22:1477, 1990.
52. Movsesian MA, Bristow MR, Krall J: Ca{−2+} uptake by cardiac sarcoplasmic reticulum from patients with idiopathic dilated cardiomyopathy. Circ Res 65:1141, 1989.
53. Gwathmey JW, et al.: The role of intracellular calcium handling in force-interval relationships of human ventricular myocardium. J Clin Invest 85:1599, 1990.
54. Regg JC, Morano I: Calcium-sensitivity

modulation of cardiac myofibrillar proteins. J Cardiovasc Pharma 14:S20, 1989.

55. Morano I, Arndt H, Gartner C, Regg JC: Skinned fibers of human atrium and ventricle: myosin isoenzyme and contractility. Circ Res 62:632, 1988.

56. Ventura C, Capogrossi MC, Spurgeon HA, Lakatta EG: Kappa-opido peptide receptor stimulation increases cytosolic pH and myofilament responsiveness to $Ca\{+2+\}$ in cardiac myocytes. Am J Physil 261:H1671, 1991.

57. Capogrossi MC, et al.: $Ca2+$ dependence of alpha-adrenergic effects on the contractile properties and $Ca2+$ homeostasis of cardiac myocytes. Circ Res 69:540, 1991.

58. Kramer BK, Smith TW, Kelly RA: Endothelin and increased contractility in adult rat ventricular myocytes. Role of intracellular alkalosis induced by activation of the protein kinase C-dependent $Na+-H+$ exchanger. Circ Res 68:269, 1991.

59. Kelly RA, et al.: Endothelin enhances the contractile responsiveness of adult rat ventricular myocytes to a calcium by a pertussis toxin-sensitive pathway. J Clin Invest 86:1164, 1991.

60. Hajjar RJ, Gwathmey JK, Briggs GM, Morgan JP: Differential effect of DP1 201–106 on the sensitivity of myofilaments to $Ca2+$ in intact and skinned trabeculae from control and myopathic human hearts. J Clin Invest 82:1578, 1988.

61. Wankerl M, et al.: Calcium sensitivity and myosin light chain pattern of atrial and ventricular skinned cardiac fibers from patients with various kinds of cardiac diseases. J Mol Cell Cardiol 22:1425, 1990.

62. D'Angelo A, et al.: Contractile properties and $Ca2+$ release activity of the sarcoplasmic reticulum in dilated cardiomyopathy. Circulation 85:518, 1992.

63. Wankerl M, et al.: Calcium sensitivity and myosin light chain pattern of atrial and ventricular stunned cardiac fibers from patients with various kinds of cardiac disease. J Mol Cell Cardiol 22:1425, 1990.

64. Perreault CL, Brozovich FV, Ransil BJ, Morgan JP: Effects of MCI-154 on $Ca\{+2+\}$ activation of skinned human myocardium. Eur J Pharm 165:305, 1989.

65. Pagani ED, et al.: Changes in myofibrillar content and MgATPase activity in ventricular tissues from patients with heart failure caused by coronary artery disease, cardiomyopathy or mitral valve insufficiency. Circ Res 63:380, 1988.

66. Cunningham MJ, Apstein CS, Weinberg EO, Lorell BH: Deleterious effect of ouabain on myocardial function during hypoxia. Am J Physiol 256:H681, 1989.

67. Chodos AP, et al.: Effects of ouabain and isoproterenol on diastolic function during low-flow ischemia in isolated rabbit hearts. Clin Res 36:267A, 1988.

68. Lorell BH, et al.: Effects of ouabain and isoproterenol on left ventricular diastolic function during low-flow ischemia in isolated, blood-perfused rabbit hearts. Circ Res 63:457, 1988.

69. Weinberg EO, Apstein CS, Vogel WM: Impaired myocardial relaxation is improved by combined beta-adrenergic stimulation and calcium channel blockade. J Mol Cell Cardiol 23(Suppl III):S.68, 1991.

70. Katz AM: Physiology of the Heart. New York, Raven Press, 1992, pp. 151–177.

71. Bittl JA, Ingwall JS: Reaction rates of creatine kinase and ATP synthesis in the isolated rat heart. J Bio Chem 260:3512, 1985.

72. Bittl JA, Balschi JA, Ingwall JS: Contractile failure and high-energy phosphate turnover during hypoxia: 31P-NMR surface coil studies in living rat. Circ Res 60:871, 1987.

73. Apstein CS, Bing OHL, Levine HJ: Cardiac muscle function during and after hypoxia: Effect of glucose concentration, mannitol and isoproterenol. J Mol Cell Cardiol 8:627, 1976.

74. Apstein CS, Gravino FN, Haudenschild CC: Determinants of a protective effect of glucose and insulin on the ischemic myocardium: Effects of contractile function, diastolic compliance, metabolism and ultrastructure during ischemia and reperfusion. Circ Res 52:515, 1983.

75. Eberli FR, et al.: Protective effect of increased glycolytic substrate against systolic and diastolic dysfunction and increased coronary resistance from prolonged global underperfusion and reperfusion in isolated rabbit hearts perfused with erythrocyte suspensions. Circ Res 68·466, 1991.

76. Owen P, Dennis S, Opie LH: Glucose flux rate regulates onset of ischemic contracture in globally underperfused rat hearts. Circ Res 66:344, 1990.

77. Gubdjarnason S, Mathes P, Ravens KG: Functional compartmentalization of ATP and creatine phosphate in heart muscle. J Mol Cell Cardiol 1:325, 1970.

78. Weiss J, Hiltbrand B: Functional compartmentation of glycolytic versus oxidative metabolism in isolated rabbit hearts. J Clin Invest 75:436, 1985.

79. Weiss JN, Lamp ST: Glycolysis preferentially inhibits ATP-sensitive $K+$ channels

in isolated guinea pig cardiac myocytes. Science 238:67, 1987.

80. Paul RJ, et al.: Preferential support of Ca++ uptake in smooth muscle plasma membrane vesicles by an endogenous glycolytic cascade. FASEB J 3:2298, 1989.

81. Han JW, Thielczek R, Varsanyi M, Herlmeyer LMG: Compartmentalized ATP synthesis in skeletal muscle triads. Biochem 31:377, 1992.

82. Entman ML, et al.: Association of glycogenolysis with cardiac sarcoplasmic reticulum. J Bio Chem 25:3140, 1976.

83. Apstein CS, Deckelbaum L, Hagopian L, Hood WBJ: Acute cardiac ischemia and reperfusion. Contractility, relaxation and glycolysis. Am J Physiol 235:H637, 1978.

84. Gordon PC, Weinberg EO, Apstein CS, Lorell BH: Glycolytic cytosolic ATP modifies lusitropic reserve in well-oxygenated rabbit hearts. Circulation 84:II-278, 1991.

85. Cunningham MJ, et al.: Influence of glucose and insulin on the exaggerated diastolic and systolic dysfunction of hypertrophied rats hearts during hypoxia. Circ Res 66:406, 1990.

86. Gaasch WH, et al.: Tolerance of the hypertrophic heart to ischemia. Circulation 81:1644, 1990.

87. Dzau VJ: Cardiac renin-angiotensin system: molecular and functional aspects. Am J Med 84:22, 1988.

88. Kanapuli SP, Kumar A: Molecular cloning of human angiotensin cDNA and evidence for the presence of its nRNA in rat heart. Circ Res 60:786, 1987.

89. Baker KM, Campanile CP, Trachte GJ, Peach MJ: Identification and characterization of the rabbit angiotensin II myocardial receptor. Circ Res 54:286, 1984.

90. Schunkert H, et al.: Increased rat cardiac angiotensin converting enzyme activity and mRNA expression in pressure overload left ventricular hypertrophy: Effects on coronary resistance, contractility and relaxation. J Clin Invest 86:1913, 1990.

91. Eberli FR, Apstein CS, Ngoy S, Lorell BH: Exacerbation of left ventricular ischemic diastolic dysfunction by pressure overload hypertrophy: Modification by specific inhibition of cardiac angiotensin converting enzyme. Circ Res 70:931, 1992.

92. Lorell BH, Weinberg EO, Ngoy S, Apstein CS: Angiotensin II directly impairs diastolic function in pressure overload hypertrophy. Circulation 82:440, 1990.

93. Mochizuki T, Eberli FR, Apstein CS, Lorell BH: Exacerbation of ischemic dysfunction by angiotensin II in red-cell perfused rabbit hearts: Effects on coronary flow, contractility, and high energy phosphate metabolism. J Clin Invest 89:490, 1992.

94. Hori M, et al.: Angiotensin II stimulates protein synthesis in neonatal rat cardiomyocytes through enhanced Na+/H+ exchange (abstract). Circulation 80:450, 1989.

95. Baker KM and Singer HA: Identification and characterization of guinea pig angiotensin II ventricular and atrial receptors: Coupling to inositol phosphate production. Circ Res 62:896, 1988.

96. Dosemeci A, et al.: Phorbol ester increases calcium current and simulates the effects of angiotensin II on cultured neonatal rat heart myocytes. Circ Res 62:347, 1988.

97. Nosek TM, Williams MF, Aeigler ST, and Godt RE: Inositol triphosphate enhances calcium release in skinned cardiac and skeletal muscle. Am J Physiol 250:c807, 1986.

98. Nabika T, Velletri PA, Lovenberg W, Beaven MA: Increase in cytosolic calcium and phosphoinositide metabolism induced by angiotensin II and [Arg] vasopressin in vascular smooth muscle cells. J Bio Chem 260:4661, 1985.

99. Gwathmey JK, Haijar R: Effect of protein kinase C activation on sarcoplasmic reticulum function and apparent myofibrillar Ca2+ sensitivity in intact and skinned muscles from normal and diseased human myocardium. Circ Res 67:744, 1990.

100. Yuan S, Sunahara FA, Sen AK: Tumor-promoting phorbol esters inhibit cardiac functions and induce redistribution of protein kinase C in perfused beating rat heart. Circ Res 61:371, 1987.

101. Moorman JR, Kirsch GE, Lacerda AE, Brown AM: Angiotensin II modulates cardiac Na+ channels in neonatal rat. Circ Res 65:1804, 1989.

102. Nishizuka Y: Studies and perspectives of protein kinase C. Science 233:305, 1986.

103. Lorrell BH, Weinberg EO, Ikenouchi H, Barry WH: Change of Indo-I [Ca2+] transients and contractility induced by angiogensin II. Circulation 82(Suppl III): III-141, 1990.

104. Mochizuki T, et al.: The effects of angiotensin in pressure overload hypertrophy are simulated by protein kinase C activation. Circulation 84(Suppl II):II–308, 1991.

105. Mochizuki T, et al.: Impairment of diastolic function by angiotensin II in pressure overload hypertrophy: Evidence for Na+/H+ exchange. Circulation 84:II-280, 1991.

106. Coleman GM, Gradinac S, Taegtmeyer H, et al.: Efficacy of metabolic support with glucose-insulin-potassium for left ventricular pump failure after aortocoronary bypass surgery. Circulation 80(Suppl I):I-91, 1989.

107. Mantle JA, Rogers WJ, Smith R, et al.: Clinical effects of glucose-insulin-potassium on left ventricular function in acute myocardial infarction: Results from a randomized clinical trial. Am Heart J 102: 313, 1981.

Chapter 2

PHYSIOLOGIC CONTROL OF RELAXATION IN ISOLATED CARDIAC MUSCLE AND INTACT LEFT VENTRICLE

Thierry C. Gillebert and Stanislas U. Sys

The cardiologist at a patient's bedside describes left ventricular (LV) function in terms of blood pressure, filling pressure, pressure-volume relation, cardiac output, and ejection fraction. This clinical approach adequately describes the cardiovascular system as a *pump*, but does not directly relate to underlying properties of the LV *myocardium* such as contractility, relaxation and compliance.

Compliance relates to the passive properties of the LV, measured during diastole. *Diastole* means separation between two contraction-relaxation cycles (Fig. 2–1), and its use should be restricted for describing passive cardiac properties such as muscular stiffness or ventricular compliance (1). Diastole starts when relaxation has been completed, which in normal circumstances is during rapid LV filling near minimum pressure. LV diastole includes the later part of rapid LV filling, slow LV filling, and atrial contraction.

Relaxation of isolated cardiac muscle relates to the processes whereby cardiac muscle after contraction returns to its initial length and tension. In the intact LV transition between contraction and relaxation occurs during LV ejection (2–3). LV relaxation encompasses the later part of LV ejection, isovolumetric LV pressure fall and the earlier part of rapid LV filling. Early LV filling is still part of active relaxation with decreasing pressures and increasing volumes and even the ability of the LV to develop active suction (4–5). Relaxation, as the manifestation of *myocardial inactivation*, has physiologic determinants such as heart rate, temperature, and neurohumoral stimulation. Impaired inactivation can result from aging, ischemia, hypertro-

phy and fibrosis, hypothyreosis, myocarditis etc. Clinical cardiologists expect indexes reflecting pathologic changes in inactivation, which might prove useful in clinical situations. The time constant of LV pressure fall τ, and the underlying assumption that isovolumetric LV pressure fall is monoexponential, were initially considered to be the rather undisturbed expression of cardiac muscle inactivation (6). However, when experimental data became available, it appeared that neither τ, nor any index of relaxation could be used to directly assess muscle inactivation. Relaxation itself, and hence its indexes, are regulated not only by inactivation but also by load and nonuniformity (1). To understand usefulness and limitations of indexes of relaxation, it is important to first understand the factors that influence relaxation under normal conditions (7). (See Chap. 13.) Therefore, a distinction between contribution of impaired inactivation, nonuniformity, and load requires detailed understanding of how these three determinants control isolated cardiac muscle relaxation and how they affect timing and pattern of LV relaxation.

This chapter analyzes conceptual aspects of isolated cardiac muscle physiology and integrates these aspects in the observed behavior of the intact LV.

CARDIAC MUSCLE RELAXATION

Load Dependence of Relaxation

In earlier work, load dependence of relaxation described cardiac muscle properties related to the extent of development and the activity of calcium-sequestering membrane systems. Load dependence initially described rapid lengthening of preloaded or afterload isotonic twitches. Iso-

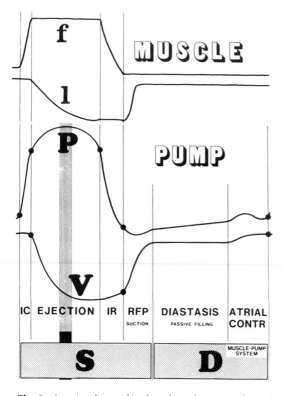

Fig. 2–1. Analogy of isolated cardiac muscle and intact LV function. Time traces of force (f) and length (l) of an afterloaded twitch with physiologic relaxation sequence are synchronized with LV pressure (P) and volume (V) curves. One heart cycle is represented and subdivided in systole and diastole. Systole encompasses contraction and relaxation. See text for details. Modified with permission from Brutsaert, D.L., and Sys, S.U.: Relaxation and diastole of the heart. Physiol. Rev. 69: 1228, 1989.

pendence focuses on the contrast between isotonic and isometric twitches and on the contrast between isotonic and isometric relaxation. Isotonic twitches are shorter than isometric twitches. Isotonic lengthening is a fast phenomenon in contrast to isometric force decline, which is slow. The result of this contrast is a separation in time, a delay of relaxation, when afterload increases from a preloaded isotonic twitch to an isometric twitch. The extent of the separation in time of relaxation of differently loaded twitches is therefore determined by time of onset and by speed of isotonic lengthening and isometric force decline. Variations in load dependence, which manifest as variations in the extent of separation in time, result from changes in the different processes underlying lengthening as well as force decline during relaxation. Isotonic and isometric relaxation are governed by the totality of processes leading to the disappearance of force-generating sites. Important processes determining number of crossbridges at any moment in time during relaxation are (1) the life-cycle of each individual crossbridge along with regulatory properties of the contractile proteins, and (2) calcium removal by the calcium-sequestering membrane systems, particularly the sarcoplasmic reticulum. These processes together underlie cardiac muscle inactivation. The interaction between load and inactivation controls onset and rate of isometric force decline and isotonic lengthening. The nonuniform distribution in time and space of load and (in)activation, at all levels of performance from the molecular to the whole organ level, is considered as a third control mechanism of myocardial performance (10).

At the ultrastructural level, control of relaxation by load, inactivation and nonuniformity can be interpreted in terms of contractile protein properties and cellular calcium homeostasis. The contribution of these processes in controlling onset and rate of relaxation seems to depend critically upon experimental conditions, particularly upon isometric versus isotonic loading conditions, neurohumoral and hormonal environment. In the following section, recent experiments will be described that give new insights into processes underlying relaxa-

tonic lengthening was shown to be very responsive to load. For example, an increase in load during relaxation induced a premature lengthening of the muscle and early termination of the twitch (8).

Subsequent studies emphasized that preloaded or afterloaded isotonic twitches were of shorter duration than an isometric twitch (9) and that this different duration of twitches also disappeared when activity of calcium-sequestering membrane systems was impaired.

More recently (1), the concept of load dependence was generalized and integrated into the triple control of relaxation by load, inactivation and nonuniformity. *Load de-*

tion in rapid lengthening and slow force decline.

Lengthening During Isotonic Relaxation

Rapid lengthening allows load-dependent relaxation to become manifest. In isotonic twitches, load is important in prematurely interrupting force generation with subsequent rapid lengthening of the muscle and abbreviation of the preloaded or afterloaded isotonic twitch. This abbreviation of the isotonic twitch is presumably induced by the imbalance between developed force and load to be carried (8). In the crossbridge model of (skeletal) muscle contraction (11), the load would put a progressively increasing strain on the remaining crossbridges which are still attached; this would cause them to rotate backwards over their full range of movement and to detach, thereby causing the myofilaments to slide back to their original positions (12). This forceful detachment of crossbridges further manifests by the subsequent abrupt isometric force decline of the afterloaded isotonic twitch (8).

The abbreviation of the isotonic twitch, induced by the imbalance between developed force and load to be carried, requires a preceding calcium sequestration by the sarcoplasmic reticulum. Its importance is derived from a variety of experimental conditions in which the sarcoplasmic reticulum is less developed, biochemically destroyed, or functionally inhibited. When sarcoplasmic reticulum is less functional, isotonic muscle lengthening is prolonged and follows the time course of force decline of an isometric twitch: twitch duration becomes almost independent of load or changes in load. As a consequence, whenever removal of the myoplasmic activating calcium has been suppressed, load dependence of mammalian cardiac muscle relaxation is diminished through impairment of rapid isotonic lengthening.

Force Decline During Isometric Relaxation

In isolated cardiac muscle, force decline during relaxation has been analyzed (13–15) after reversal of the isotonic-isometric to an isometric-isotonic relaxation sequence, in order to better mimic the relaxation sequence in the intact heart where iso(volu)metric pressure fall precedes isotonic filling. However, when extrapolating such data to the intact LV, one has to realize that myocardial segments seldom are strictly isometric between aortic valve closure and mitral valve opening: some segments develop postejection shortening while other segments develop early segment re-extension. Therefore, one has to be extremely cautious and include nonuniform LV segmental behavior when extrapolating data on physiologically sequenced force decline to LV pressure fall.

Yet, determinants of the entire process of force during relaxation cannot be derived from these studies because only peak rate of force decline was considered in those studies. We proposed phase-plane analysis of the rate of force decline as a function of instantaneous force during relaxation for analyzing the pattern of force decline (16). We will now describe influences of loading or shortening history (short-term load, within the same twitch), of muscle length and of extracellular calcium concentration on force decline during isometric relaxation in isolated cat papillary muscle.

Time Independence of Rate of Force Decline versus Force

In Figure 2–2, three pairs of isometric and afterloaded isotonic twitches are compared. Each letter A, B or C, indicates a pair of two twitches with different contraction phase (isometric versus afterloaded isotonic), but with force decline occurring at exactly the same muscle length. In each pair, the phase-plane traces during isometric relaxation coincided, indicating an otherwise identical pattern of force decline despite a shift in time of these patterns ranging from 15 msec in A to 50 msec in C. Hence, at a given muscle length during relaxation, force decline of an isometric twitch and of an afterloaded isotonic twitch with isometric-isotonic relaxation sequence followed a single pattern. The same rate of force decline was thus recorded at any given instantaneous force in pairs of twitches despite marked differences in peak force. Even more striking separation (up to 350 msec) of the time traces of force decline during relaxation were described

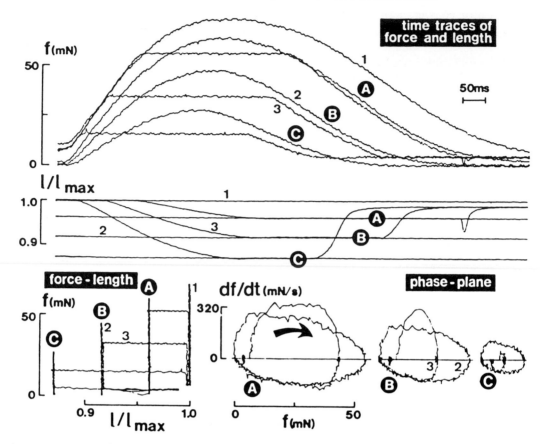

Fig. 2–2. Time independence of isometric force decline. Time tracings of force and length of three pairs (A, B, and C) of twitches are displayed along with the relations of force versus length and of df/dt versus force (phase-plane). In pair B, for instance, twitch 2 was an isometric twitch at a shorter than optimal muscle length; preload and peak developed force were typically lower than in the isometric twitch at l_{max} (twitch 1 as a reference). Twitch 3 was an afterloaded isotonic twitch during which the muscle reached the same length at peak shortening as the length during twitch 2. For force decline in twitches 2 and 3 to occur at the same muscle length, relaxation sequence in twitch 3 was made isometric-isotonic. During both isometric relaxation phases, the pattern of force decline was shifted in time (35 ms in this example) but otherwise identical. The force decline traces share a common path on the phase-plane of df/dt versus f, which suggests that, despite a different time of onset, amplitude and rate of force decline are uniquely related. Reproduced with permission from Sys, S.U., and Brutsaert, D.L.: Determinants of force decline during relaxation in isolated cardiac muscle. *Am. J. Physiol.* 257:H1490, 1989.

in the presence of coinciding phase-plane trajectories (16). The superposition of the curvilinear of phase-plane traces of rate of force decline as a function of instantaneous force shows that, at any given muscle length, rate of force decline was determined by instantaneous force, independently of the time at which this force occurred.

The relationship between force and rate of force decline during isometric relaxa-tion at any given muscle length was not in-fluenced by the way this length was reached or by the history of loading and shortening during the contraction phase of the twitch, e.g., preload or muscle length at the onset of the twitch and afterload or extent of shortening. This time-independent rate of force decline was consistent with the find-ing that force decline during late relaxation did not depend on the sarcoplasmic reticu-lum (17) and that, during the first minutes of hypoxia or reoxygenation, the only observed change of the mechanic performance was a shift in time of force decline (18). Time independence of force decline relates to the second phase of force decline only. By contrast, early isometric force decline is very sensitive to load or changes in load. Early isometric force decline slows down following a late load increase and accelerates following a late load decrease (15). This sensitivity of early isometric force decline is a manifestation of load dependence and is presumably related to changes in crossbridge life cycle or Ca^{2+} affinity of contractile proteins, induced by load changes during relaxation.

Length but not Calcium as Modulator of Terminal Force Decline

Length modulation of force decline was studied because, in isometric twitches at shorter muscle lengths, a higher rate of terminal force decline was observed for the same instantaneous force. In phase-plane analysis of isometric twitches, even after peak rate of force decline was attained, the pattern of force decline was not linear but curved. A quantitative measure of the rate of force decline near the end of relaxation could be obtained from the slope of the phase-plane trace in the origin, i.e., near the end of isometric relaxation, when developed force and rate of force decline tend toward zero. Time constants were derived alluding to the common use of a time constant to characterize pressure fall in the intact ventricle. This measure can be interpreted as a limit of time constant of a piecewise exponential approximation to force decline as developed force tends to zero or as mechanic activity of the muscle ceases, i.e., the time constant of terminal force decline. The time constant of terminal force decline was calculated from isometric twitches at different muscle lengths and different external calcium concentrations.

In addition to time independence of the relation between force and rate of overall force declining during relaxation, the rate of terminal force decline was independent of $[Ca^{2+}]_o$. Although a direct comparison with literature data is not so obvious, at least two previous papers (19, 20) led to a similar conclusion. For any given contrac-

tile state, terminal rate of force decline increased at shorter muscle lengths; the relationship between length and the time constant could appropriately be represented by a straight line. From an average of 85 ± 12 ms at l_{max}, the time constant of terminal force decline decreased by 20 ± 6 ms with every length decrease of 10% l_{max}. Increased rate of isometric relaxation at shorter lengths has been described for skeletal (21–23) and cardiac muscle (24). Apparently contradictory findings concerning the effects of length or $[Ca^{2+}]_o$ can largely be explained by the applied normalization procedure.

In summary, when myoplasmic calcium has returned to a sufficient low level during isometric relaxation, instantaneous force may become the principal opposing determinant for force decline (25). Changes in developed force and changes in length may influence the calcium-troponin interaction (actin-linked regulation) or the actinomyosin interaction (myosin-linked regulation). In a discussion of effects of altered temperature on calcium-sensitive force in myocardium and skeletal muscle (26), a clarifying section illustrated present knowledge of thin filament cooperativity or actin-linked regulation. A more rigid tropomyosin is more difficult to displace for an adjacent tropomyosin, thus reducing cooperative activation. The affinity of troponin-C for calcium increases, probably by a combination of effects of force in muscle and of binding effects of the S1 fragment of myosin or the number of crossbridges. Potential mechanisms of thick filament or myosin linked regulation are the phosphorylation of the C-protein and of the regulatory light chain of myosin (27).

Endocardial Endothelium

Growing experimental evidence has shown that the endocardial endothelium may act as a direct modulator of performance of the subjacent myocardium and as a mediator of the inotropic action of several constituents of the circulating blood (28–29). Activation of the endocardial endothelium prolongs contraction and its inactivation abbreviates contraction. The mechanisms by which the endocardium affects contraction duration are not yet clear.

Proposed mechanisms are the presence of a physicochemical barrier at the endocardial level and the release of inotropic substances, similar to the release of vasoactive substances by the vascular endothelium.

Nonuniformity of Cardiac Muscle Performance

The contention that nonuniformity may constitute an essential property of cardiac muscle is supported by several experimental observations at different levels of integration, ranging from the subcellular level to the level of the intact heart as a whole (10, 30). In most studies on myocardial and ventricular function, mechanic uniformity has been implicitly assumed. Load dependence of relaxation, however, becomes even more pronounced when segmental muscle length is controlled instead of total muscle length (31). On the other hand, load dependence of relaxation was shown to be manifest even in the presence of marked nonuniformities (32, 33).

To study patterns of nonuniformity, four individual, longitudinal segments of isolated cat papillary muscle were demarcated by three glass microelectrode tips, inserted laterally into the core of the muscle, to divide the muscle into four adjacent segments: two segments in the central part of the papillary muscle, one including the basal, so-called damaged end and a last segment including the tendon end. The mechanic behavior of these segments, i.e., their length changes, was studied at rest and during contraction and relaxation of muscle-isometric twitches along the ascending limb of the force-length relation and at different $[Ca^{2+}]_o$. Different behavior was found, not only between central and end segments, but also within the central segments and within the end segments. We therefore attempted to quantify nonuniformity along the muscle in the above mentioned conditions.

Nature of Nonuniformity in Isolated Papillary Muscle

Nonuniformity of segmental kinetics is qualitatively illustrated in Figure 2–3. From the segment kinetics, two types of nonuniformity can be distinguished in longitudinal muscle mechanics. The first type

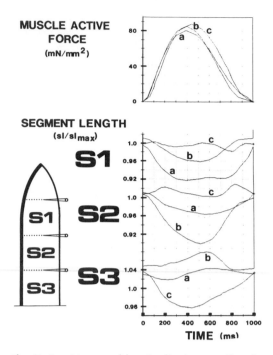

Fig. 2–3. Nature of longitudinal nonuniformity in isolated papillary muscle. The upper panel shows force versus time traces of an isometric twitch under the same conditions of length and $[Ca^{2+}]_o$ obtained from different muscles labelled a, b and c. These three muscles were selected because of their similar twitch contraction phase: comparable rate of force development (mN/mm²/s) and comparable peak twitch force (mN/mm²). The lower panel shows the time course of directly measured length of the three nontendinous muscle segments, evidencing different types of nonuniformity (see text). Reproduced with permission from Brutsaert DL, and Sys SU: Ventricular function: Is the total more than the sum of the parts? Circulation 83:1444, 1991.

of nonuniformity was observed when one particular segment, e.g., S_1, was compared in the three different muscles. In twitch of muscle a, S_1 substantially shortened, reaching peak shortening at the time of peak twitch force; S_1 shortened less and reached its shortest length at a later time during twitch of muscle b; finally, an irregular pattern of S_1 length change was observed in twitch of muscle c. This illustrates nonuniformity (of any particular segment) among different muscles: the pattern of length change of any particular segment was not a priori predictable from muscle to muscle. The second type of nonuniformity was observed when all segments within a given muscle were considered, i.e., by comparing the behavior of S_1, S_2, and S_3 in the isometric twitch of, e.g., muscle a. Substantial differences in these patterns of length change illustrate nonuniformity among the different segments within a given muscle. Despite the remarkable similarity of the force traces during the three isometric twitches, both types of nonuniformity demonstrate wide variation in segmental kinetics. It is, of course, most tempting to reverse this proposition: despite or perhaps through nonuniformity at the segmental scale, papillary muscles manage to produce almost predictable uniform patterns of force versus time during isometric twitches: a principle of uniformity through nonuniformity, similar to "order through fluctuations" (34) or "homogeneity out of heterogeneity" (35). This proposal is supported by predictable mechanic responses of the muscle as a whole after perturbations such as load clamps or quick stretches and by force-controlled predictable rate of force decline during relaxation, in the presence of unpredictable nonuniformities of longitudinal segment kinetics (16, 30).

Among possible sources of nonuniformity in cardiac muscle are geometry and architecture, electric excitation, and the activation-contraction and inactivation-relaxation coupling (10). Controllable sources of nonuniform segment kinetics specific for isolated papillary muscle such as the pattern of electric excitation or the cross-sectional area of the different segments did not contribute to the eventual nonuniform segment kinetics. Differences in collagen content and/or organization (36) are still under investigation. Regional differences in excitation-contraction coupling may be related to the action potential or to calcium handling: differences in calcium current, in sarcoplasmic reticulum distribution; calcium release, or calcium reuptake; and in calcium extrusion are still debatable. A particular role may be attributed to the sensitivity of the contractile proteins. Contractile protein sensitivity may be nonuniform, not only in space (37, 38), but also in time. In a shortening muscle segment, the decrease in length corresponds to a decrease in instantaneous passive force. Because measured force is total force, segment shortening results in a shift of load from passive (preload) to active (afterload) To shorten for the same, or, manifestly, for a larger amount, a stiffer segment such as S_1 must therefore be stronger, or have more force potential. When, during isometric twitches, a (strong) segment is capable to shorten, decreasing length may diminish the sensitivity and thereby decrease strength. This would constitute a stabilizing effect (39).

Segment Behavior During Contraction and Relaxation

As a consequence of changes in calcium availability and calcium sensitivity (40–42) isometric twitches at different muscle lengths and at different $[Ca^{2+}]_o$ showed marked variations in amplitude and in time course. To compare these twitches with respect to segment length changes, we used phase-slicing by force as an analyzing technique (43). The resulting averaged length of each segment progressively shortened during the isometric contraction phase. Longitudinal nonuniformity, quantified by the variation coefficient of segment lengths, progressively increased. The increase in variation coefficient during isometric contraction appeared to run in parallel with the increase in force. Because force development is approximately linearly related to time during most of the contraction phase, we cannot conclude whether nonuniformity increased with force development or with time. During relaxation, the degree of nonuniformity among the segments was markedly higher than at peak force. The maximal value of variation coefficient was observed when force had declined to approximately 75% of its peak during relaxation: during the first quarter of isometric relaxation, nonuniformity increased further. As a function of time (instead of force), the further increase in nonuniformity during the first quarter of isometric relaxation appears to be continuous with the increase in nonuniformity during the contraction phase; it may relate to the delay in time between peak force and minimal segment length (31, 44). This further increase might also be related to the previously described knee, shoulder or give (11, 21, 45, 46) during isometric relaxation. As still another explanation, this increase could be indeed due to inherent instability in the muscle during early relaxation, as evidenced by load dependence of relaxation (1). Finally, during the second half of relaxation, the original state of the muscle underwent progressive restitution.

Comments

Changes in load dependence of relaxation can be, both conceptually and experimentally, separated into two classes. Diminished load dependence can result from a slower or a delayed calcium reuptake by the sarcoplasmic reticulum and hence be manifested by a slower or a delayed lengthening during isotonic relaxation. Diminished load dependence can also result from an accelerated or an earlier disappearance of the actino-myosin interactions or force-generating crossbridges and hence be manifested by an accelerated or an earlier force decline during isometric relaxation. It is therefore important that changes of load dependence be interpreted separately on both the lengthening traces during isotonic relaxation and on the force decline traces of isometric relaxation. Nonuniformity of load and inactivation results from regional variations in the contraction phase, in onset and rate of inactivation, and in the distribution and decay of force developed force. This physiologic nonuniformity is important in modulating normal ventricular relaxation. It is expected to influence the manifestation of load dependence of relaxation in cardiac muscle in vitro and in vivo.

LEFT VENTRICULAR RELAXATION

Efficient relaxation and adequate diastolic function should result in high LV filling rates at low filling pressures, even during exercise when stroke volume and heart rate are increased. This physiologic goal is achieved by rapid, complete relaxation and by a compliant LV chamber, in the presence of sufficient LV filling time. This goal is ideally achieved in the long-distance runner through accelerated relaxation and through the development of an enlarged ventricle (47, 48). In the next section, we will discuss control of onset, control of rate, and control of extent in view of *triple control*

of relaxation and load dependence. Thereafter, we will briefly focus on the distinction between incomplete relaxation and impaired diastolic function.

Control of Onset of Relaxation

Physiologic and pharmacologic interventions influence duration of contraction and determine when, during the cardiac cycle, relaxation manifests and induces LV pressure fall.

Load

Different aspects of load affect timing of relaxation. Selective, beat-to-beat increases in preload slightly delay force decline of isolated cardiac muscle (49) and pressure fall of the intact ejecting LV (50). Effects of preload are of limited magnitude, though, when compared to effects of afterload. Beat-to-beat increases in afterload delay force decline in isolated cardiac muscle (1, 2, 8, 49) and delay pressure fall in the intact ejecting LV (1, 3, 51) (Fig. 2–4). Preload and afterload are the manifestation of *contraction load*, or load during muscular contraction. Its increase consistently delays relaxation.

When load is increased during early relaxation, such as during later LV ejection (*relaxation load*), effects are opposite, and force decline (pressure fall) occurs prematurely (1, 2, 3, 8, 51) (Fig. 2–5). (See Chap. 13).

Effects of systolic load on the onset of relaxation regulate the duration of LV ejection. For example, the systolic LV pressure waveform (52) is the manifestation of changing load during ejection, and modulated LV ejection duration, hence, to some minor extent, also peak-systolic LV volume. This modulation implies that the systolic pressure waveform influences peak length-tension relation of isolated cardiac muscle (15) and pressure-volume relation of the intact LV (53). As a consequence, a given state of contractility manifests as a family of closely related pressure-volume relations instead of as a unique pressure-volume relation.

The effects of beat-to-beat LV pressure increases should be considered distinct from the more complicated effects of steady-state increases in LV pressure as

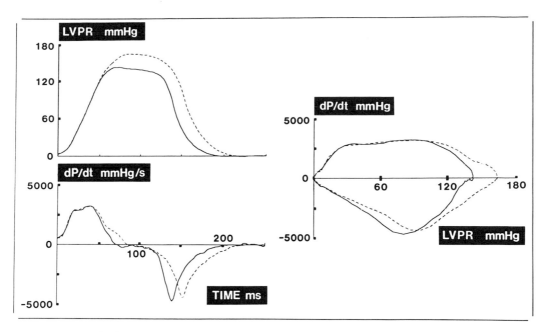

Fig. 2–4. Control of LV relaxation by load: Early pressure increase. The left panels represent LV pressure-time tracings (upper left, LVPR mmHg versus time ms) and their first derivatives (lower left, dP/dt mmHg/s versus time ms). The right panel represents phase-plane tracings of dP/dt versus LVPR. Phase-plane tracings are read clockwise from the left: pressure rise is above the 0 line, peak pressure at the right end of the panel, and pressure fall below the 0 line. Two tracings are superposed, a control tracing (solid line) and a test tracing (dashed line).

The early pressure increase (dashed line) prolongs LV ejection and delays LV pressure fall. On the phase plane, tracing initial acceleration of LV pressure fall (on the right) is less steep, so that control and test curve converge toward peak − dP/dt. Peak − dP/dt is somewhat lower in this example, less negative. Late LV pressure fall, after peak − dP/dt, projects slightly above control, which indicates a slightly slower course of late LV pressure fall.

produced by methoxamine, phenyleph-rine, aortic occlusion, or volume loading. These effects include prolonged changes in diastolic LV volume and fiber length (54), which alter contractility and inactivation. Steady-state increases in LV pressure, however, also consistently delay LV pressure fall.

Inactivation

Heart rate has a predominant influence on timing of relaxation. Increasing stimulation frequency in isolated cardiac muscle increases contractility, i.e., increased velocity of force development, shortening. Contraction duration, however, becomes shorter, and relaxation is induced earlier. Increasing heart rate in the intact heart has similar effects: positive dP/dt increases and LV ejection time decreases. For example,

when heart rate increases from 70 to 100 bpm, time from end-diastole to aortic valve closure decreases from mean 406 msec to 342 msec or a decrease of 16%. This computation is based on Weissler's formula for systolic time intervals (55). The formula relates left ventricular ejection time (LVET) to heart rate (HR) as LVET − 415 − (HR × 1.6). We assumed, in addition, a normal ratio pre-ejection time/ejection time of 0.34 (56). However, remaining time for pressure fall and filling decreases much more from mean 451 msec to 258 msec, or a decrease of 43%.

The *interaction between load and inactivation* is illustrated by the Frank-Starling law (Fig. 2–6, upper panel). When preload or end-diastolic LV volume increases, stroke work also increases. This increased stroke work is achieved by both a sarcomere-length-dependent increase in contractility

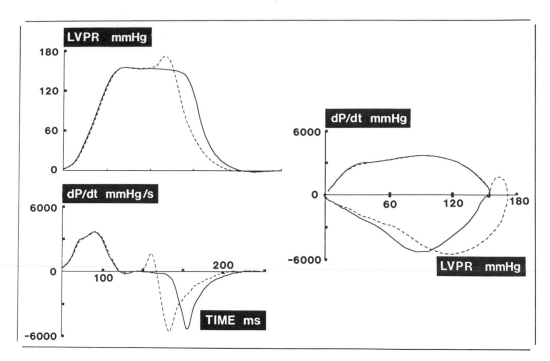

Fig. 2–5.   Control of LV relaxation by load: Late pressure increase. Same settings and abbreviations as in Figure 2–4. The late pressure increase (dashed line) abbreviates LV ejection and induces an earlier onset of LV pressure fall. On the phase plane tracing, initial acceleration of LV pressure fall (on the right) is steeper so that control and test curve diverge in their initial part. Peak − dP/dt is slightly increased. Pressure fall after peak − dP/dt is projected above control, which indicates a slower course of late LV pressure fall. Of note, control and test tracings coincide near terminal LV pressure fall at the left end of the tracing.

manifesting in the figure as a steeper pressure increase and by a delayed relaxation manifesting as a prolonged ejection duration.

Various *inotropic influences* on the myocardium can have different effects on LV ejection duration and on timing of relaxation. Catecholamines and increasing heart rate markedly abbreviate LV ejection duration, whereas calcium, digoxin, or phosphodiesterase inhibitors only slightly abbreviate this interval.

Effects of *ischemia* on twitch duration in isolated cardiac muscle depend on experimental conditions (57). Load dependence and separation in time between isometric and isotonic twitches decrease (1, 2). Profound hypoxia abbreviates twitch duration (58). Hypoxia at higher experimental temperatures (59) or intermediate levels of hypoxia (60) prolong twitch duration. Reoxygenation systematically prolongs twitch duration (18, 61). This manifests, for example, in the postejection shortening of LV segments typically observed during postischemic reperfusion. In experimental and clinical studies on ischemia of the in vivo LV myocardium, data on duration of ejection are obviously neglected in published presentation of data.

The influence of the *endocardial endothelium*, this tiny structure that separates the myocardium from the LV cavity, also affects onset of relaxation in a rather selective way (Fig. 2–6, lower panel). An intact endocardial endothelium prolongs LV ejection duration, whereas endocardial inactivation as induced by high power, high frequency, continuous wave ultrasound abbreviates LV ejection duration (62). Effects of endocardial endothelium on contraction duration are independent from changes in contractility, as defined by changes in rate of pressure rise or changes in rate of LV

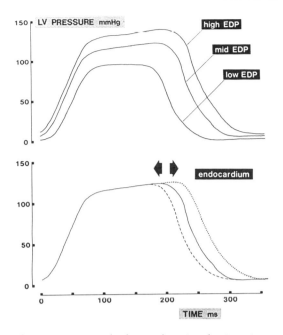

Fig. 2–6. Control of LV relaxation by inactivation. Upper panel: Frank-Starling law. Three LV pressure tracings are superimposed, corresponding to a steady-state low, mid, and high end-diastolic pressure (EDP). When EDP increases from low to high, the generated stroke work increases according to the Frank-Starling law. This increased stroke work is achieved through an increased contraction velocity, manifesting by a steeper pressure rise, and through an increased contraction duration, manifesting as a delayed LV pressure fall. Lower panel: Endocardial modulation. Three superimposed LV pressure (mmHg) tracings are shown. The solid line is a control tracing. The dotted line represents endocardial activation obtained here by selective increase of alpha-1 activity. The dashed line represents a condition where endocardial effects were impaired with an intraventricular source of high power, high frequency, continuous wave ultrasound. The panel illustrates selective effects of endocardial endothelium on timing of LV pressure fall, without alteration of pressure rise or early ejection. Modified with permission from Gillebert, T.C. et al.: Intracavitary ultrasound impairs left ventricular performance: presumed role of endocardial endothelium. Am. J. Physiol. *263*, H857, 1992; and Gillebert, TC, and Brutsaert DL: Regulation of left ventricular pressure fall. Eur Heart J 11(I):124, 1990.

ejection (62, 63). Of note, while the intact vascular endothelium has a predominantly vasodilating effect, the intact endocardial endothelium seems to have an overall effect, which delays onset of relaxation.

Nonuniformity

Asynchronous wall movements during isovolumic relaxation, also modulate timing of LV pressure fall. When early re-extension and outward bulging develop in a LV wall segment, further ejection is prevented and premature pressure fall is initiated (Fig. 2–7). Later, during the course of isovolumic LV pressure fall, the still-shortening segments of the LV wall displace blood into the bulging segment (64), which is obviously inefficient from a hemodynamic point of view. If, for example, early segmental re-extension is induced experimentally by selective injection of isoproterenol in a coronary branch, premature bulging and premature pressure fall are elicited (65, 66).

Control of Rate of Relaxation

From discussions on relaxation in isolated cardiac muscle, it became evident that relaxation manifests as isometric force decline (isovolumetric LV pressure fall) and as isotonic lengthening (isotonic LV filling). Isometric and isotonic relaxation have a distinct regulation. When discussing extent of relaxation, we will consider regulation of LV filling by late relaxation; in this section on rate of relaxation we will describe rate of LV pressure fall.

A relaxation which manifests early is faster, and a relaxation whose manifestation is delayed is slower. This general rule can be applied in most circumstances of physiologic regulation of relaxation.

Load

A delayed relaxation due to increased systolic LV pressures, i.e. an increased *contraction load*, will be slower (67–69) accordingly. In the healthy heart this influence appears to be minimal (70). A recent clinical study on patients with heart failure (71) however highlighted that the effect of systolic LV pressures on the time constant τ becomes critical when heart function is impaired. This means that in severely diseased hearts a slight increase in LV systolic pressure will induce a marked slowing of relaxation.

The link between timing and rate of relaxation is not observed when selective

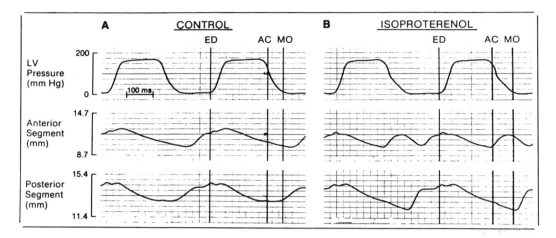

Fig. 2–7. Control of LV relaxation by nonuniformity. Tracings of LV pressure, anterior and posterior segment lengths. Vertical lines denote timing of end-diastole (ED), aortic valve closure (AC), and mitral valve opening (MO). During control period (left panel), both segments shorten synchronously and have minimal length change during isovolumetric LVP fall (AC to MO). After injection of 10 ng of isoproterenol into the mid-left anterior descending coronary artery (right panel), anterior segment develops early lengthening during LVP fall. Posterior segment is not directly stimulated but has increased shortening during LVP fall. There is a regional intraventricular unloading effect whereby the posterior wall shortens and shifts blood into the expanding anterior wall during LVP fall. This increase in nonuniformity is associated with an earlier onset (shorter interval ED-AC) and slower overall rate (longer interval AC-MO) of LVP fall. Modified with permission from Gillebert, T.C., and Lew, W.Y.W.: Nonuniformity and volume loading independently influence isovolumic relaxation rates. Am. J. Physiol. *257*:H1927, 1989.

changes in *relaxation load* occur, such as during late LV ejection. Late-ejection increases in LV pressure, referred to as late load clamps, induce a premature onset but a slower overall course of LV pressure fall (70, 72). Premature onset is presumably related to the imbalance between number of interacting crossbridges and load to be carried. Slower course is presumably related to delayed inactivation of remaining crossbridges (70). In experimental circumstances in which very abrupt and late pressure increases are induced, the premature onset of pressure fall can be followed by an acceleration of pressure fall (73), limited, however, to the initial phase in which peak $-dP/dt$ is measured (49). Both early onset and acceleration of initial pressure fall may be related to sarcoplasmic reuptake of calcium because these effects are less important after administration of caffeine (73). They could be the manifestation of segmental early re-extension and isotonic acceleration of relaxation. The physiologic relevance of initial acceleration of LV pressure fall, which can be elicited only by very abrupt and late LV pressure increases, is

unclear. The different studies analyzing systolic load clamps illustrate the effects of the systolic pressure waveform (52) on rate of LV pressure fall. Rate of LV pressure fall is responsive to even subtle alterations in systolic pressure waveform, and this responsiveness increases as ejection proceeds (70). As a consequence, pharmacologic agents that alter systolic pressure waveform, such as vasoactive drugs, influence rate of LV pressure fall even if they do not exert any direct cardiac effect. Pathophysiologic conditions such as hypertension, valvular heart diseases, cardiac hypertrophy or congestive heart failure can also be associated with altered systolic pressure waveform and can influence rate of LV pressure fall, in addition to their well-known effects on muscle inactivation, nonuniformity, and global load.

Inactivation

The general rule linking timing and rate of relaxation applies in most circumstances of regulation of relaxation by inactivation like regulation by heart rate, hormonal influences, inotropic effects. It typically applies in case of modulation of cardiac function by the endocardial endothelium (Fig. 2–6): delayed relaxation, as induced for example by slight and selective alpha-1 agonist activity is slightly slower, while premature relaxation as induced by ultrasonic inactivation of the endocardium is slightly faster (62, 63).

Nonuniformity

Another exception to the rule linking timing and rate of relaxation is nonuniformity. Asynchronous wall movements occurring during LV pressure fall are associated with slower LV pressure fall, even if pressure fall occurs earlier, such as when it is induced by regional ischemia or regional inotropic stimulation (Fig. 2–7) (64–66). Interaction between load and nonuniformity was addressed in a recent study (74). The magnitude of load and nonuniformity in determining the rate of LV pressure fall is comparable. LV pressure increases slow down LV pressure fall but does not alter nonuniformity. Regional inotropic stimulation with a constant dose of isoproterenol injected into the left anterior descending artery induces a given extent of nonuniformity and a given slowing of LV pressure fall, regardless of the prevailing loading conditions. Load and nonuniformity are therefore two important factors that modulate the rate of LV pressure fall, but by independent mechanisms.

Control of Extent of Relaxation

In physiologic circumstances, relaxation is completed during early filling. Slower relaxation can alter indices of early filling such as peak early filling rate or Doppler E wave. Relaxation is completed somewhat later during LV filling and does not result in higher filling pressures or dyspnea at rest. Relaxation could, however, become incomplete when heart rate increases, e.g., during exercise. LV filling pressures then increase, reflecting still ongoing relaxation during the major part of LV filling, in addition to increased venous return and decreased filling duration. During exercise, cardiac output can therefore become critically dependent on relaxation rate and extent. When relaxation is slowed, but also

when compliance is decreased or filling time is inappropriately reduced, diastolic pressures increase, inducing dyspnea. The relevance of extent of relaxation is illustrated with some representative experimental data.

Load

A recent study (75) investigated the effects of acute coronary occlusion on shifts of the pressure-volume curve during LV filling. It compared shifts at low and high LV filling pressures. Coronary occlusion induced a rightward shift of the curve at low, and a rightward and upward shift at high filling pressures. One could therefore wonder whether incomplete relaxation in the presence of coronary occlusion would occur mainly when filling pressures are elevated. However, changes in LV pressure-volume curves during coronary occlusion were superposable to changes seen during passive filling of the nonischemic ventricle, indicating that the observation just illustrated the curvilinear morphology of the passive LV pressure-volume relation and was unrelated to changes in extent of relaxation.

Inactivation

With regard to the extent of relaxation, previous work by Grossman, Paulus, and coworkers (76) highlighted essential differences between demand ischemia and primary ischemia. Demand ischemia (coronary stenosis, ischemia induced by rapid pacing, and analysis of immediate postpacing condition, seen in Fig. 2–8 left panel) induces an upward shift of the pressure-volume relation during left ventricular filling (lower limb of the pressure-segment length loop), while primary ischemia (occlusion of a coronary artery, Fig. 2–8 right panel) displaces the portion of the loop to the right, similarly to what would be induced by volume loading. This indicates an incomplete relaxation (rigor bridges?) in the former experimental condition only. This incomplete relaxation manifests even at normal heart rates.

The relationship among hypertrophy, fibrosis, and hemodynamic behavior was recently analyzed in early canine experimental hypertension (77). Pressure fall was

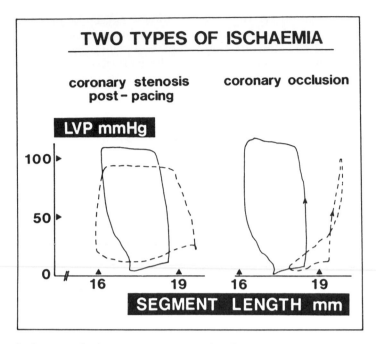

Fig. 2–8.   Control of extent of relaxation: experimental ischemia. Pressure-segment length loops from the anterior left ventricular wall. Two curves are superposed, a control curve (solid line) and a curve during myocardial ischemia (dashed line).

Left panel: Ischemia is induced by rapid atrial pacing in the presence of critical coronary narrowing. The test tracing was recorded at the same paced heart rate as the control tracing, immediately after rapid pacing for several minutes. When compared to control, systolic shortening is reasonably well preserved but LV filling and segment re-extension occur at higher filling pressures. This manifests as an upward shift of the lower limb of the pressure-segment length loop and reflects incomplete relaxation.

Right panel: Ischemia is induced by occlusion of the left anterior descending coronary artery. The segment develops akinesia. LV filling and segment reextension occur at higher segmental lengths but not at higher segmental pressures. This manifests as a rightward shift of the lower limb of the pressure-segment length loop. Relaxation is completed during early filling and the lower limb of the loop mainly reflects the passive pressure-segment length relation (segmental compliance). Modified with permission from Paulus, W.J. et al.: Different effects of two types of ischemia on myocardial systolic and diastolic function. Am J Physiol *248*:H719, 1985.

slower and filling pattern impaired, reflecting a slower relaxation. Chamber stiffness and passive elastic stiffness were unchanged, reflecting both a complete relaxation during the later part of LV filling and still-normal passive LV properties. The study confirmed that impaired relaxation is the hallmark of early hypertension, and elegantly dissociated ongoing relaxation from passive, diastolic LV compliance in their effects on LV filling.

Nonuniformity

An important experimental issue is to know whether nonuniformity could explain incomplete relaxation and elevation of LV filling pressures in demand ischemia. Segmental dyssynchrony could explain why LV filling pressures increase during demand ischemia and not during primary ischemia. Experimental findings, however (78) indicated that the extent of nonuniformity was similar in demand and primary ischemia so that incomplete relaxation in demand ischemia was presumably not caused by nonuniformity.

Relaxation and Diastolic Function

Discussion on diastole is beyond the scope of the present article, which analyzes relaxation. Diastole is, however, briefly presented to differentiate between incomplete relaxation and impaired diastolic function. Diastolic function is one of the several determinants of LV filling and relates to actual LV volume, LV compliance, right ventricular interaction, and pericardial constraint. (See Chap. 4.) LV compliance, for instance, is related to passive LV properties, in the absence of myocardial bactivation. LV compliance is typically decreased in concentric LV hypertrophy, as a consequence of an increased radius-to-wall-thickness ratio and in severe hypertrophy as a consequence of increased myocardial fibrosis (79). In contrast to the hypertensive LV or the LV in aortic valve diseases, the LV of patients with mitral regurgitation does not exhibit a decreased compliance (80).

Recent literature extensively focused on the role and function of the collagen network and the effects on LV compliance (81). Collagen provides strength and stiffness to the myocardium. Furthermore, the organization of the collagen provides a structural framework for the myocytes and, as part of this support, collagen fibers provide myocyte-to-myocyte connections (referred to as collagen struts) that are thought to be important in tethering the cells. Structural changes in the collagen matrix and increased myocardial fibrosis have been described as induced by mechanic stress, aldosterone, diabetes mellitus, uremia and parathormone. These changes are particularly relevant in LV hypertrophy (myocardial fibrosis), after myocardial infarction (ventricular remodeling), and in dilated cardiomyopathy.

In addition to relaxation and compliance disturbances, it is necessary to assess the extent to which filling duration is impaired. This can be especially important in patients with congestive heart failure and in subjects with decreased exercise tolerance.

ASSESSMENT OF RELAXATION AND DIASTOLIC FUNCTION

Various clinical indexes relate to distinct aspects of relaxation, filling, and compliance. Cardiologists look at the LV as a pump and not primarily as a muscle. They subdivide the cardiac cycle into phases separated by valve opening and closure. We therefore suggest the following subdivision of indexes, as related to relaxation, LV filling, and passive LV properties.

Relaxation

1. **Onset** of relaxation, or duration of excitation-contraction coupling and contraction, e.g., LV ejection duration, time from end-diastole to peak $-$ dP/dt.
2. **Rate** of relaxation as derived mainly from LV pressure fall, e.g., peak $-$ dP/dt (early LV pressure fall), time constant τ (late LV pressure fall), isovolumic relaxation time.
3. **Pattern** of early LV filling and LV pressure course during active, early LV filling. LV early filling has multiple determinants besides muscle inactivation such as elastic recoil forces, viscoelastic effects, LV filling pressures, diastolic left atrial pressures, LV stiffness, ventricular interaction, and pericardial constraint (82). The most frequently used index is peak LV filling rate. The Doppler E wave of the mitral valve occurs simultaneously with peak filling rate, but gives distinct information, being closely related to LV and left atrial pressure differences after mitral valve opening (83, 84).

Diastole

4. Passive **compliance**, e.g., shifts in late LV filling pressures, LV or myocardial stiffness, LV pressure waveform during atrial contraction, Doppler flow across the mitral value (A wave) and in the pulmonary vein during atrial contraction.

Duration of Filling

5. LV filling **duration** is a distinct clinical index of diastolic function. It depends on heart rate and on duration of the time interval from end-diastole to mitral valve opening. This interval is determined mainly by onset of relaxation and, to a lesser extent, by rate.

SUMMARY

Relaxation in isolated cardiac muscle is regulated by triple control through load, inactivation, and nonuniformity, manifesting as load dependence. Load dependence describes different contributions of load and inactivation on control of isometric and isotonic relaxation and can be interpreted in terms of contractile protein properties and cellular calcium handling.

From the extrapolation of triple control to onset, rate, and extent of relaxation in the intact LV, a distinct regulation of isometric pressure fall and isotonic filling becomes evident. Slower relaxation manifests as slower LV pressure fall and impaired initial LV filling. Incomplete relaxation is residual active force in ventricular muscle fibers throughout filling, manifesting as increased filling pressures.

Diastolic function relates to passive muscular and ventricular properties and can be evaluated only when relaxation has been completed. Diastolic dysfunction is a stiffer LV and manifests as filling disturbances and increased filling pressures.

REFERENCES

1. Brutsaert DL, Sys SU: Relaxation and diastole of the heart. Physiol Rev 69:1228, 1989.
2. Brutsaert DL, Housmans PR, Goethals MA: Dual control of relaxation. Its role in the ventricular function in the mammalian heart. Circ Res 47:637, 1980.
3. Ariel Y, Gaasch WH, Bogen DK, McMahon TA: Load-dependent relaxation with late systolic volume steps: servo-pump studies in the intact canine heart. Circulation 75: 1287, 1987.
4. Sabbah HN, Stein PD: Pressure-diameter relations during early diastole in dogs. Incompatibility with the concept of passive left ventricular filling. Circ Res 45:357, 1981.
5. Udelson JE, Bacharach SL, Cannon RO, Bonow RO: Minimum left ventricular pressure during beta-adrenergic stimulation in human subjects. Evidence for elastic recoil and diastolic "suction" in the normal heart. Circulation 82:1174, 1990.
6. Weiss JL, Frederiksen JW, Weisfeldt ML: Hemodynamic determinants of the time course of fall in canine left ventricular pressure. J Clin Invest 58:751, 1976.
7. Lew WYW: Evaluation of left ventricular diastolic function. Circulation 79:1393, 1989.
8. Brutsaert DL, De Clerck NM, Housmans PR, Goethals MA: Relaxation of ventricular cardiac muscle. J Physiol (London) 283: 469, 1978.
9. Lecarpentier YC, et al.: Nature of load dependence of relaxation in cardiac muscle. Am J Physiol 237:H455–H460, 1979.
10. Brutsaert DL: Nonuniformity: A physiologic modulator of contraction and relaxation of the normal heart. J Am Coll Cardiol 9:341, 1987.
11. Huxley AF, Simmons RM: Mechanical transient and the origin of muscular force. Cold Spring Harb Symp Quart Biol 37: 669–680, 1973.
12. Housmans PR, Brutsaert DL: Three step yielding of load clamped mammalian cardiac muscle. Nature 262:56, 1976.
13. Tamiya K, et al.: Maximum rate of tension fall during isometric relaxation at end-systolic fiber length in canine papillary muscle. Circ Res 40:584, 1977.
14. Wiegner AW, Bing OHL: Isometric relaxation of rat myocardium at end-systolic fiber length. Circ Res 43:865, 1978.
15. Gillebert TC, Sys SU, Brutsaert DL: Influence of loading patterns on peak length-tension relation and on relaxation in cardiac muscle. J Am Coll Cardiol 13:483, 1989.
16. Sys SU, Paulus WJ, Claes VA, Brutsaert DL: Post-reextension force decay of relaxing cardiac muscle. Am J Physiol 253:H256, 1987.
17. Hoerter J, Mazet F, Vassort G: Perinatal growth of the rabbit cardiac cell: possible implications for the mechanisms of relaxation. J Mol Cell Cardiol 13:725, 1981.
18. Sys SU, Housmans PR, Van Ocken ER, Brutsaert DL: Mechanisms of hypoxia-induced decrease of load dependence of relaxation in cat papillary muscle. Pfluegers Arch 401:368, 1984.
19. Parmley WW, Sonnenblick F: Relation between mechanics of contraction and relaxation in mammalian cardiac muscle. Am J Physiol 216:1084, 1969.
20. Mattiazzi A, Garay A, Cingolani HE: Critical evaluation of isometric indexes of relaxation in rat and cat papillary muscles and load ventricular strips. J Mol Cell Cardiol 18:749, 1986.
21. Edman KAP, Flitney FW: Laser diffraction studies of sarcomere dynamics during "isometric" relaxation in isolated muscle fibres of the frog. J Physiol 329:1, 1982.
22. Hill DK: Resting tension and the form of a twitch of rat skeletal muscle at low temperature. J Physiol 221:161, 1972.
23. Jewell BR, and Wilkie DR: The mechanical properties of relaxing muscle. J Physiol 152:30, 1960.
24. Chemla D, et al.: Relationship between inotropy and relaxation in rat myocardium. Am J Physiol 250:H1008, 1986.
25. Sys SU, Brutsaert DL: Determinants of force decline during relaxation in isolated

cardiac muscle. Am J Physiol 257:H1490, 1989.

26. Sweitzer NK, Moss RL: The effect of altered temperature on Ca^{2+}-sensitive force in permeabilized myocardium and skeletal muscle. Evidence for force dependence of thin filament activation. J Gen Physiol 96(6):1221, 1990.

27. Lin L-E, McClellan G, Weisberg A, Winegrad S: A physiological basis for variation in the contractile properties of isolated rat heart. J Physiol 441:73, 1991.

28. Brutsaert DL, Meulemans AL, Sipido KR, Sys SU: Effects of damaging the endocardial surface on the mechanical performance of isolated cardiac muscle. Circ Res 62:358, 1988.

29. Brutsaert DL: Role of endocardium in cardiac overloading and failure. Eur Heart J 11(Suppl G):8, 1991.

30. Brutsaert DL, Sys SU: Ventricular function: Is the total more than the sum of the parts? Circulation 83:1444, 1991.

31. Donald TC, et al.: Effect of damaged ends in papillary muscle preparations. Am J Physiol 238:H14, 1980.

32. Poggesi C, Reggiani C, Ricciardi L, Minelli R: Factors modulating the sensitivity of the relaxation to the loading conditions in rat cardiac muscle. Pfluegers Arch 394:338, 1982.

33. Lecarpentier YC, et al.: Real-time kinetics of sarcomere relaxation by laser diffraction. Circ Res 56:331, 1985.

34. Prigogine I, Stengers I: La nouvelle alliance. Gallimard, Paris, 1979.

35. Katz AM, Katz PB: Homogeneity out of heterogeneity. Circulation 79:712, 1989.

36. Ohayon J, Chadwick RS: Effects of collagen microstructure on the mechanics of the left ventricle. Biophys J 54:1077, 1988.

37. Edman KAP, Reggiani C, Schiaffino S, Te Kronnie G: Maximum velocity of shortening related to myosin isoform composition in frog skeletal muscle fibre. J Physiol 395:679, 1988.

38. Josephson RK, Edman KAP: The consequence of fibre heterogeneity on the force-velocity relation of skeletal muscle. Acta Physiol Scand 132:341, 1988.

39. Morgan DL: From sarcomeres to whole muscles. J Exp Biol 115:69, 1985.

40. Allen DG, Kentish JC: The cellular basis of the length-tension relation in cardiac muscle. J Mol Cell Cardiol 17:821, 1985.

41. Babu A, Sonnenblick EH, Gulati J: Molecular basis for the influence of muscle length on myocardial performance. Science 240:74, 1988.

42. Hofmann PA, Fuchs F: Effects of length

and crossbridge attachment on calcium-binding to cardiac troponin-C. Am J Physiol 253:C90, 1987.

43. Sys SU, Brutsaert DL: Nonuniformity in isolated cardiac muscle. Proc 9th Internat Conf Cardiovasc System Dynamics Soc, Halifax, Canada, p. 51–54, 1988.

44. Huntsman LL, Joseph DS, Oiye MY, Nichols GL: Auxotonic contractions in cardiac muscle segments. Am J Physiol 237:H131, 1979.

45. Edman KAP: The role of non-uniform sarcomere behaviour during relaxation of striated muscle. Eur Heart J 1(Suppl. A):49, 1980.

46. Krueger JW, Pollack GH: Myocardial sarcomere dynamics during isometric contraction. J Physiol 251:627, 1975.

47. Schaible TF, Scheuer J: Cardiac adaptations in chronic exercise. Prog Cardiovasc Dis 27:297, 1985.

48. Gillebert TC, Rademakers FE, Brutsaert DL: Left Ventricular Function in the Athlete: Analysis of Relaxation. *In* Sportscardiology: Exercise in Health and Disease. Edited by Fagard R, Bekaert I. The Hague (Netherlands), Martinus Nyhoff Publishers, 1986.

49. Gillebert TC, Brutsaert DL: Regulation of left ventricular pressure fall. Eur Heart J 11(I):124, 1990.

50. Gaasch WH, Carroll JD, Blaustein AS, Bing OHL: Myocardial relaxation: effects of preload on the time course of isovolumetric relaxation. Circulation 73:1037, 1986.

51. Noble MIM: The contribution of blood momentum to left ventricular ejection in the dog. Circ Res 23:663, 1968.

52. Murgo JP, Westerhof N: Arterial reflections and pressure waveforms in humans. *In* Ventricular/Vascular Coupling: Clinical, Physiological and Engineering Aspects. Edited by Yin FCP. New York, Axel Springer-Verlag, 1987.

53. Maughan WL, Sunagawa K, Brukhoff D, Sagawa K: Effects of arterial impedance on the end-systolic pressure-volume relation. Circ Res 54:595, 1984.

54. Lew WYW: Time-dependent increase in left ventricular contractility following acute volume loading in the dog. Circ Res 63:635, 1988.

55. Weissler AM, Harris LC, White GD: Left-ventricular ejection-time index in man. J Appl Physiol 18:919, 1963.

56. Weissler AM, Harris LC, Schoenfeld CD: Bedside techniques for the evaluation of ventricular function in man. Am J Cardiol 23:577, 1969.

57. Paulus WJ: Disturbed cardiac muscle inacti-

vation in pacing induced angina and in hypertrophic cardiomyopathy. Ph. D Thesis, University of Antwerp, Belgium, 1984.

58. Tyberg JV, et al.: Effects of hypoxia on mechanics of cardiac contraction. Am J Physiol 218:1780, 1970.

59. Frist WH, Palacios I, Powell WS, Jr.: Effects of hypoxia on myocardial relaxation in isometric cat papillary muscle. J Clin Invest 61:1218, 1978.

60. St. John Sutton MG, Ritman EL, Paradise NF: Biphasic changes in maximal relaxation rate during progressive hypoxia in isometric kitten papillary muscle and isovolumic rabbit ventricle. Circ Res 47:516, 1980.

61. Bing OHL, Brooks WW, Messer JV: Prolongation of tension on reoxygenation following myocardial hypoxia: a possible role for mitochondria in muscle relaxation. J Mol Cell Cardiol 8:205, 1976.

62. Gillebert TC, et al.: Intracavity ultrasound impairs left ventricular performance: presumed role of endocardial endothelium. Am J Physiol 263:857, 1992.

63. De Hert SG, Gillebert TC, Brutsaert DL: Alteration of left ventricular endocardial function by intracavitary high power ultrasound interacts with volume, inotropic state and alpha-adrenergic stimulation. Circulation 87:000, 1993.

64. Kumada T, et al.: Effects of coronary occlusion on early ventricular diastolic events in conscious dogs. Am J Physiol 237:H542, 1979.

65. Illebekk AJ, Lekven J, Kiil F: Left ventricular asynergy during intracoronary isoproterenol infusion in dogs. Am J Physiol 239:H594, 1980.

66. Lew WYW, Rasmussen CW: Influence of nonuniformity on rate of left ventricular pressure fall in the dog. Am J Physiol 257:H222, 1989.

67. Raff GL, Glantz SA: Volume loading slows left ventricular isovolumic relaxation rate. Evidence of load-dependent relaxation in the intact dog heart. Circ Res 48:813, 1981.

68. Karliner JS, et al.: Pharmacologic and hemodynamic influences on the rate of isovolumic left ventricular relaxation in conscious dogs. J Clin Invest 60:511, 1977.

69. Gaasch WH, et al.: Myocardial relaxation II: Hemodynamic determinants of rate of LV isovolumic pressure decline. Am J Physiol 239:H1, 1980.

70. Gillebert TC, Lew WYW: Timing of abrupt systolic pressure increases and the rate of left ventricular pressure fall. Am J Physiol 261:H805, 1991.

71. Eichhorn EJ, et al.: Are contraction and relaxation coupled in patients with and without congestive heart failure? Circulation 85:2132, 1992.

72. Hori M, et al.: Loading sequence is a major determinant of afterload-dependent relaxation in intact canine heart. Am J Physiol 249:H747, 1985.

73. Zile MR, Gaasch WH: Load-dependent left ventricular relaxation in conscious dogs. Am J Physiol 261:H691, 1991.

74. Gillebert TC, Lew WYW: Nonuniformity and volume loading independently influence isovolumic relaxation rates. Am J Physiol 257:H1927, 1989.

75. Applegate RJ: Load dependence of left ventricular diastolic pressure-volume relations during short-term coronary artery occlusion. Circulation 83:661, 1991.

76. Paulus WJ, et al.: Different effects of two types of ischemia on myocardial systolic and diastolic function. Am J Physiol 248:H719, 1985.

77. Douglas PS, Tallant B: Hypertrophy, fibrosis, and diastolic dysfunction in early canine experimental hypertension. J Am Coll Cardiol 17:530, 1991.

78. Takahashi T, Levine MJ, Grossmann W: Regional diastolic mechanics of ischemic and nonischemic myocardium in the pig heart. J Am Coll Cardiol 17:1203, 1991.

79. Hess OM, Felder L, Krayenbuehl HP: Diastolic function in valvular heart disease. Herz 16:124, 1991.

80. Corin WJ, et al.: Left ventricular passive diastolic properties in chronic mitral regurgitation. Circulation 83:797, 1991.

81. Weber KT: Cardiac interstitium in health and disease: the fibrillar collagen network. J Am Coll Cardiol 13:1637, 1989.

82. Gilbert JC, Glantz SA: Determinants of left ventricular filling and of the diastolic pressure-volume relation. Circ Res 64:827, 1989.

83. Nishimura RA, Housmans PR, Hatle LK, Tajik AJ: Assessment of diastolic function of the heart: background and current applications of Doppler Echocardiography. Part II. Clinical studies. Mayo Clin Proc 64: 181, 1989.

84. Thomas JD, Weyman AE: Echocardiographic Doppler evaluation of left ventricular diastolic function. Circulation 84:977, 1991.

Chapter 3

THE ENERGETICS OF RELAXATION

Gerd Hasenfuss, Christian Holubarsch, Louis A. Mulieri,
Edward M. Blanchard, and Norman R. Alpert

Myothermal measurements using sensitive antimony-bismuth thermopiles provide information on the entire metabolic energy turnover during isometric contraction and relaxation of heart muscle. They are equivalent to oxygen consumption measurements regarding overall metabolism (1, 2). The advantage in using the myothermal technique for assessing energy flux is that heat measurements give the exact time course of rapid changes and allow differentiation of heat evolution into the energy turnover of the contraction and relaxation phase of the cardiac cycle (3). Moreover, total heat liberated by the muscle can be partitioned into the heat evolution of the contractile proteins, the excitation-contraction coupling system, the recovery system, and basal metabolism. These measurements, in conjunction with the mechanical performance, provide quantitative information on the extent and rate of the reactions involved in crossbridge interaction, excitation-contraction coupling, recovery, and basal metabolism. We emphasize energetics of crossbridge interaction and excitation-contraction coupling processes in human (control and volume-overload), rabbit (control, pressure-overload and hyperthyroid) and rat (control and hypothyroid) myocardium. The power of using different types of myocardium across and within species is that it presents a more global picture and allows for a better analysis of the relationship between the energetic and mechanic variables.

THERMODYNAMIC CONSIDERATIONS

The systolic and diastolic contractile performance of the heart is critically dependent on the characteristics of the myosin-actin crossbridge cycle and the time course of activation and deactivation of the actomyosin system. The primary events that occur in contraction and relaxation involve (1) the release of calcium into the cytosol followed by its removal and (2) the myosin-actin crossbridge cycle, in which the myosin crossbridge head attaches to actin, rotates in a manner that develops force or causes shortening, and then detaches from the actin filament to start another cycle. There is an obligatory hydrolysis of one high-energy phosphate bond with each crossbridge cycle (4). Calcium is removed from the cytosol predominantly by calcium ATPases of the sarcoplasmic reticulum with a stoichiometry of 2 Ca^{2+} per high-energy phosphate bond hydrolyzed (5). In addition, calcium is removed by the sarcolemmal Na^+-Ca^{2+}-exchanger, which is energetically linked to the Na^+-K^+-ATPpase (net 1 Ca^{2+}/high-energy phosphate bond) and by the sarcolemmal Ca^{2+}-ATPase (1 Ca^{2+}/high-energy phosphate bond) (6). In all of these events, the bond energy residing in the terminal phosphate bond of ATP is the primary source of energy. Hydrolysis of ATP is tightly coupled to the resynthesis of ATP from ADP by the creatine phosphotransferase reaction which results in a virtually instantaneous resynthesis of the hydrolyzed ATP. From an energetic perspective, the hydrolysis of creatine phosphate is the reaction that must be considered. According to Woledge and Reilly, the enthalpy change for phosphocreatine hydrolysis is considered to be 35 KJ/mol (7). In a closed system, the total enthalpy change is equal to the heat liberated and the work performed. The enthalpy change is the result of the sum of all the enthalpy changes that occur in all the reactions coupled to the contraction-relaxation cycle.

MYOTHERMAL MEASUREMENTS

Definition of Heat Terms

Under steady state isometric conditions with no external work performed, all of the energy turned over by the muscle is liberated as heat by the end of the twitch. The total heat is composed of total activity-related heat and resting heat. The total activity-related heat is divisible into initial and recovery components. Initial heat is composed of the tension-dependent heat and tension-independent heat. Tension-dependent heat results from high-energy phosphate hydrolysis by cycling cross-bridges. Tension-independent heat reflects high-energy phosphate hydrolysis by sarcoplasmic reticulum calcium pumps, predominantly, and, to a lesser extent, high-energy phosphate hydrolysis by sarcolemmal calcium pumps, by sarcolemmal sodium-potassium ATPases, and other ATP-utilizing pumps (8). During steady-state conditions, tension-independent heat mainly reflects the amount of calcium removed (by sarcoplasmic reticulum calcium ATPases) and, therefore, the amount released during the isometric twitch (8, 9). Resting heat rate results from high-energy phosphate hydrolysis and resynthesis by systems that maintain concentration gradients and protein metabolism (10).

Thermal Measurements

Changes in muscle temperature were measured with 14-junction, Hill-type thermopiles fabricated by vacuum deposition of bismuth and antimony junctions on mica substrates (11). Thermopiles had a temperature sensitivity between 1.08 and 1.32 μV/m°C. Average heat loss coefficient was 0.54 mcal/°C·s. Thermopile output was amplified by an Ancom chopper amplifier (Model 15C-3A, Ancom, Ltd., Cheltenham, UK). Isometric force was measured by a cantilever beam force transducer (12). Temperature and force signals were displayed on an oscilloscope and simultaneously recorded on a chart recorder (Gould-Brush, Model 2400, Gould, Cleveland,

Ohio). The heat loss coefficient and sensitivity of the thermopile were determined as previously described (11).

Experimental Protocol

Muscle strip preparations were performed from various types of myocardium as will be described. To perform the heat and mechanical measurements, the muscles were mounted on the thermopile in contact with the active region and connected to the force gauge. The muscle and thermopile were then submerged in Krebs-Ringer solution at 21 to 22°C, and the muscles were stimulated end-to-end at intervals of 5 to 6 seconds 20% above threshold. After an equilibration period of 90 to 120 minutes, the muscles were stretched gradually (0.5 to 0.1 mm) until maximum twitch force was reached, this length is designated l_{max}. When steady-state conditions were reached at l_{max}, the chamber was drained and temperature and tension signals were recorded during repetitive stimulation (Fig. 3–1). Following the recording of steady-state force and temperature records, stimulation was stopped and the muscle temperature was allowed to cool to its baseline resting level, which was recorded. The physical cool-off time constant was obtained by heating the muscle from this baseline temperature with a 10^6 Hz sine wave current passed end-to-end through the muscle, recording the cool-off after stopping the current and fitting a least-squares monoexponential function to the record. The strategy for partitioning initial heat into tension-dependent heat and tension-independent heat involves the incubation of the muscle in Krebs-Ringer solution containing 2,3-butanedione monoxime or manitol to selectively inhibit the cross-bridge cycle without influencing the thermal counterparts of the excitation-contraction coupling processes. This allows the tension-independent heat to be obtained. By subtracting the tension-independent heat from the initial heat, the tension-dependent heat is obtained (8, 9). Following measurements of heat and tension, muscle length at l_{max} was measured and blotted weight of this segment was obtained. Cross-sectional area for normalization of force

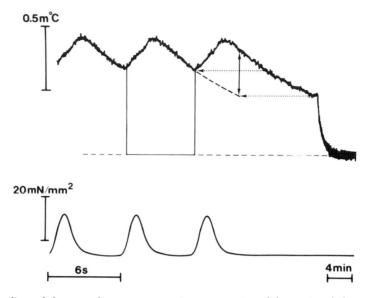

Fig. 3–1. Recording of the muscle temperature (upper trace) and force signal (lower trace) from an isometrically contracting human papillary muscle strip. The vertical arrow at the end of the isometric twitch in the upper tracing indicates the temperature difference between the evolving temperature record and the extrapolated temperature signal (dashed line) of the preceding twitch for the calculation of initial heat. The dashed line is obtained by translating the falling temperature curve after the stimulus is stopped (horizontal arrows). Please note that heat liberation occurs without delay simultaneously with the development of isometric force and that during the relaxation of the isometric twitch the temperature signal is still in the rising phase. Reproduced with permission from Hasenfuss, G. Mulieri, L.A., Blanchard, E.M. Holubarsch, C.H., et al.: Energetics of isometric force development in control and volume-overload human myocardium. Comparison with animal species. Circ, Res, 68:836, 1991

values was calculated as the ratio of blotted weight to muscle length (l_{max}).

Thermal Analysis

Initial heat was calculated by measuring the temperature difference, at the time of complete twitch relaxation, between the evolving temperature record and the falling baseline of the previous twitch that would have occurred if the stimulation had been terminated (Fig. 3–1). This was corrected for heat loss by the single time constant method of Hill (13). The corrected temperature record was then multiplied by the heat loss coefficient and the cool-off time constant and divided by the blotted muscle weight. Tension-independent heat was calculated from the temperature records measured with force inhibited by 2,3-butanedione monoxime or mannitol (see previous text) by the same method used for initial heat calculations. Tension-dependent heat was obtained by subtracting ten-sion-independent heat from initial heat. Average tension-independent heat rate was obtained as the ratio of tension-independent heat and twitch-time (time from the beginning of the isometric twitch to complete relaxation).

The average crossbridge force-time integral was calculated using the following assumptions (9):

1. The force-time integral developed by the muscle results from the summation of the force-time integrals of all individual crossbridge cycles in a muscle length of one half-sarcomere (1.2 μm (14)) (equation 1).
2. During each crossbridge cycle one high energy bond is hydrolyzed (4). Therefore, tension-dependent heat liberated by a muscle length of one half-sarcomere during the isometric twitch is the product of the enthalpy of hydrolysis of one high energy bond and the number of crossbridge cycles (equation 2).

3. Tension-dependent heat liberated by a muscle length of one half-sarcomere is obtained from tension-dependent heat liberated by the entire muscle times the ratio of half-sarcomere-length to muscle length (equation 3). Crossbridge force-time integral (fti) is calculated by dividing the force-time integral of the isometric twitch (FTI) by the number of crossbridge cycles (n) in a muscle length of one half-sarcomere (equation 4).

$$FTI = n \times fti \qquad (1)$$

$$TDH_{hs} = n \times \Delta H_{pCr} \qquad (2)$$

$$TDH_{hs} = THD \times hs/l_{max} \qquad (3)$$

from (2) and (3) $n = TDH \times hs/l_{max} \times \Delta H_{pCr}$

fti =

$$FTI \times l_{max} \times \Delta H_{pCr}/TDH \times hs \qquad (4)$$

where fti = crossbridge force-time integral; FTI = muscle force-time integral; n = number of crossbridge cycles during one twitch in a muscle length of one half-sarcomere; TDH = tension-dependent heat of the muscle; ΔH_{pCr} = enthalpy of hydrolysis of one molecule of phosphocreatine, obtained from the molar enthalpy of phosphocreatine hydrolysis (-35 KJ/mole) (7) and Avogadro's number; hs = length of one half-sarcomere (1.2 um (14)); TDH_{hs} = tension-dependent heat liberated from a muscle length of one half-sarcomere.

Statistical Analysis

Data are expressed as mean ± SEM. To evaluate the statistical significance of differences between the various groups, one-way analysis of variance followed by the Student-Newman-Keuls test was used, or the modified t test and Bonferroni method was applied. A value of $p < 0.05$ was accepted as statistically significant.

Myocardial Tissue and Muscle Preparation

The myothermal measurements were performed in control and volume-overload human myocardium, in control, pressure-overload and hyperthyroid rabbit myocardium, and in control and hypothyroid rat myocardium.

Human Myocardium

Volume overload human myocardium (n = 10 muscle preparations) was obtained from papillary muscles excised during mitral valve replacement surgery in five patients with severe mitral regurgitation. Control myocardium was obtained from papillary muscle tissue of one patient with mitral stenosis (n = 2 muscle strip preparations) undergoing mitral valve replacement surgery and from subepicardial biopsies obtained during coronary artery bypass surgery from three patients with coronary artery disease (n = 4 muscle strip preparations). Biopsies were cut from the anterolateral wall of the left ventricle immediately after complete cardioplegia (15).

The excised myocardium was immediately submerged in a special protective solution at room temperature and oxygenated by bubbling with 95% O_2–5% CO_2 (14). For the muscle strip preparation, we used a new, recently described method, by which it is possible to obtain thin ventricular muscle strips from larger pieces of human myocardium (14).

Rabbit Myocardium

Control myocardium was obtained from 11 albino New Zealand rabbits (2 to 2.5 kg in weight). Pressure-overload myocardium was obtained from 10 rabbits in which right ventricular pressure-overload was induced by surgical constriction of the pulmonary artery (67% decrease of diameter) for 2 weeks (16, 17). Hyperthyroid myocardium was obtained from eight rabbits in which hyperthyrosis was induced by a daily intramuscular injection of 0.2 mg/kg body wt of l-thyroxine for 14 days. Right ventricular papillary muscles were prepared as described (17).

Rat Myocardium

Control rat myocardium was obtained from seven Wistar-Kyoto rats (180 to 250 g in weight). Hypothyroid myocardium was obtained from seven of these rats in which hypothyrosis was induced by adding 0.8 mg/mL propylthiouracil to the drinking water over a period of 3 weeks. Left ventricular papillary muscle strips were prepared as described (18).

RESULTS

Mechanical Measurements

Human Myocardium

In volume overload, compared to control human myocardium, peak twitch tension was reduced by 55%, tension-time integral was reduced by 52%, and maximum rates of tension rise and fall were reduced by 18% and 20%, respectively (Table 3–1, Fig. 3–2). Time to peak tension and time to 50% relaxation tended to be increased by 9% and 24%, respectively in the volume-overload myocardium.

Rabbit Myocardium

Peak twitch tension was not significantly different in the three types of rabbit myocardium (Table 3–1, Fig. 3–2). Compared to control, the tension-time integral was not significantly altered in pressure-overload myocardium, but was reduced by 43% in hyperthyroid myocardium. Maximum rate of tension rise was reduced by 41% in pressure-overload and increased by 68% in hyperthyroid compared to control myocardium. Maximum rate of tension fall was increased by 32% in hyperthyroid myocardium and was not significantly altered in

pressure-overload compared to control myocardium. Time to peak tension and time to 50% relaxation were reduced in hyperthyroid myocardium by 48% and 20%, respectively, and increased in pressure-overload myocardium by 41% and 28% compared to control myocardium, respectively.

Rat Myocardium

Peak twitch tension and tension-time integral were not significantly different in control and hypothyroid myocardium (Table 3–1, Fig. 3–2). In hypothyroid myocardium, maximum rate of tension rise was reduced by 26%, whereas maximum rate of tension fall was not significantly different from that of control myocardium. Time to peak tension and time to 50% relaxation were prolonged by 46% and 22% in hypothyroid compared to control myocardium, respectively. The tension-time integral can be divided into a contraction and relaxation tension-time integral (Fig. 3–3). The tension-time integral for relaxation was greater than that for contraction in all species and types of myocardium.

Myothermal Measurements

Human Myocardium

In volume-overload compared to control myocardium, initial heat and tension-dependent heat were reduced by 74% and 73%, respectively (Table 3–2, Figure 3–2). Tension-independent heat and tension-independent heat rate tended to be reduced

Table 3–1. Mechanical Data

Myocardium	Peak Twitch Tension (mN/mm^2)	Tension-time Integral (mN·s/mm^2)	$+ \dfrac{dT/dt}{T}$ (s^{-1})	$- \dfrac{dT/dt}{T}$ (s^{-1})	Time to Peak Tension (ms)	Time to 50% Relaxation (ms)
Human control	44.0 ± 11.7	74.8 ± 20.5	1.55 ± 0.12	0.93 ± 0.14	1100 ± 65	937 ± 54
Human volume-overload	19.9 ± 3.7*	35.6 ± 6.3*	1.27 ± 0.06*	0.74 ± 0.06*	1194 ± 21	1160 ± 106
Rabbit control	46.1 ± 2.6	47.6 ± 4.2	2.80 ± 0.14	1.18 ± 0.06	674 ± 21	596 ± 34
Rabbit pressure-overload	41.7 ± 5.0	55.4 ± 6.8	1.65 ± 0.13*	1.12 ± 0.14	950 ± 38*	765 ± 67*
Rabbit hyperthyroid	37.8 ± 4.0	27.3 ± 3.9*	4.70 ± 0.20*	1.56 ± 0.13*	354 ± 9*	475 ± 43*
Rat control	56.4 ± 4.4	29.9 ± 2.9	6.33 ± 0.23	1.91 ± 0.08	257 ± 5	331 ± 7
Rat hypotyroid	44.7 ± 3.3	32.2 ± 2.7	4.69 ± 0.11*	1.89 ± 0.06	374 ± 17*	404 ± 25*

$+ \, dT/dt/T$ = maximum rate of tension rise; $- \, dT/dt/T$ = maximum rate of tension fall; * = p < 0.05 versus control myocardium of the same species.

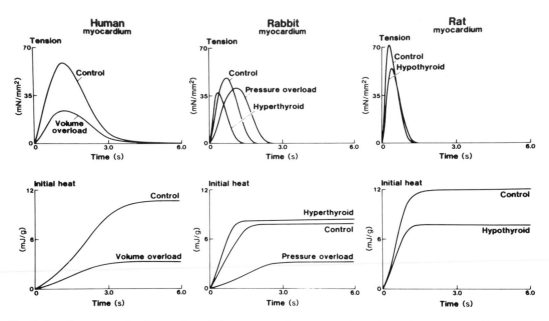

Fig. 3–2. Representative isometric twitch myograms (upper panels) and simultaneous initial heat evolution (lower panels) in human, rabbit, and rat myocardium. Please note that initial heat liberation occurs without delay simultaneously with the development of isometric force and that initial heat evolution continues during the relaxation phase of the isometric twitch. Reproduced with permission from Hasenfuss, G. Mulieri, L.A., Blanchard, E.M, Holubarsch, C.H., et al.: Energetics of isometric force development in control and volume-overload human myocardium. Comparison with animal species. Circ Res 68:836, 1991

in volume-overload compared to control myocardium. Average crossbridge force-time integral was increased by 85% in the volume-overload myocardium.

Rabbit Myocardium

Initial heat and tension-dependent heat were reduced by 55% and 54%, respectively, in pressure-overload, and not significantly different in hyperthyroid compared to control myocardium (Table 3–2, Fig. 3–2). Tension-independent heat and tension-independent heat rate were reduced by 59% and 69%, respectively, in pressure-overload and not significantly different from control in hyperthyroid myocardium. Average crossbridge force-time integral was increased by 164% in pressure-overload and decreased by 47% in hyperthyroid myocardium

Rat Myocardium.

Initial heat and tension-dependent heat were reduced by 44% and 45%, respectively in hypothyroid compared to control

myocardium (Table 3–2, Fig. 3–2). Tension-independent heat and tension-independent heat rate tended to be reduced in the hypothyroid compared to control myocardium. Average crossbridge force-time integral was increased by 100% in hypothyroid compared to control myocardium. Across species and types of myocardium, initial heat was lowest in volume-overload human myocardium and highest in control rat myocardium (Fig. 3–4). The tension-independent heat portion of initial heat amounted to between 9% and 19% of initial heat in the various types of myocardium. Initial heat can be divided into the portions released during contraction and relaxation (Fig. 3–5). Initial heat for relaxation was significantly greater than that for contraction in control and volume-overload human myocardium as well as in control and hypothyroid rat myocardium.

Relationship Between Mechanical and Myothermal Parameters

Including the different types of myocardium within and across species, there was

Tension-time integral

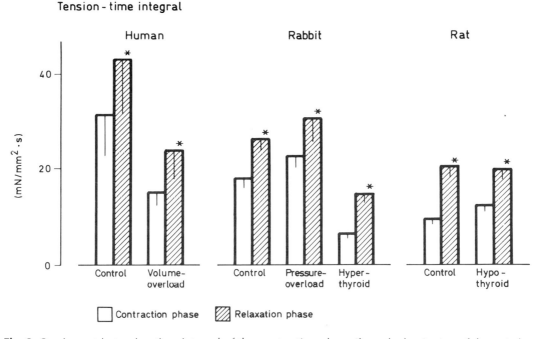

Fig. 3–3. Isometric tension-time integral of the contraction phase (from the beginning of the twitch to time at peak tension) and the relaxation phase (from the time at peak tension to complete relaxation). * = p < 0.05

a close inverse correlation between tension-independent heat rate and time to 50% relaxation and a positive correlation between tension-independent heat rate and maximum rate of tension fall (Fig. 3–6). Furthermore, there was an inverse correlation between average crossbridge force-time integral and tension-independent heat rate in the different types of myocardium (Fig.

3–7). To compare the energy cost of tension generation during the contraction and relaxation phase of the isometric twitch, initial heat was normalized for tension-time integral. The ratio of initial heat to tension-time integral of the relaxation phase was significantly greater than that of the contraction phase in the control human and the control rat myocardium (Fig. 3–8). In

Table 3–2. Myothermal Data

Myocardium	Initial Heat (mJ/g)	Tension-dependent Heat (mJ/g)	Tension-indepndent Heat (mJ/g)	Tension-independent Heat Rate (mW/g)	Crossbridge Force-time Integral (pN/s)
Human control	7.98 ± 2.26	7.23 ± 2.22	0.75 ± 0.19	0.18 ± 0.05	0.52 ± 0.07
Human volume-overload	2.05 ± 0.25*	1.92 ± 0.25*	0.39 ± 0.04	0.09 ± 0.01	0.96 ± 0.10*
Rabbit control	7.65 ± 0.84	6.60 ± 0.75	1.00 ± 0.17	0.48 ± 0.08	0.36 ± 0.02
Rabbit pressure-overload	3.42 ± 0.54*	3.05 ± 0.46*	0.41 ± 0.08*	0.15 ± 0.03*	0.95 ± 0.11*
Rabbit hyperthyroid	8.69 ± 1.21	6.52 ± 0.88	1.35 ± 0.33	0.65 ± 0.13	0.19 ± 0.01*
Rat control	10.07 ± 0.88	9.11 ± 0.75	0.96 ± 0.17	0.68 ± 0.13	0.16 ± 0.01
Rat hypothyroid	5.64 ± 0.54*	5.02 ± 0.59*	0.63 ± 0.08	0.43 ± 0.05	0.32 ± 0.02*

* = p < 0.05 versus control myocardium of the same species.

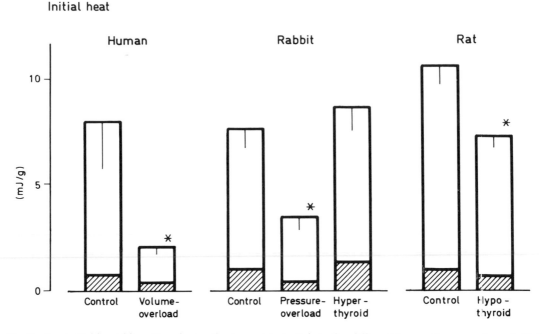

Fig. 3–4. Initial heat liberation during the isometric twitch in the different types of myocardium. Initial heat is partitioned into its two components, tension-dependent heat and tension-independent heat. Tension-dependent heat (open portion of the bars) results from high-energy phosphate hydrolysis of contractile proteins. Tension-independent heat (hatched area of the bars) results from high-energy phosphate hydrolysis of excitation-contraction coupling processes. * = $p < 0.05$ for initial heat versus control myocardium of the same species.

the hyperthyroid rabbit, myocardium, the ratio of initial heat to tension-time integral of the relaxation phase tended to be lower than that of the contraction phase (borderline significance), whereas in the other types of myocardium both ratios were similar.

DISCUSSION

In this chapter, we use initial heat to investigate the energy turnover of isometrically contracting human, rabbit, and rat myocardium. The sensitive antimony-bismuth thermopiles allow evaluation of initial heat evolution simultaneously with the mechanical performance on a beat-to-beat basis. Moreover, because the delay between the actual production of heat and the change in thermopile output are below 10 ms (11) and thus negligible in relation to the time scale of the isometric twitch (Table 3–1), the heat measurements enable differ-

entiation between the energy liberation during the contraction and relaxation phase of the isometric twitch. In addition, initial heat was partitioned into its two components, tension-dependent heat and tension-independent heat, to relate cross-bridge behavior and excitation-contraction coupling to relaxation parameters of the isometric twitch. As is shown in Figure 3–4, there are considerable differences in initial heat liberated in the various types of myocardium throughout the isometric twitch. These differences quantitatively result from differences in tension-dependent heat, i.e., high-energy phosphate hydrolysis by contractile proteins, which in the various types of myocardium makes up between 81% and 91% of initial heat. Assuming that one high-energy phosphate bond is hydrolyzed during each cross-bridge cycle (4), differences in tension-dependent heat indicate that considerable differences exist in the number of cross-

Initial heat

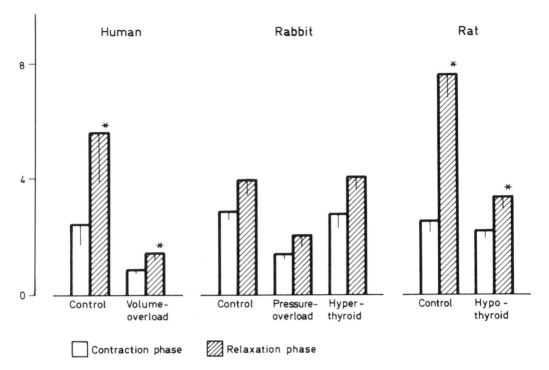

Fig. 3–5. Initial heat liberation during the contraction phase (from the beginning of the twitch to time at peak tension) and relaxation phase (from the time at peak tension to complete relaxation) of the isometric twitch. * = $p < 0.05$

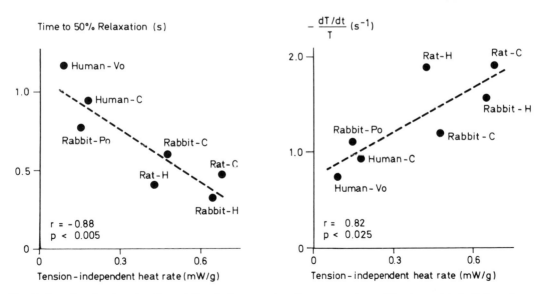

Fig. 3–6. Graphs showing the relation between relaxation parameters of the isometric twitch and average tension-independent heat rate in the various types of myocardium. Tension-independent heat rate reflects the average rate of calcium removal. The linear regression lines were calculated from average values of the different groups. $-dT/dt/T$ = maximum rate of tension fall.

Crossbridge force-time integral

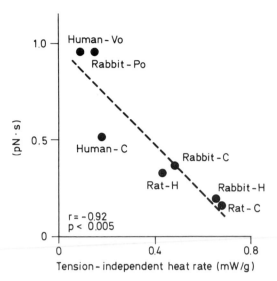

Fig. 3–7. Graph showing the relationship between average cross-bridge force-time integral and tension-independent heat rate. The linear regression line was calculated from the average values in the different groups.

bridges activated during the isometric twitch in the various types of myocardium. The remaining 9 to 19% of initial heat, i.e., tension-independent heat, results from high-energy phosphate hydrolysis by excitation-contraction coupling processes. This includes high-energy phosphate hydrolysis of sarcoplasmic reticulum Ca^{2+}-ATPases, sarcolemmal Ca^{2+}-ATPases, sarcolemmal Na^+-K^+-ATPases, and other ATP-utilizing ion pumps. The major portion of tension-independent heat results from high-energy phosphate hydrolysis of sarcoplasmic reticulum Ca^{2+}-ATPases to remove calcium from the cytosol (3, 8, 9). Therefore, from the tension-independent heat values we calculated the amount of calcium cycled using the assumption that there is a coupling ratio of 2 Ca^{2+} per high-energy phosphate bond hydrolyzed (2, 5, 8) and that the enthalpy of creatine phosphate hydrolysis is 35 KJ/mol (7). In addition, from the amount of sodium calculated to be necessary for depolarization (19), we assumed that 0.13 mJ/g of tension-independent heat is associated with sodium removal. Accordingly, the amount of calcium cycled during

the isometric twitch was calculated to be between 15 nmol/g wet weight in the volume-overload human and 70 nmol/g in the hyperthyroid rabbit myocardium. Fabiato estimated from biochemical data that the amount of calcium necessary to activate the contractile apparatus of mammalian myocardium to 70% was 54 nmol/g (20). Tension-independent heat rate reflecting the average rate of calcium removal amounted to between 0.09 mW/g in volume-overload human myocardium and 0.68 mW/g in control rat myocardium.

Relaxation of the myocardium may depend on kinetics of calcium removal and/or kinetics of crossbridge cycling (21). To investigate the possible role of rate of calcium removal on relaxation of the myocardium, tension-independent heat rate was correlated with relaxation parameters of the isometric twitch. Across the different types of myocardium, there was a significant positive correlation between tension-independent heat rate and maximum rate of tension fall and a significant inverse correlation between tension-independent heat rate and time to 50% relaxation. This may suggest that rate of calcium removal is a major determinant of myocardial relaxation under those conditions. However, we also found a significant inverse correlation between tension-independent heat rate and the average crossbridge force-time integral across the different types of myocardium. Assuming that differences in crossbridge force-time integral result from different rate constants of crossbridge detachment (22), the close inverse correlation between tension-independent heat rate and crossbridge force-time integral indicates that, in types of myocardium with high rates of calcium removal, crossbridge attachment is short, whereas it is prolonged in types of myocardium with slow calcium removal. From an energetics point of view, increased crossbridge force-time integral means increased economy of isometric force development because a higher crossbridge force-time integral is obtained per unit of high-energy phosphate hydrolyzed. On the other hand, prolonged crossbridge attachment time may reduce the shortening velocity and relaxation rate of the muscle. Therefore, the abbreviated crossbridge force-time integral in conjunction with a

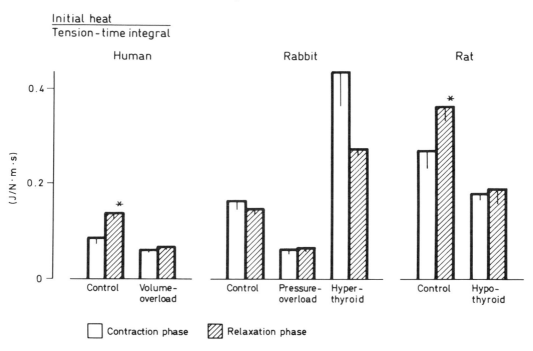

Fig. 3—8. Ratio of initial heat to tension-time integral of the contraction phase (from the beginning of the twitch to time at peak tension) and relaxation phase (from the time at peak tension to complete relaxation) of the isometric twitch (see values in Figs. 3–3 and 3–5). * = $p < 0.05$. Note the considerable differences in these ratios between the various types of myocardium, which are caused by differences in cross-bridge force-time integral (see discussion).

fast excitation-contraction coupling system enables high shortening velocity, high rates of relaxation and high heart rates in the rat and hyperthyroid rabbit myocardium, but the economy of force production is low. In contrast, in the human myocardium, in particular in the case of volume overload, increased crossbridge force-time integral in conjunction with a slow excitation-contraction coupling system is favorable from an energy economy point of view, but at the expense of reduced shortening velocity, reduced rate of relaxation, and reduced maximum heart rate.

The observed relationship between excitation-contraction coupling and contractile protein system suggests coordinated genetic changes in contractile and excitation-contraction coupling processes across species and coordinated restructuring due to hormonal and hemodynamic stresses. On a molecular level, changes in contractile protein behavior and excitation-contraction coupling systems seem to be controlled by different genetic mechanisms. Altera-

tions in contractile protein behavior seem to be regulated by qualitative changes, i.e., expression of different myosin heavy chain isoforms or different troponin T isoforms in the various types of myocardium (9, 17, 18, 23, 24). In contrast, alterations in excitation-contraction coupling with respect to calcium removal seem to be regulated predominantly by quantitative changes in the number of sarcoplasmic reticulum Ca^{2+}-ATPases expressed (25–28). Alterations of the excitation-contraction coupling and contractile protein system occurring in the hormonally or hemodynamically stressed myocardium are considered to be adaptational. One might speculate that changes in excitation-contraction coupling processes or kinetics of the crossbridge cycle exceeding a certain level may cause myocardial failure (29). Alternatively, failure in the coordination of both systems may cause the deleterious step from coordinated hypertrophy to myocardial failure.

There is considerable controversy in the literature regarding the energy dependence of tension generation during relaxation. In 1964, Monroe showed that, in the isovolumic contracting dog heart, a sudden reduction of volume at peak pressure with a concomitant decrease of the pressure-time integral by about 50% reduced oxygen consumption by only about 10% (30). Similar findings were obtained by Suga et al.; compared to oxygen consumption of entire isovolumic contractions, in quick-release contractions at end-systole, oxygen consumption was reduced by only about 10% (31, 32). Elzinga et al. found that oxygen consumption of isovolumic contractions and that of quick-release contractions at peak systolic pressure were not significantly different (33). These findings might indicate that tension generation during relaxation is considerably less energy-dependent than during contraction. Cooper and Hiasano and Cooper on the other hand observed 36% reduction of oxygen consumption in similar quick-release experiments (34, 35).

To compare energetics of contraction with those of relaxation, isometric tension-time integral and initial heat were analyzed separately from the beginning of the twitch to peak tension development (contraction phase) and from peak tension to complete relaxation (relaxation phase). In all types of myocardium investigated, tension-time integral of relaxation was significantly greater than that of contraction (Fig. 3–3). Tension generation during relaxation was associated with a considerable amount of initial heat liberation during the relaxation phase of the isometric twitch (Figs. 3–1 and 3–5). Initial heat liberation during relaxation was significantly greater than that during contraction in the human and the rat myocardium. In all types of rabbit myocardium, initial heat of the relaxation phase tended to be greater than that of the contraction phase, but the difference did not reach statistical significance. When initial heat liberation during contraction and relaxation was normalized for the tension-time integral of the contraction and relaxation phase, respectively, the ratio of initial heat to tension-time integral of relaxation was significantly greater than that of contraction in the control human and control rat myocardium, whereas it was not significantly different in the other types of myo-

cardium. This shows that, dependent on the species and type of myocardium, the energy expenditure per unit of tension-time integral during relaxation may even exceed that during the contraction phase of the isometric twitch. We did not partition initial heat of relaxation into its tension-dependent and tension-independent portions. However, because initial heat of relaxation was between three and eight times higher than the tension-independent heat liberated during the total isometric twitch, the major portion of initial heat of relaxation results from high-energy phosphate hydrolysis of cycling crossbridges. This clearly demonstrates that, under isometric conditions, tension generation is energy-dependent at all phases of the cardiac cycle, including the relaxation phase.

SUMMARY AND CONCLUSIONS

In human, rabbit, and rat myocardium, significant amounts of heat are liberated during the relaxation phase of the isometric twitch, which can be attributed to high-energy phosphate hydrolysis of contractile proteins. The quantity of energy turnover during the relaxation phase relative to that during the contraction phase depends on the species and, within species, on the hormonal status or hemodynamic stress that was imposed on the heart.

Considerable differences in mechanical parameters of the isometric twitch and the function of the excitation-contraction coupling and contractile protein system exist in the various types of myocardium investigated. The mechanical parameters of relaxation are closely related to the function of the excitation-contraction coupling system (rate of calcium removal), which in turn is in close relation with the behavior of the individual crossbridge cycle. This indicates coordinated genetic changes in excitation-contraction coupling and contractile protein system across species and coordinated restructuring of both systems following hormonal or hemodynamic stresses. Inadequate restructuring or failure in the coordination of both systems may be the cause of the transition from coordinated hypertrophy to myocardial failure. Further studies are warranted to investigate the function of the excitation-contraction coupling and contractile protein system in the transition from the compensated to the failure state.

REFERENCES

1. Coulson RL, Rusy BF: A system of assessing mechanical performance, heat production and oxygen utilization in isolated perfused whole hearts. Cardiovasc Res 7:859, 1973.
2. Alpert NR, Mulieri LA, Hasenfuss G: Myocardial chemo-mechanical energy transduction. *In* The Heart and Cardiovascular System. Edited by HA Fozzard et al. New York, Raven Press, 1992.
3. Alpert NR, Mulieri LA: The effect of regional myocardial heterogeneity on the economy of isometric relaxation. *In* Diastolic Relaxation of the Heart. Edited by W Grossman, BH Lorell. Boston, Martinus Nijhoff, 1987.
4. Huxley AF: Muscle structure and theories of contraction. Prog Biophys Chem 7:255, 1957.
5. Tada M, Imei M: Regulation of calcium transport by the ATPase phospholamban system. J Mol Cell Cardiol 15:565, 1983.
6. Carafoli E: The homeostasis of Ca in heart cells. J Mol Cell Cardiol 17:203, 1985.
7. Woledge RC, Reilly PJ: Molar enthalpy change for hydrolysis of phosphorylcreatine under conditions in muscle cells. Bio phys J 54:97, 1988.
8. Alpert NR, Blanchard EM, Mulieri LA: Tension-independent heat in rabbit papillary muscle. J Physiol (London) 414:433, 1989.
9. Hasenfuss G, Mulieri LA, Blanchard EM, et al.: Energetics of isometric force development in control and volume-overload human myocardium. Comparison with animal species. Circ Res 68:836, 1991.
10. Loiselle DS: Cardiac basal and activation metabolism. *In* Cardiac Energetics. Edited by R Jacob, H Just, C Holubarsch. Darmstadt, Steinkopff Verlag, Darmstadt, 1987.
11. Mulieri LA, Luhr G, Trefry J, Alpert NR: Metal-film thermopiles for use with rabbit right ventricular papillary muscles. Am J Physiol 233:C146, 1977.
12. Hamrell BB, Panaanan R, Trono J, Alpert NR: A stable, sensitive, low-compliance capacitance force transducer. J Appl Physiol 38:190, 1975.
13. Hill AV: Recovery heat in muscle. Proc R Soc (Biol) 127:297, 1939.
14. Mulieri LA, Hasenfuss G, Ittleman F, et al. Protection of human left ventricular myocardium from cutting injury with 2,3 butanedione monoxime. Circ Res 65:1441, 1989.
15. Mulieri LA, Leavitt BJ, Hasenfuss G, et al.: Contraction frequency dependence of twitch and diastolic tension in human dilated cardiomyopathy. *In* Cellular and Molecular Alterations in the Failing Human Heart. Edited by G Hasenfuss, C Holubarsch, H Just, NR Alpert. Darmstadt, Steinkopff Verlag, 1992.
16. Hamrell BB, Alpert NR: The mechanical characteristics of hypertrophied rabbit cardiac muscle in the absence of congestive heart failure. Circ Res 40:20, 1977.
17. Alpert NR, Mulieri LA: Increased myothermal economy of isometric force development in compensated cardiac hypertrophy induced by pulmonary artery constriction in the rabbit. Circ Res 50:491, 1982.
18. Holubarsch C, Goulette R, Litten RZ, et al.: The economy of isometric force development, myosin isoenzyme pattern and myofibrillar ATPase activity in normal and hypothyroid rat myocardium. Circ Res 56:78, 1985.
19. Langer GA: Sodium exchange in dog ventricular muscle. J Gen Physiol 50:1221, 1967.
20. Fabiato A: Calcium-induced release of calcium from the cardiac sarcoplasmic reticulum. Am J Physiol 245:C1, 1983.
21. Brutsaert DL, Stanislas US: Relaxation and diastole of the heart. Physiol Rev 69:1228, 1989.
22. Brenner B: Effect of Ca^{2+} on crossbridge turnover kinetics in skinned single rabbit psoas fibers: Implications for regulation of muscle contaction. Proc Natl Acad Sci 85:3265, 1988.
23. Swynghedauw B: Developmental and functional adaptation of contractile proteins in cardiac and skeletal muscles. Physiol Rev 66:710, 1986.
24. Anderson PAW, Malouf NN, Oakely AE, et al.: Troponin T isoform expression in humans: A comparison among normal and failing adult heart, fetal heart and adult and fetal skeletal muscle. Circ Res 69:1226, 1991.
25. Arai M, Otsu K, MacLennan DH, et al.: Effect of thyroid hormone on the expression of mRNA encoding sarcoplasmic reticulum proteins. Circ Res 69:266, 1991.
26. Lompre AM, Lambert F, Lakatta EG, Schwartz K: Expression of sarcoplasmic reticulum Ca^{2+}-ATPase and calsequestrin genes in rat heart during ontogenic development and aging. Circ Res 69:1380, 1991.
27. Mercadier JJ, Bouveret P, Gorza L, Schiaffino S, et al.: Myosin isoenzymes in normal

and hypertrophied human ventricular myocardium. Circ Res 53:52, 1983.

28. De la Bastie D, Levitsky D, Rappaport L, Mercardier JJ, et al.: Function of the sarcoplasmic reticulum and expression of its Ca^{2+}-ATPase gene in pressure overload-induced cardiac hypertrophy in the rat. Circ Res 66:554, 1990.

29. Hasenfuss G, Mulieri LA, Leavitt BJ, et al.: Alterations of contractile function and excitation-contraction coupling in dilated cardiomyopathy. Circ Res (in press).

30. Monroe RG: Myocardial oxygen consumption during ventricular contraction and relaxation. Circ Res 14:294, 1964.

31. Suga H: Ventricular Energetics. Physiol Rev 70:247, 1990.

32. Yasumura Y, Nozaw T, Futki S, Tanaka N, Suga H: Time-invariant oxygen cost of mechanical energy in dog left ventricle: Consistency and inconsistency of time-varying elastance model with myocardial energetics. Circ Res 64:763, 1989.

33. Elzinga G, Duwel CMB, Mast F, Westerhof N: Mechanical determinants of myocardial energy turnover. *In* Cardiac Energetics. Basic Mechanisms and Clinical implications. Edited by B Jacob, H Just, C Holubarsch. Darmstadt, Steinkopff Verlag, 1987.

34. Cooper G: Myocardial energetic during isometric twitch contractions of cat papillary muscle. Am J Physiol 236:H244, 1979.

35. Hisano R, Cooper G: Correlation of force-length area with oxygen consumption in ferret papillary muscle. Circ Res 61:318, 1987.

Chapter 4

THE LEFT VENTRICULAR DIASTOLIC PRESSURE-VOLUME RELATION, RELAXATION, AND FILLING*

Hideo Shintani and Stanton A. Glantz

Changes in diastolic function affect not only filling of the left ventricle but systolic function as well (1–11). Growing awareness of the importance of diastolic function has been accompanied by progress in sophisticated new technologies and approaches to observe cardiac function, including Doppler echocardiography, the cardiac volume conductance catheter, digital angiography, and magnetic resonance imaging (MRI). Until the 1970s, the left ventricle was considered an isolated shell in which the left ventricular diastolic pressure-volume relationship depended only on the myocardium's material properties and the left ventricle's wall thickness and geometry. According to this view, the relationship between diastolic pressure and volume could change only in response to chronic changes in the cardiac muscle's material properties, such as scarring after infarction (12), or changes in cardiac geometry due to hypertrophy. Consequently, the diastolic pressure-volume relationship was considered unique over the short term. A practical application of this assumed uniqueness was that left ventricular diastolic pressure was used as a surrogate for volume in evaluating systolic function.

However, in the early 1970s, studies of patients with coronary artery disease contradicted this simplistic view of the diastolic pressure-volume relationship (13–17). In these patients, the left ventricular diastolic pressure-volume curve shifted upward temporarily immediately after cardiac pacing-induced angina and then returned to prepacing values. Later, other investigators (18, 19) observed that vasodilator and vasoconstrictor drugs, which change the vascular loading conditions of the left ventricle, also produced acute reversible shifts in the left ventricular diastolic pressure-volume curve. In the process of explaining these clinical observations, we have learned that many factors can affect left ventricular filling and the diastolic pressure-volume relationship acutely.

The original concept that the pressure within the left ventricle is determined by the balance between the forces caused by pressures within the ventricular cavity that expand the ventricle and forces caused by elasticity of the myocardium that resist this expansion remains the centerpiece of our understanding of the diastolic pressure-volume relationship. However, it is now clear that changes in active relaxation of the myocardium, mechanical interaction between the ventricles, the pericardium, so-called diastolic suction, pulmonary-cardiac contact pressure, myocardial viscoelasticity, and engorgement of the coronary vasculature all play some role in determining the left ventricular pressure-volume relationship during diastole (Fig. 4–1). The questions are: "How large an effect does each of these factors have on the left ventricular diastolic pressure-volume relationship?" and "When during diastole does each of them act?" The answers are that during early diastole the rate of relaxation is, and diastolic suction may be, important. During late diastole (and at end-diastole), the extent of relaxation and ventricular interaction modulated by the pericardium is important. The other factors—pulmonary-cardiac contact pressure, viscoelasticity of the myocardium, and engorgement

* This chapter is a revised and updated version of "Determinants of Left Ventricular Filling and of the Diastolic Pressure-Volume Relation" by J. Gilbert and S. Glantz (*Circ. Res.* 64:827–852, 1989).

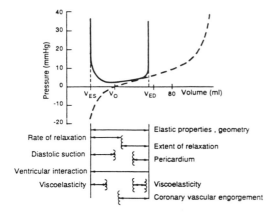

Fig. 4–1. Several different factors affect the diastolic pressure during diastole, with different factors being important at different times. The myocardium's elasticity and geometry (size and wall thickness) are important throughout diastole, the other effects are superimposed on the pressure because of the myocardial elasticity. During early diastole, active relaxation and the recoil effect of elastic energy which may be stored in the myocardium from the previous systole (so-called "diastolic suction") determine the atrioventricular pressure gradient and ventricular filling rate. The dashed line shows the purely elastic pressure-volume curve of the myocardial shell in the absence of the component caused by active relaxation from the previous beat, the negative pressures here reflect the elastic energy which combines with the relaxation component to determine the observed pressure. Late in diastole, ventricular interaction and the pericardium become important. Viscoelastic properties of the myocardium play a small role during rapid filling and during atrial contraction, and diastole. The different factors are listed below the curve, with an indication of when they are important in determining the diastolic pressure. Wavy lines indicate the approximate boundary when each factor is important. V_{ES}, end-systolic volume, V_{ED}, end-diastolic volume, V_O, equilibrium volume. Gilbert, J.C. and Glantz, S.A.: Determinants of left ventricular filling and of the diastolic pressure-volume relation. Circ. Res. 64:827, 1989; with permission of the American Heart Association.

of the coronary vasculature—are less important in determining the left ventricular diastolic pressure-volume relationship.

GEOMETRY, MUSCLE ELASTICITY, AND THE BASIC PRESSURE-VOLUME RELATIONSHIP

The diastolic pressure-volume relationship results from forces acting both *within*

and *on* the myocardium. The forces acting on the myocardium, in turn, result from the pressure *within* the left ventricle and the other cardiac chambers and from the constraining forces exerted *on* the epicardium by the pericardium and the lungs. The forces acting within the myocardium result from the fact that the myocardium is an elastic material so that the muscle itself develops a resisting force as it extends. The physical relationships that govern these forces provide the framework within which we will discuss the factors that affect the diastolic pressure-volume relationship.

To understand many of the factors that affect the left ventricular diastolic pressure-volume relationship, the left ventricle can be modeled as a simple, pressurized, spherical shell (20). Three simplifying assumptions permit us to derive an equation, the *Laplace Law*, which relates wall stress to pressure, and geometry, i.e., radius and wall thickness. (*Stress*, σ, is the force per cross-sectional area of a material such as the muscle.) The assumptions are that: (1) The left ventricle is a sphere with uniform wall thickness, h, and inside radius, r; (2) The left ventricle is in static equilibrium (i.e., nothing is moving); and (3) The wall is thin, so that the stress may be considered constant through the wall. (See Chap. 9.)

To begin, cut the sphere through its center to expose the internal forces (Fig. 4–2A). The total force tending to push the lower hemisphere away from the upper hemisphere is equal to the pressure within the sphere, p, times the internal cross-sectional area, πr^2. The total force in the wall holding the two halves together equals the wall stress, σ, times the cross-sectional area of the wall. These two forces must balance:

$$p(r^2) = [(r + h)^2 - r^2] \qquad (1)$$

which simplifies to:

$$p\,r = \sigma\,h\,(2 + h/r). \qquad (2)$$

Because we assumed a thin wall, the ratio of the thickness to the internal radius is much smaller than 2, so we can neglect h/r. Solving equation (2) for the stress yields:

$$\sigma = pr/2h. \qquad (3)$$

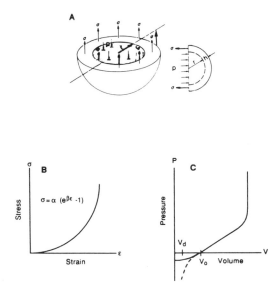

Fig. 4–2. The elastic component of the diastolic pressure-volume curve is determined by the balance of the force (pressure) in the ventricular chamber tending to push the chamber apart and force (stress) in the wall holding it together (A), combined with the relation between stress and strain (distension) of the myocardium (B). These elements are combined to derive a pressure-volume relation for the left ventricle shown by the solid line in panel C. The relation expressed in panel C provides a good description of the left ventricle's pressure-volume characteristics above the equilibrium volume, V_O, but not below V_O, when the myocardial wall is in compression and storing elastic energy (dashed line). The ability of the myocardium to store elastic energy in compression when the end-systolic volume is below the equilibrium volume gives rise to the phenomenon of so-called diastolic suction. σ, stress, p, pressure, r, radius of curvature (to the endocardium), h, wall thickness, α and β, elasticity parameters, ε, Lagrangian strain. Gilbert, J.C., and Glantz, S.A.: Determinants of left ventricular filling and of the diastolic pressure-volume relation. Circ. Res. 64:827, 1989; with permission of the American Heart Association.

Equation (3), the Laplace law for a thin-walled sphere, relates the pressure in the left ventricle and its geometry (i.e., radius and wall thickness) to the wall stress. According to the Laplace Law, the wall stress in a sphere increases in direct proportion to the internal pressure and radius and decreases in inverse proportion to the wall thickness.

The Laplace law and the elastic proper-ties of the myocardium can be used to derive the ventricular pressure-volume relationship. The Laplace law shows that, as the ventricular pressure increases, the wall stress increases, extending the muscle and thus increasing the ventricle's radius. In our assumed spherical ventricle, the radius is related directly to ventricular volume ($V = 4/3\ \pi r^3$). The next step is to relate the wall stress to ventricular volume.

The relationship between wall stress and ventricular volume depends on the elastic properties of the myocardium. As in most biologic materials, muscle becomes stiffer as it is extended, i.e., it requires greater increments of force to produce each additional increment of length. *Strain* is a normalized, dimensionless measure of the deformation of a solid such as the myocardium. The most common way of defining strain is *Lagrangian strain*, which is defined as extension from equilibrium length divided by the equilibrium length, $\epsilon = (1 - l_0)/l_0$. The *equilibrium length* is the length that a specimen of material exhibits when subjected to no external forces. This equilibrium length is usually used as the reference length for computing strains.

The elastic properties of the myocardium have been described by an exponential relationship between stress (σ) and strain (ε) (21):

$$\sigma = \alpha(e^{\beta\epsilon} - 1). \qquad (4)$$

In a purely *elastic material*, the stresses depend only on the strain (deformation), ε. The parameters α and β in equation (4) are constants and determine the precise nature of this relationship, which is shown by the curve in Figure 4–2B and described by equation (1); thus α and β are called *elastic constants.*

This one-dimensional stress-strain relationship can be extended to a pressure-volume relationship by using the spherical ventricular geometry and the Laplace Law for a sphere (22). In addition, the concept of an equilibrium length, described previously, can be generalized to an *equilibrium volume*, V_0, the volume that a shell (such as the left ventricle) exhibits when subjected to no transmural pressure.

The resulting model, however, is not a good description of the pressure-volume characteristics of the left ventricle below its equilibrium volume, V_0. As the dashed curve in Figure 4–2C shows, the actual ventricular pressure drops rapidly as chamber volume falls below V_0, whereas a simple elasticity model predicts little change in pressure (dark curve in Figure 4–2C). This difference is probably a result of two factors: First, the assumption of a "thin" wall is drastically violated at small volumes. Second, equation (4) is probably not a good description of the elastic properties of the myocardium in compression at volumes below V_0 (23–28). The rapid drop in pressure that occurs for ventricular volumes below V_0 (Fig 4–2C) is important for understanding so-called diastolic suction.

Effects of Hypertrophy

When the left ventricle is subjected to a chronic volume or pressure overload, it grows. The Laplace law provides the theoretical framework for understanding the mechanical stimulus for the changes that take place (29–31). In addition, although the changes that accompany hypertrophy often have beneficial effects in terms of helping the left ventricle maintain systolic function in the face of increased loading, this is often accomplished at the expense of increases in diastolic pressure that can eventually lead to circulatory congestion and congestive heart failure because of increases in end-diastolic pressure necessary to maintain a given end-diastolic volume (32).

Diastolic heart failure is characterized by increased resistance to diastolic filling of one or both cardiac ventricles. Although diastolic dysfunction is a relatively common problem and some degree of diastolic failure exists in most patients presenting clinically with heart failure, a substantial subset of patients has relatively pure diastolic heart failure with normal systolic function; so many have mild or asymptomatic congestive heart failure (33, 34). Diastolic heart failure can be caused by structural abnormalities that increase resistance to ventricular inflow, including extramyocardial (such as constrictive pericarditis or mitral stenosis) or intramyocardial (such as fibrosis or amyloidosis) abnormalities. There is evidence that advanced myocardial hypertrophy is associated with increased resistance to ventricular diastolic inflow because of both structural alterations and impaired relaxation of the hypertrophied myocardium. Physiologic mechanisms for impaired relaxation in advanced hypertrophy remain controversial, but can include disordered function of myocardial sarcoplasmic reticulum, subendocardial ischemia, and altered adenylate cyclase function (34–36). (See Chaps. 20 and 21.)

When the left ventricle is first subjected to a volume overload, the myocardium is strained more than usual during diastole because the difference between the volume and equilibrium volume, V_0, is increased. As a result of this increased strain, diastolic wall stress and end-diastolic pressure increase. Over time, cardiac myocytes respond by elongating and thickening in a way that effectively increases V_0 with little or no increase in wall thickness. This increase in V_0 means that the larger volume now corresponds to a lower strain, and so leads to correspondingly lower wall stress and diastolic pressure. The left ventricle appears to stop growing when it has increased V_0 to the point that end-diastolic wall stress has returned to values present before imposition of the volume overload (31). This so-called eccentric hypertrophy also occurs in response to physical training (37, 38) and in people with aortic or mitral insufficiency (39). The changes that accompany volume overload seem to be primarily those associated with changing size of the heart (and the related changes in equilibrium volume) rather than intrinsic changes in the elastic properties of the myocardium (37, 40, 41).

This situation contrasts with that observed during pressure overload (42). The conventional wisdom (29) is that in pressure overloads, the stress that the myocardium must develop during systole is increased because of the increased afterload. The left ventricle responds by developing a so-called concentric hypertrophy in which there is an increase in wall thickness with little or no change in chamber radius, presumably because of the addition of new sarcomeres in parallel with existing ones. According to this hypothesis, this increase in wall thickness allows the left ventricle to generate increased systolic pressure at a lower level of average wall stress (i.e., force development in individual sarcomeres) than would occur in the absence of hypertrophy.

In addition to the purely geometric effects associated with pressure-overload hypertrophy, the structure of the cardiac interstitum changes to increase the amount of collagen present and thus increase the elastic stiffness (41, 43–45). (See Chap. 8.) The net effect of these changes is to lead to higher diastolic pressure at any given volume. This upward shift in the diastolic pressure-volume relationship accounts partly for the increase in diastolic pressure that accompanies pressure overload and the potential for patients with pressure overload to develop congestive heart failure.

The analysis thus far has presumed that stress in the wall is determined principally by ventricular geometry and myocardial elasticity. Although this is true late in diastole, when the heart is fully relaxed, it is not true during early diastole, while the muscle is relaxing from the previous beat and is rapidly expanding, or during atrial systole. During early diastole, wall stress is composed of components caused by the relaxation from the previous systole as well as the muscle's passive elastic properties. Fortunately, the Laplace law can still be used to understand the effects of these stresses because it simply relates ventricular pressure, radius, and wall stress and thus intrinsically incorporates the state of the myocardium. Moreover, the relationship between left ventricular size, left ventricular wall thickness, and the elasticity of the myocardium is the single most important determinant of the diastolic pressure-volume relationship.

RELAXATION

The rate and extent of relaxation are two different quantities, each of which influences the left ventricular diastolic pressure-volume relationship. The extent of relaxation is the end state of the muscle after relaxation has been completed and is the more important of the two because it determines the myocardium's equilibrium length, which, in turn, determines the left ventricle's equilibrium volume. Impaired

extent of relaxation means smaller-than-normal equilibrium volumes, which lead to larger strains and higher diastolic pressures at a given end-diastolic volume. Higher pressures at the same volume result in an upward shift in the diastolic pressure-volume relationship. Thus, the extent of relaxation is important at the end of diastole. The rate of relaxation affects the diastolic pressure-volume relationship early in diastole because it affects the atrioventricular pressure gradient and therefore affects filling rate during the rapid filling phase of diastole. The rate of relaxation generally does not influence end-diastole directly because the relaxation process is over well before the time diastole ends.

Estimating Relaxation Rate

One must be able to quantify changes in left ventricular relaxation in order to study how it affects diastolic pressure. (See Chaps. 5 and 13.) The rate of relaxation can be quantified using the exponential relationship Weiss et al. (46) proposed. They quantified left ventricular relaxation rate by fitting the time course of the isovolumic pressure fall beginning at the time of dp/dt$_{min}$ and lasting through the mitral valve opening with the exponential function of time:

$$p(t) = p_0 e^{-t/T} \qquad (5)$$

where p_0 = pressure at time of dp/dt$_{min}$, t = time after dp/dt$_{min}$, and T = time constant of isovolumic pressure fall. Ventricular relaxation rate is thus quantified by a single number, T, the relaxation time constant. (The time constant equals the time required for the pressure to decay to e^{-1} = 0.37 of its original value.)

The major problem with equation (6) is the implicit assumption that if the left ventricle were allowed to relax fully without filling (as t → ∞), the pressure would fall asymptotically to zero. Zero pressure asymptote means that the isovolumic ventricle would have zero wall stress when it is fully relaxed (equation (3)). However, as shown in Figure 4–2C, the total ventricular wall stress is zero only if the left ventricle is at its equilibrium volume, V_0, and the end-systolic and equilibrium volumes are not necessarily the same (47–50). Equation (5) can be modified to take into account the effect of unequal end-systolic and equilibrium volumes by incorporating the term, p_∞, which is the pressure to which the ventricle would relax if the ventricle were held at its end-systolic volume and allowed to relax completely:

$$p(t) = (p_0 - p_\infty)\, e^{-t/T} + p_\infty \qquad (6)$$

One cannot observe p_∞ directly in situ because the mitral valve opens and the left ventricle begins filling before the muscle fully relaxes from the previous systole. However, Yellin et al. (50, 51) observed pressures as low as -13 mm Hg in dog left ventricles by preventing filling and allowing the ventricles to relax completely while being held at their end-systolic volumes. Ohtani et al. (27) improved Yellin et al.'s technique by developing a volume-clamping model that preserves the native mitral valve and apparatus intact and avoids using cardiopulmonary bypass for the surgical preparation, and observed much smaller negative left ventricular pressures (-1 to -3 mm Hg). Although these observations of negative pressures validated the hypothesis that the left ventricular end-systolic volume can be smaller than the equilibrium volume (V_0), and hence give rise to diastolic suction, this effect may be much smaller under physiologic conditions than Yellin et al. suggest.

Effects of Ischemia on the Extent of Relaxation

Slowed calcium uptake by the sarcoplasmic reticulum in response to ischemia has been proposed to explain the shifts in the diastolic pressure-volume curve after cardiac pacing-induced angina in patients with ischemic heart disease. This hypothesis led several investigators to measure the rate of relaxation in patients following production of ischemia (15, 52–60). (See Chaps. 15 and 16.) Unfortunately, although people routinely observed slowed relaxation (i.e., a larger value of T), the reduction in relaxation rate secondary to ischemia was not large enough to produce the shifts in the diastolic pressure-volume curve that had been observed at end-dias-

tole. Moreover, animal studies of the effects of global ischemia and hypoxia on myocardial stiffness (61, 62) failed to demonstrate that ischemia can cause changes in myocardial stiffness.

An experimental preparation that more closely modeled the situation that existed in the clinical studies has clarified the link between ischemia and shifts in the diastolic pressure-volume curve (63–65). In this preparation, occluders were placed on the circumflex and left anterior descending coronary arteries of open-chest open-pericardium dogs, and then tightened until flow in these two arteries was reduced by approximately 50%. The left ventricular diastolic pressure-volume curve was not affected by this decrease in flow. The hearts were then paced at approximately twice the resting heart rate. Immediately after pacing was stopped, the pressure-volume curve shifted upward, but returned to normal within one minute. Thus, in contrast to previous animal studies, reversible shifts in the diastolic pressure-volume relationship were produced that mimicked the shifts observed in patients with coronary artery disease.

These reversible shifts in the left ventricular diastolic pressure-volume relationship appear to be associated with the myocyte's ability to move calcium in and out of the cytosol, but the principal effect of impaired calcium handling ability should be on the *extent* of relaxation rather than on the *rate*. Although there is some slowing of relaxation (reflected by an increase in T) because of a reduction in the ability of the sarcoplasmic reticulum to sequester cytosolic calcium, the primary effect seems to be accumulation of calcium within the cytosol which, in turn, might lead to an increase in the number of active crossbridges during diastole.

Differences from previous experimental studies led Serizawa et al. (63, 64) to propose that there are actually two types of ischemia in the intact heart: "supply-induced" and "demand-induced." (See Chap. 17.) During supply-induced ischemia, the normally beating heart is underperfused (or perfused with a deoxygenated perfusate), which reduces systolic work, oxygen demand, and the amount of metabolic waste products produced. This is the situation that prevailed during the earlier animal studies. Under these conditions, a low coronary flow is sufficient both to supply oxygen and to remove metabolites and, consequently, there are little or no changes in the diastolic properties of the myocardium. In contrast, during "demand-induced" ischemia, such as that during pacing after coronary artery occlusion, myocardial metabolic demands increase while the supply of oxygen and the capacity to remove waste products are limited by the occlusion. As a result, the sarcoplasmic reticulum takes up calcium more slowly, and more actin-myosin crossbridges remain intact at the end of relaxation (15, 66–68). When an excess of Ca^{++} ions remains in the cytosol after a contraction, an excess of cross-bridges remains attached and the equilibrium length of the muscle is shorter than normal. Thus, inadequate supply of ATP, Ca^{++} overload, leakage of Ca^{++} from the sarcoplasmic reticulum, or perhaps even the failure of the cell to return Ca^{++} to the extracellular space are all possible mechanisms that could cause the upward shift in the diastolic pressure-volume relationship that accompanies ischemia.

The finding (65) that caffeine potentiated the changes in left ventricular diastolic properties during demand ischemia supports these explanations. An increase in the concentration of the intracellular Ca^{++} during acute ischemia and reperfusion has been proposed by several investigators (68–72). Kihara et al. (72) demonstrated that different primary mechanisms determine the systolic and diastolic responses to acute hypoxia versus ischemia. During hypoxia, changes in Ca^{++} handling probably play a major role, whereas, during ischemia, changes in Ca^{++} sensitivity of the myofilaments appear to be of primary importance.

Although the distinction between supply-induced and demand-induced ischemia provides an appealing explanation for the differences observed in different experimental models of cardiac ischemia, it does not completely explain the mechanism for upward shifts in the diastolic pressure-volume curve in people with coronary artery disease. In earlier research, the effects of pacing angina and coronary occlusion were studied separately. Newer studies compared the effects of both types of ischemia directly in the same dog (73–75) and revealed different myocardial effects of pacing angina and brief coronary occlusion. Three minutes of pacing tachycardia in the presence of two vessel-critical coronary stenoses resulted in an upward shift of the diastolic left ventricular pressure-segment length relation. In the same experimental preparation, 3 minutes of coronary occlusion caused an outward bulge of the ischemic segment during systole, accompanied by a rightward shift of the diastolic pressure-segment length relationship.

The situation with pacing-induced angina is a clear example of demand-induced ischemia. (See Chap. 16.) With the advent of percutaneous transluminal coronary angioplasty, the clinical analog of animal experiments in which a coronary artery was transiently occluded became possible (76–81). To complement the earlier studies on pacing angina (82–84), Serruys et al. (85) performed a detailed study of systolic function in patients with coronary artery disease during balloon angioplasty. In contrast to previous experimental results on brief coronary occlusions, the left ventricular diastolic pressure-radial length relation shifted upward during the balloon occlusion, then moved back toward preocclusion values after the occlusion ended.

These new experimental and clinical findings led to reassessment of the concept of upward shift and rightward shift, as specific markers of demand ischemia and supply ischemia (86). A severe reduction in systolic performance of the ischemic segment precludes a decrease in regional diastolic distensibility or, conversely, preserved systolic shortening of the ischemic segment is a prerequisite for an upward shift of the diastolic left ventricular pressure-volume relationship and, in terms of cellular physiology, the absence or presence of an inhibitory effect on the myofilaments by tissue metabolites explains such divergent myocardial effects as upward shift and outward bulge.

Recently, to make optimal demand ischemia, the extent of stenosis was controlled not to impair the left ventricular segment systolic function, and the relationship of the regional myocardial blood flow to left ventricular diastolic mechanics was studied during pacing-induced ischemia. Previous work has shown that this degree of narrowing represents a critical stenosis of approximately 90%. Regional function rather than epicardial coronary flow was used to assess the degree of the flow limitation because regional function occurs with as little as 20% reduction in subendocardial flow, and epicardial coronary artery flow might not accurately reflect subendocardial flow during ischemia. Applegate et al. (87) evaluated a more severe form of post-pacing ischemia than has been previously reported and found that, after 3 minutes of rapid atrial pacing in the presence of the critical bilateral coronary stenosis, ventricular function after cessation of pacing was characterized by moderately severe contractile depression, left ventricular dilatation, impairment of isovolumic relaxation, an upward and rightward shift in the diastolic pressure-dimension relation, and an increase in passive diastolic chamber stiffness. Although epicardial and endocardial blood flow were similar to control in the presence of bilateral coronary stenoses, both were reduced significantly after pacing-induced ischemia. These findings differ from those of previous studies. They concluded that different degrees and types of ventricular dysfunction obtained using different models of ischemia suggest that the ventricular response to ischemia should not be classified simply on the basis of whether supply or demand ischemia is present but rather on a complex interaction among the duration, extent and severity, and type of ischemia elicited. Momo-mura et al. (88) also showed that, during pacing tachycardia in the presence of the same extent of coronary stenosis, subendocardial perfusion assessed by microspheres decreased markedly in the ischemic region, possibly reflecting impaired regional myocardial relaxation and subendocardial compression because of increased left ventricular end-diastolic pressure.

Kass et al. (89) reported that the resting diastolic pressure-volume relation shifted upward and the chamber elastic stiffness apparently increased during balloon coronary occlusion in humans, but during inferior vena caval occlusion, control and ischemic end-diastolic pressure-volume relations displayed little or no difference. Simple unloading of the right heart renders ischemic end-diastolic data similar to control data. This result suggests a prominent role of pericardial or right ventricular loading constraints as opposed to primary myocardial property changes in explaining the steady-state pressure-volume shifts. Moreover, it could be speculated that factors other than changes in myocardial property may play an important role in upward shift of diastolic pressure-volume relation, because changes in relaxation rate and elastic stiffness were large enough to explain the upward shift.

The precise physiologic mechanisms for these shifts remain to be defined. The clearest evidence that impaired Ca^{++} uptake by the sarcoplasmic reticulum in the presence of hypoxia impairs myocardial relaxation is provided by studies of the load-dependence of relaxation in isolated muscle taken from different animal species (90, 91). In these studies, cat, rat, and frog papillary muscles were investigated because each species has a different amount of sarcoplasmic reticulum and, therefore relaxes differently in response to changing mechanical loading conditions. Cat myocytes are rich in sarcoplasmic reticulum and are thus sensitive to ischemia, which alters calcium energetics within the cell, whereas frog myocytes have relatively little sarcoplasmic reticulum; rat myocytes have an intermediate amount. At various times during isotonic contraction, the afterloads were increased incrementally. In the cat papillary muscle, the time course of relaxation changed when the load increased, implying that relaxation was sensitive to loading conditions. In contrast, frog heart muscle relaxation was largely independent of load; rat heart muscle was in between. Thus, cardiac relaxation appears to depend on load and the ability of the sarcoplasmic reticulum to sequester Ca^{++} and hence release actin-myosin crossbridges.

Chuck et al. (92) demonstrated that hypoxia made cat papillary muscle less sensitive to load. Hypoxia suppresses the reuptake of calcium by the sarcoplasmic reticulum (93, 94) and this action would prolong activation because it would prolong the period during which calcium remains in the vicinity of the actomyosin crossbridges. This effect could explain the observed diminution of load sensitivity. Hypoxia plus caffeine (which tends to make the sarcoplasmic reticulum permeable to calcium) made cat papillary muscle completely insensitive to load, and the force-deflection traces for the cat muscle were similar to those for frog papillary muscle. Thus, by making the cat papillary muscle hypoxic and adding caffeine, the cat muscle was effectively converted to frog heart muscle, which has little sarcoplasmic reticulum. This means that the ability of the sarcoplasmic reticulum to sequester cytosolic Ca^{++} is probably the rate-limiting step of load-dependent relaxation. Moreover, because hypoxia (or ischemia) results in more calcium remaining in the cytosol at end-diastolic, the equilibrium length would also decrease because a greater number of intact crossbridges would result in shorter muscle fibers at end-diastole because of the lack of complete relaxation. Thus, hypoxia or ischemia would cause a lessening of the extent of relaxation.

Factors That Affect the Relaxation Rate

Several factors affect the relaxation rate but do not shift the entire diastolic pressure-volume relationship because none of the changes in relaxation rate is large enough to affect ventricular pressure at end-diastole. Changes in relaxation rate do, however, affect the atrioventricular pressure gradient and thus affect the left ventricular filling rate during early diastole (95).

The extent of systolic shortening and interventions thought to influence calcium dynamics at a cellular level, such as ischemia, exogenous calcium, and norepinephrine, affect T (46, 96, 97) increased by about 20% during reperfusion after regional ischemia, but was unaffected by nitroprusside or by the ischemia itself (98). Asynchrony of left ventricular contraction induced by selective coronary occlusion, rather than regional relaxation abnormalities of the myocardium, increases the relaxation time constant (99, 100). Prolongation of T resulted from nonuniformity of the regional left ventricular contraction induced by selective injection of isoprotere-

nol (101, 102) and nonsequential electrical activation (103) supports this explanation.

Load also affects relaxation (92, 93, 104, 105). (See Chaps. 2 and 13.) Zile and Gaasch (106) recently studied load-dependent relaxation by inflating intra-aortic balloons in dogs at different points in the cardiac cycle. Load-dependent relaxation was not inhibited when left ventricular relaxation was impaired by propranolol or verapamil, but, in contrast, was attenuated by caffeine. T also decreased after administration of isoproterenol and increased after administration of propranolol, suggesting that contractility affects T. T increased by 58% as both end-diastolic pressure and mean aortic systolic pressure increased during volume loading of intact hearts in anesthetized dogs (107). Finally, T increased by 45% after administration of phenylephrine to increase afterload in anesthetized dogs (108). Early ejection slows relaxation rate, whereas late ejection accelerates it, indicating that ejection timing rather than peak left ventricular pressure is a primary determinant of ventricular relaxation rate (109). The duration of relaxation is also increased (i.e., relaxation is slowed) in filling versus nonfilling left ventricles (23). Myocardial relaxation is modulated by filling and a function of both ventricular volume and time (25, 26).

Although in all of the cases just listed, the changes in relaxation rate were large as a percentage of T, they were not large enough in magnitude (i.e., T in the range of 30 to 50 msec) to change end-diastolic pressure, because relaxation was always complete before end-diastole at normal heart rates (Fig. 4–3) (110). Ventricular relaxation is considered complete approximately 3.5 T after dp/dt_{min} because the ventricular pressure falls to 3% of its value at dp/dt_{min} after 3.5 time constants (111). Because T is typically about 40 msec in dogs and humans, the effect of relaxation is essentially over 140 msec after the time of dp/dt_{min}. This means that relaxation from the previous systole will not have any effect on end-diastolic pressure at heart rates below approximately 150 to 160 beats/min (assuming that diastole occupies 40% of the R-R interval) (112). At very high heart rates, it is possible that relaxation may

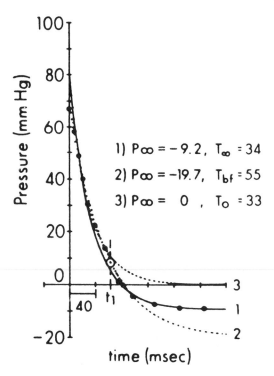

1) $P\infty = -9.2$, $T_\infty = 34$

2) $P\infty = -19.7$, $T_{bf} = 55$

3) $P\infty = 0$, $T_0 = 33$

Fig. 4–3. Curve 1 shows the time course of isovolumic relaxation when the mitral valve was occluded to prevent filling in a dog heart. Note that the fully relaxed pressure is -9.2 mmHg, indicating that the end-systolic volume is below the left ventricle's equilibrium volume. The time constant of isovolumic relaxation derived from fitting all these data to Equation (6) is 34 msec. Under normal conditions, however, one can only observe the isovolumic pressure fall before the mitral valve opens and the heart begins to fill. Curve 2 shows the resulting exponential curve obtained by fitting Equation (6) to this limited data set during isovolumic relaxation. Note that there are large errors in both the value of the time constant (55 msec isovolumic data versus the true value of 34 msec) as well as the estimated value of the pressure asymptote (-19.7 mmHg isovolumic data versus the true value of -9.2 mmHg). This problem arises because the short isovolumic period does not contain enough information to accurately extrapolate the full relaxation curve. Surprisingly, the value of the time constant obtained by assuming (incorrectly) that the heart always relaxes to zero pressure, curve 3 fitted to Equation (5), is close to the true value (34 msec, $p_\infty = 0$, vs. true value of 33 msec). Yellin, E.L., et al.: Left ventricular relaxation in the filling and nonfilling intact canine heart. *Am. J. Physiol.* *250*:H620, 1986.

not be complete before the next systole begins.

Hypertrophy and Relaxation

Although so-called physiologic hypertrophy, which accompanies increased physical activity, and volume overload hypertrophy do not appear to affect left ventricular relaxation (38, 113), pressure overload hypertrophy (114, 115), and hypertrophic cardiomyopathy (116–119) reduce the rate and extent of relaxation. The reduced rate and extent of relaxation combine to reduce significantly the rate of left ventricular filling during early diastole. These changes in relaxation appear to be caused by changes in the way the sarcoplasmic reticulum handles calcium; the whole process slows in the presence of pressure overload hypertrophy (120) or hypertrophic cardiomyopathy (36, 71, 121).

Myocardial ischemia also plays a role in modulating left ventricular relaxation in the presence of pressure overload hypertrophy, even in the absence of coronary artery disease. Pressure overload hypertrophy is associated with a substantial decrease in capillary density (41) and coronary vasodilator reserve (122, 123). Thus, in dogs with pressure overload hypertrophy, pacing tachycardia (which increases myocardial oxygen demand) can reduce subendocardial perfusion and produce metabolic evidence of ischemia (124). Studies of patients with aortic stenosis also reveal hemodynamic and metabolic evidence of ischemia in response to increased demands on the heart (59, 125), as well as histologic evidence of interstitial fibrosis compatible with ischemic injury (126). (See Chap. 20.)

The mechanics of pressure overload hypertrophy also aggravate the problems associated with ensuring adequate perfusion of the subendocardium. In thick-walled shells, the stress is highest on the inside wall, and the gradient of stress across the wall increases as the wall thickens. Thus, as the myocardium thickens to reduce the average stress in the wall, the stress near the endocardium may increase, putting additional demands on the cells located near the endocardium. The reduction of capillary density and coronary reserve in this region that accompanies pressure overload hypertrophy further reduces the capacity to deliver oxygen and remove waste products in this region, particularly when wall stresses increase in response to increased demands put on the heart as a whole.

In sum, it appears that pressure overload hypertrophy and hypertrophic cardiomyopathy affect relaxation in two ways. First, the function of the sarcoplasmic reticulum itself is depressed, slowing the uptake (and possibly the release) of calcium. This slowing of calcium uptake results in a slower relaxation and may allow changes in the resting level of calcium within the sarcomeres and so affect the extent of relaxation as well. Second, these forms of hypertrophy appear to be associated with at least transient subendocardial ischemia, and the ischemia itself affects rate and extent of relaxation.

Implications for Systolic Function

The original clinical studies of pacing-induced angina documented the effects on the diastolic pressure-volume relationship of the entire left ventricle and led to the search for relaxation abnormalities as the cause. However, coronary artery disease is a regional disease, in which the regions of the heart that are served by obstructed vessels are affected and the regions served by unobstructed vessels are not affected. Thus, if the mechanism for shifts in the left ventricular diastolic pressure-volume curve during ischemia is a reduction in the equilibrium length of the ischemic muscle because of changes in the extent of relaxation, it should be possible to show stiffening of the muscle in regions served by obstructed arteries and normal diastolic properties in the regions perfused by patent arteries. Angiographic studies of regional wall motion in patients who had coronary artery disease have demonstrated this point (127, 128). In regions served by an obstructed coronary artery, the diastolic pressure-segment length curve shifted upward after pacing-induced angina. In parts of the heart perfused by normal coronary arteries, the resulting increase in diastolic pressure led to higher stresses and therefore greater strain (extension) of the normal myocardium, which moved up a single diastolic pressure-segment length curve

(Fig. 4–4). This observation confirmed that there are regional changes in muscle stiffness during ischemia in patients who experienced pacing-induced angina.

The results of Sasayama et al. (127) also have important implications for how the heart maintains overall systolic function in the face of the reduced systolic function of the ischemic myocardium. As shown in Figure 4–4, the muscle outside the ischemic region is stretched longer than normal in response to the increase in diastolic pressure due to the stiffening of the ischemic myocardium. Because muscle develops more systolic force when it is stretched (according to the Frank-Starling mechanism), the surrounding normal muscle will increase systolic performance and help compensate for the loss of systolic function in the ischemic region.

This work is the clinical analog of experimental studies conducted by Theroux et al. (129), who permanently occluded the circumflex coronary artery in dogs and then studied the animals in the conscious state after they had recovered from the surgery. As expected, in the region served by an occluded coronary artery, both the end-diastolic segment length (measured with implanted ultrasonic crystals) and systolic shortening decreased. The end-diastolic segment length decreased by 30% below preocclusion lengths, with a concomitant reduction in systolic function. Systolic function was also reduced near the ischemic region, as demonstrated by a 12% decrease in segment shortening. In contrast, segment lengths increased in the normal myocardium far from the ischemic region of the left ventricle, resulting in an 8% increase in systolic function after 4 weeks. These results can be explained using basic mechanics and the Frank-Starling mechanism without resorting to a "zone of injury" near the ischemic area or compensatory hyperfunction remote from the injured area. Because all the myocardium must remain connected, the normal myocardium near the ischemic region is mechanically constrained by its attachments to the (stiffer) ischemic myocardium (130). Thus, the stiffer myocardium cannot be stretched to normal end-diastolic lengths, the sarcomeres cannot move up as far on their individual Frank-Starling curves, and the muscle

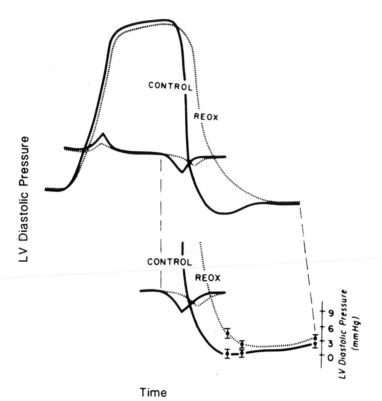

Time

Fig. 4–4. The rate, but not extent, of left ventricular relaxation is slowed during reoxygenation after fifteen minutes of hypoxia. Reoxygenation caused the pressure curve to be delayed and the relaxation time constant to be prolonged. The minimum diastolic pressure was also higher during reoxygenation. Nevertheless, the effects of ischemia on left ventricular relaxation rate die out before the end of diastole and do not affect subsequent beats. Modified from Blaustein, A.S., and Gaasch, W.H.: Myocardial relaxation iii. Reoxygenation mechanics in the intact dog heart. Circ. Res. 49:633, 1981, with permission of the American Heart Association.

near the ischemic region develops less systolic force. However, for the left ventricle to fill to its normal end-diastolic volume, muscle farther from the stiff region must stretch more than normal and will therefore develop greater force during systole. Thus, compensatory lengthening in the normal muscle caused by the mechanical forces acting in the myocardial shell tends to reduce the global severity of regional ischemia on systolic function.

Both the extent and rate of relaxation are important determinants of the atrioventricular pressure gradient. The extent of relaxation determines the equilibrium length of the muscle fibers and thus the equilibrium volume of the left ventricle. The relationship between the equilibrium and end-systolic volumes determines the initial atrioventricular pressure gradient just before the ventricle begins to fill. The rate of relaxation determines how quickly the pressure gradient decays. Thus, both rate and extent of relaxation affect filling rate during early diastole.

VENTRICULAR DIASTOLIC SUCTION

Under some conditions, at end-systole the muscle fibers are compressed to lengths shorter than their equilibrium length, resulting in a left ventricular end-systolic volume smaller than the equilibrium volume. (See Chap. 5.) This condition stores elastic energy in the muscle that is released during relaxation, resulting in an elastic recoil of the ventricle. Under some experimental conditions, negative ventricular pressures can be observed as evidence for this elastic recoil, and because a negative ventricular pressure during diastole would tend to suck blood into the ventricle from the atrium the condition is often called *ventricular diastolic suction.*

Experimental studies have provided the best evidence that negative pressures occur in relaxed left ventricles when end-systolic volume is less than equilibrium volume (131–135). Yellin et al. (50, 51, 109, 136) conducted the most elegant experiments demonstrating diastolic suction. They implanted a modified Star-Edwards prosthetic valve in the mitral orifice of dogs, which allowed them to prevent left ventricular filling by rapidly occluding the mitral orifice during systole. They recorded pressures as low as −13 mm Hg in the first beat after occlusion and −28 mm Hg during subsequent beats. Subsequently, Ohtani et al. (27) demonstrated less negative (−1 to −3 mmHg) diastolic suction using their newly developed left ventricular volume clamp model. They implanted a modified Bjork-Shiley mitral valve in beating dog heart while preserving the native mitral valve and apparatus and without cardiopulmonary bypass. The negative left ventricular pressures as an evidence of diastolic suction recorded in this model were less negative than those of Yellin's. The reasons for the difference remains unclear.

Clinical studies seldom directly demonstrate diastolic suction by revealing negative diastolic pressures because, when the left ventricular pressure falls below the left atrial pressure, the mitral valve opens and blood flows into the ventricle. This filling causes the left ventricular volume to increase above V_0, so that the condition that allows negative pressures to be observed is eliminated. However, the manifestations of a smaller end-systolic than equilibrium volume are observed occasionally in humans (137), particularly when partial occlusion of the mitral orifice impairs normal filling. Udelson et al. (28) observed development of negative left ventricular pressure in normal human heart during isoproterenol infusion and rapid atrial pacing. Partial occlusion occurs in patients with mitral stenosis, and negative diastolic pressures as low as −7 mm Hg have been observed in these patients (138, 139). If mitral flow had been prevented altogether (as it can be in experimental animals), more negative pressures could probably be observed. Small negative left ventricular pressures similar to those reported by Ohtani et al. (27) have been observed during procedure of percutaneous transvenous mitral commissurotomy as treatment for patients with mitral stenosis.

Diastolic suction may help the heart respond to increased demands when contractility increases. Increasing contractility leads to smaller end-systolic volumes, stronger recoil forces, and thus, a larger atrioventricular pressure gradient (136, 140) and more rapid early diastolic filling (23, 25, 26, 49). This increase in filling rate maintains or even increases (141) end-diastolic volume and so maintains end-diastolic sarcomere stretch and, therefore, systolic function. The exact role and magnitude of diastolic suction in normal hearts remain controversial.

VENTRICULAR INTERACTION

The chambers of the heart interact mechanically with each other, particularly during diastole, when the pressures (and, hence, wall stresses) are low (142, 143). Acute increases in right ventricular volume cause increases in left ventricular diastolic pressure. Similarly, increases in left ventricular volume increase right ventricular diastolic pressure. Thus, in addition to ischemia, which alters relaxation, ventricular interaction also shifts the left ventricular diastolic pressure-volume curve in response to changes in the vascular loading conditions the left ventricle faces. The degree of direct ventricular interaction and its importance to the left ventricular diastolic pressure-volume relationship and the overall function of the heart depend on the mechanical forces (stresses) to which the muscle is subject and on the elasticity of the myocardium. The pericardium, which encloses the entire heart, strengthens mechanical ventricular interaction. (See Chap. 6.)

The stresses in the intraventricular septum are particularly important in ventricular interaction, because the position of the septum depends on the transseptal pressure gradient and its material properties. Shifting of the septum is an important element in mediating ventricular interaction. When the left ventricular diastolic volume is held constant and right ventricular volume increased, the left ventricular anterior-posterior dimension increases and the septum becomes flatter and moves toward the left ventricle (144–153).

Ventricular interaction has been intensively studied under pathologically altered conditions of right ventricle, such as right ventricular ischemia (154–157), right ventricular pressure or volume overload (152, 153, 158–160), increased right ventricular filling due to systemic hypoxia (161), and electrically isolated right ventricle preparation (162). Goldstein et al. (154, 155) found that the septum demonstrated reversed curvature in diastole and bulged paradoxically into the right ventricle during early systole, generating the initial peak of right ventricular pressure and reducing its volume. When contractility of its free wall is acutely depressed, right ventricular performance is dependent on left ventricular-septal contractile contributions transmitted by the septum. Calvin (157) showed that in an experimental model of right ventricular wall infarction, cardiac output is restored to baseline values by volume loading sufficient to increase the right ventricular diastolic pressure to 16 mmHg. Evidence of pericardial constraint was observed and appears to be mediated by an atrioventricular interaction in addition to the direct ventricular interaction. Belenkie et al. (159) demonstrated that neither left ventricular compliance nor contractility is substantially altered during acute pulmonary embolism. The altered left ventricular performance is caused by reduced left ventricular preload mediated by increased pericardial constraint as reflected by a decrease in transmural left ventricular end-diastolic pressure. Santamore et al. (152, 153) indicated that the left ventricular pressure-volume relation can be modified by changes in right ventricular pressure and compliance even without a change in right ventricular volume. Brilla et al. (161) reported that the shift of the end-diastolic pressure-volume curve in the early stage of acute hypoxia is predominantly a result of the influence of increased right ventricular filling. Damiano et al. (162) demonstrated importance of left ventricular contraction for right ventricular developed pressure and volume outflow analyzing double-peaked waveforms for right ventricular pressure and pulmonary arterial blood flow obtained by a unique electrically isolated right ventricular free wall preparation. Goto et al. (158) found that changes in left ventricular geometry during acute right ventricular pressure overload are associated with nonuniform regional changes in systolic shortening in the left ventricular minor axis. All these studies supported the conclusion that right ventricular function di-

rectly affects the left ventricle through ventricular interaction.

Ventricular interaction has been observed in patients given drugs that alter ventricular loading conditions and shift the diastolic pressure-volume relationship upward or downward. For example, ventricular interaction can explain the acute shifts upward or downward in the pressure-volume relationship in patients given the vasoconstrictor angiotensin or the vasodilator nitroprusside (18). This observation, confirmed by others (19, 163–165), was particularly important because it was the first evidence that hemodynamic changes other than ischemia alter the diastolic pressure-volume relationship.

Evidence for the hypothesis that ventricular interaction was responsible for the shifts in the diastolic pressure-volume relationship after giving vasodilating or vasoconstricting drugs was provided by a study in which patients were given nitroglycerine or amyl nitrate (19). The left ventricular pressure-volume curve shifted downward in the patients given nitroglycerine but not in the patients given amyl nitrate. Both drugs lower systemic arterial pressure, but nitroglycerine also reduces right ventricular filling and volume by lowering venous return. Because nitroglycerine reduced right ventricular size as well as lowering arterial pressure, left ventricular pressure also fell. Therefore ventricular interaction appeared responsible for the downward shift of the left ventricular pressure-volume curve.

Direct experimental evidence to support the hypothesis that ventricular interaction, modulated by the pericardium, was the mechanism for the shifts in the diastolic pressure-volume curve in response to vasodilation or vasoconstriction has been provided by animal studies (166). In this study, nitroprusside was administered to conscious dogs instrumented with ultrasonic crystals to determine ventricular dimensions. After administration of nitroprusside, the left ventricular pressure-dimension curve shifted downward. These shifts disappeared when the pericardium was removed. Thus, the pericardium plays an important role in modulating the upward and downward shifts in the diastolic pressure-volume relationship after acute administration of vasodilators or vasoconstrictors (167).

Direct Versus Series Interaction

So far, we have been discussing so-called direct ventricular interaction, which is a manifestation of the forces transmitted through the septum (and, to a lesser extent, via the pericardium) between the two cardiac ventricles. Two types of ventricular interaction exist, however: direct interaction—by way of mechanical forces across the septum—and series interaction—because right ventricular output becomes left ventricular input after passing through the pulmonary circulation.

The degree of direct ventricular interaction can be determined from isolated heart preparations in which the volume in one ventricle is held constant while the pressure-volume relationship of the other ventricle is determined (168–174). These experiments, although easy to interpret, require severe disruption of the normal anatomic situation in which right ventricular output becomes left ventricular input, and thus are of limited value in understanding the normally functioning heart.

Determining the degree of ventricular interaction using the intact heart reflects normal physiology and anatomy, but the results are difficult to interpret. Studies of ventricular interaction using intact hearts have reported various degrees of direct interaction (144, 147, 148, 150, 175–179). This variability is caused largely by the difficulty of determining the relative roles of direct and series ventricular interaction in the intact circulatory system. Using the traditional approach of collecting data in physiological steady-state, it is virtually impossible to separate direct from series ventricular interaction in the intact circulatory system.

To resolve this problem, Slinker and Glantz (179) used a new approach, which took advantage of the time lag between a change in right ventricular output and left ventricular input (180–182) to separate, empirically, the series (delayed) from the direct (immediate) ventricular interaction. After transiently constricting the pulmonary artery or venae cavae, they measured left and right ventricular volumes and

pressures over several seconds and found that direct interaction was about one-half as important as series interaction in determining left ventricular end-diastolic size with the pericardium on. Removing the pericardium decreased the importance of direct interaction to about one-fifth that of the series effect, supporting the view that the pericardium modulates ventricular interaction.

The relationship of direct to series interaction also depends on the stiffness of the ventricular walls. In hypertrophied hearts with thickened ventricular walls (resulting from 3 months of renal hypertension), direct interaction at end-diastole was only about one tenth as important as series interaction in determining left ventricular size with the pericardium on (150). Removing the pericardium had very little effect on the relative importance of direct versus series interaction in these hypertrophied hearts because the thicker myocardium (and particularly the intraventricular septum) carried a relatively greater proportion of the wall stress than the normal hearts.

Implications for Systolic Function

Diastolic ventricular interaction is important for maintaining systolic function in response to changes in loading conditions, such as those associated with vasodilation. For instance, the downward shift in the left ventricular diastolic pressure-volume curve, such as that which occurs after acute administration of the vasodilator nitroprusside, is a critical factor in maintaining stroke volume (183). Specifically, Figure 4–5 shows data from a patient before and after being given nitroprusside (18). During the control condition, the end-diastolic pressure was 16 mm Hg, and the end-diastolic volume was 194 mL, with a stroke volume of 118 mL. After administration of nitroprusside, the diastolic pressure-volume curve shifted downward, so that the end-diastolic pressure fell to 9 mm Hg, but, because the curve shifted, end-diastolic volume fell only slightly, to 176 mL, and stroke volume remained essentially constant at 114 mm Hg. Now, suppose that no ventricular interaction and no pericardium existed, so that the left ventricular diastolic

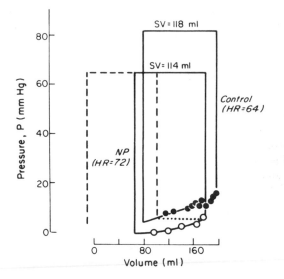

Fig. 4–5. Data from one patient showing that shifts in the left ventricular diastolic pressure-volume curve help maintain stroke volume (SV) in response to changes in loading conditions after administration of the vasodilator sodium nitroprusside (NP). Because of the shift in the curve, stroke volume was maintained despite large reductions in end-diastolic pressure. Had the left ventricle moved down the control pressure-volume curve, the end-diastolic volume would have been less than the stroke volume before administering the drug, yielding a negative end-systolic volume (dashed line), which is impossible. By shifting downward, the left ventricle could exhibit a lower end-diastolic pressure with little change in end-diastolic volume, thereby making it possible to maintain stroke volume near the control level (solid line). Reproduced from Tyberg, J.V., et al.: The relationship between pericardial pressure and right atrial pressure: an intraoperative study. Circulation 73:428, 1986, with permission of the American Heart Association.

pressure volume curve moved down a unique pressure-volume curve and the end-diastolic volume fell as end-diastolic pressure fell. If this had happened, the end-diastolic volume would have dropped to about 94 mL, making it impossible to maintain stroke volume near its original value of 118 mL. But because the entire pressure-volume curve shifted downward, stroke volume was maintained in the presence of a lowered end-diastolic pressure. Thus, ventricular interaction is important for maintaining systolic function.

THE PERICARDIUM

The pericardium surrounds the heart, reducing friction between the heart and the surrounding tissues and providing a barrier against infection. Its attachments to the mediastinum help restrain the heart from excessive motion within the chest when body position changes. When the heart's volume increases, the heart presses on the pericardium, which, in turn, presses back on the epicardium and constrains the heart's expansion (184). Because it constrains the whole heart and is stiffer than the myocardium, the pericardium increases the mechanical interaction between the four cardiac chambers (185, 186), and even affects the end-diastolic coronary pressure-flow relationship (187). Thus, an increase in the size of one ventricle causes the pressure-volume relationship of the other ventricle to shift upward because of the constraint of the pericardium. (See Chap. 6.)

How the Pericardium Affects the Left Ventricular Diastolic Pressure-Volume Relationship

The pericardium modulates the pressure-volume relationship, both because it exerts normal stresses perpendicular to the epicardium and because it has a steeper stress-strain relationship than the myocardium does. The effect of the pericardium on the diastolic pressure-volume relationship depends on the magnitude of the normal stress exerted by the pericardium on the epicardium, which, in turn, depends on the elastic properties of the pericardium (i.e., its stress-strain relation). At small pericardial volumes, pericardial stress is low and the pericardial stress-strain curve is fairly flat, so that large changes in strain (volume) result in only small changes in stress (pressure). Thus, at small pericardial volumes, the pericardium exerts only small normal stresses on the epicardium and the effect of the pericardium on ventricular diastolic pressure is small. However, when heart volume increases acutely above normal end-diastolic volumes, the pericardium is stretched and is moved up its increasingly steeper stress-strain curve (Fig. 4–6). On steeper portions of the curve, small increases in strain (volume) result in large in-

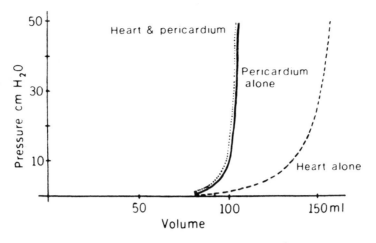

Fig. 4–6. Pressure-volume relations of the heart and pericardium, together and alone. The heart without the pericardium has a pressure-volume relation that is far to the right (less stiff) of the curve of the heart with pericardium. The combined heart plus pericardium is virtually the same as the pericardium alone, indicating that the stiffness of the pericardium dominates the curve for the ventricle alone, particularly along the steeper portion of the pericardium's stress-strain curve. Reproduced with permission from Hort, W.: Herzbeutel und herzgroesse. Arch Kreislaufforsch 44:21, 1964.

creases in stress (pressure). Thus, the normal stress exerted on the epicardium is large, and the pericardium contributes substantially to ventricular diastolic pressure. This increased stress means that a higher absolute left ventricular pressure is required to achieve a given left ventricular volume.

The key to assessing how much the pericardium influences the left ventricular diastolic pressure-volume relationship under physiologic conditions is determining where the pericardium normally operates on its pressure-volume curve. Answering this question is difficult, and it has been the subject of considerable debate.

Several investigators have assessed the effect of the pericardium by comparing the left ventricular diastolic pressure-volume relationships before and after removing the pericardium (87, 144, 148, 150, 166, 179, 188–190). At high left ventricular filling pressures (above about 10 mm Hg), pericardial stiffness clearly increases left ventricular diastolic pressures (142, 144, 174, 189, 191–195). This effect becomes more pronounced as left ventricular filling pressure and end-diastolic volume increase (196, 197). In contrast, Stokland et al. (190) reported only a slight (4%) increase in left ventricular myocardial chord lengths after

they increased blood volume and opened the pericardium of open chest dogs, and Tyson et al. (98) reported little effect of the pericardium in conscious, chronically instrumented dogs with low diastolic pressures. Therefore, although the constraining effect of the pericardium contributes significantly to the upward shift of the left-ventricular pressure-volume curve under the conditions of acute cardiac dilation, there is only a minimal effect at normal diastolic pressures.

The Atria and The Right Ventricle

The pericardium increases mechanical coupling, not only between the two cardiac ventricles, but also between the ventricles and the atria. In a study using postmortem dog hearts in which the mitral and tricuspid valves were removed and the orifices plugged with disks, Maruyama et al. (188) found the effect of left atrial pressure was about one fourth that of right ventricular pressure in determining left ventricular pressure with the pericardium around the heart. When the pericardium was removed, neither the right nor the left ventricular diastolic pressure-volume relationship was affected by a 22 mm Hg increase in right or left atrial pressure alone. The pericardium's role in strengthening the interaction between the atria and ventricles is not surprising because the atria have thinner walls, are more easily distended, and therefore are more tightly coupled with the pericardium than either of the ventricles. Although the left atrium and ventricle were isolated from one another in the Maruyama et al. (188) study, their results can still indicate a tighter coupling between the pericardium and the cardiac chambers even when the atrioventricular valves are open. For example, during diastole, while the mitral valve is open, the left atrium and left ventricle form, in essence, a single chamber, which is influenced by the presence of pericardium. The pericardium surrounding the atria is essential for modulating the mechanical coupling between them and the ventricles. The influence of the pericardium on the left and right ventricular filling was compared by measuring left and right ventricular pressure-segment length relations by Assanelli et al. (199) They found that, at the higher end-diastolic pressure, the pericardium was responsible for a larger proportion of right ventricular end-diastolic pressure than of left ventricular end-diastolic pressure. The pericardium has differing effects on right and left ventricular end-diastolic pressure-segment length relations, despite the fact that the effective pericardial surface is similar over both ventricles.

Assessing Pericardial Constraint in Patients

Although knowing pericardial pressure is important in assessing pericardial constraint and hence ventricular function during diastole, it is seldom possible to measure pericardial pressure in patients directly. However, because the right ventricle and and atria have thinner walls than the left ventricle and, hence, are more closely coupled with the pericardium, right ventricular or atrial pressure has been proposed as a substitute for direct measurement of pericardial pressure (62, 193, 194, 200).

In a comparative study between patients with tamponade who underwent pericardiocentesis and open-chest dogs with large pericardial effusions, Smiseth et al. (201) concluded that right ventricular pressure

was a useful approximation of pericardial pressure. Likewise, Tyberg et al. (202) found that the pericardial pressure was similar in magnitude to the mean right atrial pressure in patients over a wide range of these pressures (-4 to $+20$ mm Hg). These investigators concluded that, in normal hearts during diastole when the right atrioventricular valve is open, right atrial and ventricular pressures can be used to approximate pericardial pressure. Influence of the pericardium on left ventricular diastolic and systolic function was studied in patients with heart failure of varying severity and diverse etiology (203). The occurrence of pericardial constraint, which was characterized by a rise in right atrial pressure and pulmonary capillary wedge pressure, was independent of the degree of reduced maximum oxygen consumption and the severity of heart failure.

There are clearly limits to approximating pericardial pressure with right atrial or ventricular diastolic pressure (150, 204, 205). One example is when the right ventricle stiffens as a result of right ventricular hypertrophy (148). Another example is in patients with cor pulmonale or pulmonary hypertension (206). In both cases, right atrial pressures may be much higher than pericardial pressures. During pericardial drainage to treat cardiac tamponade, pericardial pressure falls considerably below right atrial pressure (182, 207). These low pericardial pressures are most likely to occur because, in patients with large chronic pericardial effusions, the pericardium is stretched well above its normal capacity. Thus, removing the pericardial fluid would result in a very loosely fitting (or even collapsed) pericardium and no pericardial constraint. Under normal conditions, however, the right atrial pressure can probably be used as a reasonable approximation for pericardial pressure during diastole.

Pericardial Adaptation to Ventricular Hypertrophy

The pericardium adapts to chronic increases in heart size by increasing its mass (size) (208) and, as the pericardium expands over time, its effect on the left ventricular diastolic pressure-volume relationship decreases. This changing role of the pericardium was demonstrated by Lewinter and Pavalec (209), who compared left ventricular diastolic pressure-segment relations before and after removing the pericardium in dogs during the early (7 to 9 days) and late (34 to 50 days) stages of hypertrophy after imposing a chronic left ventricular overload. Removing the pericardium early after creating the volume overload reduced the right and left ventricular end-diastolic pressures and increased dimensions at matched levels of left ventricular end-diastolic pressure greater than 10 mm Hg. Hence, shortly after creating the volume overload, the heart had expanded against the pericardium, which led to an increase in diastolic left ventricular pressure. In contrast, later, after left ventricular mass increased, neither left ventricular end-diastolic dimension nor right ventricular end-diastolic pressure changed when the pericardium was removed, indicating that the pericardium had expanded and was exerting less of a constraining force on the heart. Thus, when the pericardium hypertrophies along with the heart, the pericardium plays a smaller role in determining the left ventricular diastolic pressure-volume relationship than in normal hearts (150, 205, 209–211). The influence of the pericardium changes because, as the heart increases in size, the pericardium is stressed chronically. The pericardium responds to this increased stress by increasing its size. When this happens, the enlarged pericardium would operate on a flatter portion of its stress-strain curve; the constraining forces are smaller and the influence of the pericardium on the heart is less than its influence before the hypertrophy.

Another effect of myocardial hypertrophy is that the relative importance of the pericardium and of direct ventricular interaction is less when the ventricular wall thickens. For example, in normal dog hearts, Slinker and Glantz found that removing the pericardium decreased the relative importance of direct versus series ventricular interaction in dogs from about one half to one fifth. In hearts that had hypertrophied in response to 3 months of renal hypertension, the importance of di-

rect interaction was less, becoming only about one tenth as important as series interaction with the pericardium on and essentially zero without the pericardium (150, 205). As the ventricular walls thicken in response to the pressure overload, the thicker walls become less distensible, and more of the ventricular pressure is balanced by the elasticity of the myocardium as opposed to the pericardium.

Implications for Systolic Function

By restricting the expansion of the heart, and thus restricting extension of the sarcomeres that make up the myocardium, the pericardium can affect left ventricular systolic function by means of the Frank-Starling mechanism under certain pathologic conditions. Thus, approximately accounting for pericardial constraint may allow many changes in left ventricular systolic performance, thought to represent changes in contractility or to be explained on the basis of preload changes and the Frank-Starling mechanism (212). For example, right ventricular infarction can precipitate a low cardiac output syndrome. Although a reduction in right ventricular systolic function plays a role by reducing right ventricular output and left ventricular input, ventricular interaction, mediated by the pericardium, is also important. Goldstein et al. (213, 214) produced right ventricular infarction in dogs by infusing mercury into the coronary circulation. Immediately after the infarct, the right ventricle attempted to dilate within the pericardium, increasing pericardial pressure, increasing left ventricular diastolic pressure, and inhibiting filling. The associated lower left ventricular end-diastolic volumes impaired systolic function because of the Frank-Starling mechanism. When the pericardium was opened, and the right ventricle was free to dilate without competing with the left ventricle within the pericardium, the left ventricle could expand and increase end-diastolic volume, stroke volume, and cardiac output.

PULMONARY-CARDIAC CONTACT PRESSURE

The observation that blood pressure and cardiac output fell in patients ventilated with positive end-expiratory pressure (PEEP) stimulated interest in the effect of the lungs on cardiac function (215–219). Just as the ventricles and the pericardium interact with each other because they are in physical contact, so the heart and lungs interact mechanically because they are in physical contact. Like the pericardium, the lungs affect the left ventricle's diastolic pressure-volume curve by exerting a normal stress on the heart. The contact pressure, which is on the order of a few mm Hg, has little direct mechanical effect during systole. However, during diastole, when pressures are low, inflating the lungs can increase pressure outside the heart and lower the left ventricular transmural pressure at any given absolute left ventricular pressure. This lower transmural pressure can reduce end-diastolic volume and cardiac output because of the Frank-Starling mechanism. This mechanical interaction between the heart and lungs explains the reduction in cardiac output that occurs during PEEP.

Lung hyperinflation or positive pressure ventilation with more than 10 cm H_2O (8 mm Hg) PEEP reduces both ventricles' diastolic size because of the direct compressive force the lungs apply to the heart (175, 180, 191, 192, 217, 230–234). Fewell et al. (227) directly observed the effect of mechanical compression of the heart by hyperinflated lungs by attaching flat balloon pressure transducers to the epicardium of both left and right ventricles of dog hearts. Cardiac transmural pressures were calculated as the difference between ventricular and balloon pressures. They determined transmural pressures during 0 and 12 cm H_2O PEEP with the chest open, with the chest closed and evacuated, and with the pericardium intact and removed. With the chest closed and the pericardium intact, *absolute* left and right ventricular end-diastolic pressures increased from 4 to 7 mm Hg and from 3 to 6 mm Hg respectively, when PEEP was increased from zero to 12 cm H_2O (Figure 4–6). In contrast, left and right ventricular end-diastolic *transmural* pressures and volumes both fell. This difference between absolute and transmural end-diastolic pressure was not caused by the pericardial constraint because the pericardium simply transmits the pressure exerted by the lungs and removing it does not alter the effect of pulmonary-cardiac contact pressure. This fact was demonstrated in the open-chest dogs in which the lungs were held away from the heart to prevent the lungs from pressing on the heart. Although end-diastolic volume increased about 11% when the lungs were held away from the heart, there was no change in either cardiac output or ventricular end-diastolic pressure during PEEP. Lung hyperinflation or positive pressure ventilation with more than 10 cm H_2O PEEP decreases right and left end-diastolic volumes due to mechanical compression of the heart by the hyperinflated lungs. Heart rate does not change; therefore cardiac output drops because of the Frank-Starling mechanism (234, 235). The reduction in cardiac output appears to be primarily a mechanical effect of the lungs pressing on the heart, which occurs independently of changes in myocardial contractility, or neural and humoral effects.

VISCOELASTIC PROPERTIES OF THE MYOCARDIUM

So far, we have seen that the primary determinants of left ventricular filling and of the diastolic pressure-volume relationship are the myocardium's intrinsic mechanical characteristics—the geometry of the ventricular cavity (particularly wall thickness), the elasticity of the myocardium, and the extent and rate of relaxation—and the external forces acting on the left ventricle through ventricular interaction, the pericardium, and pulmonary-cardiac contact pressure. In addition to these major factors, there are two additional factors that make a small contribution to the diastolic pressure: *viscoelasticity* of the myocardium and *coronary vascular engorgement*.

Like most biologic materials, the myocardium is viscoelastic (236, 237) so that stresses in the heart wall depend on the rate at which it deforms (strain rate, $\dot{\epsilon}$) as well as on the magnitude of the deformation (strain, ϵ). This dependence means that the diastolic pressure depends on the filling rate as well as on the ventricular volume and that the diastolic pressure at a given volume increases as filling rate increases.

Because viscous forces increase with filling rate, these forces are greatest during the rapid filling phase in early diastole and atrial systole. However, elastic recoil or restoring forces are almost most significant during rapid filling. Therefore, it is difficult to separate changes in the diastolic pressure-volume relationship during early diastole caused by myocardial viscoelasticity from the changes caused by active relaxation. Although there is no doubt that viscous forces contribute to diastolic pressure, particularly during rapid filling and atrial systole, this contribution is probably small.

The fact that viscous forces are greatest at the same time as filling is greatest during active relaxation (or atrial systole) makes separating viscoelastic from relaxation effects difficult. Pasipoularides et al. (238) proposed a mathematical method to separate viscoelastic from relaxation effects. They subtracted a component of pressure assumed to be caused by relaxation calculated on the basis of the monoexponential model of isovolumic pressure fall (equation 6), and then examined the residual pressure for evidence of viscoelastic (i.e., rate-dependent) effects. In so doing, they assumed that the isovolumic ventricle would relax to a zero pressure asymptote ($p_\infty = 0$), an assumption demonstrated to be invalid. Although Pasipoularides et al. admitted that a nonzero pressure asymptote could alter their results by shifting the passive pressure-volume curve up or down, they argued that this would have a negligible effect on the passive stiffness-stress relation in their model. Using this method to evaluate patients with normal hearts who had undergone cardiac catheterization, they concluded that in hearts in the "basal" state, the strain rate-dependent (viscoelastic) effects were minimal. This conclusion is supported by Fioretti et al. (239), who reasoned that viscous effects in early diastole are overshadowed by relaxation effects. The confounding effects of relaxation are not present late in diastole during atrial systole, when the ventricle is fully relaxed. Thus viscoelastic effects probably do play a role in increasing left ventricular pressure during atrial systole.

In summary, whether or not they are measurable, viscous forces increase continuously as a function of filling rate. The difficulty in interpreting these strain rate-de-

pendent effects is that the strain rates are highest in early diastole, when filling is fastest and when active relaxation from the previous beat is taking place. Most of the effects that have been attributed to viscoelasticity during rapid filling are probably from active relaxation. However, viscous forces may make an identifiable contribution to left ventricular pressure during atrial systole.

CORONARY VASCULAR ENGORGEMENT

It has been hypothesized that increasing coronary artery pressure stiffens the network of coronary arteries that permeate the myocardium and so stiffens the left ventricular wall, analogous to the way that erectile tissue stiffens when it is engorged with blood. This resultant stiffening of the left ventricular wall would be reflected in the diastolic pressure-volume relationship just as if the muscle itself became stiffer. The effect of coronary vascular engorgement on ventricular stiffness would be most evident late in diastole, when the coronary arteries are maximally perfused. Although myocardial stiffening as a result of vascular engorgement has been demonstrated in isolated heart preparations, the effect is small in most normal hearts, so it does not contribute appreciably to the diastolic pressure-volume relationship. In abnormal hearts, vascular engorgement can have a substantial effect on chamber stiffness. (See Chap. 7.)

If increasing coronary arterial perfusion pressure causes the myocardium to stiffen, then reducing perfusion pressure should have the opposite effect. By reducing coronary arterial perfusion pressure to zero in isovolumic dog hearts, Gaasch and coworkers (240, 241) observed that diastolic wall thickness decreased by 7% and diastolic pressure decreased by 23%. In addition, Gaasch and Bernard (240) found that during reactive hyperemia (after coronary artery ligation and reperfusion), wall thickness was 10% greater than the control (before ligation), indicating a stiffened myocardium.

Other similar studies have not demonstrated changes in chamber stiffness as a function of coronary perfusion pressure (61, 242–245). The lack of observed changes in chamber stiffness in these studies may have resulted from either measuring diastolic pressures and flows at a single left ventricular volume or too small a change in the coronary perfusion pressure to obtain much effect.

The mechanism of the coronary erectile effect has not been fully established. Because the effect correlates closely with changes in intramyocardial blood volume and left ventricular wall volume, it is possible that coronary venous pressure may be a significant determinant of the coronary erectile effect. Watanabe et al. studied effects of coronary venous pressure on left ventricular diastolic distensibility in blood-perfused left ventricular isovolumic dog heart (246). They demonstrated that increased coronary venous pressure decreases left ventricular diastolic distensibility with increasing left ventricular wall volume, and this mechanism appears to act independently of diastolic ventricular interaction caused by right ventricular enlargement.

The main problem encountered in studies designed to determine whether the myocardium stiffens because of coronary vascular engorgement is to decouple metabolic effects (changes in the myocardium caused by changes in coronary blood flow or perfusate) from hydraulic (erectile) effects. Many studies have compared the way in which myocardial stiffness changes when coronary flow is stopped (ischemia) with the way in which it changes when the coronary arteries are perfused with a hypoxic perfusate (hypoxia). In both cases, oxygen supply to the heart is reduced, and this affects cell metabolism, calcium flux, active relaxation and, perhaps, myocardial stiffness. Therefore hypoxia or ischemia tends to mask a possible erectile effect by the effects of the ischemia or hypoxia. This masking is further complicated by the small nature of the erectile effect itself. For example, Vogel et al. (247) perfused isolated rabbit hearts with various normoxic and hypoxic media and found that changes in the diastolic pressure-volume curve were directly related to changes in wall thickness associated with the different perfusates, independent of the effects of ischemia per se.

The problem of decoupling erectile (hydraulic) from metabolic effects was directly addressed in studies (248, 249) that used a rapid freeze-clamp method to stop metabolism 10 seconds after stopping coronary arterial perfusion and measured left ventricular equatorial cross-sectional area, diastolic wall thickness, developed pressure, and high energy phosphate metabolism in isovolumic rat and hamster hearts. Ten seconds of ischemia were not sufficient to cause measurable changes in metabolism but did reduce left ventricular diastolic wall thickness by 4% and left ventricular epicardial cross-sectional area by 8%. Thus, these results demonstrated an erectile effect independent of metabolic effects within the first 10 seconds of ischemia.

Theoretical work has also demonstrated that coronary vascular engorgement has a small effect on left ventricular stiffness. Huyghe (250) did a theoretical analysis of the beating left ventricle and intramyocardial coronary circulation using a nonlinear, finite element analysis which showed that diastolic ventricular stiffness increased slightly, by 10%, when coronary perfusion pressure was increased from 45 to 120 mm Hg. Also, Huyghe et al. (251) recently reported a theoretical analysis of a porous medium finite element model of the passive ventricle, including torsion about the axis of symmetry. They showed that the ventricular model stiffens following an increase of the intracoronary blood volume. At a given left ventricular volume, pressure increased by 33% when raising the intracoronary blood volume from 9 to 14 mL/100 g left ventricle. Thus, both experimental and theoretical investigation has shown that increasing coronary perfusion pressure increases the apparent stiffness of the diastolic left ventricle, but the effect is small.

CONCLUSION

It is now well established that the traditional view of the diastolic left ventricle as an isolated shell in which filling pressure and volume are uniquely related is incorrect. The diastolic pressure-volume relationship changes in response to changes in the heart's operating environment. The diastolic pressure-volume relationship depends on the balance between the pressure in the left ventricle and the stresses in the myocardium. These stresses, in turn, depend on the size and thickness of the ventricle and the elasticity of the myocardium. Thus, when the left ventricle contracts to a volume smaller than its equilibrium volume, elastic energy is actually stored in the myocardium. This stored energy is manifested as so-called diastolic suction, which increases the atrioventricular pressure gradient and speeds filling during early diastole. In addition to these factors, there are two major categories of factors that can acutely change the diastolic pressure-volume curve.

The first category of factors includes those that alter the extent of relaxation from the previous systole, such as demand-induced ischemia. This type of ischemia impairs active uptake of calcium from the cytosol, which yields a higher resting concentration of calcium in the sarcomeres during diastole and a smaller apparent equilibrium volume for the ventricle. This smaller equilibrium volume means that the strains (and, hence, stresses) within the wall of the heart are higher for any given volume of the left ventricle than before ischemia, so pressure is higher at any given volume.

The second category of factors that alter the diastolic pressure-volume curve includes those that alter the external mechanical environment in which the left ventricle resides, in particular, the other cardiac chambers, the pericardium, and contact pressure with the lungs. Interventions such as vasodilation and vasoconstriction alter the forces that these other components exert on the left ventricle. Because the pressure within the left ventricular cavity represents the net effect of the forces within the myocardium and those outside it, changes in these external forces are reflected in pressure changes within the left ventricle at any given volume, and therefore shift the diastolic pressure-volume curve.

These changes in the diastolic pressure-volume curve have several important implications for systolic function. First, when the end-systolic volume is below the left ventricle's equilibrium volume, the myocardial wall is put into compression and stores elastic energy during systole (just as compressing a spring stores energy). This energy is released when the myocardium relaxes and acts to reduce the ventricular pressure, thus increasing the atrioventricular pressure gradient during early diastole. Increasing the atrioventricular pressure gradient causes the ventricle to fill more rapidly, which helps maintain end-diastolic volume and, by means of the Frank-Starling mechanism, systolic function. Second, shifts in the diastolic pressure-volume relationship in response to vascular loading changes are essential in helping the left ventricle maintain stroke volume during vasodilation because these shifts maintain end-diastolic volume even though left ventricular end-diastolic pressure falls during vasodilation. Finally, the fact that filling pressure and volume are not uniquely related means that end-diastolic pressure cannot be used as a surrogate for end-diastolic volume when assessing systolic function.

REFERENCES

1. Mirsky I: Assessment of diastolic function: suggested methods and future considerations. Circulation 69:836, 1984.
2. Grossman W, Lorell BH (eds.): Diastolic Relaxation of the Heart. Boston, Martinus Nijhoff, 1988.
3. Gilbert JC, Glantz SA: Determinants of left ventricular filling and of the diastolic pressure-volume relation. Circ Res 64: 827, 1989.
4. Little WC, Downes TR: Clinical evaluation of left ventricular diastolic performance. Prog Cardiovasc Dis 32:273, 1990.
5. Mirsky I, Pasipoularides A: Clinical assessment of diastolic function. Prog Cardiovasc Dis 32:291, 1990.
6. Stauffer JC, Gaasch WH: Recognition and treatment of left ventricular diastolic dysfunction. Prog Cardiovasc Dis 32:319, 1990.
7. Zile MR, Gaasch WH: Mechanical loads and the isovolumic and filling indices of left ventricular relaxation. Prog Cardiovasc Dis 32:333, 1990.
8. Sys SU, Brutsaert DL: Physiologic aspects of relaxation and the myocardium. Herz 15:345, 1990.
9. Little WC, Downes TR, Applegate RJ: Invasive evaluation of left ventricular diastolic performance. Herz 15:362, 1990.
10. Brutsaert DL, Sys SU: Relaxation and

diastole of the heart. Physiol Rev 69:1228, 1989.

11. Carroll JD, Carroll EP: Diastolic function in coronary artery disease. Herz 16:1, 1991.

12. Hood WB Jr, Bianco JA, Kumar K, Whiting RB: Experimental myocardial infarction iv. reduction of left ventricular compliance in the healing phase. J Clin Invest 49:1316, 1970.

13. Bristow JD, van Zee BE, Judkins MP: Systolic and diastolic abnormalities of the left ventricle in coronary artery disease, studies in patients with little or no enlargement of ventricular volume. Circulation 17:219, 1970.

14. Dwyer EM, Jr: Left ventricular pressure-volume alterations and regional disorders of contraction during myocardial ischemia induced by atrial pacing. Circulation 42:1111, 1970.

15. McLaurin LP, Rolett EL, Grossman W: Impaired left ventricular relaxation during pacing-induced ischemia. Am J Cardiol 32:751, 1973.

16. McCann LL, Parker JO, Butler J: Left ventricular pressure-volume relationship during myocardial ischemia in man. Circulation 48:775, 1973.

17. Barry WH, Booker JZ, Alderman EL, Harrison DC: Changes in diastolic stiffness and tone of the left ventricle during angina pectoris. Circulation 49:255, 1974.

18. Alderman EL, Glantz SA: Acute hemodynamic interventions shift the diastolic pressure-volume curve in man. Circulation 54:662, 1976.

19. Ludbrook PA, Byrne JD, McKnight RC: Influence of right ventricular hemodynamics on left ventricular diastolic pressure-volume relations in man. Circulation 59:21, 1979.

20. Stillwell GK: The law of laplace: some clinical applications. Mayo Clin Proc 48:863, 1973.

21. Glantz SA: A three-element model describes excised cat papillary muscle elasticity. Am J Physiol 228:284, 1975.

22. Glantz SA, Kernoff RS: Muscle stiffness determined from canine left ventricular pressure-volume curves. Circ Res 37:787, 1975.

23. Nikolic S, et al.: Passive properties of canine left ventricle: Diastolic stiffness and resting forces. Circ Res 62:1210, 1988.

24. Yellin EL, Nikolic S, Frater RWM: Left ventricular filling dynamics and diastolic function. Prog Cardiovasc Dis 32:247, 1990.

25. Nikolic S, et al.: Effect of early diastolic loading on myocardial relaxation in the intact canine left ventricle. Circ Res 66:1217, 1990.

26. Nikolic S, et al.: Diastolic viscous properties of the intact canine left ventricle. Circ Res 67:352, 1990.

27. Ohtani M, Nikolic S, Glantz SA: A new approach to in situ left ventricular volume clamping in dogs. Am J Physiol 261:H1335, 1991.

28. Udelson JE, Bacharach SL, Cannon RO, Bonow RO: Minimum left ventricular pressure during β-adrenergic stimulation in human subjects, evidence for elastic recoil and diastolic "suction" in the normal heart. Circulation 82:1174, 1990.

29. Grossman W, Jones D, McLaurin LP: Wall stress and patterns of hypertrophy in the human left ventricle. J Clin Invest 56:56, 1975.

30. Grossman W: Cardiac hypertrophy: useful adaptation or pathologic process? Am J Med 69:576, 1980.

31. Florenzano F, Glantz SA: Left-ventricular mechanical adaptations to chronic aortic regurgitation in intact dogs. Am J Physiol 252:H969, 1987.

32. Lorell BH: Cardiac hypertrophy: the consequences for diastole. J Am Coll Cardiol 9:1189, 1987.

33. Grossman W: Diastolic dysfunction and congestive heart failure. Circ Res 81(Suppl III):III1, 1990.

34. Gaasch WH: Congestive heart failure in patients with normal left ventricular systolic function: a manifestation of diastolic dysfunction. Herz 16:22, 1991.

35. Warren SE, Grossman W: Therapeutic approaches affecting diastolic ventricular function. Herz 16:33, 1991.

36. Bonow RO: Left ventricular diastolic function in hypertrophied cardiomyopathy. Herz 16:13, 1991.

37. Rippe JM, et al.: Studies of systolic mechanics and diastolic behavior on the left ventricle in the trained racing greyhound. Basic Res Cardiol 77:619, 1982.

38. Fagard R, et al.: Assessment of stiffness of the hypertrophied left ventricle of bicyclists using left ventricular inflow doppler velocimetry. J Am Coll Cardiol 9:1250, 1987.

39. Grossman W, McLaurin LP, Stefadouros MA: Left ventricular stiffness associated with chronic pressure and volume overloads in man. Circ Res 35:793, 1974.

40. Nomura S: Diastolic property of left ventricle under experimental volume overload. Jpn Circulation J 50:426, 1986.

41. Michel JB, et al.: Morphometric analysis

of collagen network and plasma perfused capillary bed in the myocardium of rats during evolution of cardiac hypertrophy. Basic Res Cardiol 81:142, 1986.

42. Peterson KL, et al.: Diastolic left ventricular pressure-volume and stress-strain relations in patients with valvular aortic stenosis and left ventricular hypertrophy. Circulation 58:77, 1978.

43. Hess OM, et al.: Diastolic function and myocardial structure in patients with myocardial hypertrophy: special reference to normalized viscoelastic data. Circulation 63:360, 1981.

44. Thiedemann KU, Holubarsch C, Medugorac I, Jacob R: Connective tissue content and myocardial stiffness in pressure overload hypertrophy: a combined study of morphologic, morphometric, biochemical, and mechanical parameters. Basic Res Cardiol 78:140, 1983.

45. Weber KT, et al.: Collagen remodeling of pressure-overloaded, hypertrophied nonhuman primate myocardium. Circ Res 62: 757, 1988.

46. Weiss JL, Frederiksen JW, Weisfeldt ML: Hemodynamic determinants of the timecourse of fall in canine left ventricular pressure. J Clin Invest 58:751, 1976.

47. Rushmer RF, Crystal DF, Wagner C: The functional anatomy of ventricular contraction. Circ Res 3:633, 1953.

48. Rushmer RF: Cardiac Diagnosis. Philadephia and London, W.B. Saunders Co., 1956.

49. Sonnenblick EH: The structural basis and importance of restoring forces and elastic recoil for the filling of the heart. Eur Heart J 1(Suppl A):107, 1980.

50. Yellin EL, et al.: Left ventricular relaxation in the filling and nonfilling intact canine heart. Am J Physiol 250:H620, 1986.

51. Meisner JS, et al.: Development and use of a remote-controlled mitral valve. Ann Biomed Eng 14:339, 1986.

52. Mann T, Brodie BR, Grossman W, McLaurin LT: Effect of angina on the left ventricular diastolic pressure-volume relationship. Circulation 55:761, 1977.

53. Mann T, Goldberg S, Mudge GH, Grossman W: Factors contributing to altered left ventricular diastolic properties during angina pectoris. Circulation 59:14, 1979.

54. Grossman W, Mann JT: Evidence for impaired left ventricular relaxation during acute ischemia in man. Eur J Cardiol 7(Suppl):239, 1978.

55. Stein PD, Sabbah HN, Mazilli M, Anbe DT: Effect of chronic pressure overload on the maximal rate of pressure fall of the right ventricle. Chest 78:10, 1980.

56. Bourdillon PD, Paulus WJ, Serizawa T, Grossman W: Effects of verapamil on regional myocardial diastolic function in pacing-induced ischemia in dogs. Am J Physiol 251:H834, 1986.

57. Sasayama S, et al.: Analysis of asychronous wall motion by regional pressure-length loops in patients with coronary artery disease. J Am Coll Cardiol 4:259, 1984.

58. Carroll JD, et al.: The differential effects of positive inotropic and vasodilator therapy on diastolic properties in patients with congestive cardiomyopathy. Circulation 74:815, 1986.

59. Fifer MA, Bourdillon PD, Lorell BH: Altered left ventricular diastolic properties during pacing-induced angina in patients with aortic stenosis. Circulation 74:675, 1986.

60. Raya TE, et al.: Serial changes in left ventricular relaxation and chamber stiffness after large myocardial infarction in rats. Circulation 77:1424, 1988.

61. Palacios I, Johnson RA, Newell JB, Powell WJ, Jr: Left ventricular end-diastolic pressure-volume relationship with experimental acute global ischemia. Circulation 53: 428, 1976.

62. Smiseth OA, et al.: Ventricular diastolic pressure-volume shifts during acute ischemic left ventricular failure in dogs. J Am Coll Cardiol 3:966, 1984.

63. Serizawa T, Carabello BA, Grossman W: Effect of pacing-induced ischemia on left ventricular diastolic pressure-volume relations in dogs with coronary stenoses. Circ Res 46:430, 1980.

64. Serizawa T, Vogel WM, Apstein CS, Grossman W: Comparison of acute alterations in left ventricular relaxation and diastolic chamber stiffness induced by hypoxia and ischemia. J Clin Invest 68:91, 1981.

65. Paulus WJ, Serizawa T, Grossman W: Altered left ventricular diastolic properties during pacing-induced ischemia in dogs with coronary stenosis potentiation by caffeine. Circ Res 50:218, 1982.

66. Nayler WG, Williams A: Relaxation in heart muscle: some morphological and biochemical considerations. Eur J Cardiol 7(Suppl):35, 1978.

67. Carroll JD, Hess OM, Hirzel HO, Krayenbuehl HP: Exercise-induced ischemia: the influence of altered relaxation on early diastolic pressures. Circulation 67(3):521, 1983.

68. Nayler WG, Poole-Wilson PA, Williams A: Hypoxia and calcium. J Mol Cell Cardiol 11:683, 1979.

69. Jennings RB, Reimer KA, Steenbergen C: Myocardial ischemia and reperfusion: role of calcium. *In* Control and Manipulation of Calcium Movement. Edited by JR Parratt. New York, Raven Press, 1985, pp. 273–302.
70. Steenbergen C, Murphy E, Levy L, London RE: Elevation in cytosolic free calcium concentration early in myocardial ischemia in perfused rat heart. Circ Res 60: 700, 1987.
71. Gwathmey JK, et al.: Abnormal intracellular calcium handling in myocardium from patients with end-stage heart failure. Circ Res 61:70, 1987.
72. Kihara Y, Grossman W, Morgan PJ: Direct measurement of changes in intracellular calcium transients during hypoxia, ischemia, and reperfusion of the intact mammalian heart. Circ Res 65:1029, 1989.
73. Paulus WJ, et al.: Different effects of two types of ischemia on myocardial systolic and diastolic function. Am J Physiol 248: H719, 1985.
74. Momomura S, et al.: The relationships of high energy phosphates, tissue pH, and regional blood flow to diastolic distensibility in the ischemic dog myocardium. Circ Res 57:822, 1985.
75. Carlson RE, Kavanaugh KM, Buda AJ: The effect of different mechanisms of myocardial ischemia on left ventricular function. Am Heart J 16:536, 1988.
76. Serruys PW, et al.: Left ventricular performance, regional blood flow, wall motion, and lactate metabolism during transluminal angioplasty. Circulation 70:25, 1984.
77. Wijns W, et al.: Effect of coronary occlusion during percutaneous transluminal angioplasty in humans on left ventricular chamber stiffness and regional diastolic pressure-radius relations. J Am Coll Cardiol 7:455, 1986.
78. Carlson EB, Hinohara T, Morris KG: Recovery of systolic and diastolic left ventricular function after a 60-second coronary arterial occlusion during percutaneous transluminal coronary angioplasty for angina pectoris. Am J Cardiol 60:460, 1987.
79. Bertrand ME, et al.: Left ventricular systolic and diastolic function during acute coronary artery balloon occlusion in humans. J Am Coll Cardiol 12:341, 1988.
80. Kern MJ, Deligonul U, Labovitz A: Influence of drug therapy on the ischemic response to acute coronary occlusion in man: supply-side economics. Am Heart J 118:361, 1989.
81. Bronzwaer JGF, Bruyne B, Ascoop CAPL,

Paulus WJ: Comparative effects of pacing-induced and balloon coronary occlusion ischemia on left ventricular diastolic function in man. Circulation 84:211, 1991.
82. Isoyama S, et al.: Acute decrease in left ventricular diastolic chamber distensibility during stimulated angina in isolated hearts. Circ Res 61:925, 1987.
83. Dawson JR, Gibson DG: Left ventricular filling and early diastolic function at rest and during angina in patients with coronary artery disease. Br Heart J 61:248, 1989.
84. Sasayama S, Nakamura Y, Kawai C: Effects of nifedipine on left ventricular distensibility, relaxation and filling dynamics during pacing-induced myocardial ischemia. Am J Cardiol 63:102E, 1989.
85. Serruys PW, et al.: Ejection, filling, and diastasis during transluminal occlusion in man: Consideration on global and regional left ventricular function. *In* Diastolic Relaxation of the Heart. Edited by Grossman W, Lorell BH. Boston, Martinus Nijhoff Publishing, 1988, pp. 255–280.
86. Paulus WJ: Upward shift and outward bulge: Divergent myocardial effects of pacing angina and brief coronary occlusion. Circulation 81:1436, 1990.
87. Applegate RJ, Walsh RA, O'Rourke RA: Comparative effects of pacing-induced and flow-limited ischemia on left ventricular function. Circulation 81:1380, 1990.
88. Momomura S, et al.: Regional myocardial blood flow and left ventricular diastolic properties in pacing-induced ischemia. J Am Coll Cardiol 17:781, 1991.
89. Kass DA, Midei M, Brinker J, and Maughan WL: Influence of coronary occlusion during PTCA on end-systolic and end-diastolic pressure-volume relations in humans. Circulation 81:447, 1990.
90. Brutsaert DL, De Clerck NM, Goethals MA, Housmans PR: Relaxation of ventricular cardiac muscle. J Physiol 283:469, 1978.
91. Chuck LHS, Goethals MA, Parmley WW, Brutsaert DL: Load-insensitive relaxation caused by hypoxia in mammalian cardiac muscle. Circ Res 48:797, 1981.
92. Chuck LHS, Parmley WW: Caffeine reversal of length-dependent changes in myocardial contractile state in the cat. Circ Res 47:592, 1980.
93. Schwartz A, et al.: Abnormal biochemistry in myocardial failure. Am J Cardiol 32: 407, 1973.
94. Brodie BR, et al.: Effects of sodium nitroprusside and nitroglycerin on tension pro-

longation of cat papillary muscle during recovery from hypoxia. Circ Res 39:596, 1976.

95. Thomas JD, and Weyman AE: Echocardiographic doppler evaluation of left ventricular diastolic function: physics and physiology. Circulation 84:977, 1991.

96. Frederikesn JW, Weiss JL, Weisfeldt ML: Time constant of isovolumic pressure fall: determinants in the working left ventricle. Am J Physiol 235(6):H701, 1978.

97. Cheng CP, et al.: Effects of loading conditions, contractile state, and heart rate on early diastolic left ventricular filling in conscious dogs. Circ Res 66:814, 1990.

98. Gaasch WH, Bing OHL: Myocardial relaxation i. Effect of nitroprusside on the tension prolongation phenomenon. Am J Physiol 237:H185, 1979.

99. Heyndrickx GR, Paulus WJ: Effect of asynchrony on left ventricular relaxation. Circulation 81(Suppl III):III41, 1990.

100. Bonow RO: Regional left ventricular nonuniformity: Effects of left ventricular diastolic function in ischemic heart disease, hypertrophic cardiomyopathy, and the normal heart. Circulation 81(Suppl III): III54, 1990.

101. Gillbert TC, Lew WYW: Nonuniformity and volume loading independently influence isovolumic relaxation rates. Am J Physiol 257:H1927, 1989.

102. Lew WYW, Rasmussen CM: Influence of nonuniformity on rate of left ventricular pressure fall in the dog. Am J Physiol 256: H222, 1989.

103. Aoyagi T, et al.: Wall motion asynchrony prolongs time constant of the left ventricular relaxation. Am J Physiol 257: H883–H890, 1989.

104. LeCarpentier YC, et al.: Nature of load dependence of relaxation in cardiac muscle. Am J Physiol 237:H455, 1979.

105. LeCarpentier YC, Martin JL, Gastineau P, Hatt PY: Load dependence of mammalian heart relaxation during cardiac hypertrophy and heart failure. Am J Physiol 242: H855, 1982.

106. Zile MR, Gaasch WH: Load-dependent left ventricular relaxation in conscious dogs. Am J Physiol 261:H691, 1991.

107. Raff GL, Glantz SA: Volume loading slows left ventricular isovolumic relaxation rate: evidence of load-dependent relaxation in the intact dog heart. Circ Res 48:813, June 1981.

108. Karliner JS, LeWinter MM, Engler R, O'Rourke RA: Pharmacologic and hemodynamic influences on the rate of isovolumic left ventricular relaxation in the normal conscious dog. J Clin Invest 60: 511, 1977.

109. Hori M, et al.: Ejection timing as a major determinant of left ventricular relaxation rate in isolated perfused canine heart. Circ Res 55:31, 1984.

110. Blaustein AS, Gaasch WH: Myocardial relaxation iii. Reoxygenation mechanics in the intact dog heart. Circ Res 49:633, 1981.

111. Weisfeldt ML, Frederiksen JW, Yin FCP, Weiss JL: Evidence of incomplete left ventricular relaxation in the dog. J Clin Invest 62:1296, 1978.

112. Weisfeldt ML, Weiss JL, Frederiksen JT, Yin FCP: Quantification of incomplete left ventricular relaxation: relationship to the time constant for isovolumic pressure fall. Eur Heart J 1(Suppl A):119, 1980.

113. Granger CB, et al.: Rapid ventricular filling in left ventricular hypertrophy: i. Physiologic hypertrophy. J Am Coll Cardiol 5:862, 1985.

114. Hanrath P, Mathey DG, Siegert R, Bleifeld W: Left ventricular relaxation and filling pattern in different forms of left ventricular hypertrophy: an echocardiographic study. Am J Cardiol 45:15, 1980.

115. Smith VE, et al.: Rapid ventricular filling in left ventricular hypertrophy: ii. Pathologic hypertrophy. J Am Coll Cardiol 5: 869, 1985.

116. Lorell BH, et al.: Modification of abnormal left ventricular diastolic properties by nifedipine in patients with hypertrophic cardiomyopathy. Circulation 65:499, 1982.

117. Alvares RF, Shaver JA, Gamble WH, Goodwin JF: Isovolumic relaxation period in hypertrophic cardiomypathy. J Am Coll Cardiol 3:71, 1984.

118. Betocchi S, et al.: Isovolumic relaxation period in hypertrophic cardiomyopathy: Assessment by radionuclide angiography. J Am Coll Cardiol 7:74, 1986.

119. Yamakado T, Nakano T: Left ventricular systolic and diastolic function in the hypertrophied ventricle. Jpn Circulation J 54:554, 1990.

120. Gwathmey JK, Morgan JP: Altered calcium handling in experimental pressure-overload hypertrophy in the ferret. Circ Res 57:836, 1985.

121. Morgan JP, Morgan KG: Calcium and cardiovascular function: Intracellular calcium levels during contraction and relaxation of mammalian cardiac and vascular smooth muscle as detected with aequorin. Am J Med 77(Suppl 5A):33, 1984.

122. Alyono D, et al.: Alterations of myocardial blood flow associated with experimental canine left ventricular hypertrophy secondary to valvular aortic stenosis. Circ Res 58:47, 1986.

123. Tomanek RJ, et al.: Morphometry of canine coronary arteries, arterioles, and capillaries during hypertension and left ventricular hypertrophy. Circ Res 58:38, 1986.

124. Bache RJ, Arentzen CE, Simon AB, Vrobel TR: Abnormalities in myocardial perfusion during tachycardia in dogs with left ventricular hypertrophy: Metabolic evidence for myocardial ischemia. Circulation 69:409, 1984.

125. Diver DJ, et al.: Diastolic function in patients with aortic stenosis: influence of left ventricular load reduction. J Am Coll Cardiol 12:642, 1988.

126. Hess OM, et al.: Diastolic stiffness and myocardial structure in aortic valve disease before and after valve replacement. Circulation 69:855, 1984.

127. Sasayama S, et al.: Changes in diastolic properties of the regional myocardium during pacing-induced ischemia in human subjects. J Am Coll Cardiol 5:599, 1985.

128. Grossman W: Why is left ventricular diastolic pressure increased during angina pectoris? J Am Coll Cardiol 5:607, 1985.

129. Theroux P, et al.: Regional myocardial function and dimensions early and late after myocardial infarction in the unanesthetized dog. Circ Res 40:2:158, 1977.

130. Janz RF, Waldron RJ: Predicted effect of chronic apical aneurysms on the passive stiffness of the human left ventricle. Circ Res 42(2):255, 1978.

131. Bloom WL: Demonstration of diastolic filling of the beating excised heart (motion picture) (Abstract). Am J Physiol 183:597, 1955.

132. Bloom WL: Diastolic filling of the beating excised heart. Am J Physiol 187:143, 1956.

133. Brecher GA: Critical review of recent work on ventricular diastolic suction. Circ Res 6:554, 1958.

134. Tyberg JV, Keon WJ, Sonnenblick EH, Urschel CW: Mechanics of ventricular diastole. Cardiovasc Res 4:423, 1970.

135. Suga H, et al.: Pressure-volume relation around zero transmural pressure in excised cross-circulated dog left ventricle. Circ Res 63:361, 1988.

136. Hori M, Yellin EL, Sonnenblick EH: Left ventricular diastolic suction as a mechanism of ventricular filling. Jpn Circulation J 46:124, 1982.

137. Roberts WC, Brownlee WJ, Jones AA, Luke JL: Sucking action of the left ventricle: demonstration of a physiologic principle by a gunshot wound penetrating only the right side of the heart. Am J Cardiol 43:1234, 1979.

138. Sabbah HN, Anbe DT, Stein PD: Negative intraventricular diastolic pressure in patients with mitral stenosis: evidence of left ventricular diastolic suction. Am J Cardiol 45:562, 1980.

139. Sabbah HN, Anbe ST, Stein PD: Can the human right ventricle create a negative diastolic pressure suggestive of suction? Cathet Cardiovasc Diagn 7:259, 1981.

140. Zile MR, Blaustein AS, Gaasch WH: The effect of acute alterations in left ventricular afterload and beta-adrenergic tone on indices of early diastolic filling rate. Circ Res 65:406, 1989.

141. Suga H, et al.: Ventricular suction under zero source pressure for filling. Am J Physiol 251:H47, 1986.

142. Janicki JS, Weber KT: Factors influencing the diastolic pressure volume relation of the cardiac ventricles. Fed Proc 39:133, 1980.

143. Bove AA, Santamore WP: Ventricular interdependence. Prog Cardiovasc Dis 23:365, 1981.

144. Glantz SA, et al.: The pericardium substantially affects the left ventricular diastolic pressure-volume relationship in the dog. Circ Res 42:433, 1978.

145. Lorell BH, et al.: Right ventricular distension and left ventricular compliance. Am J Physiol 240:H87, 1981.

146. Weber KT, Janicki JS, Shroff S, Fishman AP: Contractile mechanics and interaction of the right and left ventricles. Am J Cardiol 47:686, 1981.

147. Kingma I, Tyberg JV, Smith ER: Effects of diastolic transseptal pressure gradient on ventricular septal position and motion. Circulation 68:1304, 1983.

148. Little WC, Badke FR, O'Rourke RA: Effect of right ventricular pressure on the end-diastolic left ventricular pressure-volume relationship before and after chronic right ventricular pressure overload in dogs without pericardia. Circ Res 54:719, 1984.

149. Sunagawa K, Maughan WL, Burkhoff D, Sagawa K: Left ventricular interaction with arterial load studied in isolated canine ventricle. Am J Physiol 245:H773, 1983.

150. Slinker BK, Chagas ACP, Glantz SA: The importance of direct ventricular interaction decreases in chronic pressure over-

load hypertrophy in the dog. Am J Physiol 253:H347, 1987.

151. Piene H, Myhre ES: Position of interventricular septum during heart cycle in anesthetized dogs. Am J Physiol 260:H158, 1991.

152. Santamore WP, et al.: Contribution of each ventricular wall to ventricular interdependence. Basic Res Cardiol 83:424, 1988.

153. Santamore WP, et al.: Alterations in left ventricular compliance due to change in right ventricular volume, pressure and compliance. Cardiovasc Res 22:768, 1988.

154. Goldstein JA, et al.: Determinants of hemodynamic compromise with severe right ventricular infarction. Circulation 82:359, 1990.

155. Goldstein JA, et al.: Hemodynamic importance of systolic ventricular interaction, augmented right atrial contractility and atrioventricular synchrony in acute right ventricular dysfunction. J Am Coll Cardiol 16:181, 1990.

156. Goldstein JA, et al.: Importance of left ventricular function and systolic ventricular interaction to right ventricular performance during acute right heart ischemia. J Am Coll Cardiol 19:704, 1992.

157. Calvin JE: Optimal right ventricular filling pressures and the role of pericardial constraint in right ventricular infarction in dogs. Circulation 84:852–861, 1991.

158. Goto Y, Slinker BK, LeWinter MM: Nonhomogeneous left ventricular regional shortening during acute right ventricular overload. Circ Res 65:43, 1989.

159. Belenkie I, Dani R, Smith ER, Tyberg JV: Ventricular interaction during experimental acute pulmonary embolism. Circulation 78:761, 1988.

160. Santamore WP, Peterson JT, Johnston WE, Vinten-Johansen J. Variable non-linearity in end systolic pressure-volume relationships results from interaction between and diastolic and developed-pressure-volume relations. Cardiovasc Res 25:36, 1991.

161. Brilla C, Kissling G, Jacob R: Significance of right ventricular filling for left ventricular end-diastolic pressure-volume relationship under acute hypoxia in the dog. Basic Res Cardiol 82:109, 1987.

162. Damiano RJ, et al.: Significant left ventricular contribution to right ventricular systolic function. Am J Physiol 261:H1514, 1991.

163. Parmley WW, et al.: Acute changes in the diastolic pressure-volume relationship of the left ventricle. Eur J Cardiol 4(Suppl): 105, 1976.

164. Brodie BR, Grossman W, Mann T, McLaurin LP: Effects of sodium nitroprusside on left ventricular diastolic pressure-volume relations. J Clin Invest 59:59, 1977.

165. Ludbrook PA, Bryne JD, Kurnik PB, McKnight RC: Influence of reduction of preload and afterload by nitroglycerin on left ventricular diastolic pressure-volume relations and relaxation in man. Circulation 56:937, 1977.

166. Shirato K, et al.: Alteration of the left ventricular diastolic pressure-segment length relation produced by the pericardium: effects of cardiac distension and afterload reduction in conscious dogs. Circulation 57:1191, 1978.

167. Ross J: Acute displacement of the diastolic pressure-volume curve of the left ventricle: role of the pericardium and the right ventricle. Circulation 59(editorial):32, 1979.

168. Ullrich KJ, Riecker G, Kramer K: Das drunckvolumdiagramm des warmblueterherzens isometrische gleichgewichtskurven. Pflugers Arch 259:481, 1954.

169. Taylor RR, Covell JW, Sonnenblick EH, Ross J, Jr: Dependence of ventricular distensibility in filling of the opposite ventricle. Am J Physiol 213:711, 1967.

170. Bemis CE, et al.: Influence of right ventricular filling pressure on left ventricular pressure and dimension. Circ Res 34:498, 1974.

171. Elzinga G, van Grondelle R, Westerhof N, van den Bos GC: Ventricular interference. Am J Physiol 226:941, 1974.

172. Santamore WP, et al.: Myocardial interaction between the ventricles. J Appl Physiol 41:362, 1976.

173. Santamore WP, Shaffer TH, Hughes D: A theoretical and experimental model of ventricular interdependence. Basic Res Cardiol 81:529, 1986.

174. Janicki JS, Weber KT: The pericardium and ventricular interaction, distensibility, and function. Am J Physiol 238:H494, 1980.

175. Stool EW, Mulloins CB, Leshin SJ, Mitchell JH: Dimensional changes of the left ventricle during acute pulmonary arterial hypertension in dogs. Am J Cardiol 33: 868, 1974.

176. Molaug M, Geiran O, Kiil F: Dynamics of the interventricular septum and free ventricular walls during selective left ventricular volume loading in dogs. Acta Physiol Scand 119:81, 1983.

177. Olsen CO, et al.: Dynamic ventricular interaction in the conscious dog. Circ Res 52:85, 1983.

178. Visner MS, et al.: Alterations in left ventricular three-dimensional dynamic geometry and systolic function during acute right ventricular hypertension in the conscious dog. Circulation 67:353, 1983.

179. Slinker BK, Glantz SA: End-systolic and end-diastolic ventricular interaction. Am J Physiol 251:H1062, 1986.

180. Ruskin J, Bache RJ, Rembert JC, Greenfield JC, Jr: Pressure-flow studies in man: Effect of respiration on left ventricular stroke volume. Circulation 48:79, 1973.

181. Elzinga G, Piene H, De Jong JP: Left and right ventricular pump function and consequences of having two pumps in one heart. Circ Res 46:564, 1980.

182. Boltwood CM, Jr: Ventricular performance related to transmural filling pressure in clinical cardiac tamponade. Circulation 75:941, 1987.

183. Tyberg JV, Misbach GA, Parmley WW, Glantz SA: Effects Of The Pericardium On Left Ventricular Performance. *In* Cardiac Dynamics. Edited by Baan J, Arntzenius AC, Yellin EL. The Hague, Boston, London, Martinus Nijhoff, 1987, pp. 159–168.

184. Mirsky L, Rankin JS: The effects of geometry, elasticity, and external pressures on the diastolic pressure-volume and stiffness-stress relations: how important is the pericardium? Circ Res 44:601, 1979.

185. Santamore WP, Li KS, Nakamoto I, Johnston WE: Effects of increased pericardial pressure on the coupling between the ventricles. Cardiovasc Res 24:768, 1990.

186. Santamore WP, Shaffer T, Papa L: Theoretical model of ventricular interdependence: pericardial effects. Am J Physiol 259:H181, 1990.

187. Watanabe J, et al.: Effects of the pericardium on the diastolic left coronary pressure-flow relationship in the isolated dog heart. Circulation 75:670, 1987.

188. Maruyama Y, et al.: Mechanical interactions between four heart chambers with and without the pericardium in canine hearts. Circ Res 50:86, 1982.

189. Spadaro J, Bing OHL, Gaasch WH, Weintraub RM: Pericardial modulation of right and left ventricular diastolic interaction. Circ Res 48:233, 1981.

190. Stokland O, Miller MM, Lekven J, Illebekk A: The significance of the intact pericardium for cardiac performance in the dog. Circ Res 47:27, 1980.

191. Robotham JL, Mitzner W: A model of the effects of respiration on left ventricular performance. J Appl Physiol 46:411, 1979.

192. Robotham JL, Rabson J, Permutt S, Bromberger-Barnea B: Left ventricular hemodynamics during respiration. J Appl Physiol 47:1295, 1979.

193. Smiseth OA, et al.: The pericardial hypothesis: a mechanism of acute shifts of the left ventricular diastolic pressure-volume relation. Clin Physiol 5:403, 1985.

194. Smiseth OA, et al.: Assessment of pericardial constraint in dogs. Circulation 71:158, 1985.

195. Minczak BM, Wolfson MR, Santamore WP, Shaffer TH: Pericardial effects on diastolic ventricular interaction during development. Pediatr Res 27:547, 1990.

196. Junemann M, et al.: Quantification of effect of pericardium on LV diastolic PV relation in dogs. Am J Physiol 252:H963, 1987.

197. Lavine SJ, Campbell CA, Kloner RA, Gunther SJ: Diastolic filling in acute left ventricular dysfunction: Role of the pericardium. J Am Coll Cardiol 12:1326, 1988.

198. Tyson GS, Jr, et al.: Pericardial influences on ventricular filling in the conscious dog: An analysis based on pericardial pressure. Circ Res 54:173, 1984.

199. Assanelli D, Lew WYW, Shabetai R, LeWinter MM: Influence of the pericardium on right and left ventricular filling in the dog. J Appl Physiol 63:1025, 1987.

200. Boltwood CM, Jr, Shah PM: The pericardium in health and disease. Curr Probl Cardiol 9:1, 1984.

201. Smiseth OA, et al.: Assessment of pericardial constraint: the relation between right ventricular filling pressure and pericardial pressure measured after pericardiocentesis. J Am Coll Cardiol 7:307, 1986.

202. Tyberg JV, et al.: The relationship between pericardial pressure and right atrial pressure: an intraoperative study. Circulation 73:428, 1986.

203. Janicki JS: Influence of the pericardium and ventricular interdependence on left ventricular diastolic and systolic function in patients with heart failure. Circulation 81(Suppl III):III15, 1990.

204. Santamore WP, Constantinescu M, Little WC: Direct assessment of right ventricular transmural pressure. Circulation 75:744, 1987.

205. Slinker BK, Ditchey RV, Bell SP, LeWinter MM: Right heart pressure does not equal pericardial pressure in the potassium chloride-arrested canine heart in situ. Circulation 76:357, 1987.

206. Boltwood CM, Jr, et al.: Intraoperative measurement of pericardial constraint:

role in ventricular diastolic mechanics. J Am Coll Cardiol 8(6):1289, 1986.

207. Reddy PS, Curtiss EJ, O'Toole JD, Shaver JA: Cardiac tamponade: Hemodynamic observations in man. Circulation 58:265, 1978.

208. Freeman GL, LeWinter MM: Pericardial adaptations during chronic cardiac dilation in dogs. Circ Res 54:294, 1984.

209. LeWinter MM, Pavelec R: Influence of the pericardium on left ventricular end-diastolic pressure-segment relations during early and later stages of experimental chronic volume overload in dogs. Circ Res 50(Part 4):501, 1982.

210. Lee JM, Boughner DR: Tissue mechanics of canine pericardium in different test environments. Circ Res 49:533, 1981.

211. Lee MC, et al.: Biaxial mechanical properties of the pericardium in normal and volume overload dogs. Am J Physiol 249(Part 2):H222, 1985.

212. Tyberg JV, Smith ER: Ventricular diastole and the role of the pericardium. Herz 15:354, 1990.

213. Goldstein JA, et al.: The role of right ventricular systolic dysfunction and elevated intrapericardial pressure in the genesis of low output in experimental right ventricular infarction. Circulation 65:513, 1982.

214. Goldstein JA, et al.: Volume loading improves low cardiac output in experimental right ventricular infarction. J Am Coll Cardiol 2:270, 1983.

215. Cournand A, Motley HL, Werko L, Richards DW, Jr: Physiological studies of the effects of intermittent positive pressure breathing on cardiac output in man. Am J Physiol 152:162, 1948.

216. Powers SR, et al.: Physiologic consequence of positive end-expiratory pressure (peep) ventilation. Ann Surg 178:265, 1973.

217. Smith PK, et al.: Cardiovascular effects of ventilation with positive expiratory airway pressure. Ann Surg 195:121, 1982.

218. Dorinsky PM, Whitcomb ME: The effect of peep on cardiac output. Chest 84:210, 1983.

219. Kingma I, et al.: Left ventricular external constraint: relationship between pericardial, pleural and esophageal pressures during positive end-expiratory pressure and volume loading in dogs. Ann Biomed Eng 15:331, 1987.

220. Robotham JL, et al.: Effects of respiration on cardiac performance. J Appl Physiol 44:703, 1978.

221. Robotham JL, Wise RA, Bromberger-Barnea B: Effects of changes in abdominal pressure on left ventricular performance and regional blood flow. Crit Care Med 13:803, 1985.

222. Robotham JL, et al.: Effects of changes in left ventricular loading and pleural pressure on mitral flow. J Appl Physiol. 65:1662, 1988.

223. Scharf SM, Brown R, Tow DE, Parisi AF: Cardiac effects of increased lung volume and decreased pleural pressure in man. J Appl Physiol 47:257, 1979.

224. Scharf SM, Bianco JA, Tow DE, Brown R: The effects of large negative intrathoracic pressure on left ventricular function in patients with coronary artery disease. Circulation 63:871, 1981.

225. Fewell JE, Abendschein DR, Murray JF, Rapaport E: Continuous positive-pressure ventilation decreases right and left ventricular end-diastolic volumes in the dog. Circ Res 46:125, 1980.

226. Fewell JE, et al.: Mechanism of decreased right and left ventricular end-diastolic volumes during continuous positive-pressure ventilation in dogs. Circ Res 47:467, 1980.

227. Fewell JE, et al.: Continuous positive-pressure ventilation does not alter ventricular pressure-volume relationship. Am J Physiol 240:H821, 1981.

228. Santamore WP, Heckman JL, Bove AA: Cardiovascular changes from expiration to inspiration during IPPV. Am J Physiol 245:H307, 1983.

229. Santamore WP, Bove AA, Heckman JL: Right and left ventricular pressure-volume response to positive end-expiratory pressure. Am J Physiol 246:H114, 1984.

230. Santamore WP, Heckman JL, Bove AA: Right and left ventricular pressure-volume response to respiratory maneuvers. J Appl Physiol 57:1520, 1984.

231. Wallis TW, Robotham JL, Compean R, Kindred MK: Mechanical heart-lung interaction with positive end-expiratory pressure. J Appl Physiol 54:1039, 1983.

232. Cassidy SS, Ramanathan M: Dimensional analysis of the left ventricle during peep: Relative septal and lateral wall displacements. Am J Physiol 246:H792, 1984.

233. Olsen CO, et al.: Diminished stroke volume during inspiration: a reverse thoracic pump. Circulation 72:668, 1985.

234. Calvin JW, Baer RW, Glantz SA: Pulmonary injury depresses cardiac systolic function through starling mechanism. Am J Physiol 251:H722, 1986.

235. Marini JJ, Culver BH, Butler J: Effect of positive end-expiratory pressure on canine ventricular function curves. J Appl Physiol 51:1367, 1981.

236. Pinto JG, Fung YC: Mechanical properties

of the heart muscle in the passive state. J Biomech 6:597, 1973.

237. Glantz SA: A constitutive equation for the passive properties of muscle. J Biomech 7:137, 1974.

238. Pasipoularides A, et al.: Myocardial relaxation and passive diastolic properties in man. Circulation 74(5):991, 1986.

239. Fioretti P, Broer RW, Meester GT, Serruys PW: Interaction of left ventricular relaxation and filling during early diastole in human subjects. Am J Cardiol 46:197, 1980.

240. Gaasch WH, Bernard SA: The effect of acute changes in coronary blood flow on left ventricular end-diastolic wall thickness: An echocardiographic study. Circulation 56:593, 1977.

241. Gaasch WH, et al.: The influence of acute alterations in coronary blood flow on left ventricular diastolic compliance and wall thickness. Eur J Cardiol 7(Suppl):147, 1978.

242. Abel RM, Reis RL: Effects of coronary blood flow and perfusion pressure on left ventricular contractility in dogs. Circ Res 27:961, 1970.

243. Arnold G, et al.: The importance of the perfusion pressure in the coronary arteries for the contractility and the oxygen consumption of the heart. Pflugers Archiv 299:339, 1968.

244. Templeton GH, Wildenthal K, Mitchell JH: Influence of coronary blood flow on left ventricular contractility and stiffness. Am J Physiol 223:1216, 1972.

245. Spadaro J, et al.: Effects of perfusion pressure on myocardial performance, metabolism wall thickness, and compliance: comparison of the beating and fibrillating heart. J Thorac Cardiovasc Surg 84:398, 1982.

246. Watanabe J, et al.: Effects of coronary venous pressure on left ventricular diastolic distensibility. Circ Res 67:923, 1990.

247. Vogel WM, et al.: Acute alterations in left ventricular diastolic chamber stiffness role of the "erectile" effect of coronary arterial pressure and flow in normal and damaged hearts. Circ Res 51:465, 1982.

248. Watters TA, et al.: Hydrodynamics in the heart modulates work. Heart Vessels 4:128, 1988.

249. Bouchard A, et al.: Effects of altered coronary perfusion pressure on function and metabolism of normal and cardiomyopathic hamster hearts. J Mol Cell Cardiol 19:1011, 1987.

250. Huyghe JMRJ: Non-linear finite element models of the beating left ventricle and the intramyocardial coronary circulation. Ph.D Dissertation, 1986, pp. 5-13,5-23.

251. Huyghe JMRJ, Campen DHV, Arts T, Heethaar RM: A two-phase finite element model of the diastolic left ventricle. J Biomech 24:527, 1991.

Chapter 5

DIASTOLIC SUCTION AND THE DYNAMICS OF LEFT VENTRICULAR FILLING

Edward L. Yellin and Srdjan D. Nikolic

Ventricular opening (diastole), like its closing (systole), is an active, powerful movement and it *pulls* down blood from the upper ventricles, which in their turn propel it by their *elastic rebound* and muscular action into the lower ventricles. (emphasis added)

Leonardo da Vinci (1)

Moreover, and contrary to the general opinion, neither the heart nor anything else can dilate and distend itself so as to *draw anything into its cavity during the diastole*, unless, like a sponge it has been first compressed and is returning to its primary condition. (Emphasis added)

William Harvey (2)

HISTORICAL BACKGROUND

Pre-Harveyian physicians and natural philosophers were well aware of the power in the ventricular muscle. Being ignorant of the pump function of the heart, however, they viewed the ventricles as mixing chambers that dilated and actively filled by *sucking* in the blood (3). When William Harvey discovered the circulation of the blood, he placed the heart at the center of the circulatory system and thus, for the first time, described the role of the heart as a mechanical pump. This revolutionary discovery led Harvey to focus on active contraction and pulsatility so that he not only denied the existence of ventricular "suction," he failed to understand the passive role of the atrium as a reservoir, and he wrote, in the sentence following the above quotation; "...consequently it is by the *contraction of the auricles* that the blood is *thrown* into the ventricles..." (emphasis added). With Harvey's momentous discoveries, systole and diastole assumed new physiologic roles, and the stage was set for a vigorous controversy on whether the ventricles filled by blood being thrown into them vis a

tergo, or pulled into them, vis a fronte. For example, in 1906, in his canine studies on the phases of the cardiac cycle, Henderson observed:

> ...the absence of any *negative* pressure in some of our curves and the brevity of its duration in all others demonstrate that in these experiments the ventricles on passing into diastole exerted no *suction* sufficient to be considered as an important factor in the filling of the ventricles [emphasis added] (4).

In 1930, Katz commented:

> The current view of ventricular filling conceives the ventricles as being entirely passive, i.e., the ventricular walls are stretched by the force of the pressure head in the veins and auricles and that the energy of filling comes entirely from this pressure head ... [but] ... The idea that the ventricle plays no role in filling ignores the fact that the ventricle, like ordinary skeletal muscle is an elastic body which has one elastic state when contracted and another when relaxed (5).

Katz went on to describe the state of the heart with an elastance concept whereby the P-V relation shifts from the contractile to the relaxed state allowing a precipitous fall in pressure. He then cited Wiggers (6, 7), who showed that, if the ventricle is not fully relaxed when filling begins, the com-

Supported in part by NIH PO1 HL 37412 and HL 49614.

pletion of relaxation will facilitate filling. Armed with these concepts, and obviously aware of the interaction between relaxation and filling, Katz used a turtle heart, which had been filled from a constant head reservoir with the ability to produce a mitral valve occlusion, to demonstrate that LVP could fall below the system level during filling and could fall further still when filling was prevented. After specifically stating that the elastic state of the ventricle does not permit pressures below atmospheric, Katz went on to conclude: "The relaxing ventricle, therefore, not only can but does exert a *sucking* action to draw blood into its chamber" [emphasis added] (5). One potential source of misunderstanding is thus semantic: Henderson rules out suction in the absence of a negative pressure; Katz accepts suction if the ventricular pressure falls below the atrial despite its physical inability to develop negative pressures.

The early postwar years saw a resurgence of interest in the concept of diastolic suction and its role in ventricular filling (8, 9) (see Brecher (10) for a review). Major credit for clarifying the concept of elastic recoil and relating it to ventricular volume, contractility, and afterload belongs to Brecher and coworkers, who backed their conceptual approach with important experimental evidence (11–13). Particularly useful was their formulation of the concept

of ventricular equilibrium volume and their definition of suction: "If the pressure in the ventricle is lowered by some force below that which would exist in the ventricle in the absence of such force, then one may call this phenomenon suction" (10, 14). The pressure-volume relation of Figure 5–1 obtained by Brecher and Kissen (12) was the first to demonstrate the positive and negative portions of the passive ventricle. Note, however, that the negative portion of Figure 5–1 was obtained by aspirating saline from the passive ventricle, in contrast to a contraction below equilibrium. We will discuss this important difference in the following paragraphs.

The equilibrium volume, i.e., the volume at zero transmural pressure, is clearly shown in Figure 5–1. The negative portion of the P-V relation provides the physical basis for the concept of diastolic suction. An end-systolic volume below equilibrium provides the elastic recoil to generate negative pressures if the volume is not permitted to increase, hence, the technique of studying suction by obstructing inflow (9). Because the need to use inflow obstruction is frequently misunderstood, we would like to clarify the process. Inflow obstruction does not *create* suction, it *unmasks* the property by allowing the ventricle to relax completely in the absence of filling and thus without the subsequent increase in pres-

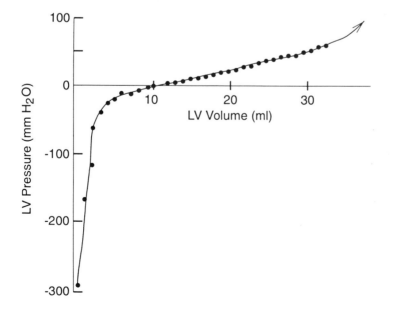

Fig. 5–1. Pressure-volume relation of the diastolic arrested canine left ventricle. The positive portion was obtained by saline infusion, the negative portion by aspiration. Adapted from Brecher, G.A., and Kissen, A.T.: Relation of negative intraventricular pressure to ventricular volume. Circ. Res. 5. 157, 1957, with permission of the American Heart Association.

sure due to stretch of passive elastic elements.

It is interesting to note that, after apparently receiving a preprint of a manuscript to be published in the January, 1958 issue of Circulation Research, Wiggers published a letter in the December 17, 1957 issue of *Science,* stating:

> Recent experimental evidence indicates that the relaxing ventricles can develop suction under certain *artificial* experimental conditions [Brecher, Circulation Research (Jan. 1958)]. Before such evidence can be used to revive the *discarded* concept that ventricular filling of the normally beating heart is aided by, or due to, aspiration, it is necessary to consider the way in which the cardiac pump operates [emphasis added] (15).

Wiggers went on to argue that, because the most rapid decline of ventricular pressure is isovolumic, with filling occurring only after ". . .the major fall of pressure. . ." had taken place:

> An aspirating force could, therefore, aid the positive left atrial pressure in transferring blood only during this short interval. . . Crucial evidence is still required that the small remnant of elastic recoil still operative at the end of relaxation can create sufficient suction to be of significance in filling the normally beating heart. Dynamically it must be shown that the concordant decline of atrial and ventricular pressure are {sic} due to a more rapid rate of ventricular relaxation than of filling from the atria (15).

Wiggers had no problem accepting the concept of suction based on the rate of ventricular relaxation and its ability to fall below the atrial pressure, but he did raise a crucial question: does suction play a significant role in ventricular filling?

In the 1960s, the role of suction took second place to the study of cardiac muscle mechanics and systolic pump function. By the end of the decade, however, Tyberg et al. (16) neatly integrated the properties of cardiac muscle with chamber function in diastole. They demonstrated the existence of negative transmural pressures by using an isolated dog heart and completely obstructing inflow to allow completion of ventricular relaxation. They related sarcomere shortening to end systolic volume by reasoning that cardiac muscle contracts to

below its rest length (17, 18), thereby storing potential energy in the form of compressed elements. They also related sarcomere shortening to the two conditions that reduce end systolic volume and increase elastic recoil: increased contractility and decreased afterload, noting also that this is precisely what happens during exercise (16). The existence of restoring forces has since been demonstrated in isolated cardiac muscle (19) as well as in isolated cardiac cells (20).

In the 1980s, the study of diastole blossomed. The advent of high-resolution echocardiography brought with it the ability to measure transmitral flow velocity waveforms noninvasively and to relate these velocity patterns to changes in chamber properties. With the realization that diastolic dysfunction frequently precedes systolic pump failure, the pendulum swung from systole to diastole. Because it is intuitively obvious that ventricular filling patterns are influenced by the active process of myocardial deactivation and by the passive elastic chamber properties, the roles of relaxation and elastic recoil assume renewed importance.

Having placed the concept of diastolic suction in an historical context, let us now place the role of diastolic ventricular suction within the context of the dynamic determinants of left ventricular filling, and offer an approach that defines suction *operationally,* using experiments from our laboratory to demonstrate its conceptual utility. Finally, we will use a computational model to analyze the role of suction in filling and to study its influence on the transmitral velocity patterns.

DYNAMICS OF LEFT VENTRICULAR FILLING

The left ventricle fills under the action of the atrioventricular pressure gradient. A useful first approximation to quantifying and conceptualizing the pressure-flow relations is given by the following equation of motion (21, 22):

$$\Delta P = (L)dQ/dt + (R)Q^2 \qquad (1)$$

where ΔP is the atrioventricular pressure difference, Q is the volume flow rate, and

(L) and (R) are inertial and resistive coefficients determined by the shape of the mitral apparatus. The first term on the right-hand side is the pressure difference due to inertia; the second term is the pressure difference required to create the kinetic energy. Because there is little or no recovery of pressure from the kinetic energy, this term can be considered a loss term; hence (R) is a resistive coefficient. Because equation (1) is often used and often poorly understood, we would like to emphasize the pertinent concepts. *For a given valvular impedance, the determinants of ventricular filling are uniquely related to the factors that determine the pressure gradient.* Thus the active and passive properties of both the atrium and the ventricle determine transmitral filling patterns because they determine the AV pressure gradient. Furthermore, the factors that determine these properties, e.g., afterload, preload, contractility, and heart rate, must also influence the filling patterns by means of their effects on the pressure gradient. Thus, regardless of how suction is defined, it acts by means of the atrioventricular pressure gradient. The

rate of ventricular relaxation influences the *rate of change* of ΔP; the ability of the ventricle to develop negative pressure, i.e., the extent of relaxation, influences the *magnitude* of ΔP.

The physiologic importance of equation (1) is that it clarifies the relation between chamber properties and flow patterns. The time-varying properties of the myocardium create the atrioventricular pressure difference that drives the flow; the pressure difference, in turn, is modulated by the impedance of the mitral apparatus; and because the passive atrial and ventricular properties change with their changes in volume, elastic effects also have a temporal influence on the characteristics of the pressure gradient, and hence on flow patterns. The mathematical characteristics of equation (1) also lead us to understand the relative roles of inertance and resistance. If inertia dominates (the normal condition, see below), then peak flow will occur out of phase with the gradient; and if resistance dominates (mitral stenosis), then peak flow and peak pressure difference will be in phase.

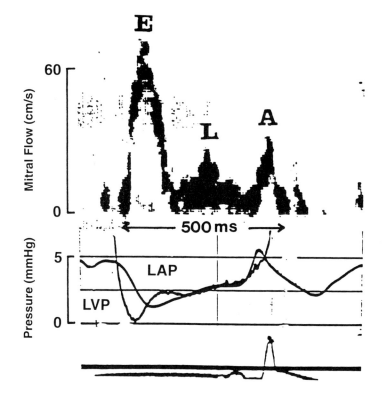

Fig. 5–2. Oscillographic record from a normal conscious dog of high fidelity left atrial and ventricular pressures with a superimposed simultaneous pulsed-Doppler recording of transmitral flow. Note, particularly, the oscillations in the AV pressure difference and the mid-diastolic L-wave of transmitral flow. LVP, LAP = left ventricular, left atrial pressure; E, L, A = Peak rapid early filling velocity, mid-diastolic peak velocity, peak velocity during atrial contraction.

These principles are illustrated in Figure 5–2, a simultaneous recording from a conscious chronically instrumented dog of transmitral flow (pulsed Doppler) and high-gain atrial and ventricular pressures (micromanometer). The oscillating pressure difference accelerates and decelerates blood during the early rapid filling phase (E-wave) and rebounds to give a slow mid-diastolic flow (L-wave). The atrial contraction produces another positive gradient to accelerate flow (A-wave); the blood is then decelerated by the fall in atrial and rise in ventricular pressure. Thus, the mitral valve closes *after* the final AV pressure crossover, indicating the inertial nature of the flow (23, 24). The simultaneous occurrence of the peak E and reversal of the AV pressure gradient seen in Figure 5–2 and elsewhere (21, 25), is another indication of the relative insignificance of resistance across a normal mitral valve.

The changes in transmitral flow caused by changes in ventricular properties in a dog with pacing-induced dilated cardiomyopathy and congestive heart failure are shown in Figure 5–3. The profound increase in chamber stiffness in this pathology leads to an increase in frequency of oscillation of the pressure gradient, thereby increasing the rates of acceleration and deceleration, and shortening the duration of early filling. In comparison to Figure 5–2, oscillation frequency increased (4.9 to 7.7/sec); time to peak flow decreased (80 to 45 msec); and duration of early filling decreased (185 to 120 msec). The pressure-flow relations of equation (1) thus exhibit the properties of an harmonic oscillator (26, 27). These are increased stiffness and inertia that tend to increase the frequency of oscillation, and increased resistance that tends to decrease the frequency and damp the oscillation.

As defined, resistance is the component of the pressure gradient caused by convective acceleration that is lost in heat. Dissipative losses can also arise from the vis-

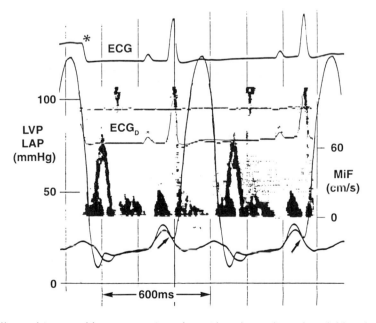

Fig. 5–3. Oscillographic record from a conscious dog with tachycardia-induced dilated cardiomyopathy and congestive heart failure. The arrows denoted the fall in LVP following an increase in volume caused by the atrial contraction; because there is no regurgitation, the pressure is assumed to be strain-rate dependent. Compare with Figure 5–2. Pressures are elevated and both pressures and flow oscillate more rapidly. ECG, ECG$_D$ = Electrocardiogram recorded on the same record as the pressures, electrocardiogram recorded on the same record as the pulsed-Doppler signal. *: denotes the onset of the synchronization signal for both recordings so that they could be superimposed. Abbreviations as in Figure 5–2. MiF = Mitral flow velocity.

cous property of strain-rate dependent force, whereby the measured pressure contains a component proportional to the rate of change of volume, i.e., the flow rate. Viscoelastic effects have been demonstrated in the dynamic pressure-volume relation of normal dogs (28, 29), but may be absent at small volumes (30). Figure 5–3 demonstrates a significant viscoelastic effect at end-diastole in a dog with dilated cardiomyopathy. The fall in LVP (arrow) while there is still inflow is caused by the dependence of force on rate of strain arising from the property of tissue viscosity (31). The classical exponential equation describing passive ventricular properties should thus include a viscoelastic component (27, 29).

$$P = P_{asy}(e^{\alpha(V - V_o)} - 1) + (ve)dV/dt \quad (2)$$

where P_{asy} is the pressure asymptote (a material property), α is the stiffness constant (a material property), V_o is the equilibrium volume, and (ve) is the viscoelastic coefficient.

Although we have thus far characterized the dynamic transmitral pressure-flow relation and the dynamically obtained diastolic P-V relation, the role of suction in ventricular filling remains to be demonstrated. Because suction, when and if it exists, apparently exerts its influence during early diastole when LVP is rapidly falling, efforts to clarify its role have tended to focus on the factors that influence relaxation (32–34). The study of relaxation, however, is confounded by the fact that the measured ventricular chamber pressure is the consequence of stresses in the wall arising from both active and passive properties. The active stress is caused by cross-bridge attachments and cycling. Passive stresses may arise from several sources: parallel elasticity, i.e., length-dependent forces caused by shortening below equilibrium volume (12, 14, 16), asynchrony of relengthening during relaxation (35–37); and torsion (38, 39) or shape change (40). Thus, the structural basis for storing energy can be in the myocardium (41) or in the myocyte (20).

To determine the time course of ventricular relaxation unaffected by stresses caused by lengthening, we developed the technique of end-systolic volume clamping in the intact canine preparation (42, 43). Two important conclusions were derived from these experiments:

1. In the absence of filling, the left ventricular pressure frequently reaches a negative asymptote (see Fig. 5–4) (42).

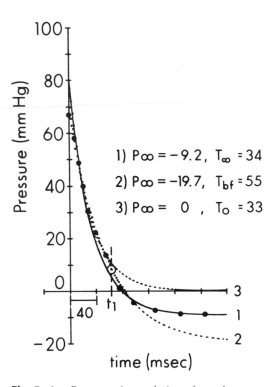

Fig. 5–4. Pressure-time relations from the onset of isovolumic relaxation to end relaxation in an anesthetized dog following clamping at end systolic volume. The filled circles, curve 1, are the actual data points; t_1 and the open circle denote the time of mitral valve opening and the onset of filling in a normal beat. Curve 2 is based on an extrapolation of the isovolumic data points assuming an exponential fit to asymptote P_∞; i.e., it is the best fit $_{(bf)}$ approach. Curve 3 is the extrapolation of the same data points as curve 2 to a zero asymptote. Thus, P_∞ of curve 1 is the true asymptote, whereas that of curve 3 is incorrect. Note also that the calculated time constant, T, depends on the method of fitting the data. The negative value of P_∞ is caused by elastic recoil and not the active decay of excitation. Reproduced with permission from Yellin, E.L., et al.: Left ventricular relaxation in the filling and nonfilling intact canine heart. Am. J. Physiol. *250*(Heart Circ Physiol 19): H620, 1986.

2. Increased contractility potentiates the degree of negativity (43).

The first effect is consistent with contraction below the equilibrium volume. The second must be caused by other mechanisms of storing elastic energy, e.g., torsion. A third important conclusion, although not as relevant to this chapter, is worth noting. The actual decline of LVP to the completely relaxed state is not truly monoexponential (42).

Further experiments with more sophisticated methods of mitral valve clamping led to the characterization of the passive pressure-volume relation in both the positive and negative planes (44, 45). It is important to note that, in contrast to Brecher's seminal studies (12) (Fig. 5–1), our measurements were dynamic; they were made in the intact heart by controlling volume and allowing relaxation to proceed to completion at different volumes (Fig. 5–5). Negative pressures were obtained, not by aspiration from the passive ventricle leading to nonphysiologic shape changes (12), but by active contraction to below equilibrium volumes (30, 44, 45). These experiments demonstrated that the active relaxation process, which is not to be confused with measured pressure, is profoundly slowed by relengthening during filling (45); that there is a relation between elastic forces and

shape (40); and again, that inotropy increases elastic recoil independent of volume (44, 45). We further determined that a logarithmic characterization of the pressure-volume relation is a more meaningful conceptualization than an exponential description (44).

$$P_p = -S_p \ln[(V_m - V)/(V_m - V_o)] \quad (3)$$

where V_m is the maximum attainable volume of the ventricle, i.e., the yield volume, S_p is a material property, and the subscript (p) refers to the positive portion of the P-V relation. The logarithmic approach to the P-V relation is the equivalent of an exponential V-P relation, and is heuristically desirable because it scales the passive ventricle to function within the natural limits of its rest and yield volumes. Differentiating:

$$S_p = (dP_p/dV)(V_m - V) \quad (4)$$

Thus, S_p is seen to be a constant defined as the chamber stiffness normalized by scaling the instantaneous volume to the operating range of the ventricle in the positive plane. Because S_p has the units of pressure, it is reasonable to conclude that it is related to the wall stress modified by a geometric factor.

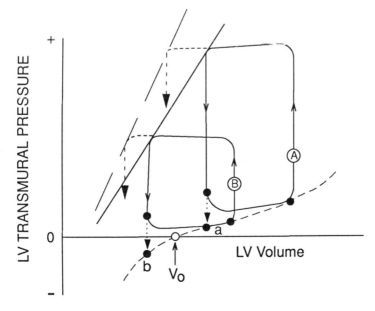

Fig. 5–5. Two pressure-volume loops illustrating the concept and role of diastolic suction. Loop A has an ESV greater than equilibrium, V_o, and can never reach a pressure lower than "a". Increased contractility (broken line and dotted loop) can reduce ESV and lead to distolic suction. Loop B has the potential ability to relax to "b" and can have the same filling volume as loop A with a lower mean LAP. Increasing contractility can lead to even greater elastic recoil.

A similar approach is followed for the negative portion of the P-V relation:

$$P_n = S_n \ln[(V - V_d)/(V_o - V_d)] \quad (5)$$

$$S_n = (dP_n/dV)(V - V_d) \quad (6)$$

where the subscript (n) denotes the negative portion of the P-V relation. Here again, S_n is seen to be a constant with the units of stress and is defined by the local stiffness normalized by the operating range of the ventricle in the negative plane. Again, when the P-V relation is determined from dynamic data, a viscoelastic component may have to be included as in equation (2). Our experiments demonstrated convincingly that the normal canine ventricle contracted to below its equilibrium volume and stored elastic energy during systole. This energy was returned during early diastole as the ventricle filled. Before discussing the role of elastic recoil and suction in the filling process, we must first decide on a suitable definition.

DEFINITION OF SUCTION

When I use a word . . . it means just what I choose it to mean. . . . When I make a word do a lot of work . . . I always pay it extra.

Humpty Dumpty to Alice (46)

The various approaches to analyzing the issue of ventricular suction fall into two categories: the ability of the ventricle to develop negative pressure, and the ability of the ventricular chamber pressure to fall below the atrial pressure. Dealing first with the latter approach, we reason as follows:

In large mammals at basal heart rates and normal rates of relaxation, there are at least 500 msec from closure of the aortic valve to the onset of atrial systole, and the ventricle is fully relaxed at that time. What would be the consequences if ventricular pressure were *not* to fall below atrial? There would be no early filling, ventricular minimum pressure would be determined solely by its compliance at its end systolic volume, and all filling would be caused by the atrial contraction. This is contrary to experience. Under *normal* conditions, there is always an early filling phase preceding the atrial contraction, and the atrial pressure is always

high enough to exceed ventricular. Therefore, under normal conditions, ventricular pressure *always* falls below atrial pressure. Under conditions of very slow and/or incomplete relaxation, one may conceive of a situation in which the atrial pressure does not reach a level high enough to open the mitral valve or to provide significant early filling before the atrial contraction. But how long can an atrial contraction alone provide a cardiac output that is consistent with life? Under normal and most abnormal conditions, it is thus reasonable to conclude that the ventricular pressure will fall below the atrial and filling will start. There is, then, little *utilitarian* value in accepting a definition of suction that relies on ventricular pressure declining to values below the atrial for filling to start. We therefore reject the argument that interprets "as incompatible with the concept of passive left ventricular filling" the observation that pressure continues to decline after relengthening starts (47).

We start by assuming that the normal myocardium relaxes to a state of zero stress in an approximately exponential manner (48):

$$P_a(t) = P_o \, e^{-t/T} \quad (7)$$

where P_a is the active pressure, P_o is the pressure at onset of isovolumic relaxation, and T is the time constant of exponential decay. We also assume that the concept of elastic recoil implies that energy is stored in a functionally parallel element so that the measured pressure, P_m, is the sum of the active pressure (equation [7]) and the passive pressure, P_p (45, 49).

$$P_m(t,V) = P_a(t) + P_p(V) \quad (8)$$

Notice that the passive pressure is a function of time as well as of volume, because the volume changes during filling. Because the measured transmural pressure is the sum of active and passive components, the *measured* pressure should not be confused with the *active* pressure (45). Relaxation to a positive value of pressure, i.e., P_m, means that filling to above the equilibrium volume has occurred and/or that some form of "diastolic tone" exists, usually caused by ischemia. Relaxation to a negative pressure, when the extraventricular pressure is zero, is caused by elastic restoring forces producing a wall stress that requires a negative intraventricular pressure for equilibrium (42). Thus, curve 1 in Figure 5–4 is the *measured* pressure and has a negative asymptote because of storage of energy in "compressed" elastic elements. If the active decay of pressure were exponential, it would be represented by curve 3, but we have found that the active decay of pressure calculated from equation [8] is not truly exponential and is influenced by relengthening (45).

We conclude that, in Humpty Dumpty's words, it is not necessary to "pay extra" in order to accept Brecher's (10, 14) approach: *diastolic suction is caused by the storage of potential energy generated by a systolic contraction to below the equilibrium volume.* But we must now ask: How does suction affect filling? Can its effect be quantified?

The most obvious consequence of suction is the ability of the stored energy to be converted by the relaxing ventricle into a lowered left atrial pressure, thereby maintaining the integrity of the lungs at the cost of a small amount of extra energy expended during systole. This is schematically shown in Figure 5–5. Elastic recoil at small end systolic volumes, arising from either decreased afterload or increased

contractility, results in a decreased left atrial pressure at the onset of filling. This mechanism assumes increasing importance during exercise, when a large stroke volume must enter the ventricle during a decreased diastolic interval (Fig. 5–6) (50). Augmented suction during increased contractility, independent of end-systolic volume, has been demonstrated in dogs (43–45) as well as in humans (51). This is a significant and intriguing finding, but its mechanism is unknown. Although it is conceivable that the wall stresses caused by stored energy may affect the relaxation rate of the ventricle, thereby enhancing early filling (33, 52), we think that this has not yet been convincingly demonstrated.

Sonnenblick (18) has advanced another intriguing hypothesis. Left ventricular elastic recoil enhances the movement of the base of the heart, thereby facilitating filling of the right ventricle and maintaining low right-sided filling pressures, of particular importance during exercise. Although this hypothesis remains speculative, we have observed a similar effect. As shown in Figure 5–7, negative left ventricular pressures during mitral valve occlusion augment the output of the right ventricle (21). We assume that this is caused by a septal shift, but the mechanism is not substantiated.

To our knowledge, the only attempt to

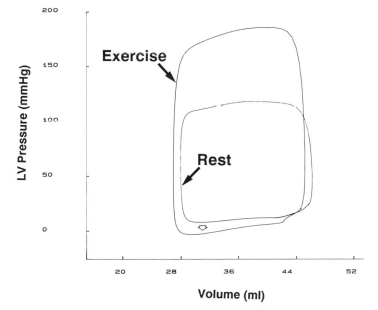

Fig. 5–6. Two pressure-volume loops from a normal conscious dog during rest and exercise. The arrow indicates the decreased LVP$_{min}$ and increased elastic recoil during exercise leading to a maintained filling volume at normal pressure despite a decreased filling time. Thus, the higher flow velocities were achieved by a higher pressure gradient due to a lower LVP, thereby maintaining the integrity of the lungs. Reproduced from Cheng C.-P., Igarashi, Y., and Little, W.C.: Mechanism of augmented rate of left ventricular filling during exercise. Circ. Res. *70*:9, 1992, with permission of the American Heart Association.

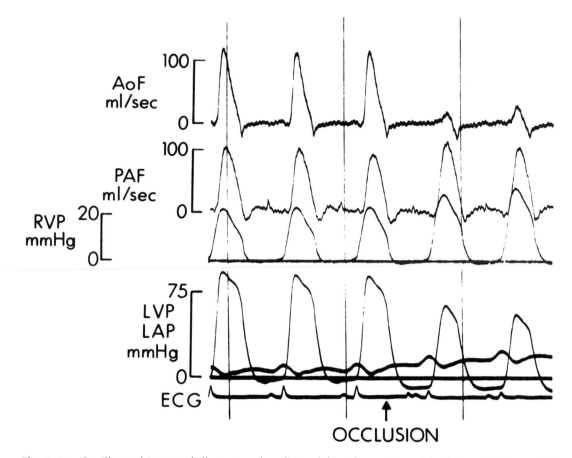

Fig. 5–7. Oscillographic record illustrating the effect of diastolic suction of the left ventricle on right ventricular filling. Following a mitral valve occlusion during systole (end systole volume clamping) left ventricular pressure became negative and pulmonary artery flow increased despite the increased left atrial pressure. The mechanism is not clear and remains open to speculation. AoF, PAF = aortic, pulmonary artery flow; RVP = right ventricular pressure; other abbreviations as in Figure 5–2. Reproduced with permission from Yellin, E.L., Nikolic, S., and Frater, R.W.M.: LV filling dynamics and diastolic function. Prog. Cardiovasc. Dis. *32*:247, 1990.

quantify the amount of filling due to suction has been a study by Suga et al. (53). They immersed an isolated canine heart in saline and measured the amount of left ventricular inflow under zero source pressure. Under these conditions, they found that 8 mL/100 g LV entered the ventricle. Although not definitive, this study clearly demonstrates both the existence and importance of diastolic suction in left ventricular filling.

In the absence of a suitable animal protocol to quantify the effect of suction on filling, we have sought to clarify the interaction of active and passive ventricular properties and their effect on filling patterns using a validated model of transmitral filling dynamics (27, 32, 54–56). The passive elastic properties of the model left ventricle allow negative strain, i.e., the ability to store elastic energy when the end-systolic volume is below equilibrium. This permits us to qualitatively and quantitatively study the dynamic determinants of ventricular filling and, in particular, the role of diastolic suction. The power of the model lies in our ability to vary individual parameters in isolation or in combination, and then to analyze the consequences of the perturbations. An example of modeling is shown in Figure 5–8.

Figure 5–8 demonstrates the influence

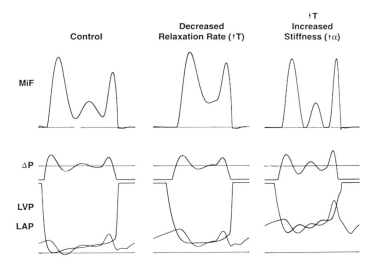

Fig. 5–8. Results of a model study examining the effects of diastolic suction under conditions of slowed relaxation (middle panel) and slowed relaxation coupled with increased chamber stiffness (right panel). Compare the normal pressure-flow patterns of Figure 5–2 with that of the control (left panel). Note, particularly, the dynamic relations between the frequency of pressure oscillations, the damping of the oscillations, and their relation to the flow patterns. See text for a detailed discussion. ΔP = atrioventricular pressure difference; T = time constant of an exponential rate of relaxation; α = stiffness constant of an exponential pressure-volume relation.

of changes in relaxation rate and chamber stiffness on the atrioventricular pressures and mitral flow patterns. The left panel (control) is the analog of Figure 5–2. Minimum LVP is zero, but it would have been negative if there were no inflow, i.e., the rise in pressure caused by filling offsets the fall in pressure caused by elastic recoil. Note the similarities between Figure 5–2 and the control panel of Figure 5–8. Similar oscillating pressure patterns produce similar oscillating flow patterns. This is a direct result of appropriate matching of active and passive properties between the in vivo heart and the model heart.

In the middle panel, *only* relaxation rate was decreased, T changed from 20 to 70 msec; diastole was shortened by 116 msec; the frequency of ΔP oscillation was unchanged but ΔP was damped; minimum LVP increased and remained constant despite filling in mid-diastole because active relaxation had not yet ceased at this large time constant; and mean LAP increased. Despite the decrease in diastolic time, filling volume increased slightly (10%) because of decreased early deceleration and increased mid-diastolic flow. Of course, this increase in filling volume was accompa-

nied by an increase in mean LAP (2 to 4 mm Hg).

In the left panel, which is the analog of Figure 5–3, the stiffness constant, α, was increased from 0.05 to 0.1/mL, with T remaining at 70 msec. The increased stiffness produced an increase in the frequency of ΔP oscillation and a decrease in the damping. Mean LAP increased even further (double that of the middle panel) despite a 25% decrease in filling volume under these conditions of increased stiffness and slowed relaxation. The increased LAP is the result of an increased stiffness, and the decreased filling is the result of the rapid deceleration of flow brought about by the increased oscillation frequency of the pressure difference, itself a consequence of increased stiffness. LVP rose after reaching a minimum and fell again in mid-diastole because the influence of relaxation dominated the effects of minimal mid-diastolic filling.

It is interesting to note that, when we did an identical model study but imposed the condition of constant filling volume, the mean LAP increased another two times to maintain the cardiac output. In the model, as in life, diastolic dysfunction can manifest itself by either a decreased cardiac output and/or an increased filling pressure. Changes in active and passive properties of the left ventricle influence not only the *patterns* of transmitral flow, but also the left atrial pressure required to maintain the filling volume. In the example shown in Figure 5–8, prolonged relaxation and increased chamber stiffness offset the ability of diastolic suction to maintain a low left atrial pressure.

It is interesting to note further that the model predicts only small physiologic changes in hemodynamic parameters with large changes in relaxation rate. For example, when T was increased from 20 to 70 msec (Fig. 5–8, middle panel), mean LAP increased from 2 to 4 mm Hg, and cardiac output was not only maintained, but increased slightly. Apparently, an isolated decrease in relaxation rate has little effect on cardiac output, despite a shortening of filling time. It is reasonable to conclude that the consistent clinical correlation between depressed filling and prolonged relaxation is caused by multiple interconnected factors. Slowed relaxation and increased chamber stiffness probably have a common structural and biochemical origin, and in combination these lead to elevated end-diastolic pressures and poor filling.

These interactions of active and passive ventricular properties and their effect on filling dynamics illustrate the complexities of evaluating the role of diastolic suction. Further, perhaps they explain the difficulties in designing in vivo experiments to give definitive answers to the question, how does diastolic suction influence ventricular filling? In summary, the left ventricle fills under the action of an atrioventricular pressure gradient. Ventricular diastolic suction arises from energy stored during systole that is recovered as elastic recoil during diastole and serves to drive down the chamber pressure, thereby providing a pressure gradient for flow at a relatively low left atrial pressure and maintaining the integrity of the lungs. Diastolic suction is particularly important in patients with mitral stenosis who have an elevated LAP even when the myocardium is normal. The loss of elastic recoil in these patients is harmful. Because LAP is low in the normal heart at rest, the physiologic value of suction is most evident during exercise.

REFERENCES

1. Da Vinci L: Corpus of the anatomical studies of Leonardo Da Vinci. *In* The Collection of Her Majesty the Queen at Windsor Castle, Vol 2. p 654. Edited by K.D. Keele and C. Pedretti. London, Johnson Reprint Co, Ltd., 1978–1980, p. 654.
2. Harvey W: An anatomical disquisition on the motion of the heart and blood in animals. *In* Classics of Medicine and Surgery. Edited by Camac CNB. New York, Dover Publications, Inc., p. 106.
3. Cohn AE: The development of the Harveian circulation. The Harvey Lectures 1927–1928. Baltimore, The Williams and Wilkins Co, 1929.
4. Henderson Y: The volume curve of the ventricles of the mammalian heart, and the significance of this curve in respect to the mechanics of the heart-beat and the filling of the ventricles. Am J Physiol 16:325, 1906.
5. Katz LN: The role played by the ventricular relaxation process in filling the ventricle. Am J Physiol 95:542, 1930.
6. Wiggers CJ: Studies on the cardiodynamic action of drugs. I. The application of optical methods of pressure registration in the study of cardiac stimulants and depressants. J Pharmacol Exper Ther, 30:217, 1927.
7. Wiggers CJ: Studies on the cardiodynamic action of drugs. II. The mechanism of cardiac stimulation by epinephrine. J Pharmacol Exper Ther, 30:233, 1927.
8. Bloom WL, Ferris EB: Elastic recoil of the heart as a factor in diastolic filling. Trans Assoc Am Physicians 69:200, 1956.
9. Fowler NO, Couves C, Bewick J: Effect of inflow obstruction and rapid bleeding on ventricular diastolic pressure. J Thorac Surg 35:532, 1957.
10. Brecher GA: Critical review of recent work on ventricular diastolic suction. Circ Res 6:554, 1958.
11. Brecher GA: Experimental evidence of ventricular diastolic suction. Circ Res 4:513, 1956.
12. Brecher GA, Kissen AT: Relation of negative intraventricular pressure to ventricular volume. Circ Res 5:157, 1957.
13. Brecher GA, Kissen AT: Ventricular diastolic suction at normal arterial pressures. Circ Res 6:100, 1958.
14. Brecher GA, Kolder H, Horres AD: Ventricular volume of nonbeating excised dog

hearts in the state of elastic equilibrium. Circ Res 19:1080, 1966.

15. Wiggers CJ: Cardiac mechanisms that limit operation of ventricular suction. Science 126:1237, 1957.

16. Tyberg JV, Keon WJ, Sonnenblick EH, Urschel CW: Mechanics of ventricular diastole. Cardiovasc Res 4:423, 1970.

17. Sonnenblick EH: The structural basis and importance of restoring forces and elastic recoil for the filling of the heart. Eur Heart J 1(Suppl A):107, 1980.

18. Sonnenblick EH, et al.: Ultrastructure of the heart in systole and diastole: Changes in sarcomere length. Circ Res 21:423, 1967.

19. Backx PMY, de Tombe PP, ter Keurs HE: Restoring forces in rat cardiac trabeculae. Circulation 78:II-68, 1988.

20. Krueger JW: Rapid relengthening in isolated cardiac cells and the origin of diastolic recoil. *In* Cardiac Mechanics and Function in the Normal and Diseased Heart. Edited by M Hori, et al. Tokyo, Springer-Verlag, 1989.

21. Yellin EL, Nikolic S, Frater RWM: LV filling dynamics and diastolic function. Prog Cardiovasc Dis 32:247, 1990.

22. Thomas JD, et al.: Physical and physiological determinants of transmitral velocity: Numerical analysis. Am J Physiol 260(Heart Circ. Physiol. 29):H1718, 1991.

23. Nolan SP, et al.: Left ventricular filling and diastolic pressure-volume relations in the conscious dog. Circ Res 24:269, 1969.

24. Laniado S, et al: Temporal relation of the first heart sound to closure of the mitral valve. Circulation 47:1006, 1973.

25. Courtois M, Kovacs SJ, Jr, Ludbrook PA: Transmitral pressure-flow velocity relation. Importance of regional pressure gradients in the left ventricle during diastole. Circulation 78:661, 1988.

26. Kovacs SJ, Jr, Barzilai B, Perez JE: Evaluation of diastolic function with Doppler echocardiography: The PDF formalism. Am J Physiol 252(Heart Circ. Physiol. 21):H178, 1987.

27. Yellin EL, Meisner JS, Nikolic SD, Keren G: The scientific basis for the relations between pulsed-doppler transmitral velocity patterns and left heart chamber properties. Echocardiography 9:313, 1992.

28. Kennish A, Yellin EL, Frater RWM: Dynamic stiffness profiles in the left ventricle. J Appl Phyisol 39:665, 1975.

29. Rankin JS, et al.: Viscoelastic properties of the diastolic left ventricle in the conscious dog. Circ Res 41:37, 1977.

30. Nickolic S, et. al.: Diastolic viscous properties of the canine left ventricle. Circ Res 67:352, 1990.

31. Stevenson-Smith W, et al.: The left ventricular end diastolic pressure may *not* be uniquely related to the end diastolic volume in heart failure. (Abstract) JACC 17:376A, 1991.

32. Ishida Y, et al.: Left ventricular filling dynamics: Influence of left ventricular relaxation and left atrial pressure. Circulation 74:187, 1986.

33. Brutsaert DL, Sys ST: Relaxation and diastole of the heart. Physiol Rev 69:1228, 1989.

34. Zile MR, Gaasch WH: Mechanical loads and the isovolumic and filling indices of left ventricular relaxation. Prog Cardiovasc Dis 32:333, 1990.

35. Lew WVW, Lewinter MM: Regional circumferential lengthening patterns in canine left ventricle. Am J Physiol 245:H741, 1983.

36. Gaasch WH, Blaustein AS, Bing OHL: Asynchronous (segmental early) relaxation of the left ventricle. J Am Coll Cardiol 5:891, 1985.

37. Bertha BG, Folts JD: Phasic mitral blood flow and regional left ventricular dimensions: possible mechanism of active assist to ventricular filling. Circulation 74:901, 1986.

38. Buchalter MB, et al.: Non-invasive quantification of left ventricular rotational deformation in normal humans using magnetic resonance myocardial tagging. Circulation 81:1236, 1990.

39. Yun KL, et al.: Alterations in left ventricular diastolic twist mechanics during acute human cardiac allograft rejection. Circulation 83:962, 1991.

40. Nikolic S, et al.: Relationship between diastolic shape (eccentricity) and passive elastic properties in the canine left ventricle. Am J Physiol 259:(Heart Circ. Physiol. 28):H457, 1990.

41. Robinson TF, Factor SM, Sonnenblick EH: The heart as a suction pump. Sci Am 254:84, 1986.

42. Yellin EL, et al.: Left ventricular relaxation in the filling and nonfilling intact canine heart. Am J Physiol 250(Heart Circ Physiol 19):H620, 1986.

43. Hori M, Yellin EL, Sonnenblick EH: Left ventricular diastolic suction as a mechanism of ventricular filling. Jpn Circ J 46(1):124, 1982.

44. Nikolic S, et al.: Passive properties of canine left ventricle: diastolic stiffness and restoring forces. Circ Res 62:1210, 1988.

45. Nikolic S, et al.: Effect of early diastolic loading on myocardial relaxation in the intact canine left ventricle. Circ Res 66:1217, 1990.

46. Carroll L: Through the Looking Glass and What Alice Found There. Berkley, University of California Press, 1983, p. 66.
47. Sabbah HN, Stein PD: Pressure-diameter relations during early diastole in dogs: incompatibility with the concept of passive left ventricular filling. Circ Res 48:357, 1981.
48. Weiss JL, Frederiksen JW, Weisfeldt ML: Hemodynamic determinants of the time-course of fall in canine left ventricular pressure. J Clin Invest 58:751, 1976.
49. Pasipoularides A, Mirsky I, Hess O: Myocardial relaxation and passive diastolic properties in man. Circulation 74:991, 1986.
50. Cheng C-P, Igarashi Y, Little WC: Mechanism of augmented rate of left ventricular filling during exercise. Circ Res 70:9, 1992.
51. Udelson JE, Bacharach SL, Cannon RO III, Bonow RO: Minimum LV pressure during beta-adrenergic stimulation in human subjects: evidence for elastic recoil and diastolic "suction" in the normal heart. Circulation 82:1174, 1990.
52. Cheng C-P, et al.: Effect of loading conditions, contractile state, and heart rate on early diastolic left ventricular filling in conscious dogs. Circ Res 66:814, 1990.
53. Suga H, et al.: Ventricular suction under zero source pressure for filling. Am J Physiol 251:H47, 1986.
54. Keren G, et al.: Inter-relationship of mid-diastolic mitral valve motion, pulmonary venous flow, and transmitral flow. Circulation 74:36, 1986.
55. Keren G, et al.: Time variation of mitral regurgitation flow in dilated cardiomyopathy. Circulation 74:684, 1986.
56. Meisner JS, et al.: Atrial contribution to ventricular filling in mitral stenosis. Circulation 84:1469, 1991.

Chapter 6

INFLUENCE OF THE PERICARDIUM AND VENTRICULAR INTERACTION ON DIASTOLIC FUNCTION

Martin M. LeWinter, Eivind E. S. P. Myhre, and Bryan K. Slinker

The two cardiac ventricles share a common interventricular septum and muscle fibers in their free walls. In addition, they are enclosed by the pericardium. As a result, the chambers of the heart interact directly during diastole. This interaction is modified by the pericardium because the diastolic volume of a ventricle, which constitutes a major determinant of the extent to which that ventricle influences or interacts with the diastolic function of the contralateral ventricle, is also a component of the total heart volume, and therefore of the extent to which the entire heart deforms the pericardium. Of course, the converse is also true, in that the influence of the pericardium on diastolic function is invariably linked to ventricular volume and, hence, ventricular interaction. These two closely coupled phenomena are discussed in separate sections, but the reader should realize that the effects of the pericardium and ventricular interaction on diastolic function are not easily separable. (See Chap. 4.)

THE NORMAL PERICARDIUM

Characteristics of the Pericardial Tissue

The major structural component of the parietal pericardium is collagen, arranged in bundles (1–3). On both light and electron microscopy, at presumptively physiologic levels of stretch, the collagen bundles appear wavy, with a complex, multilayered orientation. It is likely that the material properties of the pericardium are closely linked to these collagen bundles which, on

stretching, presumably render the pericardium easily extensible until such a point as the bundles straighten and the tissue then becomes relatively inextensible.

Studies of the material properties of isolated samples of pericardial tissue (3–8) have generally demonstrated the features described previously; i.e., at low levels of applied tension the tissue is easily extensible, but becomes inextensible relatively abruptly at higher levels of applied tension. An example of this sort of behavior is shown in Figure 6–1. In relation to the ability of the pericardium to restrain filling of the heart, it is of interest that the tensile strength of pericardial tissue is similar to that of rubber (4).

In addition to these static material properties, the pericardial tissue manifests a modest amount of stress relaxation following a rapid stretch, i.e., a gradual decrease in tension at constant length (7, 8). The converse of stress relaxation, creep, or gradual elongation following an abrupt stretch with tension subsequently held constant, appears to be negligible (7, 8). These properties suggest that, when the volume of the pericardial sac increases to a point that the tissue is rendered relatively inextensible, the pericardium should produce major resistance to additional increments in its volume, i.e., a restraining effect on the volume of the heart. This restraining effect should be mitigated to the extent that stress relaxation/creep occurs.

The relationship between pressure and volume in the pericardial sac more or less parallels the behavior that would be expected based on the isolated tissue characteristics described above (9, 10). At small volumes, the pressure-volume relation is

Supported by NIH grant no. HL35309. Dr. Slinker is an Established Investigator of the American Heart Association.

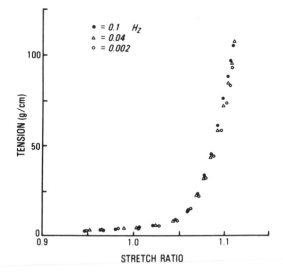

Fig. 6–1. Relation between stretch and applied tension in isolated canine parietal pericardium. Reproduced with permission from Lee MC, LeWinter MM, Freeman G, Shabetai R, Fung YC: Biaxial mechanical properties of the pericardium in normal and volume overload dogs. Am J Physiol 249:H422, 1985.

flat, but becomes steep at larger volumes with a relatively sharp transition between the flat and steep portions. This transition between a very compliant and a relatively noncompliant pericardial sac is made at hydrostatic pressures on the order of 3 to 8 mm Hg. Further, the transition is likely to be made at a heart volume at the higher end of the physiologic range, i.e., there is

relatively little pericardial reserve volume. It is important to note, however, that the pericardium has attachments to adjoining structures (for instance, a ligament connecting it to the diaphragm) and that the in situ heart and pericardium are, of course, enclosed within the cardiac fossa, consisting of the lungs and mediastinal structures surrounded by the bony thorax. These external attachments and surrounding structures undoubtedly modify the influence of the pericardium on diastolic function (11, 12). The precise details of this modification, however, are uncertain.

Although the ability of the pericardium to accommodate an increase in volume without a marked increase in pressure is limited over the short term, long-term adjustments can be prominent. Indeed, in clinical, dilated heart disease, in which total heart volume can be several times normal, some sort of chronic pericardial adaptation is mandatory. Thus, as shown in Figure 6–2, in experimental chronic cardiac dilation, the pressure-volume relation of the pericardium shifts markedly to the right and its slope decreases, indicating an increase in pericardial rest volume and compliance (9). This alteration is most likely to be related to growth of the pericardium, along with a change in the properties of the tissue itself (7, 9). As might be expected, this change in the behavior of the pericardium is associated with a change in its influence on the filling of the heart (13), as discussed in more detail as follows.

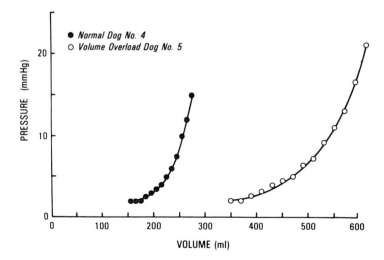

Fig. 6–2. The pressure-volume relation of the pericardium in dogs under normal conditions on the left and after a period of cardiac dilation resulting from a chronic abdominal aortic arteriovenous fistula on the right. Reproduced with permission from Freeman G, LeWinter M: Pericardial adaptations during chronic cardiac dilation in dogs. Circ Res 54: 294, 1984.

The Concept of the Pericardial Contact Pressure

Certain early studies suggested a significant restraining role for the pericardium in relation to the filling of the heart (14–17). However, other early investigations based on pericardial pressure measurements came to different conclusions (18–20). In the latter investigations, the space between the parietal and visceral pericardia was considered to be continuously fluid-filled. Accordingly, force between the two surfaces was considered in terms of a hydrostatic pressure, and measured through fluid-filled catheters inserted in the pericardial space. In these studies, the pericardial pressure was found to be near zero (similar to the adjacent intrapleural pressure) and changed little as the volume of the heart was changed. Therefore, it was concluded that the pericardium had a negligible influence on cardiac filling. Recently, however, it has become clear that the actual effective force between the parietal and visceral pericardium is best considered a contact force, analogous to the contact forces in the pleural space (21–28). To better understand this concept, Tyberg and coworkers have pointed out that if the parietal pericardium were a net with holes, it could still exert a force on the surface of the heart that restrains filling despite the fact that there would be no possibility of a hydrostatic pressure. This being the case, it is more appropriate to assess this force by making measurements with low profile, flattened balloons. Using such balloons, the magnitude of the pericardial pressure has been found to be greater than that measured with fluid-filled catheters and of a magnitude that is more consistent with observed alterations in the diastolic pressure-volume relation of the cardiac chambers following removal of the pericardium (13, 16, 21–36). Indeed, studies by Tyberg and coworkers (21–23, 26) and Boltwood et al. (24) using flat balloons implanted adjacent to the free wall of the right ventricle have revealed a magnitude of pericardial pressure similar to or slightly less than the right atrial or right ventricular diastolic pressure. Further, with increases in heart volume, the right ventricular and pericardial pressures increase with a one-to-one rela-

tionship (21–23, 26, 27). These data indicate an extremely important influence of the pericardium on right ventricular filling. Our own studies (11, 12, 25, 27) using flattened balloons of a different design are fundamentally in agreement with those of Tyberg et al., although our data suggest that the absolute level of pericardial pressure is on the order of 1 to 3 mm Hg lower.

The aforementioned marked difference in pericardial pressure measured with fluid-filled catheters and flat balloons in and of itself supports the concept of a contact pressure. Our studies of regional deformation of the in vivo pericardium (25, 27, 28) further support this notion. We have found a very dynamic deformation pattern that (1) qualitatively parallels the volume changes occurring in the adjacent chambers (atrium versus ventricle) and (2) is largely eliminated by infusion of fluid into the pericardial space, which effectively removes any contact force. Both of these features strongly support the contact force concept.

Regional variations also appear to exist in the pericardial pressure over the left and right ventricles when measured with flat balloons (26, 27). These occur during hemodynamic transients (26, 27), for instance, abrupt alterations in ventricular loading, as well as under certain steady-state conditions (27). Although it is possible that flattened balloon devices result in artifacts in pressure measurement, measurements of pericardial deformation over the right and left ventricles (12) demonstrate regional variations that are consistent with these regional variations in intrapericardial pressure. It is not clear whether regional variation in pericardial pressure influences cardiac filling, but its presence challenges the usual concept of a transmural filling pressure for the cardiac chambers. If the pericardial pressure varies by region, there is obviously no uniform transmural pressure for each of the cardiac chambers.

INFLUENCE OF THE PERICARDIUM ON THE DIASTOLIC PRESSURE-VOLUME RELATION

The most direct way to assess the effect of the pericardium on filling of the heart is to determine the relation between diastolic pressure and volume (or, as a surrogate, a dimension) before and after pericardiectomy. The extent to which this relation is shifted downward, i.e., to which pericardiectomy renders the cardiac chamber of interest more distensible, is a measure of the effective force normal to the surface of the heart, which is imposed by the parietal pericardium and which restrains the filling of the heart. An example of this downward shift is shown in Figure 6–3. It should be recalled, however, that a portion of any change in the pressure-volume relation following pericardiectomy is caused by re-

moval of the direct effect of the pericardium on the surface of the heart and a portion is indirect and related to alterations in the magnitude of diastolic ventricular interaction occurring after pericardiectomy. In general, analyses of the pressure-volume relation before and after pericardiectomy can be performed in two ways: (1) under quasistatic equilibrium conditions (e.g., at end diastole) over a specified range of diastolic pressure, or (2) over the course of a single filling cycle, from atrioventricular valve opening to atrioventricular valve closure. There has been considerable experimental assessment of the influence of the pericardium on filling under quasistatic conditions at end diastole, most of which has been performed in open-chest dogs (13, 16, 21, 29–34, 36–38). The results of these experiments have been variable, with some (16, 21, 31) suggesting an extremely important influence of the pericardium on the left ventricular end-diastolic pressure-volume relation, even at physiologic levels of filling pressure, and others (37, 38) suggesting the opposite. The reasons for these variable results are almost certainly related to methodologic differences in obtaining these data, and lie in the following areas. First, variability has been found in handling the pericardium, which in most such studies must be disrupted in some way to make measurements of left ventricular volumes and/or dimensions. It is clear that large pericardial incisions that are tightly reapproximated artifactually augment the restraining influence of the pericardium on filling of the heart (32). Second, the means by which the volume of the heart chambers is varied to generate the pressure-volume relation is critical. It is not surprising that variation of steady-state intravascular volume, for instance by infusing intravenous fluids, provides a different impression of the influence of the pericardium compared to beat-to-beat variation in volume obtained by transient obstruction of venous return to the right heart. Under the latter conditions, the normal, steady-state relationship of left and right heart volume is disturbed by the relatively selective decrease in right heart volume, and any effect of the pericardium is likely to be minimized (37). Third, the status of the surrounding structures

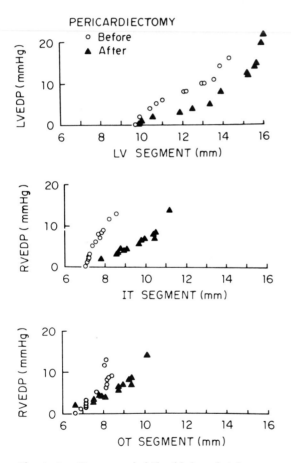

Fig. 6–3. Downward shift of left and right ventricular pressure-dimension relations following pericardiectomy in the dog. For the right ventricle, dimensions are displayed for both the inflow and outflow tracts. Reproduced with permission from Assanelli D, Lew WYW, Shabetai R, LeWinter MM: Influence of the pericardium on right and left ventricular filling in the dog. J Appl Physiol 63: 1025, 1987.

and the chest wall is likely to be an important component. Studies assessing the influence of the pericardium on filling have varied from those performed with the chest extensively opened to those performed with the chest undisturbed. As indicated previously, the pericardium has connections to adjoining structures, including the ligamentous attachment to the diaphragm. Further, under certain conditions, for example positive end-expiratory pressure, the lungs contained within the rigid thoracic cavity can add to any external pressure acting on the surface of the heart (11). We have also shown that the pericardium itself appears to be less distensible when the chest is widely opened, compared to when it is intact (12). This suggests that, when the chest is opened, the pericardial attachments and adjoining structures exert a greater stretch or "tethering" effect on the pericardial sac. Finally, methodologic differences with respect to the techniques of measurement of cardiac chamber pressures and volumes or dimensions also contribute to the variation in these studies.

With this background in mind, several studies (13, 30, 32, 34, 36, 38) have used a methodology that allows no or minimal disruption of the pericardium and protocols in which normal steady-state volume relationships between the chambers have been maintained. These studies indicate that, in the open-chest dog, the pericardium has a very modest effect on left and right ventricular diastolic pressure-volume relations at both less than physiologic and physiologic cardiac volumes. At volumes approaching the upper end of the physiologic range, this effect begins to increase in importance and increases substantially as cardiac volumes exceed the physiologic range. In contrast, with the chest and thoracic cavity undisturbed, Applegate et al. (38) have reported that the effect of the pericardium on left ventricular filling *at physiologic volumes* appears to be essentially undetectable (38). This result is consistent with our finding that the pericardium itself is more distensible when the chest cavity is intact (12). However, Applegate et al. (38) analyzed the left ventricular pressure-volume relation with the chest undisturbed before pericardiectomy, but opened after pericardiectomy. Thus, the results obtained were from both pericardiectomy and thoracotomy, not pericardiectomy alone. We are unaware of any information describing the effect of the pericardium on the *right ventricular* diastolic pressure-volume relation with an intact chest cavity.

It should also be noted that the influence of the pericardium is quantitatively different for the left and right ventricles (34, 36). This is mainly because the right ventricle is much more compliant than the left. Therefore, at any level of pericardial pressure, there is a larger proportional effect on right ventricular filling. Thus, in the open-chest, diastolic-arrested heart, the pericardium accounts for two thirds or more of the right ventricular pressure at greater than physiologic volumes, but only 30 to 40% of left ventricular pressure (36). Furthermore, if regional variations in pericardial pressure are meaningful (26, 27), this may also result in different effects on the left and right ventricles.

Little is known about the magnitude of the pericardial influence on filling of the normal human heart. Of necessity, studies involving pericardiectomy or direct pressure measurements must be confined to the operating room. One investigation using radionuclide-derived ventricular volumes and the pulmonary capillary wedge pressure as a measure of left ventricular filling pressures suggested minimal or no effect of pericardiectomy on the normal heart (39). However, this type of methodology is unavoidably crude. Measurements of pericardial pressure in patients using flattened balloon devices (22, 24) have yielded results similar to those obtained in the dog, suggesting a comparable influence. We are unaware of any methodologically acceptable direct studies of the influence of pericardiectomy on the diastolic pressure-volume relation of the human left or right ventricle.

It is also theoretically possible that the pericardium could influence nonstatic aspects of filling of the normal heart, although little data are available to date. A key determinant of the rate of ventricular filling following mitral or tricuspid valve opening is the atrioventricular pressure gradient, which is determined in a complex fashion by atrial reservoir and transport functions, ventricular relaxation rate, and the extent of elastic recoil of the ventricle (40). Immediately before atrioventricular valve opening, the atrial volume is largest and therefore, to the extent that the pericardium exerts a local contact force on the cardiac chambers, the restraining influence of the pericardium on the atrium is also largest (28). At this time, the ventricular volume is smallest, thereby resulting in a minimum influence of the pericardium on the ventricle (28). It is therefore possible that the intact pericardium could influence the atrioventricular pressure gradient by virtue of having its largest differential effect on the intracavitary atrial and ventricular pressure at the time of atrioventricular valve opening, augmenting both the gradient and early diastolic filling. A few studies (38, 41) have in fact examined the influence of the pericardium on dynamic mitral flow and left ventricular filling patterns and have not demonstrated major effects, when normalized to end-diastolic pressure or volume. However, no information is normalized to the cardiac volumes present at this time of the cycle, e.g., end-systolic volume for the ventricles, and this would seem the appropriate normalization in comparing filling patterns before and after pericardiectomy. Thus, this is an area worthy of additional investigation.

VENTRICULAR INTERACTION

In general terms, ventricular interaction refers to the influence of the performance of one cardiac chamber on the performance of other chambers. We will focus on *direct* interaction effects, as opposed to series interaction, whereby a change in the output on one side of the heart influences filling of the other side. Ventricle-ventricle interaction has received virtually all of the attention of investigators in this field, but it should be kept in mind that atrium-ventricle and atrium-atrium interactions have also been demonstrated, at least in the arrested heart (42). Ventricle-ventricle interaction occurs in both diastole and systole. For obvious reasons, we are most concerned with diastole but, as will be seen, systolic ventricular interaction may also influence filling dynamics. Finally, as discussed previously, it is important to reiterate the close links between diastolic

ventricular interaction and the influence of the pericardium on filling.

It has been recognized for many years that the level of filling pressure and volume of one ventricle influences the distensibility of the contralateral ventricle (31, 33, 43–54). The most straightforward explanation of this phenomenon is related to the fact that the interventricular septum represents a substantial portion of the surface area of each ventricle. The external force acting on this portion of the ventricle in diastole is obviously equal to the pressure in the contralateral ventricle. The net effective external force acting on each ventricle is thus a result of the combination of the pericardial pressure acting on the free wall and the pressure acting on the septum from the contralateral ventricle. In addition, continuous, shared fiber bundles connect the interventricular septum to both left and right ventricular free walls and both free walls to each other. A portion of diastolic interaction may be related to stretch and deformation of these shared fibers (52, 55, 56). Recently, Watanabe and coworkers (57) have provided evidence that right-to-left diastolic ventricular interaction may also be mediated by changes in coronary sinus pressure, which in turn is a determinant of myocardial turgor, or that portion of ventricular compliance related to the erectile effect produced by the blood contained in the coronary vasculature in the walls of the heart.

Taylor et al. (44), in their classic paper, characterized diastolic ventricular interaction in terms of the passive or fully relaxed pressure-volume relation of the ventricles. Using a left or right heart bypass preparation, the volume of one ventricle was fixed and the end-diastolic pressure-volume relation of the contralateral ventricle determined; this procedure was repeated after systematically varying the level of fixed volume. As shown in Figure 6–4, upward and leftward shifts of the pressure-volume relation were demonstrated as the volume in the fixed volume ventricle was increased. Thus, the passive compliance of a ventricle decreases in proportion to the volume of the contralateral ventricle. The change in compliance occurring for a given change in volume is a quantitative measure of direct diastolic interaction.

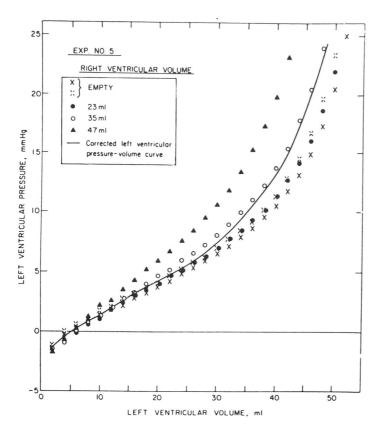

Fig. 6–4. Left ventricular diastolic pressure-volume relation at varying levels of right ventricular filling in the dog. Reproduced with permission from Taylor RR, Covell JW, Sonnenblick EH, Ross J Jr: Dependence of ventricular distensibility on filling of the opposite ventricle. Am J Physiol 213:711, 1967.

The study of Taylor et al. (44) was performed without the pericardium. Diastolic ventricular interaction is markedly amplified when the pericardium is intact (31, 33, 42, 51, 54), because changes in ventricular pressure and volume are associated with directionally similar changes in pericardial pressure, i.e., both components of the external pressure are altered. Quantifying diastolic ventricular interaction using the approach of Taylor et al. (44) and others requires the ability to fix the volume of one ventricle while varying the volume of the other ventricle. This, of course, presents considerable obstacles for quantitative assessment in the intact, beating heart. There are, however, approaches available that allow relatively selective changes in the volume of one ventricle, the best example being transient occlusion of the caval vessels, which results initially in a decrease in right heart volume out of proportion to changes in left heart volume (52–54, 58). Ultimately, of course, the left heart volume must also decrease as a function of the de-

creased right ventricular stroke volume which occurs during this maneuver (a series interaction). In any case, this approach, combined with a statistical treatment to separate direct from series interaction related to left heart underfilling caused by the decreased right ventricular stroke volume, has been used to quantify direct, diastolic ventricular interaction in the intact animal (52, 53, 58). We have also used a somewhat different approach to assess direct diastolic ventricular interaction in the intact heart with intact pericardium, namely, abrupt, single-beat hemodynamic transients (54). By using only the first beat following an abrupt intervention, this approach allows the experimental measurement of direct interaction effects without the confounding influence of series effects. An example is shown in Figure 6–5. In this case, a hemodynamic transient is produced by decreasing right heart volume during a single diastole by sucking out blood while simultaneously preventing right heart venous return (caval occlusion). This results

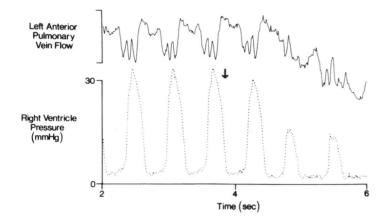

Fig. 6–5. Effects of an abrupt decrease in right heart volume on ventricular pressures and pulmonary venous flow in the dog. Reproduced with permission from Slinker BK, Goto Y, LeWinter MM: Direct diastolic interaction gain measured with sudden hemodynamic transients. Am J Physiol 256:H567, 1989.

in a sudden decrease in right ventricular end-diastolic pressure compared to the previous beat and a simultaneous, smaller decrease in left ventricular end-diastolic pressure despite the fact that left ventricular volume is unaltered at this time. Thus, left ventricular distensibility is increased by the decrease in right heart volume and pressure, i.e., direct diastolic ventricular interaction. Note that pulmonary venous flow begins to decrease as early as the very next systole, i.e., the series interaction effect occurs very rapidly. Using this approach, we have quantified these results as *right-to-left* interaction gain, or the change in left ventricular end-diastolic pressure occurring for a given change in right ventricular end-diastolic pressure. Interaction gain has averaged about 0.33 in our stud-

ies, and appears independent of the absolute level of filling pressure.

We have also made preliminary attempts to assess *left-to-right* interaction gain using hemodynamic transients, in this case either abrupt suction of blood from the left heart or an abrupt increase in afterload produced by inflating a balloon in the thoracic aorta during diastole. Our preliminary results suggest that left-to-right diastolic interaction gain is similar to right-to-left gain (59). It is also of interest that these abrupt left heart hemodynamic perturbations appear to directly influence right heart venous return (60). Thus, as shown in Figure 6–6, a small decrease in caval flow occurs in conjunction with abrupt aortic balloon inflation. The mechanism and significance of these apparent interactions between the

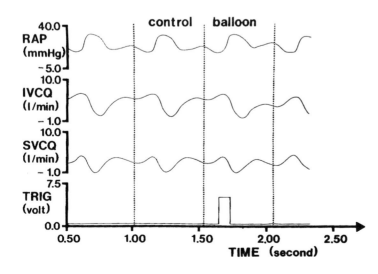

Fig. 6–6. Effect of an abrupt increase in afterload (aortic balloon inflation) on caval flow (see text). Trig channel indicates timing of balloon inflation. Note modest reduction in caval flow immediately following inflation. RAP = right atrial pressure; IVCQ, SVCQ = inferior and superior vena caval flows.

left ventricle (or left heart) and right heart venous return are unclear at present. Nonetheless, they represent a previously unappreciated, dynamic aspect of cardiac chamber (or in this case perhaps chamber-cava) interaction.

Finally, we have shown that systolic interaction can influence ventricular relaxation (61). As shown in Figure 6–7, by using an abrupt pulmonary artery constriction to increase right ventricular afterload, we have demonstrated a small but consistent augmentation in left ventricular performance on the same contraction, i.e., direct, right-to-left systolic interaction, manifested as an increase in left ventricular developed pressure and stroke volume. During relaxation, the time constant of left ventricular pressure fall (tau) is prolonged, indicating a direct effect of increased right ventricular afterload, which slows left ventricular relaxation. The mechanism of this effect is unclear but may be related to either prolongation of the time course of right ventricular contraction and relaxation, so that direct transmission of right ventricular pressure across the septum modifies left ventricular pressure during relaxation (61), or regional left ventricular lengthening inhomogeneities introduced during the beat following the pulmonary artery constriction beat (61, 62). In any case, this is another example of a dynamic, previously unrecognized manifestation of cardiac chamber interaction.

Few attempts have been made to study ventricular interaction in the normal human heart. However, Ludbrook and co-workers (63) have used nitroglycerin and amyl nitrate to assess diastolic ventricular interaction in the cardiac catheterization laboratory. The transient hemodynamic response to these drugs includes early systemic venodilation and, most likely, an asymmetric (right > left) decrease in cardiac volume, which in turn results in changes in the left ventricular pressure-volume relation consistent with an alteration in the magnitude of diastolic ventricular interaction.

INFLUENCE OF THE PERICARDIUM AND VENTRICULAR INTERACTION ON FILLING IN DISEASE STATES

Whenever the total heart volume increases, there is a possibility of an increased influence of the pericardium and diastolic ventricular interaction on cardiac filling, to the extent that any such increase in volume exceeds the capacity of the pericardium to accommodate it. As indicated previously, the pericardium has a very limited capacity to accommodate a rapidly increasing cardiac volume, i.e., its "reserve" volume is ordinarily rather small. However, with a prolonged increase in cardiac volume, we have shown that the pressure-volume relation of the pericardium becomes markedly shifted to the right and flatter, or more compliant,

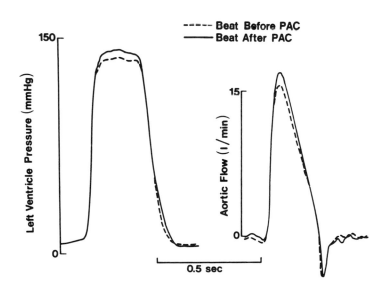

Fig. 6–7. Effect of an abrupt pulmonary artery constriction on right ventricular function, demonstrating a slowing of the rate of pressure fall in the left ventricle. Reproduced with permission from Slinker BK, Goto Y, LeWinter MM: Systolic direct ventricular interaction affects left ventricular contraction and relaxation in the intact dog circulation. Circ Res 65: 307, 1989.

than normal (9). As would be expected, this is associated with a decrease in the influence of the pericardium on filling (13). It is expected that such an alteration in the behavior of the pericardium would also tend to normalize the magnitude of diastolic ventricular interaction, because of the link between the two.

In addition to alterations in the behavior of the pericardium occurring in response to a chronic increase in the volume contained within the pericardial sac, cardiac muscle hypertrophy produces chronic alterations in the properties of the walls of the heart that can influence the magnitude of ventricular interaction. Thus, Little et al. (58) have shown that, in experimental right ventricular pressure overload (without an intact pericardium), diastolic ventricular interaction is reduced in magnitude. Slinker et al. (64) have demonstrated a similar finding in experimental left ventricular pressure overload (both with and without the pericardium).

Although most quantitative information about the effect of the pericardium and ventricular interaction on diastolic filling in the normal heart has been obtained from experimental animal studies, there is a substantial amount of clinical information available in regard to pathologic situations in which the pericardium and ventricular interaction appear to play an important role in cardiac filling. Unlike animal experiments, however, in which it is possible to more directly quantify this influence, the data in these clinical studies is largely inferential. In general, two lines of evidence suggest an enhanced role for the pericardium and ventricular interaction in these clinical studies. One, acute shifts in the diastolic pressure-volume relation in response to vasoactive drugs have been observed (65–68). In clinical studies, such shifts are almost invariably detected for single beats or over a limited range of diastolic pressure and volume, in contrast to animal experiments in which it is often possible to generate a very wide range of pressure and volume. Two, in some cases, hemodynamics suggestive of constrictive pericarditis have been observed (69–72). This, of course, suggests a situation in which the heart volume has enlarged so much that the pericardium is on an extremely steep portion of

its own pressure-volume relation. With this background in mind, we will briefly discuss some of these clinical situations.

Perhaps the earliest recognition that an alteration in diastolic ventricular interaction may have contributed to heart failure was the Bernheim syndrome (73). The basic criteria described for the Bernheim syndrome were evidence of left ventricular hypertrophy, but not failure, in association with right heart failure, which was presumed to be related to obstruction to filling caused by the hypertrophied interventricular septum. In modern terms, the Bernheim syndrome appears somewhat obscure, and the extent to which an alteration in ventricular interaction actually played a role was never clarified. There is a well-established precedent for alterations in left heart filling pressures that occur as a result of increased right ventricular loading, for instance caused by lung disease (74–76) and positive end-expiratory pressure (PEEP) (77). Particularly in the case of PEEP, there is good experimental evidence of exaggerated ventricular interaction (78, 79), and it is not unreasonable to propose that exaggerated diastolic ventricular interaction plays a role in these clinical observations.

One of the earliest clinical reports of a possible exaggerated role of the pericardium in human disease was that published by Bartle and Herman (69), describing a small group of patients with *subacute,* severe mitral regurgitation. This group of patients demonstrated elevated and equal left and right heart filling pressures, one of the classic findings of constrictive pericarditis. Accordingly, they proposed that the rapid cardiac dilation occurring in these patients resulted in major pericardial restraint of filling, accounting for these hemodynamics. In an experimental study of the *immediate* effects of acute, severe mitral regurgitation (80), we could not detect any important increase in the pericardial contact pressure and in patients studied *acutely* following the abrupt development of severe mitral regurgitation, equilibration of filling pressures is not ordinarily observed. Furthermore, equalization of left and right heart filling pressures is also not ordinarily found in patients with *chronic* left ventricular volume overload lesions. This combination of observations suggests that not enough cardiac dilation occurs immediately after imposition of acute left-sided volume overload to result in an increase in the pericardial influence on filling, but that over some relatively short period of time the heart dilates more rapidly than the pericardium, resulting in a phase resembling restrictive pericarditis. If the pericardium is ultimately able to increase its volume by growth (9), as discussed previously, this would account for the subsequent loss of the hemodynamic findings associated with pericardial constriction during chronic volume overload.

Brodie et al. (66) have reported evidence for a significant role for the pericardium and ventricular interaction in patients with *chronic* left-sided volume overload lesions, although once again hemodynamics suggestive of constrictive pericarditis are not ordinarily encountered in such patients. In this study, the vasodilator nitroprusside was administered to patients with chronic aortic regurgitation and resulted in an increase in left ventricular diastolic distensibility, manifested as a downward displacement of the relation between pressure and volume. This was ascribed to relief of the external constraints imposed by both the pericardium and the right ventricle. As with nitrates (63), this argument requires that the vasodilator produce disproportionate changes in left and right heart volume, i.e., at any left ventricular volume, the right ventricle and the total cardiac volume must be smaller during administration of nitroprusside.

One of the best recognized examples of exaggerated effects of the pericardium and ventricular interaction occurs in patients with hemodynamically significant right ventricular myocardial infarction (70–72). These individuals almost invariably have simultaneous inferior or inferoposterior left ventricular myocardial infarction. They frequently have heart failure and cardiogenic shock on the basis of extensive right ventricular involvement. When they present in this fashion, it is common to observe hemodynamics similar in many respects to constrictive pericarditis, with elevation and equalization of right and left heart filling pressures and, occasionally, a right ventricular diastolic "dip and plateau sign," Kuss-

maul's sign, and a paradoxic pulse. In conjunction with this picture, the right heart dilates markedly and rapidly, resulting in a situation in which it is not difficult to envision exhaustion of the pericardial reserve volume.

In contrast, a hemodynamic picture suggestive of pericardial constriction is not observed in patients with exclusively left ventricular myocardial infarction. This is not to say that some alteration in the influence of the pericardium and ventricular interaction on filling may not occur in these patients, but that it is not extreme enough to result in such hemodynamic findings. This is likely to be related to the fact that the thick-walled, less compliant left ventricle, along with the left atrium, which is partially extra-pericardial, simply do not dilate acutely as much as the right ventricle and atrium when a myocardial infarction has occurred. Kass and coworkers (81) have published data obtained during percutaneous transluminal coronary angioplasty which suggest that exaggerated pericardial and ventricular interaction effects may cause acute elevations in diastolic pressure immediately following a total coronary occlusion. As shown in Figure 6–8, using a conductance catheter to measure on-line ventricular volume before, during, and after angioplasty, these investigators detected a transient, upward shift of the diastolic pressure-volume relation that appeared during the time when the angioplasty balloon was inflated. This decrease in diastolic distensibility could be prevented by a transient reduction in right heart venous return produced by inflating a balloon in the inferior vena cava. This finding suggests that in the elevated left ventricular diastolic pressure that occurs during the acute, total coronary occlusion is partly caused by ventricular interaction and pericardial effects, which are relieved by a selective reduction in right heart volume. Of course, in patients with acute myocardial infarction from a coronary occlusion, the coronary occlusion has ordinarily been present for a much longer time than that which pertains to the angioplasty situation.

Finally, Janicki (82) has presented intriguing evidence that the pericardium and ventricular interaction may play a role in

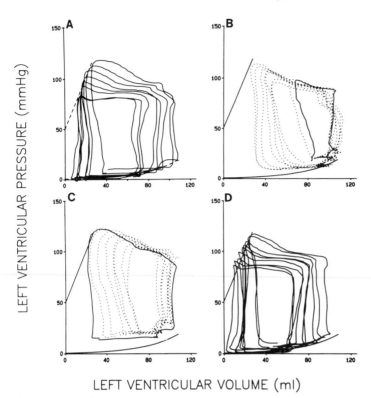

LEFT VENTRICULAR PRESSURE (mmHg)

LEFT VENTRICULAR VOLUME (ml)

Fig. 6–8. Left ventricular pressure-volume loops before, during, and after PTCA of the left anterior descending coronary artery. Panel A is a control series of pressure-volume loops obtained by partial occlusion of the inferior vena cava. Panel B was obtained during balloon inflation and demonstrates a rightward shift of the end-systolic pressure-volume relation along with an upward shift of the diastolic pressure-volume relation. Panel C was obtained immediately after balloon deflation and shows a return to normal of the end-systolic pressure-volume relation but a continuing elevation of the diastolic pressure-volume relation. Panel D is a series of pressure-volume loops recorded during partial caval occlusion following angioplasty, demonstrating a return to baseline conditions.

exercise limitation in patients with chronic, dilated heart failure with poor contractile function. It has been recognized for some time that routine measures of contractile function such as the ejection fraction are poor predictors of exercise performance in this group of patients. Janicki studied such patients during exercise with a flotation catheter in the pulmonary artery. He found that in some of these patients, as exercise progresses, the left and right heart filling pressures increase with a one-to-one relationship. This pattern of equal increases in filling pressure was correlated with both a plateau of the stroke volume and the onset of exercise-limiting symptoms. This combination of findings can be interpreted as indicating that these individuals depend more on dilation of the heart to maintain stroke volume during exercise. To the extent that the pericardium and its associated effects on ventricular interaction limit dilation of the cardiac chambers, and at the same time increase the filling pressures, this could result in exercise-limiting symptoms. Of course, many other factors may independently diminish exercise toler-

ance in these patients, for instance, the level of right ventricular function, exercise-induced abnormalities in relaxation, etc., but the possibility that the pericardium and ventricular interaction play a role is at least plausible.

In summary, then, an exaggerated effect of the pericardium and ventricular interaction on diastolic filling is very likely to play a prominent role in certain clinical syndromes in which marked and rapid dilation of the heart is associated with hemodynamic findings reminiscent of constrictive pericarditis. In other situations, a significant but less prominent role may be present when the heart dilates in response to various insults. The quantitative contribution of these effects in patients is difficult to establish, but may often be substantial and at least partly responsible for surprising and/or unexpected elevations in right or left heart filling pressures.

REFERENCES

1. Holt JP: The normal pericardium. Am J Cardiol 26:455, 1970.
2. Ishihara T, Ferrans VJ, Jones M, et al.: His-

tologic and ultrastructural features of normal human parietal pericardium. Am J Cardiol 46:744, 1980.

3. Wiegner AW, Bing OHL: Mechanical and structural correlates of canine pericardium. Circ Res 49:807, 1981.

4. Rabkin SW, Berghause DG, Bauer HF: Mechanical properties of the isolated canine pericardium. J Appl Physiol 36:69, 1974.

5. Lee JM, Boughner DR: Tissue mechanics of canine pericardium in different test environments. Circ Res 49:533, 1981.

6. Lee JM, Boughner DR: Mechanical properties of human pericardium. Differences in viscoelastic response compared with canine pericardium. Circ Res 55:475, 1985.

7. Lee MC, LeWinter MM, Freeman G, et al.: Biaxial mechanical properties of the pericardium in normal and volume overload dogs. Am J Physiol 249:H422, 1985.

8. Lee MC, Fung YC, Shabetai R, LeWinter MM: Biaxial mechanical properties of human pericardium and canine comparisons. Am J Physiol 252:H75, 1987.

9. Freeman G, LeWinter M: Pericardial adaptations during chronic cardiac dilation in dogs. Circ Res 54:294, 1984.

10. Freeman GL, Little WC: Comparison of in situ and in vitro studies of pericardial pressure-volume relation in dogs. Am J Physiol 251:H421, 1986.

11. Freeman G, LeWinter MM: Determinants of the intra-pericardial pressure in dogs. J Appl Physiol 60:758, 1986.

12. Watkins MW, Slinker BK, LeWinter MM: Regional variation of deformation in the canine pericardium. Circulation 80 (Suppl II): 178, 1989.

13. LeWinter M, Pavelec R: Influence of the pericardium on left ventricular end-diastolic pressure-segment length relations during early and later phases of experimental chronic volume overload in dogs. Circ Res 50:501, 1982.

14. Kuno Y: The significance of the pericardium. J Physiol 50:1, 1915.

15. Holt JP, Rhode EA, Kines H: Pericardial and ventricular pressure. Circ Res 8:1171, 1960.

16. Hefner LL, Coghlan HC, Jones WB, Reeves TJ: Distensibility of the dog left ventricle. Am J Physiol 201:97, 1961.

17. Bartle SH, Hermann HJ, Cavo JW, et al.: Effect of the pericardium on left ventricular volume and function in acute hypervolaemia. Cardiovasc Res 3:284, 1968.

18. Adamkiewicz A, Jacobson H: Ueber den Druck im Herzbeutel. Centralbl med Wissensch 11:483, 1873.

19. Morgan BC, Guntheroth WG, Dillard DH: Relationship of pericardial to pleural pressure during acute regurgitation and cardiac tamponade. Circ Res 16:493, 1965.

20. Kenner HM, Wood EH: Intrapericardial, intrapleural, and intracardiac pressures during acute heart failure in dogs studied without thoracotomy. Circ Res 19:1071, 1966.

21. Smiseth OA, Frais MA, Kingma I, et al.: Assessment of pericardial constraint in dogs. Circulation 71:158, 1985.

22. Tyberg JV, Taichman GC, Smith ER, et al.: The relationship between pericardial pressure and right atrial pressure: An intraoperative study. Circulation 73:428, 1986.

23. Smiseth OA, Frais MA, Kingma I, et al.: Assessment of pericardial constraint: the relation between right ventricular filling pressure and pericardial pressure measured after pericardiocentesis. J Am Coll Cardiol 7:307, 1986.

24. Boltwood GM, Skulsky A, Drinkwater DC, et al.: Intraoperative measurement of pericardial constraint: Role in ventricular diastolic mechanics. J Am Coll Cardiol 8:1289, 1986.

25. Mann D, Lew W, Ban-Hayashi E, Shabetai R, et al.: In vivo mechanical behavior of canine pericardium. Am J Physiol 251:H349, 1986.

26. Smiseth OA, Scott-Douglas NW, Thompson CR, et al.: Nonuniformity of pericardial surface pressure in dogs. Circulation 75: 1229, 1987.

27. Hoit BD, Lew WYW, LeWinter MM: Regional variation in pericardial contact pressure in the canine ventricle. Am J Physiol 255:H1370, 1988.

28. Goto Y, LeWinter MM: Nonuniform regional deformation of the pericardium during the cardiac cycle in dogs. Circ Res 47: 1107, 1990.

29. Spotnitz HM, Kaiser GA: The effect of the pericardium on pressure-volume relations in the canine left ventricle. J Surg Res 11: 375, 1971.

30. Shirato K, Shabetai R, Bhargava V, et al.: Alteration of the left ventricular diastolic pressure-segment length relation produced by the pericardium: effects of cardiac distension and afterload reduction in conscious dogs. Circulation 57:1191, 1978.

31. Glantz SA, Misbach GA, Moores WY, et al.: The pericardium substantially affects the left ventricular diastolic pressure-volume relationship in the dog. Circ Res 42:433, 1978.

32. Stokland O, Miller MM, LeKven J, Ilebekk A: The significance of the intact pericardium for cardiac performance in the dog. Circ Res 47:27, 1980.

33. Janicki JS, Weber KT: The pericardium and ventricular interaction, distensibility, and function. Am J Physiol 238 (Heart Circ Physiol 7): H494, 1980.

34. Assanelli D, Lew WYW, Shabetai R, LeWinter MM: Influence of the pericardium on right and left ventricular filling in the dog. J Appl Physiol 63:1025, 1987.

35. Santamore WP, Constantinescu M, Little WC: Direct assessment of right ventricular transmural pressure. Circulation 75:744, 1987.

36. Slinker BK, Ditchey RV, Bell SP, LeWinter MM: Right heart pressure does not equal pericardial pressure in the potassium chloride-arrested canine heart in situ. Circulation 76:357, 1987.

37. Tyson GS, Maier GW, Olsen CO, et al.: Pericardial influences on ventricular filling in the conscious dog: an analysis based on pericardial pressure. Circ Res 54:173, 1984.

38. Applegate RJ, Santamore WP, Klopfenstein HS, Little WC: External pressure of undisturbed left ventricle. Am J Physiol 258:H1079, 1990.

39. Mangano DT, Van Dyke DC, Hickey RF, Ellis RJ: Significance of the pericardium in human subjects: Effects on left ventricular volume, pressure and ejection. J Am Coll Cardiol 6:290, 1985.

40. Ishida Y, Meisner JS, Tsujioka K, et al.: Left ventricular filling dynamics: Influence of left ventricular relaxation and left atrial pressure. Circulation 74:187, 1986.

41. Hoit BD, Dalton N, Bhargava V, Shabetai R: Pericardial influences on right and left ventricular filling dynamics. Circ Res 68: 197, 1991.

42. Maruyama Y. Ashikawa K, Isoyama S, et al.: Mechanical interactions between four heart chambers with and without the pericardium in canine hearts. Circ Res 50:86, 1982.

43. Laks MM, Garner D, Swan HJC: Volumes and compliances measured simultaneously in the right and left ventricles of the dog. Circ Res 20:565, 1967.

44. Taylor RR, Covell JW, Sonnenblick EH, Ross J Jr: Dependence of ventricular distensibility on filling of the opposite ventricle. Am J Physiol 213:711, 1967.

45. Bemis CE, Serur JR, Borkenhagen D, et al.: Influence of right ventricular filling pressure on left ventricular pressure and dimension. Circ Res 34:498, 1974.

46. Elzinga G, van Grondelle R, Westerhof N, van den Bos GC: Ventricular interference. Am J Physiol 226:941, 1974.

47. Stool EW, Mullins CB, Leshin SJ, Mitchell JH: Dimensional changes of the left ventricle during acute pulmonary arterial hypertension in dogs. Am J Cardiol 33:868, 1974.

48. Santamore WP, Lynch PR, Meier G, et al.: Myocardial interaction between the ventricles. J Appl Physiol 41:362, 1976.

49. Maughan WL, Kallman CH, Shoukas A: The effect of right ventricular filling on the pressure-volume relationship of the ejecting canine left ventricle. Circ Res 49:382, 1981.

50. Lorrell BH, Palacios I, Daggett WM, et al.: Right ventricular distension and left ventricular compliance. Am J Physiol 240 (Heart Circ Physiol 9):H87, 1981.

51. Bove AA, Santamore WP: Ventricular interdependence. Prog Cardiovasc Dis 23: 365, 1981.

52. Olsen CO, Tyson GS, Maier GW, et al.: Dynamic ventricular interaction in the conscious dog. Circ Res 52:85, 1983.

53. Slinker BK, Glantz SA: End-systolic and end-diastolic ventricular interaction. Am J Physiol 251:H1062, 1986.

54. Slinker BK, Goto Y, LeWinter MM: Direct diastolic interaction gain measured with sudden hemodynamic transients. Am J Physiol 256:H567, 1989.

55. Brinker JA, Weiss JL, Lappé DL, et al.: Leftward septal displacement during right ventricular loading in man. Circulation 61: 626, 1980.

56. Kingma I, Tyberg JV, Smith ER: Effects of diastolic transseptal pressure gradient on ventricular septal position and motion. Circulation 68:1304, 1983.

57. Watanabe J, Levine MJ, Bellotto F, et al.: Effects of coronary venous pressure on left ventricular diastolic distensibility. Circ Res 67:923, 1990.

58. Little WC, Badke FR, O'Rourke RA: Effect of right ventricular pressure on the end-diastolic left ventricular pressure-volume relationship before and after chronic right ventricular pressure overload in dogs without pericardia. Circ Res 54:719, 1984.

59. Myhre ESP, Slinker BK, LeWinter MM: Influence of abrupt changes in left ventricular volume on right ventricular function. Circulation 85 (Suppl II): 38, 1991.

60. Myhre ESP, Slinker BK, LeWinter MM: Alterations in venous return related to abrupt perturbations of left ventricular pressure. Circulation (Suppl III): 82:696, 1990.

61. Slinker BK, Goto Y, LeWinter MM: Systolic direct ventricular interaction affects left ventricular contraction and relaxation in the intact dog circulation. Circ Res 65:307, 1989.

62. Goto Y, Slinker BK, LeWinter MM: Nonhomogeneous left ventricular regional

shortening during acute right ventricular pressure overload. Circ Res 65:43, 1989.

63. Ludbrook PA, Byrne JD, McKnight RC: Influence of right ventricular hemodynamics on left ventricular diastolic pressure-volume relations in man. Circulation 59:21, 1979.

64. Slinker BK, Chagas ACP, Glantz SA: Chronic pressure overload hypertrophy decreases direct ventricular interaction. Am J Physiol 253 (Heart Circ Physiol 22): H347, 1987.

65. Alderman EI, Glantz SA: Acute hemodynamic interventions shift the diastolic pressure-volume curve in man. Circulation 54: 662, 1976.

66. Brodie BR, Grossman W, Mann T, McLarinn LP: Effects of sodium nitroprusside on left ventricular diastolic pressure-volume relations. J Clin Invest 59:59, 1977.

67. Ross J Jr: Acute displacement of the diastolic pressure-volume curve of the left ventricle. Role of the pericardium and the right ventricle. Circulation 59:32, 1979.

68. Carroll JD, Lang RM, Neumann EL, Borow KM, Rafer SI: The differential effects of positive inotropic and vasodilator therapy on diastolic properties in patients with congestive cardiomyopathy. Circulation 74: 815, 1986.

69. Bartle SH, Hermann HJ: Acute mitral regurgitation in man. Hemodynamic evidence and observations indicating an early role for the pericardium. Circulation 36: 839, 1967.

70. Lloyd EA, Gersh BJ, Kennedy BM: Hemodynamic spectrum of dominant right ventricular infarction. Am J Cardiol 48:1016, 1981.

71. Baigrie RS, Hag A, Morgan CD, et al.: The spectrum of right ventricular involvement in inferior wall myocardial infarction: A clinical hemodynamic and noninvasive study. J Am Coll Cardiol 1:1396, 1983.

72. Roberts N, Harrison DG, Reimer KA, et al.: Right ventricular infarction with shock but without significant left ventricular infarction: A new clinical syndrome. Am Heart J 110:1047, 1985.

73. East T, Bain C: Right ventricular stenosis (Bernheim's Syndrome). Brit Heart J 11: 145, 1949.

74. Rao BS, Cohn KE, Eldridge FL, Hancock EW: Left ventricular failure secondary to chronic pulmonary disease. Am J Med 229: 241, 1969.

75. Jezek V, Schrijen F: Left ventricular function in chronic obstructive pulmonary disease with and without cardiac failure. Clin Sci Mol Med 45:267, 1973.

76. Sibbald WJ, Driedger AA, Myers ML, et al.: Biventricular function in the adult respiratory distress syndrome. Chest 84:126, 1983.

77. Jardin F, Fracot J, Boisante L, et al.: Influence of positive end-expiratory pressure on left ventricular performance. New Engl J Med 304:387, 1981.

78. Scharf SM, Brown R, Saunders N, et al.: Changes in canine left ventricular size and configuration with positive end-expiratory pressure. Circ Res 44:672, 1979.

79. Santamore WP, Bove AA, Heckman JL: Right and left ventricular pressure-volume response to positive end-expiratory pressure. Am J Physiol 246:H114, 1984.

80. Freeman G, LeWinter MM: Role of parietal pericardium in acute, severe mitral regurgitation in dogs. Am J Cardiol 54:217, 1984.

81. Kass DA, Midei M, Brinker J, Maughan WL: Influence of coronary occlusion during PTCA on end-systolic and end-diastolic pressure-volume relations in humans. Circulation 81:447, 1990.

82. Janicki JS: Influence of the pericardium and ventricular interdependence on left ventricular diastolic and systolic function in patients with heart failure. Circulation 81 (Suppl III):15, 1990.

Chapter 7

INFLUENCE OF THE CORONARY VASCULATURE ON LEFT VENTRICULAR DIASTOLIC CHAMBER STIFFNESS: THE ERECTILE PROPERTIES OF THE MYOCARDIUM

Carl S. Apstein

The coronary vasculature and its contents comprise approximately 15% of the left ventricular (LV) wall (1); alterations in this component of the wall are known to affect the diastolic properties of the ventricle. The normal ventricle can accommodate a substantial increase in coronary flow (e.g., during exercise) without a significant alteration in diastolic function. Pathologic alterations of coronary arterial or coronary venous pressure, however, cause major changes in LV distensibility, especially in hearts that have been damaged by ischemia or hypoxia. This influence of the coronary vasculature on LV diastolic distensibility or "elasticity" was originally described by Salisbury et al.; they ascribed these vascular effects to the "erectile" properties of the myocardium (2).

EFFECTS OF CORONARY ARTERIAL PRESSURE AND FLOW ON LEFT VENTRICULAR DIASTOLIC CHAMBER STIFFNESS

Salisbury et al. initially reported that changes in coronary perfusion pressure caused parallel changes in left ventricular diastolic pressure in isovolumetrically contracting dog hearts (2). Thus, left ventricular diastolic chamber stiffness, as estimated by ventricular diastolic pressure at constant ventricular volume, was directly related to coronary perfusion pressure. These investigators speculated that an increase in coronary blood volume within the coronary arteries and veins could alter the elasticity of the myocardial wall, and called this phenomenon an "erectile" effect of the coronary vasculature on the myocardium. Many investigators have subsequently con-

firmed an influence of coronary arterial pressure and/or flow on left ventricular diastolic properties, but others have failed to observe a significant effect. The reason for such differences, at least in part, is that some studies were performed in normal or near-normal hearts with low filling pressures, whereas others were performed in failing or abnormal hearts with high filling pressures; under such disparate conditions, the erectile effect can be minimized or maximized, respectively (Fig. 7–1).

Increases in Coronary Perfusion Pressure and Flow

Significant increases in coronary arterial pressure and flow have generally caused an increase in left ventricular diastolic chamber stiffness, i.e. a decrease in compliance or distensibility. The most marked influence of coronary arterial vascular dynamics on LV diastolic compliance was reported by Wexler et al., who simulated an acute hypertensive crisis in isolated isovolumic blood perfused rabbit hearts (3). The pericardium was removed and the right ventricle vented to remove any influence of these two structures on left ventricular diastolic distensibility. When the coronary perfusion pressure was increased from a baseline of 70 to a level of 130 mm Hg to simulate a hypertensive crisis, coronary flow increased by 50%, from 2 to 3 ml/min/g, left ventricular wall thickness increased by 20%, and isovolumic LVEDP increased by 10 mm Hg, indicating a significant increase in LV diastolic chamber stiffness. When the coronary artery perfusion pressure was reduced to a normal range (70 mm Hg), diastolic distensibility increased immediately,

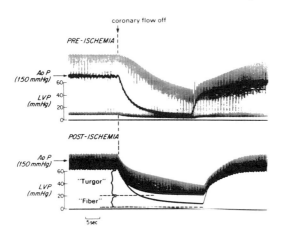

Fig. 7–1. The effect of an acute decrease in coronary perfusion pressure on left ventricular diastolic pressure-volume relations. The upper panel shows the left ventricular pressure tracing from an isolated rabbit heart with the intraventricular balloon held at constant volume. During the control period, coronary perfusion pressure was adjusted to 150 mm Hg. In the "normal heart" labeled preischemia, the transient reduction in coronary perfusion pressure was followed by a 5 mm Hg decrease in left ventricular diastolic pressure. The lower panel shows the result of a similar experiment in an "injured heart" (caused by 90 minutes of severe ischemia followed by reperfusion); post-ischemia, the decrease in perfusion pressure resulted in a 42 mm Hg decrease in left ventricular diastolic pressure (turgor component).

indicating that the effects of coronary artery hypertension were rapidly reversible. The imposition of a hypertensive coronary artery perfusion pressure caused a parallel upward shift of the left ventricular diastolic pressure-volume curve, without a change in slope. This parallel shift in the position of the diastolic pressure-volume curve would not qualify to be characterized as an increase in "stiffness" because the slope was unchanged. Nonetheless, a higher diastolic pressure was required to achieve a given diastolic volume, i.e., the ventricle was more resistant to filling when the coronary perfusion pressure was elevated (Fig. 7–2). Wexler et al. suggested that the acute coronary vascular engorgement associated with coronary arterial hypertension, and the associated increase in left ventricular diastolic chamber stiffness, may contribute to the development of acute pulmonary

edema in patients with a "hypertensive crisis."

Many studies have reported a significant interaction among an increase in coronary artery pressure and flow, intramyocardial blood volume and left ventricular wall thickness, and increased left ventricular diastolic stiffness (4–6). For example, Gaasch and Bernard demonstrated that postischemic hyperemia significantly increased diastolic wall thickness (7). Coronary vasodilation has also been demonstrated to increase left ventricular diastolic chamber stiffness (5, 8).

Other investigators have reported conflicting results regarding the influence of an increased coronary arterial pressure on left ventricular diastolic properties. Olsen and colleagues (9) reported a leftward shift in the left ventricular diastolic pressure-dimension curve in arrested dog hearts on right ventricular bypass when the coronary artery pressure was increased from 40 to 120 mm Hg, noting that the greatest changes occurred below the autoregulatory range (<80 mm Hg). Alderman and Glantz (10) showed in humans that the left ventricular pressure-volume curve shifted upward and to the left when aortic pressure was increased to hypertensive levels by an angiotensin infusion. They speculated that external mechanical loading conditions (right-left ventricular interaction and pericardial restraint) and the viscoelastic properties of the myocardium were the key factors altering the left ventricular diastolic pressure-volume relation. This reasoning, however, does not rule out a direct effect of the hypertensive coronary vasculature on passive myocardial properties as suggested by the studies of Wexler et al. (3). Similarly, Sarnoff et al. (11) observed that an increase in aortic outflow resistance was associated with an increase in left ventricular end-diastolic pressure relative to end-diastolic segment length, suggesting an increase in left ventricular diastolic chamber stiffness as a result of the increased coronary perfusion pressure.

In contrast to these studies, Abel and Reis (12) reported no change in isovolumic LVEDP in an intact balloon-in-LV canine model on right ventricular bypass when coronary perfusion pressure was either decreased to ischemic levels, or increased to

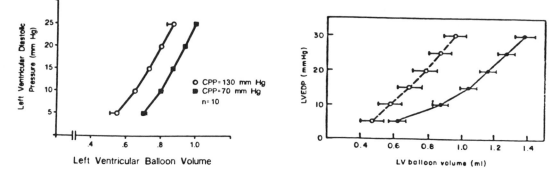

Fig. 7–2. Effect of coronary arterial perfusion on left ventricular diastolic distensibility. Panel A shows the influence of a hypertensive coronary arterial pressure on left ventricular diastolic distensibility in an isolated blood perfused rabbit heart as assessed by the position of the diastolic pressure-volume filling curve. A hypertensive coronary perfusion pressure of 130 mm Hg was associated with a significant leftward shift of the diastolic pressure-volume curve indicating an increase in diastolic chamber stiffness in comparison with a normal coronary perfusion pressure of 70 mm Hg. (Reproduced with permission from Wexler LF, et al.: Coronary hypertension and diastolic compliance in isolated rabbit hearts. Hypertension 13:598, 1989. Panel B illustrates the effect of a marked decrease in coronary perfusion pressure on left ventricular diastolic chamber stiffness. The open circles represent a left ventricular diastolic pressure-volume curve in an isolated buffer perfused rabbit heart at a coronary perfusion pressure of 100 mm Hg. The closed circles represent the diastolic pressure-volume curve measured after two minutes of total zero-flow global ischemia. The curve obtained during ischemia was shifted significantly to the right ($P < 0.001$ at all points compared to controls by paired t-test). Thus, complete cessation of coronary arterial flow results in a marked increase in LV diastolic distensibility. Reproduced with permission from Vogel WM, et al.: Acute alterations in left ventricular diastolic chamber stiffness: Role of the "erectile" effect of coronary arterial pressure and flow in normal and damaged hearts. Circ Res 51:465, 1982.

150 mm Hg. Templeton et al. (13) reported no change in either position or slope of the LV diastolic pressure-volume curve in isovolumic dog hearts when coronary perfusion pressure was increased; however, only a modest increase in coronary perfusion pressure, from 60 to 95 mm Hg, was imposed. This result is consistent with the studies of Wexler et al., who did not find a statistically significant effect on left ventricular diastolic chamber stiffness when coronary perfusion pressure was altered between 70 and 100 mm Hg; a larger increment of coronary perfusion pressure change was required to significantly affect LV diastolic chamber stiffness (3). Similarly, Arnold et al. (14) increased coronary perfusion pressure from 60 to 120 cm H_2O in an isolated isovolumic heart with an initial LVEDP of only 2 mm Hg; LVEDP was not significantly altered by this change in coronary perfusion pressure.

Decreases in Coronary Perfusion Pressure and Flow

Decreases in coronary perfusion pressure and flow have been shown to increase left ventricular diastolic distensibility, but the extent of such an effect depends on the magnitude of the change in coronary perfusion pressure. Farhi et al. (15) decrementally decreased circumflex coronary perfusion pressure in conscious dogs. The diastolic portion of the pressure-segment length curve was unchanged when the decrements in circumflex pressure were within the autoregulatory range, i.e., the pressure decrements were unassociated with changes in coronary blood flow or systolic function. Such mild reductions in circumflex pressure, to pressures above 50 mm Hg, had no effect on the position of diastolic pressure-segment length curve. Greater reductions in coronary perfusion pressure, however, were associated with a marked and progressive movement of the diastolic pressure-segment length curve downward and to the right, indicating greater distensibility of the underperfused segment (15). Similarly, Palacios et al. (16) decreased coronary perfusion pressure from 80 to 50 mm Hg and saw no change in isovolumic LVEDP in the dog. These results are consistent with those of Wexler et al. (3), in which alterations of coronary perfusion pressure between 70 and 100 mm Hg did not significantly influence global left ventricular diastolic chamber stiffness.

However, with a more marked reduction of coronary perfusion pressure and flow, such as occurs after a coronary occlusion or with the onset of zero-flow ischemia, there is a collapse of the coronary vasculature, left ventricular wall thickness decreases, and the coronary turgor contribution to diastolic chamber stiffness decreases acutely. These events are associated with a significant increase in left ventricular diastolic distensibility, i.e. an acute decrease in diastolic chamber stiffness (2, 17–23). For example, total global ischemia in isolated hearts causes an immediate decrease in left ventricular diastolic wall thickness and an increase in ventricular diastolic compliance manifested as a shift to the right with a decrease in slope of the diastolic pressure-volume curve (23). Myocardial wall thickness is an important determinant of ventricular diastolic compliance. The decrease in diastolic wall thickness that occurs with cessation of coronary perfusion is probably related to a decrease in the volume in the coronary vascular compartment. Thus, cessation of coronary perfusion, probably increases diastolic distensibility by decreasing the volume of the vascular compartment, thereby decreasing wall thickness (23).

Similarly, several investigators have reported an increase in the compliance of the ischemic segment of myocardium after coronary artery ligation, in which compliance was defined as the diastolic segment-length at a given diastolic pressure, i.e., the diastolic pressure-segment length curve shifted to the right after a coronary occlusion (24–28). This early increase in regional diastolic compliance after a coronary occlusion may be caused, at least partly, by the loss of volume in the coronary vascular bed distal to the site of the occlusion, resulting in a loss of the coronary "erectile" effect in the ischemic region.

In summary, modest decreases in coronary perfusion pressure, to a level of approximately 50 mm Hg, do not appear to significantly alter left ventricular diastolic compliance, but more substantial decreases, especially after complete coronary occlusions or the imposition of zero-flow global ischemia, are associated with an immediate and marked increase in left ventricular diastolic distensibility caused by the loss of coronary "turgor" and the "erectile" contribution to diastolic wall stiffness. This influence of alteration in coronary perfusion on diastolic chamber stiffness appears to be amplified in hearts damaged by ischemia, hypoxia, or other agents (29).

Two considerations complicate the assessment of left ventricular diastolic properties with decreases of coronary perfusion pressure and flow. First of all, the timing of such measurements is critical. The post-ischemic reperfusion state is associated with significant coronary hyperemia, an increase in diastolic wall thickness, and an increase in diastolic chamber stiffness as discussed previously. Therefore, measurements of ventricular diastolic properties must be precise in their timing when coronary pressures and flows are rapidly changing, e.g., during coronary angioplasty. Secondly, the metabolic consequences of the tissue ischemia, which occurs when coronary flow is reduced, can confound assessment of the direct vascular effects on myocardial distensibility. When a decrease in coronary perfusion is partial rather than complete, myocardial oxygen "demand" can persist. An increase in myocardial oxygen demand in the setting of a fixed low level of coronary perfusion can result in "demand ischemia" whose effect is to increase left ventricular diastolic chamber stiffness, and potentially mask the loss of the vascular "erectile" effect (30).

EFFECTS OF CORONARY VENOUS PRESSURE CHANGES ON LEFT VENTRICULAR DIASTOLIC DISTENSIBILITY

The influence of coronary venous pressure on LV diastolic properties has received relatively little attention despite its importance. Recently, Watanabe et al. (31) demonstrated that increases in coronary venous pressure markedly increased left ventricular wall volume and decreased left ventricular diastolic distensibility. Watanabe et al. increased coronary venous pressure over a range of 0 to 30 mm Hg in isolated canine hearts. An increase in coronary venous pressure from 0 to 30 mm Hg was associated with a 3 to 4% increase in diastolic LV wall thickness and a decrease in LV diastolic distensibility as manifested by an increase in isovolumic LVEDP. The increase in isovolumic LVEDP attributable to the 30 mm Hg coronary venous pressure increase was approximately 6 mm Hg (Fig. 7–3). These investigators attributed the decrease in ventricular distensibility seen at the higher coronary venous pressures to the "erectile" effect first postulated by Salisbury as discussed previously.[2]

Watanabe et al. also compared the effects on left ventricular diastolic distensibility of comparable increases in coronary venous and coronary arterial pressure. As noted, when the coronary venous pressure was increased from 0 to 30 mm Hg, isovolumic LVEDP increased by approximately 6 mm Hg. However, when mean coronary arterial pressure was increased by 30 mm Hg, from 80 to 110 mm Hg, there was no significant effect on isovolumic LVEDP consistent with the studies of Wexler et al. (3) and Farhi et al. (15), showing no influence of small alterations in coronary perfusion pressure on ventricular diastolic distensibility. Thus, a pressure increase in the coronary veins had a greater effect on diastolic distensibility than a similar pressure increase in the coronary arteries. This result suggests that the coronary erectile effect is related to intramyocardial blood volume in the coronary microcirculation; the coronary venous pressure may transmit effectively to the microcirculation through the low resistance of the venous system, in contrast to the higher resistance of the arterial system (31).

SUMMARY

In summary, numerous studies have documented an important influence of the coronary vasculature on left ventricular diastolic distensibility. Alterations of coronary arterial pressure within a "physiologic" range of approximately 50 to 110 mm Hg have a minimal effect on left ventricular diastolic chamber stiffness, but an increase to the "hypertensive" range of 130 mm Hg significantly increased diastolic chamber stiffness, as have substantial in-

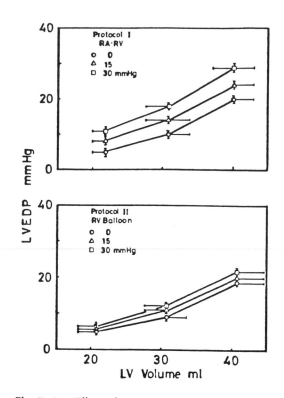

Fig. 7–3. Effect of coronary venous pressure on left ventricular diastolic distensibility. In these experiments, coronary venous pressure was increased by increasing the height of a blood reservoir connected to a cannula that opened in both the RA and RV of a canine heart. The top panel shows that an increase in the RA-RV diastolic pressure over a range of 0 to 30 mm Hg was associated with a parallel upward shift of the LV diastolic pressure volume curve. An increase in RA and RV diastolic pressures increases intracavitary as well as coronary venous pressures. The lower panel reports experiments to assess the effect of an intracavitary increase in RV diastolic pressure. In the lower panel, an RV balloon was inflated over a pressure range of 0 to 30 mm Hg and the effect on the LV diastolic pressure-volume relation was measured. Distension of the RV balloon in the lower panel had much less of an effect than that which occurred when both the RV cavity and coronary venous pressures were increased, as shown in the upper panel. Thus, the difference between the upper and lower panels indicates the influence of an increase in coronary venous pressure on left ventricular diastolic distensibility. Reproduced with permission from Watanabe J, et al.: Effects of coronary venous pressure on left ventricular diastolic distensibility. Circ Res 67:923, 1990.

creases in coronary flow such changes are more prominent in injured hearts than in normal hearts. Increases in coronary venous pressure may also cause a reduction in left ventricular diastolic distensibility. A common mechanism for both the arterial and venous pressure effects appears to be an increase in volume in the intramyocardial vascular compartment, increasing diastolic wall thickness and decreasing chamber distensibility by a mechanism of coronary vascular "turgor." Similarly, marked decreases in coronary arterial pressure and flow cause an immediate increase in diastolic distensibility.

These vascular-myocardial interactions may contribute importantly to clinical pathophysiology. For example, the elevation in right atrial and right ventricular diastolic pressures that occurs with right sided heart failure, by increasing coronary venous pressure, would have the effect of decreasing left ventricular distensibility by means of coronary venous "erectile effect." Thus, vasodilators and diuretics, by decreasing right-sided diastolic pressures, would also decrease coronary venous pressure, and secondarily cause an increase in left ventricular distensibility. This action would tend to decrease any pulmonary congestion present and increase left ventricular filling. Similarly, the coronary arterial hypertension that occurs in a "hypertensive crisis" undoubtedly makes a significant contribution to left ventricular diastolic chamber stiffness and may contribute significantly to pulmonary congestion. Correction of the hypertensive state and restoration of a normal systemic and coronary arterial pressure can thus contribute to the relief of pulmonary congestion by improving LV diastolic distensibility.

REFERENCES

1. Morgenstern C, Holjes U, Arnold G, Lochner W: The influence of coronary pressure and coronary flow on intracoronary blood volume and geometry of the left ventricle. Pflugers Arch. 340:110, 1973.
2. Salisbury PF, Cross CE, Rieben PA: Influence of coronary artery pressure upon myocardial elasticity. Circ Res 8:794, 1960.
3. Wexler LF, et al.: Coronary hypertension and diastolic compliance in isolated rabbit hearts. Hypertension 13:598, 1989.
4. Morgenstern C, Holijes U, Arnold G, Lochner W: The influence of coronary pressure and coronary flow on intracoronary blood volume and geometry of the left ventricle. Pflugers Arch 340:101, 1973.
5. Scharf SM, Bromberger-Barnea B: Influence of coronary flow and pressure on cardiac function and coronary vascular volume. Am J Physiol 224:918, 1973.
6. Cross CE, Rieben PA, Salisbury PF: Influence of coronary perfusion and myocardial edema on pressure-volume diagram of left ventricle. Am J Physiol 201:102, 1961.
7. Gaasch WM, Bernard SA: The effect of acute changes in coronary blood flow on left ventricular end-diastolic wall thickness: An echocardiographic study. Circulation 56:593, 1977.
8. Verrier ED, Bristow JD, Hoffman JIE: Coronary vasodilation shifts the diastolic pressure-dimension curve of the left ventricle. J Mol Cell Cardiol 18:579, 1986.
9. Olsen CO, et al.: The coronary pressure-flow determinants of left ventricular compliance in dogs. Circ Res 49:856, 1981.
10. Alderman EL, Glantz SA: Acute hemodynamic interventions shift the diastolic pressure volume curve in man. Circulation 54:662, 1976.
11. Sarnoff SJ, Mitchell JH, Gilmore JP, Remensnyder JP: Homeometric regulation in the heart. Circ Res 8:1077, 1960.
12. Abel RM, Reis RL: Effects of coronary blood flow and perfusion pressure on left ventricular contractility in dogs. Circ Res 27:961, 1970.
13. Templeton GH, Wildenthal K, Mitchell JH: Influence of coronary blood flow on left ventricular contractility and stiffness. Am J Physiol 223:1216, 1972.
14. Arnold G, et al.: The importance of the perfusion pressure in the coronary arteries for the contractility and the oxygen consumption of the heart. Pflugers Arch 229:339, 1968.
15. Farhi ER, Canty JMJ, Klocke FJ: Effects of graded reductions in coronary perfusion pressure on the diastolic pressure-segment length relation and the rate of isovolumic relaxation in the resting conscious dog. Circulation 80:1458, 1989.
16. Palacios I, Johnson RA, Newell WJJ: Left ventricular end-diastolic pressure volume relationships with experimental acute global ischemia. Circulation 53:428, 1976.
17. Bourdillon PD, Poole-Wilson PA: The effects of verapamil, quiescence, and cardioplegia on calcium exchange and mechani-

cal function in ischemic rabbit myocardium. Circ Res 50:360, 1982.

18. Gaasch WH, et al.: The influence of acute alterations in coronary blood flow on left ventricular diastolic compliance and wall thickness. Eur J Cardiol 7:147, 1978.

19. Momomura S, et al.: The relationship of high energy phosphate, tissue pH, and regional blood flow to diastolic distensibility in the ischemic dog myocardium. Circ Res 57:822, 1985.

20. Olson CO, et al.: The coronary pressure-flow determinants of left ventricular compliance in dogs. Circ Res 49:856, 1981.

21. Serizawa T, Vogel WM, Apstein CS, Grossman W: Comparison of acute alterations in left ventricular relaxation and diastolic chamber stiffness induced by hypoxia and ischemia: Role of myocardial oxygen supply-demand imbalance. J Clin Invest 68:91, 1981.

22. Shine KL, Douglas AM, Ricchiuti N: Ischemia in isolated ventricular septae: Mechanical events. Am J Physiol 231:1225, 1976.

23. Vogel WM, et al.: Acute alterations in left ventricular diastolic chamber stiffness: Role of the "erectile" effect of coronary arterial pressure and flow in normal and damaged hearts. Circ Res 51:465, 1982.

24. Forrester JS, Diamond G, Parmley WW, Swan HJC: Early increase in left ventricular compliance after myocardial infarction. J Clin Invest 51:598, 1972.

25. Tyberg JV, et al.: An analysis of segmental ischemic dysfunction utilizing the pressure length loop. Circulation 49:748, 1974.

26. Theroux P, Franklin D, Ross JJ, Kemper WS: Regional myocardial function during acute coronary artery occlusion and its modification by pharmacologic agents in the dog. Circ Res 35:895, 1974.

27. Vokonas PS, Pirzada FA, Hood WBJ: Experimental myocardial infarction. XII. Dynamic changes in sequential mechanical behavior of infarcted and non-infarcted myocardium. Am J Cardiol 37:853, 1976.

28. Pirzada FA, et al.: Experimental myocardial infarction XII. Sequential changes in left ventricular pressure-length relationships in the acute phase. Circulation 53:970, 1976.

29. Vogel WM, Briggs LL, Apstein CS: Separation of inherent diastole myocardial fiber tension and coronary vascular "erectile" contributions to wall stiffness of rabbit hearts damaged by ischemia, hypoxia, calcium paradox and reperfusion. J Mol Cell Cardiol 17:57, 1985.

30. Apstein CS, Grossman W: Opposite initial effects of supply and demand ischemia on left ventricular diastolic compliance: The ischemia-diastolic paradox. J Mol Cell Cardiol 19:119, 1987.

31. Watanabe J, et al.: Effects of coronary venous pressure on left ventricular diastolic distensibility. Circ Res 67:923, 1990.

Chapter 8

MYOCARDIAL COLLAGEN AND LEFT VENTRICULAR DIASTOLIC DYSFUNCTION

Joseph S. Janicki and Beatriz B. Matsubara

Cardiac myocytes and the coronary microcirculation are surrounded and supported by the interstitial collagen matrix. This matrix is part of a structural continuum that includes the valve leaflets and chordae tendineae. It consists of predominantly type I fibrillar collagen. In addition to providing a supporting network for cardiac muscle cells and blood vessels (1), the matrix:

1. Coordinates the transmission of force generated by myocytes to the ventricular chamber (2)
2. Serves as an important determinant of myocardial relaxation, diastolic stiffness (3), and ventricular size (4, 5)
3. Opposes myocardial edema (4)
4. Prevents ventricular aneurysm and rupture (6–8)
5. Together with the other components of the interstitium, serves as a medium between the circulatory and lymphatic systems and myocytes through which oxygen, electrolytes, macromolecules, and metabolic waste products must diffuse.

Hence, the collagen matrix with its multiple functions is an important component of the interstitium and myocardium.

In view of this multifunctional role, it is not surprising to find that a modification of the collagen matrix, in turn, alters myocardial mechanical properties and ventricular structure and function. In general, the matrix can be modified by either an increase in interstitial collagen concentration caused by a reactive fibrosis (i.e., newly synthesized collagen fibers and thickening of

existing fibers) and/or a reparative fibrosis (i.e., scars), or a degradation of collagen characterized by a reduction in collagen concentration and a disruption and disappearance of fibrillar collagen. A reactive growth or remodeling of the myocardial interstitial collagen matrix is associated with the following conditions: genetic hypertension, activation of the renin-angiotensin-aldosterone system, excess circulating mineralocorticoids, and aging (3, 9). Consequent to this type of remodeling and also to infarct-related scarring is an increase in myocardial passive and ventricular diastolic stiffness.

Collagen matrix degradation results in myocardial edema, ventricular dilation, muscle fiber slippage and realignment, wall thinning, and a decrease in ventricular diastolic stiffness (4, 5, 10–12). It is also responsible in part for "stunned" myocardium (13) and the change in shape and dilation of the involved region during the early phase of healing after myocardial infarction (7, 8).

The interstitial collagen network and its relation to diastolic function will be the focus of this chapter. In particular, our current understanding of alterations of the collagen matrix and its effect on myocardial passive properties and on ventricular diastolic size and stiffness will be reviewed. It is important, however, to first provide a description of the ultra- and microstructure of this extracellular collagen matrix and its relation to myocytes, muscle fibers, and the coronary blood vessels.

THE MYOCARDIAL INTERSTITIAL COLLAGEN MATRIX

Included in the interstitium of the myocardium are: connective tissue, ground

This work was supported in part by NHLBI Grant Nos. RO1-HL-31701 and RO1-HL-46461 and American Heart Assoc. Grant-In-Aid No. 901397.

substance consisting of glycosaminoglycans and glycoproteins, nerves, and blood vessels. The connective tissue consists predominantly of collagen and, to a much lesser extent, fibronectin (14–16), laminin (16), and elastin (17).

Biochemistry

Tissue collagen concentration is usually measured biochemically by determining the concentration of hydroxyproline, which is found exclusively in collagen. In the normal rat, the concentration of hydroxyproline in the left ventricle is typically between 2.5 and 3.0 µg/mg dry weight. It can also be estimated using morphometric/morphologic techniques (18, 19), whereby the percentage of tissue occupied by collagen is obtained. In the normal rat left ventricle, the collagen volume fraction ranges from 2.0 to 4.0%. Although hydroxyproline concentration and collagen volume fraction values correlate well with one another (18, 20), the morphometric/morphologic approach provides additional information regarding structure, location, and distribution of collagen in a transmural section of myocardium. It also permits the separation of collagen into interstitial and perivascular components and the exclusion of scars.

The types of collagen present in the interstitium of the myocardium are I, III, and V. Even though the relative proportions of these types appear to be species-dependent (21), type I is by far the dominant one. For example, in nonhuman primates, myocardial collagen was found to consist of 85% type I, 11% type III, and 3% type V collagen (20). The ratio of type I to type III collagen may influence collagen fiber size. Type I enriched tissues contain larger-diameter collagen fibers than do tissue with a high amount of type III collagen (22). In addition, it has been suggested that larger-diameter fibers are the ones that are able to sustain high-stress levels. However, in the myocardium, fibers that surround large bundles of myocytes (15, 16), as well as fibers in the endomysium (15, 16, 23), appear to be a copolymerization of types I and III collagen molecules.

The messenger RNA for collagen types I and III is contained within the fibroblasts (24, 25), which represent 70% of the heart's total cell population (26). The synthesis rate of collagen for the right and left ventricles has been measured in dogs as 0.56% of total ventricular collagen per day (27). If an equilibrium is to exist between collagen synthesis and degradation, then, assuming a similar degradation rate, the half-life of collagen is around 90 days.

Little is known regarding the latent collagenase system within the myocardium, which has been identified using specific antibody and immunohistochemical labeling (28) and histochemical techniques (29). Mammalian collagenases are zinc-containing proteases that can be activated with sulfhydryl-active compounds (30). Cleavage of the collagen molecule results in soluble peptides, which are then suitable substrates for a variety of other tissue proteases (31). Recently, myocardial collagen fiber disruption and degradation were observed following the infusion of disulfide reagents to an isolated rat heart (32). Presumably, this was the result of collagenolytic activity.

Structural Organization

The structural organization of the collagen matrix of the myocardium is depicted in Figure 8–1. The three major components of this network have been named the epimysium, perimysium, and endomysium in accordance with skeletal muscle terminology (33). The epimysium is the sheath of collagenous connective tissue that surrounds the entire muscle. It consists of collagen fibers several micrometers in diameter. The perimysium includes the tendinous extensions of the epimysium, which arborize to form weaves of collagen around groups of myocytes. Collagen fibers, referred to as strands, join adjacent weaves. Not shown in Figure 8–1 are the coiled perimysial fibers, which form an array in parallel with the myocytes and epimysial weave. At the light microscopic level, portions of the perimysial weave and the larger-diameter, coiled perimysial fibers are usually evident between rows of muscle fibers (Fig. 8–2). The endomysium is the collagen network at the level of the myocyte. It consists of a meshwork of fibers that surround individual myocytes and of fibers or struts that connect myocytes to

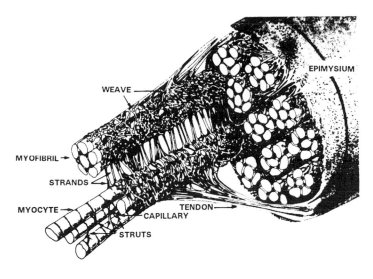

Fig. 8–1. Schematic representation of the myocardial extracellular matrix and its epimysial, perimysial (i.e., tendon, weave and strands), and endomysial (i.e., struts) elements. Reproduced with permission from Weber KT, Clark WA, Janicki JS, Shroff SG: Physiologic versus pathologic hypertrophy and the pressure-overloaded myocardium. J Cardiovasc Pharmacol 10:S37, 1987.

neighboring myocytes and capillaries (Figs. 8–1 and 8–3). These struts insert into the basal lamina to the Z band of the sarcomere and are thought to play an important role in the efficient transduction of generated force to the ventricular chamber (2, 34).

As mentioned previously, indirect immunofluorescence techniques have revealed the presence of collagen types I, III, and V in the perimysial collagen surrounding bundles of myocytes and coronary blood vessels (15, 16). In the endomysium, type III is dominant and type I is rarely detected. Type V and fibronectin tend to accumulate around each myocyte. Fibronectin also appears around blood vessels and in the vicinity of capillaries.

Mechanical Properties

Collagen is a relatively stiff material with a high tensile strength. However, its influence on the stress-strain relation of a composite material, such as the myocardium, depends on many factors including its concentration, fibril and fiber diameter, degree of crosslinking, spatial alignment, crimp properties, and collagen types. In general, tissue designed to have a high tensile strength has an elevated collagen content and larger-diameter collagen fibers that have a greater percentage of covalent crosslinks. Collagen fibers oriented in the same direction as the local stresses contribute significantly to the elasticity of the com-

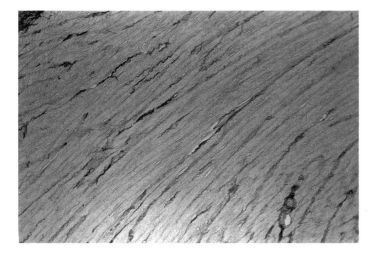

Fig. 8–2. Normal myocardium stained with collagen-specific Sirius red, demonstrating typical amounts of collagen. At this magnification ($\times 150$), coiled perimysial fibers and segments of the perimysial weave are apparent.

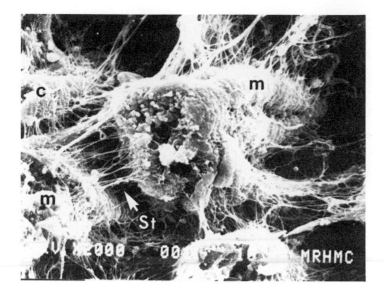

Fig. 8–3. Normal nonhuman primate heart, indicating the complex network of collagen surrounding myocytes and the numerous struts (St) that join adjacent myocytes (m) to one another and to neighboring capillaries (c). Reproduced with permission from Weber KT, et al.: Collagen in the hypertrophied pressure-overloaded myocardium. Circulation 75:I-40, 1987.

posite material as opposed to a negligible influence from those aligned perpendicular to the stress direction. This was nicely demonstrated by Weigner et al. (35), who found strips of pericardium to exhibit the greatest stiffness when most of its collagen fibers were oriented parallel to the direction of the elongating force. In papillary muscle, the orientation of the epimysial collagen fibers changes with stretch. At a muscle length at which resistance to elongation increases significantly, the collagen fibers become predominantly oriented parallel to the major axis of the muscle (23).

The crimp property of collagen refers to the amount to which a collagen fiber is coiled or, equivalently, the amount to which the fiber extends following the application of a low stress. Beyond this length, the stress required for further elongation increases exponentially. Coiled perimysial fibers oriented parallel or oblique to the long axes of myocytes that undergo focal straightening as the myocardium is stretched, have been observed throughout the myocardium (23, 36). Finally, tissue containing type I collagen (e.g., tendons) has a higher modulus of elasticity than that with predominantly type III collagen (e.g., uterus).

Based on the mechanical properties of collagen, its structural arrangement and the coiled nature of the perimysial fibers, the passive mechanical relationship be-

tween muscle and coiled perimysial fibers could be conceptualized as two springs in parallel with different mechanical properties (Fig. 8–4). The spring representing collagen fibers would exhibit a nonlinear elastic behavior whereby, for low strains, it would contribute little to the overall stiffness of the system until the fibers begin to straighten. At these low strains, the system

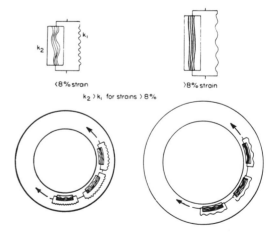

Fig. 8–4. The relationship between myocardial interstitial fibrillar collagen and cardiac muscle can be conceptualized as two springs arranged in parallel. Because of the crimp property of collagen, the muscle spring (k_1) at low strains is stiffer than the spring representing collagen (k_2). As strain is increased, the collagen spring becomes dominant.

stiffness would reflect the properties of the spring representing muscle. However, as the system is further lengthened, the collagen spring would become progressively stiffer and more contributory to the passive mechanical properties of the system. Thus, in terms of the passive pressure-volume relationship of the ventricle, the presence of fibrillar collagen shifts the curve upwards and to the left in a nonparallel fashion or results in a stiffer ventricle. (See Chap. 9.) Conversely, the degradation of myocardial collagen would be expected to shift the pressure-volume curve to the right or to reduce ventricular stiffness (see subsequent text).

MYOCARDIAL FIBROSIS AND LEFT VENTRICULAR DIASTOLIC FUNCTION

Reactive Fibrosis

Interstitial fibrillar collagen is reactively remodeled in genetic hypertension (19, 37,40), in LV pressure overload secondary to activation of the renin-angiotensin-aldosterone system (9, 16, 20, 41, 42), and with excess circulating mineralocorticoids (9, 43). Although ventricular loading is the primary determinant of myocyte growth, it should be stressed that its role in promoting nonmyocyte growth is negligible. Rather, it is the elevated level of circulating aldosterone that is responsible for the reactive fibrosis seen in renovascular, perinephritic and hyperaldosteronal hypertension (9). In genetic hypertension, elevated levels of circulating renin, angiotensin II and aldosterone have not been reported. However, this does not rule out the involvement of the myocardial tissue renin-angiotensin-aldosterone system, particularly in view of the fact that abnormal accumulations of interstitial collagen are prevented and regressed with the chronic administration of angiotensin converting enzyme inhibitors (19) but not with long-term hydralazine therapy (40).

Generally, the remodeling of the collagen matrix is observed at both the light and electron microscopic levels (Fig. 8–5) and consists of an increase in the concentration of collagen related to fibroblast proliferation (44, 45) and a sustained (4 weeks) elevation in the collagen synthesis rate from 0.6 to 4.0% per day (27). Remodeling of the peri- and endomysial components includes a thickening of collagen fibrils, fibers and tendons; an increase in the density of the weave and network surrounding myocytes; newly formed fibers; an expansion of the area occupied by perivascular collagen; and occasional microscopic scars (39–42, 46).

In renovascular and perinephritic hypertension, the myocardial collagen remodeling process is progressive. Beyond 4 weeks of experimentally induced hypertension, collagen concentration is significantly elevated and newly formed perimysial fibers are evident. As the hypertrophic process continues, further increases in collagen concentration are modest despite the appearance of patchy areas of reactive (i.e., unrelated to myocyte necrosis) fibrosis extending over muscle fibers. Late in the hypertrophic process, some of these areas become extended to the point where they completely encircle muscle (Fig. 8–5C). In many of these isolated muscle areas, cell necrosis may be present (42, 46).

In view of the strength and inextensibility of collagen, an increase in the concentration and content of this material within the myocardium would be expected to have an influence on myocardial stiffness and LV diastolic function. Indeed, several studies have reported both collagen concentration and myocardial or LV diastolic stiffness to be increased in hypertrophied myocardium. Bing et al. (47) noted that hypertrophied papillary muscles had an increased diastolic stiffness several days following the constriction of the aortic arch in rats. Thiedemann et al. (38) and Holubarsch et al. (48) have argued that the myocardial collagen increase in response to various forms of left ventricular pressure overload in the rat explained the greater diastolic stiffness found in the papillary muscle. Borg et al. (49) have observed a more extensive collagen weave separating myocyte groups in the hamster heart compared to that of the rat and suggested that this difference may account for the twofold difference in ventricular stiffness between these two species. Other studies have clearly demonstrated a relation between increased myocardial and ventricular stiffness and collagen concentration in nonhuman primates with experimental

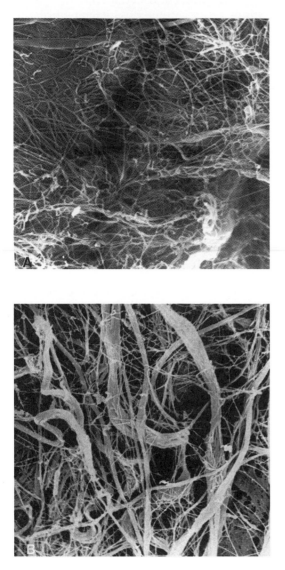

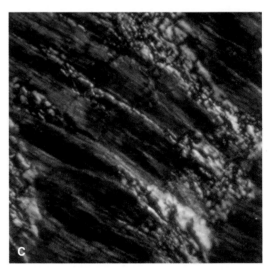

Fig. 8–5. *A,* Normal perimysial tendons and weave in nonhuman primate left ventricular myocardium (×6000). Reproduced with permission from Abrahams C, Janicki JS, Weber KT: Myocardial hypertrophy in the macaque fascicularis: Structural remodeling of the collagen matrix. Lab Invest 56:676, 1987. *B,* Collagen remodeling in nonhuman primate left ventricular myocardium with 4 weeks of perinephritic hypertension (×6000). The number and thickness of perimysial tendons are increased and the weave is denser. Reproduced with permission from Abrahams C, Janicki JS, Weber KT: Myocardial hypertrophy in the macaque fascicularis: Structural remodeling of the collagen matrix. Lab Invest 56:676, 1987. *C,* Collagen remodeling in nonhuman primate with 88 weeks of perinephritic hypertension. Tissue stained with collagen-specific Sirius red and viewed under polarized light (×100). In addition to an increased number and thickness of coiled perimysial fibers, patchy areas of reactive fibrosis overlying muscle fibers are present.

hypertension (20); rats with renovascular (42), perinephritic (50), or genetic (19, 40) hypertension; and rats with myocardial fibrosis secondary to perinephritis and/or isoproterenol (50), renovascular hypertension and isoproterenol (50) or coronary embolization (51).

The pertinent results from these studies, which are summarized in Table 8–1, indicate a strong correlation between collagen concentration and myocardial and ventricular stiffness. Two exceptions, however, require further comment. Holubarsch and coworkers (48) reported finding, in 40-

week-old spontaneously hypertensive rats (SHR), a negligible (i.e., 6% relative to 40-week-old Wistar-Kyoto rats) increase in papillary muscle stiffness despite a highly significant 36% increase in hydroxyproline. Importantly, however, the corresponding 12% expansion of the nonmyocyte space did not reach the level of statistical significance. Thus, their observed alterations in passive elastic properties correlated better with the interstitial space increase (i.e., morphometric assessment) than with the increment in hydroxyproline, a biochemical determination that

Table 8–1. **Experimentally Induced Myocardial Reactive Fibrosis, Hypertrophy, and Diastolic Stiffness**

A: Papillary or Trabecular Muscle Studies

Reference	Species	Model	Stiffness % Inc	LVH % Inc	Hpro % Inc	Nonmyocyte Space % Inc
Bing et al. (47)	Rat	AAC-4	50	40	31	—
Holubarsch et al. (48)	Rat	GBT-4	17*	53	13*	19*
		GBT-8	42	84	24	40
		SHR-40	6*	44	36	12*
		SHR-80	40	90	73	59

B: Left Ventricle Studies

Reference	Species	Model	Stiffness % Inc	LVH % Inc	Hpro % Inc	CVF % Inc
Weber et al. (20)	Primate	PN-4	−36	34	29	78
		PN-33	23	41	37	93
		PN-88	23	38	15	61
Doering et al. (42)	Rat	RHT-4	29	17	—	117
		RHT-8	42	21	—	72
Jalil et al. (50)	Rat	PN-10	27	24	—	140
		RHT-ISO-9	172	39	—	573
		PN-ISO-14	80	53	—	817
Narayan et al. (40)	Rat	SHR-36	24	27	—	174
Brilla et al. (19)	Rat	SHR-14	32	33	—	64
		SHR-26	41	41	—	150

* Not significantly different from control.
Abbreviations: %Inc = percent increase relative to appropriate control; LVH = left ventricular hypertrophy; Hpro = hydroxyproline; CVF = collagen volume fraction; AAC-4 = aorta arch constriction for 4 weeks; GBT = Goldblatt renovascular hypertension for 4 (GBT-4) and 8 (GBT-8) weeks; SHR = spontaneous hypertension for 14 (SHR-14), 26 (SHR-26), 36 (SHR-36), 40 (SHR-40) and 80 (SHR-80) weeks; PN = perinephritic hypertension for 4 (PN-4), 10 (PN-10), 33 (PN-33) and 88 (PN-88) weeks; RHT = abdominal aorta constriction plus unilateral renal ischemia for 4 (RHT-4) and 8 (RHT-8) weeks; RHT-ISO-9 = RHT for 8 weeks followed by isoproterenol (ISO) for 10 days; PN-ISO-14 = PN for 10 weeks followed by ISO for 10 days and sacrifice 3 weeks later.

includes collagen constituents such as that localized in and around blood vessels that neither significantly change the extracellular space nor alter myocardial elastic properties.

Weber et al. (20) found the myocardium to be less stiff than normal at large strains after 4 weeks of experimental perinephritic hypertension in nonhuman primates despite a 29 and 78% increase in hydroxyproline concentration and interstitial collagen volume fraction, respectively. However, after 35 and 88 weeks, the myocardium was clearly stiffer than that of controls, without further substantial increases in collagen concentration. An explanation for this transient disassociation between myocardial stiffness and fibrosis was provided by the active remodeling of fibrillar collagens, which took place over the time period of this study (46). At 4 weeks, type III collagen rose significantly from 11 to 16% or more and there was a disproportionate amount of newly formed thin perimysial fibers, which in all likelihood were type III collagen fibers that do not contribute significantly to the elastic properties of the myocardium. There was also evidence of disrupted collagen with expansion of many intermuscular spaces and muscle fiber slippage. As will be seen, these changes indicate collagen degradation and early wound healing, which typically decreases myocardial and ventricular stiffness. The subsequent abnormal elevation of stiffness (Table 8–1) was related to the restoration of a normal proportion of type III collagen relative to type I and the progressive collagen remodeling discussed earlier. That is:

1. At 35 and 88 weeks, previous evidence of myocardial edema was absent.
2. A greater number of interstitial spaces contained thick perimysial fibers.
3. Areas containing a fibrous meshwork which extended over and sometimes encircled muscle fibers were evident (46).

Thus, when considering the relation between myocardial fibrillar collagen and mechanical behavior, other properties of the collagen matrix, such as the proportion of collagen types I and III and collagen distribution, appear to be important. A full understanding of their role, however, most await further investigation.

It is also apparent from Table 8–1 that significant increases in ventricular weight also occurred in these various models of LV pressure overload. Accordingly, one could argue that myocyte enlargement is responsible for the abnormal stiffness. This possibility, however, has been discounted by several recent studies. Bing and co-workers (52) prevented the increase in collagen content with β-amino proprionitrile, which normally occurred with cardiac hypertrophy secondary to chronic aortic constriction, and concluded that elevations in resting tension depend on an increase in collagen content but not hypertrophy. Narayan et al. (40), using hydralazine, were able to prevent myocyte hypertrophy but not the abnormal accumulation of collagen in SHR. They found that the excess collagen produced an abnormal passive myocardial stiffness which was similar to that measured in the untreated SHR with hypertrophy but significantly greater than the stiffness obtained in the genetic control. Brilla and colleagues (19) reported a return to normal passive stiffness in SHR following a complete regression of collagen concentration to that found in control WKY rats using the angiotensin-converting enzyme inhibitor lisinopril. Finally, Gelpi et al. (53) and Douglas and Tallant (54) found no change in myocardial collagen concentration and LV diastolic chamber compliance in dogs with stable peri-

nephritic hypertension despite significant hypertrophy.

Physiologic versus Pathologic Hypertrophy

The heart has the ability to adapt quickly to stress by altering the ratios of the various proteins involved in its function. The degree of cellular hypertrophy can be thought of as adaptive or physiologic as long as these proteins remain in proper balance for physiologic functioning of the myocyte. On the other hand, a disproportionate increase in the structural proteins relative to myocyte enlargement which leads to diastolic dysfunction could be considered pathologic. As discussed previously, the experimentally induced, abnormal accumulation of myocardial collagen has been shown to be responsible for an increase in diastolic LV stiffness and, hence, pathologic hypertrophy. This also appears to be the case clinically. In athletes with a significant increase in LV mass and presumably physiologic hypertrophy, diastolic function is normal at rest and enhanced during exercise (55, 56). By contrast, as shown in Table 8–2, hypertensive patients with an increase in LV mass less than that seen in the athletes are found to have significant diastolic dysfunction (57). In view of the fact that collagen concentration is increased in humans with systemic hypertension (37) and that diastolic abnormalities in hypertensive patients are not closely related to increases in LV mass (58, 59), it is reasonable to assume that this impaired diastolic function is the result of excessive myocardial collagen. Similarly, in patients with aortic stenosis, the elevated levels of myocardial collagen appear to be responsible for the adverse alterations in LV diastolic properties (60).

Myocyte Necrosis and Reparative Fibrosis

The reparative collagen remodeling following myocyte necrosis is distinctly different from the reactive fibrosis associated with genetic hypertension, activation of the renin-angiotensin-aldosterone system, and excess mineralocorticoids. As described previously, reactive fibrosis consists of a thickening of existing fibrillar collagen, an increase in collagen matrix density, and the addition of new fibrillar collagen. Return-

Table 8–2. Diastolic Dysfunction in Patients with Moderate Hypertension

	Normal	Athlete	Hypertension
LV mass (g)	185 ± 50	386 ± 58*	289 ± 47*
Iso relax period (ms)	63 ± 11	57 ± 8	96 ± 22*
Peak rate dimen inc (cm/s)	15 ± 4	17 ± 3	11 ± 4
Peak rate post wall thin (cm/s)	9 ± 2	10 ± 1	7 ± 2*

* $p < 0.01$ from control

Abbreviations: Iso relax = isovolumic relation; dimen inc = dimension increase; post wall thin = posterior wall thinning.

Adapted with permission from Shapiro LM, McKenna WJ: Left ventricular hypertrophy: relation of structure to diastolic function in hypertension. Br Heart J 51:637, 1984.

ing to Figure 8–4, the net effect of this reactive remodeling would be an increase in the stiffness of the spring representing collagen. In contrast, reparative fibrosis is a confluent area of replacement collagen or scar whereby the collagen content in the necrotic area can increase by as much as 500% (61). In the nonischemic regions, the collagen concentration typically remains normal. As the collagen content of the scar increases, so does its stiffness. (See Chap. 18.) The orientation of collagen fibers within a scar corresponds to that of the muscle fibers that had previously occupied the space (62). Therefore, a scar can be thought of as linking undamaged muscle fibers. Depicted in Figure 8–6 is the mechanical analog of this replacement fibrosis. It is represented by a very stiff spring placed in series with the parallel collagen-muscle springs unit that was described in Figure 8–4.

Replacement of muscle with the much stiffer collagen would be expected to increase myocardial and LV chamber passive stiffness. This is indeed the case. Diastolic dysfunction has been reported postinfarction (63), following coronary embolization (51), and in association with isoproterenol-induced endomyocardial fibrosis (64). In these studies, myocardial stiffness increased 30 (64) to 200% (63) as a result of significant replacement fibrosis, which raised collagen volume fraction to levels ranging from 12 to 25% (51, 64) and hydroxyproline per g LV dry weight in the infarcted region to 14.5 mg (63).

Collagen Remodeling in the Senescent Myocardium

The aging human myocardium is characterized by an increase in the proportion of interstitial collagen in contrast to the

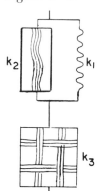

$k_3 > k_2$ and k_1
for all strains

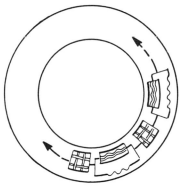

Fig. 8–6. The relationship among myocardial interstitial fibrillar collagen, cardiac muscle, and a replacement scar can be conceptualized as two springs (i.e., muscle spring [k_1] and interstitial collagen spring [k_2]) arranged in parallel coupled in series with the scar spring (k_3). For all strains, the spring representing the scar is much stiffer than the other two springs and therefore behaves as a nonextensible coupling bar between interstitial collagen-muscle spring units.

functional parenchyma (65, 66). The fibrosis is either reparative, reactive, or both. The fibrotic replacement of lost myocardium is usually of vascular origin and is prevalent in the subendocardial zone. The interstitial fibrosis, which does not replace myocytes but instead encircles them, consists of a uniformly distributed, fine network of fibrillar collagen. In the elderly heart, this increased prominence of the interstitium not only occurs in the left ventricle but also in the right ventricle and both atria and takes place with little increase in ventricular mass (65, 67). This pattern of interstitial remodeling is similar to that seen with pressure overload secondary to activation of the renin-angiotensin-aldosterone system or excess mineralocorticoids and suggests that circulating hormones may be an active participant in the aging process of the heart. (See Chap. 25.)

Although it is not known whether the fibrosis in the senescent human heart is sufficient to cause diastolic dysfunction, the marked elevations in myocardial collagen seen in the senescent rat are considered responsible for an increased myocardial stiffness (68, 69). In addition, the heart in the aged is known to be stiffer, with a slower relaxation rate. Diastolic function, as measured by filling parameters, has been found to be significantly altered, with decreased early filling and an increased atrial contribution to late filling (59, 67). Thus, there is strong evidence to hypothesize a cause-and-effect relation between collagen remodeling of the senescent myocardium and abnormal diastolic ventricular function.

INADEQUATE MYOCARDIAL COLLAGEN MATRIX AND LV DIASTOLIC FUNCTION

Immunohistochemical labeling indicates that a latent collagenase system coexists with the collagen matrix (28). Thus, once activated, a relatively rapid degradation of the collagen matrix is possible. If myocardial collagenase is similar to other mammalian collagenases, it can be activated by sulfhydryl-active compounds such as oxidized glutathione (GSSG). In the cascade of events involved with the dissolution of collagen, collagenase activity is the rate-limiting step. By cleaving collagen molecules, it causes a denaturing of the molecule, which then becomes substrate for several other proteases (31).

Functional Consequences of Collagen Degradation

O'Brien and Moore (70), in the nonliving heart with rigor and following a 90-minute incubation in a solution of collagenase, observed that the pressure-volume curve significantly shifted to the right (Fig. 8–7B). This collagenase-induced increase in ventricular distensibility was not obtained after incubation in saline, elastase, or trypsin. More recently, Matsubara et al. (4) have obtained similar results using the in vivo model of presumed myocardial collagenase activation described by Caulfield and Wolkowicz (5). This model consisted of two infusions of oxidized glutathione (25 mg/3H, IV) which are separated by one week.

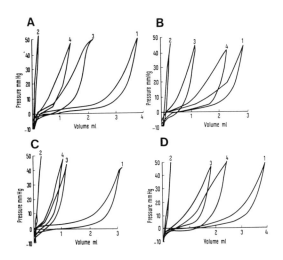

Fig. 8–7. Pressure-volume curves in the arrested rabbit heart as a function of time after isolation (curves 1, 2, 3 and 4 = 10, 60, 62 and 150 min, respectively, after isolation). *A,* saline control; *B,* curve 4 obtained after 90-minute collagenase incubation; *C,* curve 4 obtained after 90-minute elastase incubation; and *D,* curve 4 obtained after 90 min trypsin incubation. The shift to the right following collagenase incubation (i.e., curve 4) represents a significant decrease in ventricular stiffness. An equivalent shift is not seen following incubation in saline, elastase, or trypsin. Reproduced with permission from O'Brien LJ, Moore CM: Connective tissue degradation and distensibility characteristics of the non-living heart. Experientia 22:845, 1966.

Three weeks after the last infusion, the time when total hydroxyproline is expected to reach a minimum (5), the left ventricle was found to be markedly dilated. For any level of end diastolic pressure, the volume of the ventricle was 70% greater following collagen degradation. In addition, the ventricle became more distensible particularly at larger filling volumes (Fig. 8–8). It is of interest to note that this dilation was not accompanied by an increase in LV mass. Thus a rearrangement or slippage of muscle fibers must have also occurred as a consequence of collagen degradation. (See Chap. 18.)

As can be seen in Figure 8–9, infusions with GSSG, as described, resulted in the disappearance of perimysial coiled fibers and strands at the light microscopic level (see Fig. 8–2 for normal) and of the endo-

mysial network surrounding myocytes as well as struts at the scanning electron microscopic level (see Fig. 8–3 for normal). Also of note is the appearance of numerous widened interstitial spaces following collagen degradation. These are far in excess of that which would be expected to accompany tissue fixation, and in all likelihood represent myocardial interstitial edema. Thus, another function attributable to myocardial collagen is the retardation of myocardial edema. That is, the struts and strands impart a structure and stiffness to the interstitial space. Expansion of this space is constrained by these fibrillar collagen tethers and, accordingly, further accumulation of fluid is counteracted by the resulting increase in interstitial pressure. On removal of these constraints, the compliance of the interstitial space is markedly in-

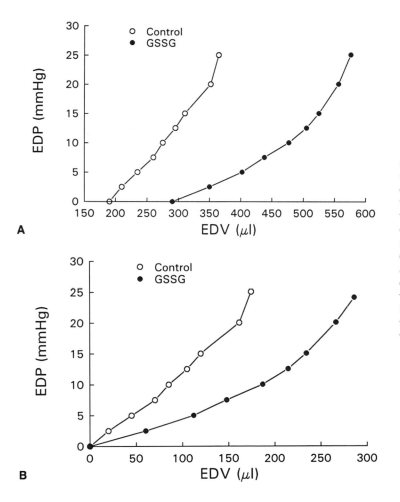

A

B

Fig. 8–8. Left ventricular diastolic pressure (EDP)-volume (EDV) curves for control and oxidized glutathione (GSSG)-treated rat hearts. The hearts were isolated and supported in cross-circulation with another rat. GSSG-induced myocardial collagen degradation results in a dilated ventricle (*A*) with decreased stiffness (*B*). In *B*, EDV was normalized by subtracting EDV at an EDP of 0 mm Hg from all subsequent volume values.

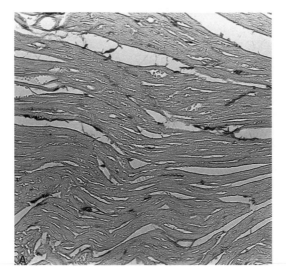

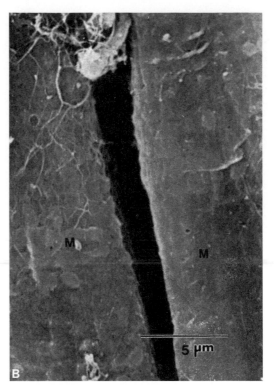

Fig. 8–9. *A,* Oxidized glutathione (GSSG)-induced myocardial collagen degradation in rat heart. Numerous widened interstitial spaces are apparent and Sirius red stain indicates perimysial fibers and strands are markedly reduced (*A,* ×150). *B,* In rats, collagen struts and the collagen network around myocytes are essentially dissolved following in vivo infusions with the disulfide compound, 5,5′-dithio(2-nitrobenzoic acid). Reproduced with permission from Caulfield JB, Wolkowicz PE: Mechanisms for cardiac dilatation. Heart Failure 6:138, 1990.

Fig. 8–4.

creased so that relatively larger amounts of fluid can accumulate without significant increases in interstitial pressure.

Myocardial interstitial edema brings about an increase in the stiffness of the myocardium and ventricle (71, 72). At otherwise constant conditions, Cross et al. (71) reported LV diastolic dysfunction following an increment in myocardial fluid amounting to 4 to 5% of heart weight. Thus, for a 100 g LV, an edema of 4 to 5 g of fluid alters the passive properties of the myocardium. This increment in weight is equivalent to only a 0.7% increase in water content (73). In the case of collagen degradation, the degree to which stiffness is reduced is indirectly related to the amount of accompanying interstitial edema. That is, without edema, the distensibility of the ventricle following collagen degradation would have been greater than that depicted in Figure 8–8.

Pathophysiologic Significance of Inadequate Myocardial Collagen

Myocardial collagen damage can occur even after short periods of ischemia. Occlusions of the left anterior descending coronary artery, which cause depression of myocyte function but not necrosis (i.e., "stunned" myocardium), result in regions of collagen damage (13, 74), particularly in the endomysium. Collagenase, activated by either oxygen-free radicals acting like a disulfide compound or GSSG itself, may have caused this collagen breakdown; the concentration of GSSG is known to be elevated in ischemic regions (75). Such damage would be expected to cause regional dilation with increased compliance and myocardial edema, which in turn could account for the paradoxic expansion and thinning of the "stunned" myocardium.

With prolonged ischemia leading to myocyte necrosis, near complete loss of portions of the collagen matrix can occur in the infarcted area (5). As a result, the region is noted to thin and expand outward during systole. Before healing, which was discussed earlier, this area devoid of collagen is prone to rupture, particularly if the infarct is transmural (7, 8).

Indications of an inadequate myocardial collagen matrix have been found in patients with dilated cardiomyopathy (10). Thick coiled perimysial fibers were rare. Numerous widened interstitial spaces were present, with conspicuous reduction or disruption of lateral connections of collagen between muscle fibers. As seen experimentally, absence or disruption of muscle bundle to muscle bundle tethers and other elements of the collagen matrix leads to ventricular dilation, wall thinning, and interstitial edema. In addition, muscle fiber slippage and a sphericalization of the ventricle are likely to occur. Thus it appears that collagen breakdown plays a major role in bringing about the dilatation, the change in shape, and the increase in distensibility of the cardiomyopathic left ventricle.

A similar statement could be made regarding the heart in end-stage heart failure. For it to become dilated with an increase in compliance, degradation of the myocardial collagen matrix must occur. Experimentally, chronic supraventricular tachycardia is widely used to create a model of heart failure. Within 3 weeks of rapid pacing, both ventricles are significantly dilated and wall thickness reduced. Histologic changes characteristic of collagen degradation, including reduced collagen concentration, significant myocardial edema, and disrupted fibrillar collagen tethers, are apparent within 6 hours of rapid ventricular pacing (11) and, with continued rapid pacing, persist for weeks (11, 12). After 3 weeks of rapid pacing, Spinale et al. (12) found hydroxyproline concentration to be significantly reduced. However, with a longer duration of rapid pacing (i.e., 5.0 ± 1.4 weeks), interstitial collagen concentration is markedly increased because of the compensatory activation of the renin-angiotensin-aldosterone system (11). After 3 weeks of rapid pacing, LV regional chamber stiffness did not differ significantly from control, despite the reduction in collagen concentration (12). This, in all likelihood, was caused by the offsetting effects of the rather large 8% increase in myocardial water content.

Finally, it should be noted that there is evidence of a transient collagen degeneration early in the hypertrophic remodeling process associated with pressure overload. Within the first 4 weeks of both perinephritic (20) and renovascular (42) hypertension, histologic examination of cardiac tissue revealed regions of diminished collagen with collagen fiber disruption and edematous-appearing intermuscular spaces. In the case of perinephritic hypertension, a transient increase in type III collagen and reduction in myocardial stiffness were also reported. This sequence resembles that which accompanies inflammation and wound healing.

SUMMARY

The myocardial collagen matrix is an active participant in determining ventricular architecture and diastolic function, and myocardial structural integrity and mechanical properties. The matrix consists of epimysial, perimysial, and endomysial components which are intimately related to the myocyte, myofibril, and muscle fiber as well as the coronary vasculature. Consisting primarily of collagen types I and III, this material exhibits a high tensile strength that, even though normally present in relatively small amounts, plays an important role in the behavior of the ventricle during diastole. Removal of less than half of the normal amount of collagen results in myocardial edema and a dilated ventricle with increased compliance. Collagen degradation of this magnitude and similar myocardial and ventricular histologic and functional alterations are evident during ischemia, with or without muscle cell necrosis, in dilated cardiomyopathy, and in end-stage heart failure. Thus it appears that a chronic change in the shape and size of the heart must be accompanied by alterations in the interstitial collagen matrix. The hypertrophic response of the myocardium to an abnormal stress includes an early stage which resembles inflammation, collagen degradation, and wound healing. However, with activation of the renin-angiotensin-aldosterone system or when circulating levels of mineralocorticoids are elevated, the collagen remodeling component of the hypertrophic process is progressive and includes a restoration of the collagen types to their normal proportions, an increase in collagen concentration, thickening of existing fibrillar collagen, and the addition of new collagen at all levels of the matrix. The consequences of the remodeling of the collagen matrix are an adverse alteration of the passive mechanical properties of the myocardium and LV diastolic dysfunction. This pathophysiologic aspect of the hypertrophic process is independent of the concomitant remodeling of the myocyte. Thus an alteration in the extracellular matrix, which results in an abnormal accumulation of interstitial collagen, is a major distinguishing factor between physiologic and pathologic hypertrophy.

REFERENCES

1. Borg TK, Caulfield JB: The collagen matrix of the heart. Fed Proc 40:2037, 1981.
2. Robinson TF, Factor SM, Sonnenblick EH: The heart as a suction pump. Sci Am 254:84, 1986.
3. Weber KT, Clark WA, Janicki JS, Shroff SG: Physiologic versus pathologic hypertrophy and the pressure-overloaded myocardium. J Cardiovasc Pharmacol 10:S37, 1987.
4. Matsubara BB, Henegar JR, Janicki JS: Structural and functional role of myocardial collagen. Circulation 84:II-212, 1991.
5. Caulfield JB, Wolkowicz PE: Mechanisms for cardiac dilatation. Heart Failure 6:138, 1990.
6. Dawson R, Milne G, Williams RB: Changes in the collagen of rat heart in copper-deficiency-induced cardiac hypertrophy. Cardiovasc Res 16:559, 1982.
7. Factor SM, Robinson TF, Dominitz R, Cho S: Alterations of the myocardial skeletal framework in acute myocardial infarction with and without ventricular rupture. Am J Cardiovasc Pathol 1:91, 1986.
8. Campbell SE, Diaz-Arias A, Weber KT: Ventricular rupture and fibrillar collagen degradation. Circulation 84:II-558, 1991.
9. Weber KT, Brilla CG: Pathologic hypertrophy and cardiac interstitium: fibrosis and renin-angiotensin-aldosterone system. Circulation 83:1849, 1991.
10. Weber KT, et al.: Inadequate type I collagen fibers in dilated cardiopathy. Am Heart J 116:1641, 1988.
11. Weber KT, et al.: Fibrillar collagen and remodeling of dilated left ventricle. Circulation 82:1387, 1990.
12. Spinale FG, et al.: Collagen remodeling and changes in LV function during development and recovery from supraventricular tachycardia. Am J Physiol 261:H308, 1991.
13. Zhao M, et al.: Profound structural alterations of the extracellular collagen matrix in postischemic dysfunctional ("stunned") but viable myocardium. J Am Coll Cardiol 10:1322, 1987.
14. Ahumada GG, Saffitz JE: Fibronectin in rat heart: A link between cardiac myocytes and collagen. J Histochem Cytochem 32:383, 1984.
15. Shekhonin BV, Domogatsky SP, Idelson GL, Koteliansky VE: Participance of fibronectin and various collagen types in the formation of fibrous extracellular matrix in cardiosclerosis. J Mol Cell Cardiol 20:501, 1988.
16. Contard F, et al.: Specific alterations in the distribution of extracellular matrix components within rat myocardium during the development of pressure overload. Lab Invest 64:65, 1991.
17. Robinson TF, Cohen-Gould L, Factor SM: The skeletal framework of mammalian heart muscle: arrangement of inter- and pericellular connective tissue structures. Lab Invest 49:482, 1983.
18. Pickering JG, Boughner DR: Fibrosis in the transplanted heart and its relation to donor ischemic time: Assessment with polarized light microscopy and digital image analysis. Circulation 81:949, 1990.
19. Brilla CG, Janicki JS, Weber KT: Cardioprotective effects of lisinopril in rats with genetic hypertension and left ventricular hypertrophy. Circulation 83:1771, 1991.
20. Weber KT, et al.: Collagen remodeling of the pressure-overloaded, hypertrophied nonhuman primate myocardium. Circ Res 62:757, 1988.
21. Medugorac I.: Characterization of intramuscular collagen in the mammalian left ventricle. Basic Res Cardiol 77:589, 1982.
22. Parry DAD, Craig AS: Collagen fibrils during development and maturation and their contribution to the mechanical attributes of connective tissue. *In* Biochemistry and Biomechanics. Vol II. Edited by M. E. Nimmi. Boca Raton, CRC Press, Inc., 1988.
23. Robinson TF, et al.: Structure and function of connective tissue in cardiac muscle: Collagen types I and III in endomysial struts and pericellular fibers. Scanning. Microsc 2:1005, 1988.
24. Eghbali M, et al.: Collagen mRNAs in isolated adult heart cells. J Mol Cell Cardiol 20:267, 1988.
25. Eghbali M, et al.: Localization of types I, III, IV collagen mRNAs in rat heart cells

by in situ hybridization. J Mol Cell Cardiol 21:103, 1989.

26. Grove D, Zak R, Nair KG, Aschenbrenner V.: Biochemical correlates of cardiac hypertrophy. IV. Observations on the cellular organization of growth during myocardial hypertrophy in the rat. Circ Res 25:473, 1969.

27. Bonnim CM, Sparrow MP, Taylor RR: Collagen synthesis and content in right ventricular hypertrophy in the dog. Am J Physiol 241:H708, 1981.

28. Montfort I, Perez-Tamayo R: The distribution of collagenase in normal rat tissues. J Histochem Cytochem 23:910, 1975.

29. Chakraborti A, Eghbali M: Collagenase activity in the normal rat myocardium: An immunohistochemical method. Histochemistry 92:391, 1989.

30. Tschesche H, Macartney HW: A new principle of regulation of enzymic activity: Activation and regulation of human polymorphonuclear leukocyte collagenase via disulfide-thiol exchange as catalyzed by the glutathione cycle in a peroxidase-coupled reaction to glucose metabolism. Eur J Biochem 120:183, 1981.

31. Woessner JF Jr.: Matrix metalloproteinases and their inhibitors in connective tissue remodeling. FASEB J 5:2145, 1991.

32. Caulfield JB, Wolkowicz P: Inducible collagenolytic activity in isolated perfused rat hearts. Am J Pathol 131:199, 1988.

33. Caulfield JB, Borg TK: The collagen network of the heart. Lab Invest 40:364, 1979.

34. Robinson TF, et al.: Morphology, composition and function of struts between cardiac myocytes of rat and hamster. Cell Tissue Res 249:247, 1987.

35. Wiegner AW, Bing OHL, Borg TK, Caulfield JB: Mechanical and structural correlates of canine pericardium. Circ Res 49:807, 1981.

36. Factor SM, et al.: The effects of acutely increased ventricular cavity pressure on intrinsic myocardial connective tissue. J Am Coll Cardiol 12:1582, 1988.

37. Pearlman ES, et al.: Muscle fiber orientation and connective tissue content in the hypertrophied human heart. Lab Invest 46:158, 1982.

38. Thiedemann KU, Holubarsch C, Medugorac I, Jacob R: Connective tissue content and myocardial stiffness in pressure overload hypertrophy: A combined study of morphological, morphometric, biochemical, and mechanical properties. Basic Res Cardiol 78:140, 1983.

39. Caulfield JB: Alterations in cardiac collagen with hypertrophy. Perspect Cardiovasc Res 8:49, 1983.

40. Narayan S, et al.: Myocardial collagen and mechanics after preventing hypertrophy in hypertensive rats. Am J Hypertens 2:675, 1989.

41. Abrahams C, Janicki JS, Weber KT: Myocardial hypertrophy in the macaque fascicularis: Structural remodeling of the collagen matrix. Lab Invest 56:676, 1987.

42. Doering CW, et al.: Collagen network remodeling and diastolic stiffness of the rat left ventricle with pressure overload hypertrophy. Cardiovasc Res 22:686, 1988.

43. Brilla CG, et al.: Remodeling of the rat right and left ventricles in experimental hypertension. Circ Res 67:1355, 1990.

44. Morkin E, Ashford TP: Myocardial DNA synthesis in experimental cardiac hypertrophy. Am J Physiol 215:1409, 1968.

45. Skosey JL, Zak R, Martin AF: Biochemical correlates of cardiac hypertrophy. V. Labeling of collagen, myosin and nuclear DNA during experimental myocardial hypertrophy in the rat. Circ Res 31:145, 1972.

46. Pick R, Janicki JS, Weber KT: Myocardial fibrosis in nonhuman primate with pressure overload hypertrophy. Am J Pathol 135:771, 1989.

47. Bing OHL, Matsushita S, Fanburg BL, Levine HJ: Mechanical properties of rat cardiac muscle during experimental hypertrophy. Circ Res 28:234, 1971.

48. Holubarsch C, et al.: Passive elastic properties of myocardium in different models and stages of hypertrophy: A study comparing mechanical, chemical, and morphometric parameters. Perspect Cardiovasc Res 7:323, 1983.

49. Borg TK, Ranson WF, Moshlehy FA, Caulfield JB: Structural basis of ventricular stiffness. Lab Invest 44:49, 1981.

50. Jalil JE, et al.: Fibrillar collagen and myocardial stiffness in the intact hypertrophied rat left ventricle. Circ Res 64:1041, 1989.

51. Carroll EP, Janicki JS, Pick R, Weber KT: Myocardial stiffness and reparative fibrosis following coronary embolization in the rat. Cardiovasc Res 23:655, 1989.

52. Bing OHL, Fanburg BL, Brooks WW, Matsushita S: The effect of the lathyrogen β-amino proprionitrile (BAPN) on the mechanical properties of experimental hypertrophied rat cardiac muscle. Circ Res 43:632, 1978.

53. Gelpi RJ, et al.: Changes in diastolic cardiac function in developing and stable perinephritic hypertension in conscious dogs. Circ Res 68:555, 1991.

54. Douglas PS, Tallant B: Hypertrophy, fibrosis, and diastolic dysfunction in early canine experimental hypertension. J Am Coll Cardiol 17:530, 1991.

55. MacFarlane N, et al.: A comparative study of left ventricular structure and function in elite athletes. Br J Sp Med 25:45, 1991.

56. Nixon JV, et al.: Effects of exercise on left ventricular diastolic performance in trained athletes. Am J Cardiol 68:945, 1991.

57. Shapiro LM, McKenna WJ: Left ventricular hypertrophy: relation of structure to diastolic function in hypertension. Br Heart J 51:637, 1984.

58. Shahi M, et al.: Regression of hypertensive left ventricular hypertrophy and left ventricular diastolic function. Lancet 336:458, 1990.

59. Szlachcic J, Tubau JF, O'Kelly B, Massie BM: Correlates of diastolic filling abnormalities in hypertension: A doppler echocardiographic study. Am Heart J 120:386, 1990.

60. Hess OM, et al.: Diastolic function and myocardial structure in patients with myocardial hypertrophy. Specialized reference to normalized viscoelastic data. Circulation 63:360, 1981.

61. Jugdutt BI, Amy RWM: Healing after myocardial infarction in the dog: changes in hydroxyproline and topography. J Am Coll Cardiol 7:91, 1986.

62. Whittaker P, Boughner DR, Kloner RA: Analysis of healing after myocardial infarction using polarized light microscopy. Am J Pathol 134:879, 1989.

63. Lerman RH, et al.: Myocardial healing and repair after experimental infarction in the rabbit. Circ Res 53:378, 1983.

64. Jalil JE, et al.: Fibrosis-induced reduction of endomyocardium in the rat after isoproterenol treatment. Circ Res 65:258, 1989.

65. Klima M, Burns TR, Chopra A: Myocardial fibrosis in the elderly. Arch Pathol Lab Med 114:938, 1990.

66. Kitzman DW, Edwards WD: Age-related changes in the anatomy of the normal human heart. J Gerontol 45:M33, 1990.

67. Pearson AC, Gudipati CV, Labovitz AJ: Effects of aging on left ventricular structure and function. Am Heart J 121:871, 1991.

68. Anversa P, et al.: Effects of age on mechanical and structural properties of myocardium of Fischer 344 rats. Am J Physiol 256:H1440, 1989.

69. Weisfeldt ML, Loeven WA, Schock NW: Resting and active mechanical properties of trabeculae carnae from aged male rats. Am J Physiol 220:1921, 1971.

70. O'Brien LJ, Moore CM: Connective tissue degradation and distensibility characteristics of the non-living heart. Experientia 22:845, 1966.

71. Cross CE, Rieben PA, Salisbury PF: Influence of coronary perfusion and myocardial edema on pressure-volume diagram of left ventricle. Am J Physiol 201:102, 1961.

72. Vogel WM, Cerel AW, Apstein CS: Postischemic cardiac chamber stiffness and coronary vasomotion: the role of edema and effects of dextran. J Mol Cell Cardiol 18:1207, 1986.

73. Laine GA, Allen SJ: Left ventricular myocardial edema: lymph flow, interstitial fibrosis, and cardiac function. Circ Res 68:1713, 1991.

74. Whittaker P, Boughner DR, Kloner RA, Przyklenk K: Stunned myocardium and myocardial collagen damage: differential effects of single and repeated occlusions. Am Heart J 121:434, 1991.

75. Romero FJ, et al.: Myocardial glutathione alterations in acute coronary occlusion in the dog. Free Radic Res Commun 4:27, 1987.

Part Two

THE EVALUATION OF DIASTOLIC FUNCTION: METHODS AND LIMITATIONS

Chapter 9

PASSIVE ELASTIC PROPERTIES OF THE LEFT VENTRICLE
William H. Gaasch

Left ventricular (LV) end-diastolic pressure can be altered profoundly by various factors, some of which are not related to the contractile (i.e., systolic) state of the myocardium (1). Thus, an elevated LV diastolic pressure, which is commonly taken as evidence of heart failure, may be seen in the presence of normal or abnormal systolic function. Indeed, diastolic dysfunction, alone or in association with systolic dysfunction, has been increasingly recognized as a cause of cardiac dyspnea and occasionally as a cause of congestive heart failure. In patients with coronary or hypertrophic heart disease, dyspnea as well as pulmonary rales, radiographic evidence of pulmonary venous congestion, and even atrial or ventricular gallops indicate abnormalities of the diastolic properties of the left ventricle, not necessarily abnormalities of systolic function (2, 3). In heart failure caused by diastolic dysfunction, the pathophysiology, treatment, and prognosis differ from what is seen in systolic dysfunction (Chap. 26.) For these reasons, it is important to assess quantitatively the diastolic properties of the left ventricle (4, 5).

The passive diastolic pressure-volume relation of the left ventricle is determined by the volume of the chamber, the wall thickness (or myocardial mass), and the material properties of the wall. Thus, under steady-state conditions, the major determinants of the pressure volume relation are the geometry (LV volume and mass) and the intrinsic properties of the wall (myocardial stiffness). During abrupt hemodynamic interventions, and in some disease states, the influence of several dynamic factors may be superimposed on the passive pressure-volume relation (6, 7). These factors, which include the process of

relaxation, right ventricular and pericardial effects, and others are discussed elsewhere in this text. The purpose of this chapter is to present a clinically relevant and mathematically proper approach to the assessment of the passive elastic properties of the fully relaxed ventricle. Special emphasis will be placed on normalization of the diastolic pressure-volume relationships.

TERMINOLOGY AND DEFINITIONS

Throughout this chapter, we will differentiate between LV chamber stiffness and myocardial stiffness. The pathophysiology of pulmonary venous hypertension and congestion is best understood by examining the factors responsible for alterations in *chamber stiffness* (derived from LV diastolic pressure-volume data). By contrast, insight into myocardial functional and structural defects can best be provided by assessing *myocardial stiffness* (derived from the stress-strain characteristics of the LV wall).

Distensibility refers to the change in volume of a hollow elastic structure relative to the change in pressure (dV/dP); under most circumstances the terms distensibility and compliance are used interchangeably.

Chamber stiffness (dP/dV) is the inverse of distensibility or compliance; it can be defined as the pressure change induced by a unit change in volume. This parameter, which may be considered an operative or instantaneous measure of stiffness is directly related to diastolic pressure. The modulus of chamber stiffness (k_c) is defined as the slope of the linear relation between dP/dV and the pressure; this assumes that the P-V relation is exponential. A preload-dependent change in stiffness can occur as a consequence of a change in operating (i.e., end diastolic) pressure. Such stretch-related alterations in dP/dV may occur with little or no change in the chamber stiffness constant (Fig. 9–1).

Stress is defined as force per unit cross-sectional area of a material; the units employed are dynes or grams per square centimeter. In a structure with complex geometry, such as the left ventricle, multiple components of stress can be considered (i.e., circumferential, meridional, radial). Because midwall fibers at the equator of the ventricle are primarily oriented circumferentially, a midwall circumferential stress is commonly used to approximate myocardial fiber stress in the intact heart.

Strain is defined as the deformation of a material that is produced by the application of a force (stress); it is usually expressed as a percentage change from the unstressed dimension. Lagrangian strain (ϵ_L) is defined as $(l - l_o)/l_o$, where l_o is the length corresponding to a state of zero stress and l is the instantaneous length. Natural strain (ϵ_N) is defined as $\log_e (l/l_o)$; this is a more appropriate definition for use with biologic materials where large deformations are en-

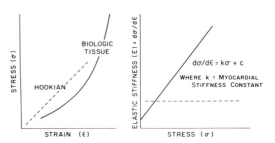

Fig. 9–2. Stress-strain curves and stiffness-stress relations for biologic material are contrasted with those from Hookian material. The stress-strain relation of biologic tissue is curvilinear (panel on the left) and the slope of any tangent to this line represents myocardial elastic stiffness ($d\sigma/d\epsilon$); if the stress-strain relation is linear and the slope of this line represents the elastic stiffness of the tissue, stiffness is constant (panel on the right). Note that material that obeys Hooke's law is characterized by a linear stress-strain relation and that elastic stiffness is independent of stress.

countered. Lagrangian and natural strains are related as follows:

$$\epsilon_N = \log(l/l_o)$$
$$= \log (1 + [l - l_o]/l_o)$$
$$= \log (1 + \epsilon_L)$$

For small deformations, ϵ_N is approximately equal to ϵ_L.

Myocardial stiffness (E) is defined as a change in stress (σ) with respect to a change in strain (ϵ); stiffness (E) = $d\sigma/d\epsilon$. It should be recognized that this definition is based on a uniaxial state of stress as occurs in a papillary muscle; these parameters must be modified for the left ventricle, which is under a three-dimensional state of stress and strain (Fig. 9–2).

These definitions and methods (see subsequent text) are well suited to a clinical assessment of the diastolic properties of the left ventricle, but future research efforts will probably utilize more detailed mathematical modeling and finite element analysis. Clinical measures of LV volume, mass, and geometry as well as myocardial and pericardial structure do not provide a sufficiently accurate data base on which to use finite element analysis. The primary application of such analyses is in the research laboratory.

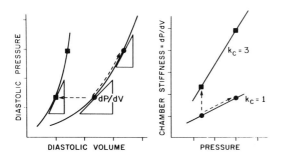

Fig. 9–1. Schematic diagram of left ventricular pressure-volume curves (left) and chamber stiffness-pressure relations (right). The slope of a tangent to the pressure-volume curve (dP/dV) represents chamber stiffness at a given diastolic pressure; with a progressive increase in volume, stiffness progressively increases (preload-dependent change in stiffness). A leftward shift of the pressure-volume curve also causes increased chamber stiffness. If the diastolic pressure-volume curve is exponential, the relation between chamber stiffness (dP/dV) and pressure is linear; the slope of the linear relation represents a chamber stiffness constant (k_c).

PRESSURE-VOLUME RELATIONS AND CHAMBER STIFFNESS

The diastolic pressure-volume (P-V) relation is generally of an exponential form and may be represented by the expression:

$$P = be^{k_c V} \qquad (1)$$

where P = LV cavity pressure, V = LV cavity volume, and b and k_c are curve-fitting parameters. This exponentiality results in a linear relation between instantaneous or operating chamber stiffness (dP/dV) and pressure:

$$dP/dV = k_c(be^{k_c V}) = k_c P \qquad (2)$$

where the curve-fitting parameter (k_c) represents a simple modulus or index of chamber stiffness. Operating chamber stiffness, therefore, can change through an alteration in operating pressure (i.e., a preload or strain dependent change) or through an alteration in k_c (i.e., a shift to a new curve). Calculated values for dP/dV or k_c can provide useful information when used during pharmacologic or other short-term interventions in a single heart (4). However, they can be limited in comparisons of the mechanical properties of hearts of different size. For this reason, attempts have been made to normalize chamber stiffness parameters for LV chamber volume or wall volume (i.e., LV mass).

NORMALIZATION

From a clinical viewpoint, a major reason to evaluate chamber stiffness is to better understand the hemodynamics of congestive heart failure. Therefore, an initial step in any evaluation of the mechanisms underlying elevated LV diastolic pressure is an evaluation of the distensibility or compliance of the LV chamber. In this fashion, non-normalized parameters (i.e., indices of chamber stiffness) can provide relevant clinical information that can be related to left atrial and pulmonary venous hypertension and congestion. For example, a given increase in central blood volume in a patient with concentric LV hypertrophy causes a greater increment in LV diastolic pressure than the same volume increase in a normal subject. Thus, an increased chamber stiffness in the patient with a small hypertrophic heart is associated with a greater change in pressure per unit change in volume than is seen in a patient with a normal ventricle. However, the increased chamber stiffness can be masked if the stiffness parameter is normalized for the small chamber volume (the result might indicate normal or near-normal stiffness). Normalization for LV mass or some other factor could likewise be misleading if the purpose of the analysis is to define the mechanisms underlying pulmonary venous hypertension and congestion in such a ventricle.

When the expression dP/dV is normalized for chamber volume, the result (VdP/dV) more closely reflects LV wall stiffness (which is determined by the thickness of the wall and the intrinsic stiffness of a unit of myocardium). In effect, the chamber size has been removed as a determinant of the diastolic properties of the ventricle. It follows, therefore, that differences in VdP/dV may not reflect differences in dP/dV; the implications of a high value for chamber stiffness are different from those of normalized stiffness. Levine illustrated this by considering and comparing the stiffness of small hypertrophic hearts with that of dilated cardiomyopathic hearts (8). If the ventricle is considered as a whole, dP/dV of the hypertrophic heart is greater than that of the dilated one. However, VdP/dV may be nearly equal in the two hearts. Recognizing that these disparities are caused by the normalization process, it appears that the preferred method depends on the purpose of the analysis. If the purpose of a diastolic pressure-volume analysis is to assess the passive properties of the LV wall or the myocardium, a volume normalization can be useful, although calculation of a myocardial stiffness constant would be more appropriate (see subsequent text). On the other hand, if the purpose of the analysis is to better understand the dynamics of pulmonary venous hypertension and congestive failure, the non-normalized measure of chamber stiffness is more meaningful. As is shown in Table 9–1, venous congestion may be the consequence of hypertrophy (i.e., hypertrophic cardiomyopathy) or an inappropriately small ventricle (i.e., heart size mismatch follow-

Table 9–1.   Left Ventricular Stiffness Parameters and Congestive Heart Failure

	dP/dV	VdP/dV	V/M	k	CHF
Normal LV: acute volume load	↑	○– ↑	○– ↑	○	+
Concentric LV hypertrophy	↑	↑	↓	○	+
Hypertrophic cardiomyopathy	↑ ↑	○– ↑	↓ ↓	○– ↑	+
Compensated MR or AI	↓	○	○	○	–
Decompensated MR or AI	↑	↑ ↑	↑	↑	+
Patient—ventricular mismatch	↑	○– ↑	○– ↑	○	+
Infarction and/or fibrosis	↑	↑	○– ↑	↑	+
Restrictive cardiomyopathy	↑ ↑	↑	↓	↑	+

Abbreviations:
   V/M = ratio of left ventricular volume to mass
     k = myocardial stiffness constant
   CHF = congestive failure or left atrial hypertension
     ○ = normal or unchanged
     + = present
     – = absent
   MR = mitral regurgitation
    AI = aortic insufficiency

ing cardiac transplantation). In either case, stiffness indices that are normalized might give misleading results. Changes in left atrial and pulmonary venous pressure correlate best with changes in dP/dV (Table 9–1). Certainly, hemodynamic studies during volume infusion, negative lower body suction, and even exercise should incorporate raw pressure-volume data and the primary analysis should emphasize non-normalized data; under some circumstances, both normalized and non-normalized parameters can be used.

CONCEPT OF CHAMBER AND MYOCARDIAL STIFFNESS

The intrinsic physical properties of the LV chamber and the myocardium are described by calculating stiffness constants from chamber P-V and myocardial stress-strain data (5, 9). Neither chamber nor myocardial stiffness constants alone, however, provide a complete assessment of the diastolic properties of the left ventricle. For this reason, the appropriate definition of the physical properties of the diastolic ventricle requires determination of both chamber and myocardial stiffness parameters.

It is common practice to curve-fit diastolic P-V or stress-diameter (σ-D) data from minimum pressure (or stress) to end diastole, in exponential or power form, and to use the exponent as an index of chamber or myocardial stiffness. Such an approach can be limited for several reasons. First, a limited number of pressure-volume coordinates are available, especially when angiographic data are obtained at rapid heart rates; considerable scatter of these coordinates is often observed. Second, events that occur during the very early diastolic (i.e., rapid filling) period are not incorporated in the analysis. Third, the exponent is size-dependent and normalization for size can provide misleading results (see previous text). Despite these limitations, chamber and myocardial stiffness constants can be used to describe clinically relevant changes in the diastolic properties of the left ventricle.

This section includes a rationale and an approach for developing indices of chamber and myocardial stiffness that are suitable for application in the clinical setting (9). Applying the theory of elasticity and assuming a spherical geometry for the LV, chamber stiffness (dP/dV) may be expressed in the form

$$dP_T/dV \sim E_s/V(1 + V/V_W) \qquad (3)$$

where E_S = myocardial stiffness based on endocardial stress and strain differences, V = cavity volume or size, V_W = wall volume or mass, and P_T = transmural pressure. A similar expression is obtained if one assumes a cylindric geometry for the LV.

It is readily observed from equation 3 that chamber stiffness is dominated by factors such as cavity size (V), elasticity of the myocardium (E_S), and the wall volume (V_W) or mass.

If the volume factor is normalized to cavity size,

$$dP_T/(dV/V) = V(dP_T/dV)$$
$$\sim E_S/(1 + V/V_W) \qquad (3a)$$

it suggests that the parameter V(dP/dV) is directly related to myocardial stiffness (E_S) and that the relation $V(dP_T/dV)$ versus P_T may yield an index of stiffness. By normalizing for volume, the chamber size is effectively removed as a determinant of stiffness and the relation primarily reflects the contribution of the LV wall. As a result, the chamber stiffness of a normal adult heart would be equal to that of a normal child's heart.

Alternatively, the volume factor can be normalized to wall volume (V_W),

$$P_T = Ae^{\alpha(V/V_W)} \qquad (3b)$$

where A and α are curve filling parameters. Because $dP_T/(dV/V_W) = \alpha P_T$, the α has been employed as a normalized chamber stiffness constant; the relation $V_W(dP_T/dV)$ versus P_T yields a dimensionless index of stiffness. However, if the purpose of such normalization is to remove wall volume (mass) as a contributing factor, it does not accomplish this; indeed, the procedure magnifies the contribution of wall mass (9).

The above relations indicate that normalized chamber stiffness is directly proportional to myocardial elastic stiffness (E_S) and inversely proportional to the volume/mass ratio (V/V_W). It appears, therefore, that normalized chamber stiffness and myocardial stiffness may not always change in the same direction. For example, a large ventricle with an increased V/V_W could have normal chamber stiffness despite an increase in myocardial stiffness. On the other hand, chamber stiffness may be increased if the V/V_W is low, despite the presence of a normal myocardial stiffness (Table 9–1). This concept is important in understanding chamber and myocardial

properties in patients with myocardial and/or valvular heart disease.

CONCEPT OF PASSIVE FILLING PRESSURE

Before proceeding with stiffness calculations, it is appropriate to address certain dynamic interactions that occur in early diastole and to introduce the concept of a passive filling pressure (10). The interplay of relaxation and passive filling is most striking during early diastole. In theory, therefore, the "relaxation pressure" should be subtracted from the measured intracavitary pressure and the resultant passive pressure should be used in the stiffness calculations. In this section, the measured intracavitary pressure is assumed to be a transmural pressure. (See Chap. 4.)

The passive filling pressure (P_p) is assumed to be the difference between the measured cavity pressure (P_m) and the active (i.e., relaxation) pressure decay (P_r):

$$P_p = P_m - P_r \qquad (4)$$

where the value for P_r is derived by extrapolating pressure-time coordinates from the LV isovolumic relaxation period:

$$P_r = P_o e^{-t/T} \qquad (5)$$

where P_o is the initial pressure at peak negative dP/dt, t the time, and T the isovolumic relaxation time constant. This form, however, does not permit the presence of negative pressures, which may occur in a variety of circumstances. It may be preferable, therefore, to use the expression:

$$P_r = a + be^{-ct} \qquad (6)$$

where a, b, and c are curve fitting parameters and t is time. Relaxation pressure (P_r) is then subtracted (equation 4) from the measured cavitary pressure to obtain the passive filling pressure.

INDEXES OF MYOCARDIAL STIFFNESS

Depending on the specific data that are available, two methods for obtaining indexes of myocardial stiffness can be proposed. If stress-diameter (σ-D) data are provided, one can consider curve fits in the form $\sigma = BD_m^\beta$. Hence, myocardial stiffness is given by:

$$E = Kd\sigma/d\epsilon$$
$$= Kd\sigma/(dD_m/D_m) = KD_m(d\sigma/dD_m)$$
$$= K\beta(BD_m^\beta)$$
$$= K\beta(\sigma) = k\sigma \qquad (7)$$

The constant K is a geometric factor that depends on the assumed geometry of the left ventricle (11), D_m is the midwall short axis diameter of the ventricle, E is myocardial elastic stiffness, σ_p = passive stress difference, and k = βK, which may be considered an index of myocardial stiffness.

In the event that pressure-volume (P-V) data are available, an alternative method for assessing LV wall stiffness is to assume curve fits in the form of $P = CV^\gamma$.

$$VdP/dV = \gamma(CV^\gamma) \qquad (8)$$
$$= \gamma P$$

where γ is an index of wall stiffness. If wall thickness is normal, γ can be used as an index of myocardial stiffness.

Although it is true that the curve fits in these expressions have their limitations, they provide indices of stiffness, which are useful for semiquantitative studies. These indices are dimensionless and therefore can be used to compare the mechanical properties of ventricles with different size and shape.

REGIONAL STIFFNESS

Several simple methods are available for analyzing regional myocardial stiffness; such methods are particularly adaptable to problems related to pacing-induced angina or ischemia. (See Chap. 16.) The approach described here relies on combined pressure and echocardiographic data (10, 12). Assuming that the LV may be represented by a cylindric annulus at the site where measurements are made, the stress difference (σ_c) may be expressed in the form

$$\sigma_c = P_p(D_m^2 - h^2)^2/2hD_m^3 \qquad (9)$$

and myocardial stiffness (E_c) may be expressed in the form

$$E_c = (3/4) \, d\sigma_c/d\epsilon_c = (3/4) \, D_m d\sigma_c/dDm \qquad (10)$$

where D_m = midwall diameter, h = wall thickness, $d\epsilon_c$ = incremental midwall strain (dD_m/D_m), P_p = passive filling pressure, and the subscript "c" denotes the cylindrical model geometry (10).

If the stress-diameter ($\sigma_c - D_m$) data are curve-fitted in the power form $\sigma_c = AD_m^\delta$, it follows that

$$E_c = (3/4) \, \delta AD_m^\delta = (3/4) \, \delta\sigma_c = k_c\sigma_c \qquad (11)$$

where $k_c = 3\delta/4$. Thus, k_c may be used as an index of regional myocardial stiffness.

Alternatively, if pressure and regional thickness data are available, the concept of a radial myocardial stiffness (E_R), may be used to obtain

$$E_R = -dP_T/d\epsilon_R = -dP_T/(dh/h) \qquad (12)$$

where $d\epsilon_R = dh/h$ is the incremental radial strain and P_T is the transmural filling pressure (12).

Curve-fitting the pressure-thickness ($P_T - h$) data in the form $P_T = Bh^{-\theta}$, we obtain

$$E_R = -(-\theta Bh^{-\theta}) = \theta(Bh^{-\theta}) = \theta P_T \qquad (13)$$

and θ may be used as an index of regional myocardial stiffness.

CLINICAL CONSIDERATIONS

These theoretic concepts and mathematical methods have been applied in various clinical conditions, including hypertensive heart disease, coronary heart disease, hypertrophic and dilated cardiomyopathy, and valvular heart disease (4, 9). The results provide a basis for understanding the mechanisms underlying pulmonary venous hypertension and congestion. For example, the major factors that affect the diastolic pressure-volume relation in pressure overload hypertrophy are increased LV wall thickness (and mass) and increased interstitial connective tissue; in late stages, especially in the presence of pump failure, ischemia and impaired relaxation also play a role. (See Chaps. 20 and 21.) In coronary heart disease, the loss of myocardial mass, scarring and fibrosis, and eventually regional hypertrophy with geometric changes, contribute to diastolic dysfunction. (See Chaps. 18 and 19.) In these and other forms of heart disease, an assessment of the passive properties of the ventricle provides insights into the factors responsible for many of the signs and symptoms of congestive heart failure.

REFERENCES

1. Braunwald E, Ross J Jr: The ventricular end-diastolic pressure: Appraisal of its value in the recognition of ventricular failure in man. Am J Med 34:147, 1963.
2. Stauffer JC, Gaasch WH: Recognition and treatment of left ventricular diastolic dysfunction. Prog Cardiovasc Dis 32:319, 1990.
3. Gaasch WH: Congestive heart failure in patients with normal left ventricular systolic function: A manifestation of diastolic dysfunction. Herz 16:22, 1991.
4. Gaasch WH, Levine HJ, Quinones MA, Alexander SK: Left ventricular compliance: mechanisms and clinical implications. Am J Card 38:645, 1976.
5. Mirsky I: Assessment of passive elastic stiffness of cardiac muscle: mathematical concepts, physiologic and clinical considerations, directions for future research. Prog Cardiovasc Dis 18:277, 1976.
6. Brutsaert DL, Sys SU: Relaxation and diastole of the heart. Physiol Rev 69:1228, 1989.
7. Gilbert JC, Glantz SA: Determinants of left ventricular filling and of the diastolic pressure-volume relationship. Circ Res 64:827, 1989.
8. Levine HJ: Compliance of the left ventricle. Circ 46:426, 1972.
9. Villari B, et al: Effect of aortic valve stenosis (pressure overload) and regurgitation (volume overload) on left ventricular systolic and diastolic function. Am J Cardiol 69:927, 1992.
10. Mirsky I, Pasipoularides A: Clinical assessment of diastolic function. Prog Cardiovasc Dis 32:291, 1990.
11. Mirsky I, Rankin JS: The effects of geometry, elasticity, and external pressures on the diastolic pressure-volume and stiffness-stress relations. How important is the pericardium? Circ Res 44:601, 1979.
12. Bourdillon PD, et al: Increased regional myocardial stiffness of the left ventricle during pacing-induced angina in man. Circulation 67:316, 1983.

Chapter 10

INTRAVENTRICULAR PRESSURE TRANSIENTS DURING RELAXATION AND FILLING

Michael Courtois and Philip A. Ludbrook

Intracardiac diastolic pressure measurements provide the clinician with important information for patient diagnosis and subsequent clinical management. In an effort to enhance our understanding of diastolic function in the normal and dysfunctional heart, we have undertaken a comprehensive characterization of the regional diastolic pressure transients that occur within the left and right ventricles during both the early and late filling phases, and during isovolumic relaxation. If the exact nature of diastole is to be elucidated, these regional intracardiac diastolic pressure transients must be empirically delineated, controlled for in experiments, and accounted for by theories.

REGIONAL DIASTOLIC PRESSURE GRADIENTS IN THE LEFT VENTRICLE

The presence of an intrachamber left ventricular early diastolic pressure gradient was first described by Ling et al. (1) in 1979. They reported 2 to 5 mm Hg pressure gradients between the mid-left ventricle and the apex in eight dogs. The apical pressure signal (Fig. 10–1, upper panel) is characterized by a sharp, relatively deep decline in pressure during early diastole, followed by an early, sharp upturn, followed by the distinctive oscillatory F-wave. This contrasts with the pressure signal recorded at the midventricular level. Here the pressure signal is characterized by a relatively shallow decline that reaches its nadir relatively late compared to the corresponding apical signal, then begins to increase gradually while exhibiting little or no oscillatory behavior. Ling et al. also consistently recorded a 2 to 3 mm Hg reversed pressure gradient (where apical pressure exceeded midventricular pressure) during late rapid filling, also illustrated in Figure 10–1. Ling et al. speculated that a reversed *intraventricular* pressure gradient of this magnitude should be expected to occur during deceleration of rapid diastolic inflow. The accuracy of this speculation was later supported by the observation by Van de Werf et al. (2) that a reversed *transmitral* pressure gradient was temporally associated with the deceleration of early LV diastolic inflow as measured by an electromagnetic flow velocity catheter positioned at the level of the mitral annulus (Fig. 10–2). Because blood accelerated during the early diastolic filling phase returns to near-zero velocity before systolic ejection, a force of comparable magnitude to the accelerative force must be exerted to decelerate flow. Thus, reversed gradients are physiologic events that may be observed during deceleration of flow across all four cardiac valves (2–5).

We subsequently extended both of these observations by comparing sequential measurements of LV apical, midventricular, and basal pressure to left atrial pressure in dogs (6). In this way, we characterized the relationship of the measured *transmitral* pressure gradient, considered to be the driving force for early diastolic filling (7), to regionally sampled LV pressures (Fig. 10–3). As the site of pressure measurement is moved from apex toward base, important regional pressure differences are recorded during the early phase of diastolic filling: minimum diastolic pressure and the time to reach it increases; the maximum forward (LAP>LVP) transmitral pressure gradient decreases; the slope and height of the left ventricular rapid filling pressure wave decrease; the timing of the

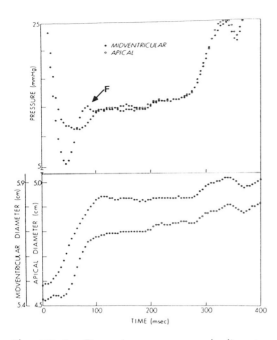

Fig. 10–1. Dynamic pressure and diameter curves obtained in a dog at the midventricular and apical levels from a representative diastole. Reproduced with permission from Ling D, Rankin JS, Edwards CH, McHale PA, Anderson RW: Regional diastolic mechanics of the left ventricle in the conscious dog. Am J Physiol 236(Heart Circ Physiol 5):H323–H330, 1979.

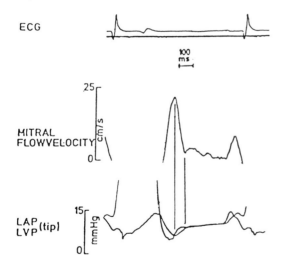

Fig. 10–2. Pressure-flow recording in a dog. Horizontal lines demonstrate temporal association of deceleration of early diastolic flow to reversed transmitral pressures. Modified with permission from Van de Werf, Minten J, Carmeliet P, De Geest H, Kesteloot H: The genesis of the third and fourth heart sounds: A pressure-flow study in dogs. J Clin Invest 73:1400, 1984.

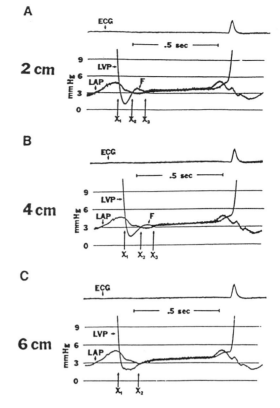

Fig. 10–3. Records of transmitral pressure recorded with the LV micromanometer positioned 2, 4, and 6 cm from the apex. Reproduced with permission from Courtois M, Kovács SJ Jr, Ludbrook PA: The transmitral pressure-flow velocity relationship: The importance of regional pressure gradients in the left ventricle. Circulation 78:661, 1988.

second crossover of atrial and ventricular pressures occurs later; and the magnitude of the reversed (LVP>LAP) gradient decreases. These differences in the magnitude of transmitral pressure gradients as a function of sampling site within the LV are summarized in Table 10–1.

Ling et al. (1) speculated that the observed early diastolic gradients might be related in some manner to the hydrodynamics of intracavitary blood flow. Stimulated by additional new evidence (8–10) indicating that the LV contributes to the process of early diastolic filling by the mechanism of ventricular suction, we speculated that the early diastolic pressure gradient pattern might be related to recoil of the ventricular walls following storage of elastic

Table 10–1.   Transmitral Pressure Variables Measured at 2, 4, and 6 cm From the Ventricular Apex

Variable	Distance from Apex		
	2 cm	4 cm	6 cm
X_1 (mm Hg)	6.7 ± 1.4	6.7 ± 1.4	6.7 ± 1.5
HR (beats/min)	88 ± 23	89 ± 23	87 ± 22
AoM (mm Hg)	96 ± 13	97 ± 13	96 ± 13
LVP_{min} (mm Hg)	1.6 ± 0.7	2.3 ± 0.6	3.1 ± 0.8*†
RFW_{slope} (mm Hg/sec)	74 ± 13	37 ± 13†	26 ± 5†
ETP_{max} (mm Hg)	3.6 ± 1.3	3.0 ± 1.1	2.1 ± 0.7†
LVP_{min}-F (mm Hg)	3.8 ± 0.7	2.7 ± 0.7	1.9 ± 0.4†
X_1-X_2 interval (msec)	71 ± 9	82 ± 10†	96 ± 13*†
X_1-X_3 interval (msec)	175 ± 17	175 ± 20	179 ± 15‡
ARP (mm Hg·msec)	101 ± 41	68 ± 37†	40 ± 33†
A wave$_{slope}$ (mm Hg/sec)	26 ± 10	19 ± 7†	16 ± 4†
A wave$_{peak}$ (mm Hg)	8.2 ± 2.0	7.8 ± 2.3	7.6 ± 2.0†
t-LVP_{min} (msec)	31 ± 3	32 ± 3	50 ± 17†
LVED (mm Hg)	8.1 ± 2.0	7.6 ± 2.2	7.4 ± 2.0†

Reproduced with permission from Courtois M, Kovács SJ Jr, Ludbrook PA: The transmitral pressure-flow velocity relationship: The importance of regional pressure gradients in the left ventricle. Circulation 78:661, 1988.
Data are mean ± SD; n = 11 dogs.
X_1, first crossover point of transmitral pressures; HR, heart rate; AoM, mean aortic pressure; LVP_{min}, minimum left ventricular pressure; RFW_{slope}, slope of left ventricular rapid-filling pressure wave; ETP_{max}, maximum early transmitral pressure gradient; LVP_{min}-F, height of the rapid-filling pressure wave from minimum left ventricular pressure to the peak of the F wave; X_1-X_2, time interval between the first and second crossovers of transmitral pressures; X_1-X_3, time interval between first and third crossovers of transmitral pressures; ARP, area of reversed pressure gradient where left ventricular pressure exceeds left atrial pressure; A wave$_{peak}$, peak pressure of the left ventricular A wave; A wave$_{slope}$, upslope of left ventricular A wave; t-LVP_{min}, time interval between first crossover of transmitral pressures and minimum left ventricular pressure.
* $p < 0.05$ vs. 4 cm group; † $p < 0.05$ vs. 2-cm group.
‡ Values at this position do not include data points from two animals in which no detectable reversal of gradient was observed.

energy at end-systole (6). Because pressure during early diastole begins to increase following minimum left ventricular pressure first near the apex and last near the base, we argued that this implies that blood is being decelerated by impacting with the ventricular wall first near the apex, and last near the base. As surmised from the simultaneous recording of apical and midventricular pressures (Fig. 10–4), filling is completed first in the apex, as indicated by the timing of the peak of the apical F wave. During the same interval, filling near the base is still ongoing as indicated by the continuing increase in pressure at that location. Thus, filling appears to be completed first near the apex and last near the base. This deduction from the pressure signal is consistent with Ling's observation that the apical diameter increased more rapidly and reached diastasis significantly earlier than did the midventricular diameter (1)

(Fig. 10–1, lower panel). The observation that the apical region fills first appears consistent with a model of diastolic function that treats the apex as a prominent source of recoil during early diastole, contributing to the process of filling by actively drawing blood from the mid- and basal levels of the heart into the apical region.

The fall in pressure following the peak of the F wave recorded in the apical region suggests that during the rapid filling phase the apex of the LV may "overfill." This may be caused by rapid early elastic recoil of the LV apex imparting sufficient inertia to the blood to transiently overfill the ventricular apex, which empties partially back into the basal region. We have observed this early diastolic overfilling of the LV apex with contrast ventriculography in both dog and human LVs at heart rates evidencing a distinct diastatic phase. Frame-by-frame analysis shows, in at least some subjects, that

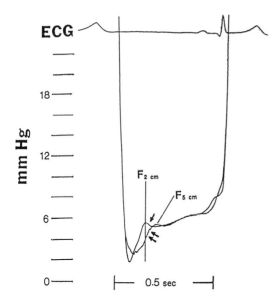

Fig. 10–4. Simultaneous regional left ventricular pressures recorded with a dual micromanometer catheter with 3 cm spacing between the sensors. Maximum early diastolic pressure is reached first near the apex, as indicated by the peak of the F wave recorded from a transducer located 2 cm from the apex (F_{2cm}), then begins to decay (single arrow) At the same time as pressure near the apex (2 cm) is falling, pressure measured by a transducer located 5 cm from the apex indicates that pressure is still increasing (double arrow), resulting in a substantially delayed F wave (F_{5cm}). This pattern of regional diastolic pressure buildup and decay suggests that regional differences in filling exist in the left ventricle. During the atrial filling phase, pressure in the base (a-wave) rises well before the apical a-wave. Thus, some finite time is required for the atria filling wave to propagate the length of the ventricular cavity. Reproduced with permission from Courtois M, Kovács SJ Jr, Ludbrook PA: The transmitral pressure-flow velocity relationship: The importance of regional pressure gradients in the left ventricle. Circulation 78:661, 1988.

during the late portion of the early diastolic filling phase, the LV apex appears to lose volume.

In addition to finding that both forward and reversed transmitral pressure gradients during early diastole are a function of LV pressure sampling site, we also found that the *late* diastolic pressure wave associated with atrial contraction is dependent on catheter position (6). The initial upstroke of the left ventricular a-wave is recorded

first near the base of the heart, and last near the apex. This difference in the timing of the apical and basal a-wave can be seen clearly in Figure 10–4. This pattern is consistent with a model of passive ventricular filling. Thus, recording the pressure impact of the blood entering the ventricle first near the base of the heart, and last near the apex is predictable as some period of time would be required for the pressure wave to propagate from base to apex. In addition, the observation that the regional pressure wave pattern recorded during atrial contraction is exactly opposite to the pattern recorded during rapid filling, during which the upstroke of the left ventricular rapid filling pressure wave occurs first near the apex and last near the base of the heart, again suggests that a mechanism other than passive filling is exerted during early diastole.

Small but statistically significant differences were also noted in the upslope of the LV a-wave and in LV end-diastolic pressure. These differences are summarized in Table 10–1.

REGIONAL DIASTOLIC PRESSURE GRADIENTS IN THE RIGHT VENTRICLE

To determine whether diastolic pressure gradients also occur in the right ventricle (RV), we measured RV regional pressures with use of micromanometers in 6 anesthetized closed-chest dogs (5). As in the LV, minimum RV pressure was consistently less if RV pressure was measured near the apex than in the inflow tract near the tricuspid valve (Fig. 10–5).

However, unlike the LV, the lowest minimum pressure was usually recorded in the RV outflow tract (Fig. 10–6), resulting in a significantly increased RA-RV outflow tract pressure gradient compared with the RA-RV apex pressure gradient. Analysis of contrast right ventriculograms revealed marked narrowing of the RV outflow tract at end-systole in all six animals, suggesting that an end-systolic deformation in this region is a likely mechanism for production of low early diastolic pressure in this region (5). According to this scenario (11), blood continues to leave the ventricle after muscle contraction has ceased, thereby causing the shape of the outflow tract to distort.

RV APEX & INFLOW TRACT

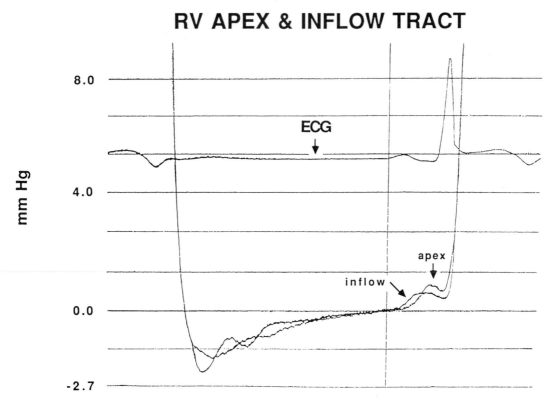

Fig. 10–5.   Simultaneous RV apex and inflow tract intraventricular pressures recorded in a dog using micromanometric catheters. During early diastole, minimum RV pressure was consistently less when measured near the apex than in the inflow tract near the tricuspid valve. During the atrial filling phase, pressure in the inflow tract (a-wave) rises well before the apical a-wave. Reproduced with permission from Courtois M, Barzilai B, Gutierrez F, Ludbrook PA: Characterization of regional diastolic pressure gradients in the right ventricle. Circulation 82:1413, 1990.

RV APEX & OUTFLOW TRACT

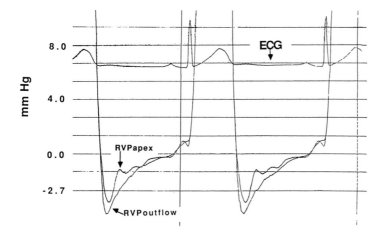

Fig. 10–6.   Record of simultaneous RV apex and outflow tract pressures obtained with micromanometric pressure sensors. A lower minimum pressure is reached in the outflow tract compared with that recorded in the apex. Reproduced with permission from Courtois M, Barzilai B, Gutierrez F, Ludbrook PA: Characterization of regional diastolic pressure gradients in the right ventricle. Circulation 82:1413, 1990.

This causes elastic energy to be stored in the myocardi᷁ ᷁, leading to recoil of the outflow tract walls during early diastole, and accounting for the low pressure recorded during early diastole in this region. In addition, storage of elastic energy in the RV outflow tract may also result from the active contraction of muscle fibers to lengths below equilibrium for that region of the heart (10).

A third possible mechanism contributing to the generation of low early diastolic pressure in the RV outflow tract may be the motion of the heart during systole. During contraction, as blood is propelled cranially, the heart is propelled caudally, stretching the great vessels. Subsequently, during early diastole, as the heart returns toward its presystolic position, the upward motion of the closed pulmonary valve may cause a local drop in pressure in the region under the closed valve leaflets. Thus, factors other than the unique architecture of the RV outflow tract may contribute to the generation of relatively low early diastolic pressure in this region. This is consistent with recent measurements made in our laboratory in the canine LV using a dual sensor micromanometric catheter. In some dogs (3 of 9), the proximal sensor, positioned in the LV just inside the aortic valve, recorded a minimum pressure as low as, or lower than, that recorded in the LV apex.

Although the largest relative RA-RV early diastolic pressure gradient is usually recorded in the outflow tract, the dimensions of this region are small compared to the overall size of the RV. Thus, in reality, the contribution of the outflow tract to total RV filling is probably minor.

During right atrial contraction, the regional RV pressure gradient pattern was similar to the LV pattern: The RV a-wave ascent occurred earlier in the inflow tract and later in the apex (Fig. 10–5).

RELATIONSHIP OF THE EARLY DIASTOLIC TRANSMITRAL PRESSURE GRADIENT TO SYSTOLIC FUNCTION

The traditional concept of early diastolic left ventricular filling is based on Starling's law of the heart (12), which portrays the relaxing ventricles as being distended during early diastole by venous pressure.

Thus, early filling is thought to be determined primarily by filling load (atrial pressure) and the rate of ventricular relaxation. (See Chap. 13.) However, as discussed previously, evidence has accumulated over the past decades indicating that ventricular ejection is also an important determinant of subsequent early diastolic filling. The results of several studies indicate that the ventricle exerts a suction effect that actively draws blood into the ventricular chamber (13–15) and that the magnitude of this suction effect is related to the degree to which end-systolic volume is below the equilibrium volume of the ventricle (9–11). Thus, early diastolic function is strongly related to myocardial shortening (16, 17). (See Chap. 5.)

Because myocardial shortening is determined primarily by LV contractility and the load against which the LV is ejecting (afterload), we undertook a study in 16 normal dogs (18) to evaluate the extent to which these two factors, along with filling load and relaxation rate, contribute to the determination of the early diastolic transmitral pressure gradient. The peak early diastolic transmitral pressure gradient was measured from simultaneous high gain recordings of LA and LV apical pressures; filling load was estimated as LA pressure at the time of mitral valve opening (X_1); myocardial relaxation was approximated by $T_{1/2}$, an index of the rate of LV isovolumic pressure decline; LV contractility was estimated by the peak rate of change of LV pressure during isovolumic contraction ($+dP/dt$); and LV afterload was approximated by aortic diastolic pressure (Ao_{dias}).

As previously reported (19), peak early diastolic filling velocity (E), as measured by transesophageal Doppler echocardiography, was shown to correlate significantly with the peak early diastolic transmitral pressure gradient ($r = 0.716$; $p < 0.002$; Fig. 10–7). (See Chap. 12.)

In this group of animals, the magnitude of the transmitral pressure gradient did not correlate significantly with either X_1 ($r = -0.253$; NS) or $T_{1/2}$ ($r = -0.296$; NS) alone, or when both were entered together as independent variables with E as the dependent variable in a multiple regression analysis ($R = 0.319$; NS).

In comparison, although the major de-

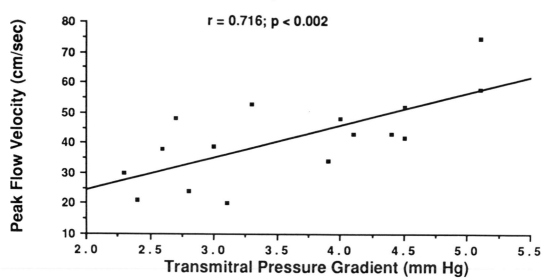

Fig. 10–7. Plot of the early diastolic transmitral pressure gradient versus peak early diastolic flow velocity recorded in 16 dogs.

terminants of myocardial shortening ($+dP/dt$ and Ao_{dias}) did not individually correlate with the transmitral pressure gradient ($r = 0.478$, NS; and $r = -0.362$, NS, respectively), when $+dP/dt$ and Ao_{dias} were entered together as independent variables in a multiple regression analysis with the transmitral pressure gradient as the dependent variable, the relationship was highly significant ($R = 0.759$; $p < 0.004$).

In this study, X_1 and $T_{1/2}$, either alone or together, were not significantly related to the transmitral pressure gradient. Common among studies identifying X_1 as a significant factor contributing to peak early diastolic flow is the large magnitude of the change in LA loading conditions produced by the various interventions employed (7, 19–21). It may be that, within the relatively normal range of LA loading found in our study, X_1 did not exert a significant influence on early diastolic filling dynamics. Because our anesthetic regimen included premedication of the dogs with morphine sulfate (1 mg/kg, subcutaneously), an agent known to increase venous capacitance and thereby reduce preload (22), factors related to systolic shortening and subsequent ventricular recoil may have dominated the determination of the early diastolic transmitral pressure gradient.

Although $T_{1/2}$ was also found to be unre-

lated to the transmitral pressure gradient, this should not be interpreted to indicate that the rate of myocardial inactivation is unrelated to early diastolic filling. As has been shown, dramatically slowed rates of myocardial relaxation are often associated with certain myocardial disease states (23), indicating that a state of residual cross-bridge attachment may exist at the time of mitral valve opening. Such a condition would certainly lead to a decrease in the magnitude of the early diastolic transmitral pressure gradient, and a subsequent reduction in the rate of early diastolic filling. Enhancement of the rate and extent of myocardial inactivation under conditions such as exercise may also lead to increased recoil and filling (24). Again, the results of this study indicate that, for this group of normal animals, myocardial shortening is an important determinant of the transmitral pressure gradient and the early diastolic filling rate.

Systolic Dysfunction and Intraventricular Pressure Gradients

Assuming the early diastolic *intraventricular* pressure gradients to be causally related to recoil of the left ventricular walls, we hypothesized that any condition that interferes with the normal sequence of regional contraction might be expected to alter the normal *intraventricular* diastolic pressure gradient pattern. Such an alteration might contribute to changes in intraventricular flow and the formation of mural thrombus that have been observed to occur in cardiac disorders affecting systolic function such as acute myocardial infarction and dilated cardiomyopathy (25–29). To determine whether acutely induced regional left ventricular systolic mechanical dysfunction is accompanied by changes in the pattern of the early diastolic intraventricular pressure gradient, we carried out an experiment (30) in nine dogs in which the intraventricular pressure gradient was measured across the mid- to apical region of the LV with a dual sensor micromanometric catheter with 3 cm spacing between the sensors. Myocardial ischemia was induced by inflation of an angioplasty balloon in the proximal left anterior descending coronary artery. Severe LV apical systolic wall dysfunction was found to result in the loss of the early regional intraventricular pressure gradient in the apical region. Figure 10–8 illustrates this loss in one animal.

We concluded from these data that systolic dysfunction, engendered by extensive anterior myocardial ischemia, is associated with the attenuation, loss, or even reversal of the maximum *intraventricular* pressure gradient during the rapid filling phase of diastole. These changes are probably related to the loss of actively contracting myocardium available to store and release energy in the form of elastic recoil. Thus acute regional myocardial ischemia, by diminishing the amount of ventricular myocardium available for contraction and subsequent elastic recoil in one region of the ventricle, may result in the loss or diminution of the diastolic intraventricular pressure gradient in that region. This in turn, could lead to the creation of an area of "pocket" in the ventricular cavity where the regional intraventricular pressure gradient that normally aids filling is reduced or absent. In such a region, blood flow would be diminished. This is consistent with reports indicating that certain cardiac disorders affecting systolic function are associated with abnormal regional *intraventricular* flow patterns (i.e., regional slow flow or stasis) and

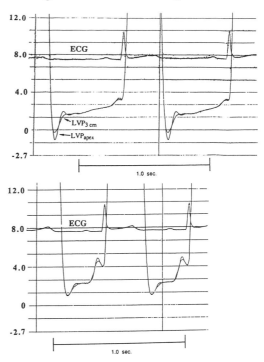

Fig. 10–8. Simultaneous intraventricular pressures recorded in a dog using a dual-sensor micromanometric catheter (3 cm spacing). Upper panel: Pressures at baseline. For this animal, ejection fraction was 48%, and the maximum early diastolic intraventricular pressure gradient = 0.9 mm Hg. Lower panel: After left anterior descending coronary artery occlusion, ejection fraction declined to 29%, LV minimum and end-diastolic pressures increased, and the normal early diastolic intraventricular pressure gradient was lost. Reproduced with permission from Courtois M, Kovacs SJ Jr, Barzilai B, Ludbrook PA: The physiologic early diastolic intraventricular pressure gradient is lost during acute myocardial ischemia. Circulation 81:1688, 1990.

the formation of mural thrombus in specific locations within the ventricle (26, 27).

Measurement of the Atrioventricular Pressure Gradient

In their influential paper, Ishida et al. (7) demonstrated a fundamental principle of left ventricular early diastolic filling dynamics: peak early diastolic flow rate across the mitral valve is directly related to the magnitude of the early diastolic atrioventricular pressure gradient. (See Chap. 5.) Although this relationship has subsequently been verified by a number of investigators, the strengths of the reported relationships have varied. One factor potentially contributing to this variation may be that no standardized method for measuring the peak atrioventricular pressure gradient has been established. Ishida et al. measured the transmitral pressure gradient at the time of peak early diastolic filling rate (7). Courtois et al. found the peak early diastolic transmitral pressure gradient to occur just before minimum LV pressure measured in the apical region (6). Takagi et al. measured the transmitral pressure gradient during early diastole as the difference between the peak of the pulmonary wedge V wave and minimum LV pressure (21). Related to this, Nikolic et al. found the difference between minimum LV pressure at the apex and minimum LV pressure at the base to be proportional to the magnitude of LV elastic recoil forces (31). Because the pressure-flow relationship during early diastole is considered central to understanding the process of ventricular filling, we undertook a systematic analysis of the relationship between various regionally- and temporally-derived measurements of early diastolic transmitral and intraventricular pressure gradients and their relationship to peak early diastolic filling rate (32).

Figure 10–9 illustrates the various *transmitral* and *intraventricular* pressure gradient measurements that we employed.

Two *noninstantaneous* transmitral pressure gradients were measured: pressure at the first crossover of LA and LV pressures (X_1) minus minimum LV apical pressure $[X_1\text{-apical}]$; and X_1 minus minimum mid-LV pressure $[X_1\text{-mid}]$. Two *instantaneous* transmitral pressure gradients were measured: the maximum LA to LV apical early diastolic transmitral pressure gra-jy-dient $[MAX_{apex}]$; and the minimum LA to mid-LV transmitral pressure gradient $[MAX_{mid}]$. In addition, two *intraventricular* gradients were measured: one instantaneous (maximum early diastolic pressure gradient between the apical and mid-LV sensors $[MIVP]$); and one noninstantaneous (minimum mid-LV pressure minus minimum apical pressure $[\text{mid-apex}]$). Correlations of these six measured gradients with peak early diastolic flow velocity as measured by transesophageal Doppler echocardiography are presented in Table 10–2. As shown, the peak flow velocity-transmitral pressure gradient relationship is significantly affected by the method of pressure gradient measurement. Surprisingly, noninstantaneous transmitral pressure gradients correlate as strongly or more strongly with peak flow velocity than do instantaneous gradients. In fact, one of the instantaneously measured gradients (MAX_{mid}) demonstrated no significant relationship to peak early diastolic flow velocity. Transmitral pressure gradients measured between X_1 and minimum LV pres-

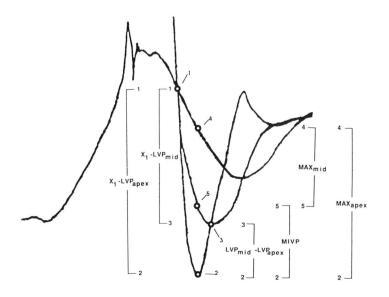

Fig. 10–9. Simultaneous recordings of left atrial, mid-LV, and LV apical pressures made with micromanometers illustrating various early diastolic transmitral and intraventricular pressure gradients measured simultaneously and nonsimultaneously. Reproduced with permission from Courtois M, Mechem CJ, Barzilai B, Ludbrook PA: The early diastolic pressure-flow relationship is dependent on pressure sampling sites and timing factors. Coronary Artery Disease 3: 331, 1992.

Table 10–2. Correlations of Various Measures of Early Diastolic Intracardiac Pressure Gradients with Peak Early Diastolic Transmitral Filling Rate

X1-apex	X1-mid	MAXapex	MAXmid	MIVP	Mid-apex
0.80**	0.77**	0.71**	0.42	0.68**	0.59*

Reproduced with permission from Courtois M, Barzilai B, Fischer AE, Ludbrook PA: Left ventricular postextrasystolic contraction augments early diastolic filling. Coronary Artery Disease 1:257, 1990.
$2n = 15$; * $p < 0.05$; ** $p < 0.01$

sure appear to reflect the total LA and LV energy available for powering early diastolic filling.

The significance of this finding is not clear. It may be that instantaneously measured pressure gradients are significantly influenced by some as yet unidentified factor, such as intra-atrial pressure gradients, which are discussed later in this chapter.

Other Factors Influencing the Assessment of the Early Diastolic Pressure-flow Relationship

As noted previously, we have documented that intracardiac pressure gradients measured during early diastole and their relationship to early diastolic flow are affected by both regional and temporal factors. In addition, several other variables can potentially influence these measured gradients and thus influence the early diastolic transmitral pressure-flow relationship.

Nonhomogeneity

Both *transmitral* and *intraventricular* pressure gradients display significant linear relationships with peak early diastolic transmitral flow (Table 10–2). If the magnitude of these gradients changes homogeneously in response to an intervention that alters early diastolic flow, one would expect that, for any given change in early diastolic flow, these gradients would change proportionally. Given the known complexity of diastolic function, it is hardly surprising that such a straightforward relationship appears not to be the case.

We have previously shown that, in the first normal sinus beat following a short-coupled premature ventricular contraction (PVC), peak early diastolic transmitral flow is significantly augmented (33). Figure

10–10 is a representative recording of transmitral flow velocity in a dog before and after an electrically induced premature ventricular contraction. Figure 10–11 is a recording of simultaneous aortic, left atrial, and two regional (mid-LV and apical) LV pressure signals from a dual sensor micromanometric catheter (3 cm spacing) recorded in a dog before and after a single electrically induced PVC. Before the PVC (single arrow), the X_1 minus minimum mid-LV pressure gradient is approximately 3.9 mm Hg (4.8−0.9), the X_1 minus minimum LV apical pressure gradient is 5.3 mm Hg (4.8−(−0.5)), and the mini-

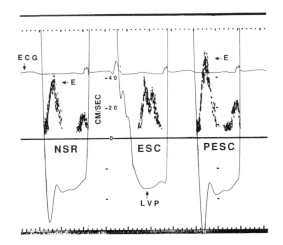

Fig. 10–10. Record of time-velocity profiles following normal sinus (NSR), extrasystolic contraction (ESC), and postextrasystolic contraction (PESC). Postextrasystolic contraction resulted in a significant increase in the maximum velocity of transmitral flow reached during early diastolic filling as measured by the peak of the Doppler E-wave. Reproduced with permission from Courtois M, Kovács SJ Jr, Ludbrook PA: The physiologic early diastolic intraventricular pressure gradient is lost during acute myocardial ischemia. Circulation 81:1688, 1990.

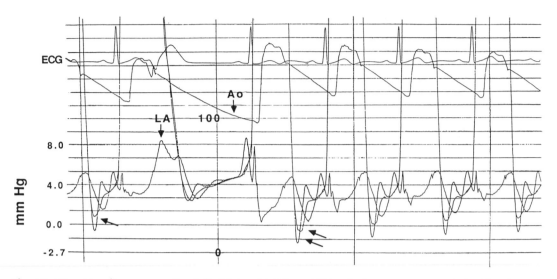

Fig. 10–11. Simultaneous aortic, left atrial, mid-LV, and LV apical pressures recorded with micromanometers in a dog before (single arrow) and after (double arrow) an electrically induced extrasystole.

mum mid-LV minus minimum LV apical pressure gradient is 1.4 mm Hg. Following the first normal systolic contraction after the PVC (double arrows), X_1 changes minimally, and minimum pressure at both LV intracavitary levels decreases. This results in a transmitral pressure gradient increase between X_1 and minimum LV pressure at the midventricular level to approximately 5.2 mm Hg (4.7–(−0.5)), representing a +33% change over baseline; an increase in the transmitral pressure gradient measured between X_1 and minimum LV apical pressure to approximately 6.4 mm Hg (4.7–(−1.7)), representing a +21% change over baseline; and a *decrease* in the *intraventricular* pressure gradient to 1.2 mm Hg, representing a −14% change from baseline. Thus, it appears that in terms of the development of the pressure gradient that determines peak early diastolic flow, the heart may not necessarily respond to a particular intervention in a uniform manner—certain regions of the LV myocardium may contribute differentially, depending on the type and circumstances of the intervention. Certain interventions may effect non-homogeneous changes in regionally measured transmitral and intraventricular pressure gradients in such a way that they may be nonuniform, or in some cases even opposite in direction to changes in early diastolic flow. Such

complexity is hardly surprising, and its full understanding requires further investigation.

Respiration

Another factor affecting the measured intracardiac pressure gradients is respiration. As shown in Figure 10–12, the intraventricular pressure gradient is significantly reduced during the inspiratory portion of the *positive pressure* respiratory cycle. This effect is even more dramatic following coronary occlusion, when the gradient is seen to actually reverse during inspiration with the midventricular minimum pressure falling below that of the apical signal (Fig. 10–13). This phenomenon is probably a result of various intrathoracic effects, including pressure changes and the physical compression of the heart by the expanding lungs (34, 35). Accordingly, most hemodynamic measurements should ideally be made during apnea, or, when this is not practical, at a specific phase of the respiratory cycle, or carefully averaged over one or more entire cardiac cycles.

Intra-atrial Pressure Gradients

In addition to intraventricular position, timing, nonhomogeneity, and respiratory artifacts, another source of variation that

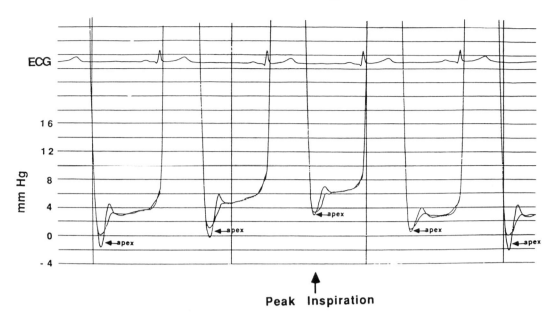

Fig. 10–12. Simultaneously recorded mid-LV and LV apical pressures demonstrating the effect of respiration on the intraventricular pressure gradient.

could potentially impact on transmitral pressure gradient measurement is intra-atrial pressure gradients. As shown in Figure 10–14, the timing and shape of the

right atrial V wave are particularly sensitive to changes in measurement position. We have routinely found in dogs that the V wave, as measured in the low RA near the

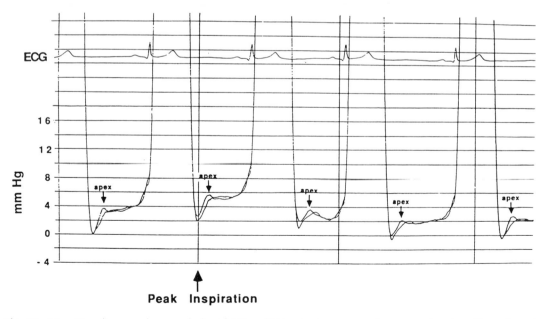

Fig. 10–13. Simultaneously recorded mid-LV and LV apical pressures demonstrating the effect of respiration on the intraventricular pressure gradient during acute occlusion of the left anterior descending coronary artery. At peak inspiration, the mid to apex gradient is seen to be substantially reversed.

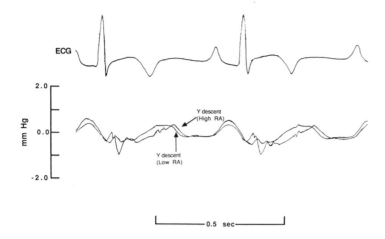

Fig. 10–14. Simultaneous high right atrial and low right atrial pressures recorded with micromanometers demonstrating differences in shape and timing of the V-wave. Reproduced with permission from Courtois M, Mechem CJ, Barzilai B, Ludbrook PA: The early diastolic pressure-flow relationship is dependent on pressure sampling sites and timing factors. Coronary Artery Disease 3:331, 1992.

tricuspid valve, begins to rise earlier, features a more rounded shape, reaches its peak earlier, and begins its Y descent earlier compared to pressure measured in the high RA near the orifice of the superior vena cava. In the normal heart, the atrial V wave is thought to result primarily from "pulling down" of the atrioventricular valve ring during ventricular systole. In the case of the RA, this piston-like action drops RA pressure which causes blood to be drawn rapidly from the vena cavae into the RA. This blood is then decelerated by impacting on the closed tricuspid valve. As shown in Figure 10–15, when pressure and flow are measured at the same level (low superior vena cava), the upslope of the V

wave is seen to be clearly related to deceleration of vena cava flow. Thus, because the upslope of the V wave primarily reflects deceleration of the blood entering the atrium, it is reasonable to expect the appearance of the V wave, first near the valve, and later in the high RA. Likewise, when the A-V valve opens, it is reasonable to expect pressure in the low RA near the A-V valve to drop somewhat earlier than in the region of the high RA. Similar subtle positionally related variations in the shape of the atrial V wave most likely exist in the LA as well. These regional differences, especially in the timing and slope of the Y descent, may also be an important source of uncontrolled error in certain measure-

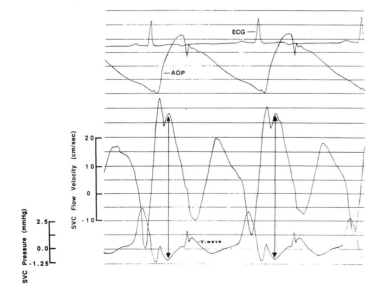

Fig. 10–15. Pressure and flow velocity recorded simultaneously at the same position in the low superior vena cava. Horizontal lines illustrate the temporal association of the occurrence of the V wave with deceleration of flow.

ments of the early diastolic transmitral pressure gradient.

ISOVOLUMIC RELAXATION

The rate of pressure fall during the isovolumic relaxation phase has been variously modeled in an effort to determine a reliable time constant of ventricular relaxation. (See Chaps. 4 and 5.) No systematic study has yet been performed to determine whether regional pressure gradients exist within the LV during the isovolumic relaxation phase. However, observations from several laboratories indicate that distinct changes in ventricular shape occur during this phase, and that these shape changes are often associated with the flow of blood from one region of the ventricle to another. Using contrast ventriculography, Altieri et al. observed regional outward wall motion during the isovolumic relaxation phase in 83% of a consecutive series of patients who underwent cardiac catheterization for evaluation of chest pain, 59% of them with, and 41% of them without significant coronary artery disease (36). Using magnetic resonance tagging, Rademakers et al. demonstrated that 50% of the apical counterclockwise twisting motion that occurs during systole is undone during isovolumic relaxation (37). McInerney et al. using Compton backscatter imaging, detected inward displacements in the lateral epicardial free walls coincident with outward displacements in other regions during isovolumic relaxation (38). Consistent with these changes in ventricular conformation, an intraventricular high velocity (100 cm/sec) apically-directed flow wave has also been shown to exist, especially in hyperdynamic hearts that exhibit some degree of cavity obliteration (39). The driving force for this intracavity flow wave is probably generated by intraventricular pressure gradients created by asynchronous relaxation and/or elastic recoil of the wall segments surrounding the obliterated cavity (39). Thus, because fluid dynamic theory predicts that flow is generated by the presence of regions of differential pressure, it may be anticipated that intraventricular pressure gradients do exist between adjacent regions within the left ventricular chamber during the isovolumic relaxation phase.

For example, in three of the six animals in which we conducted a careful examination of regional pressure gradients in the *right* ventricle, a gradient was noted during the isovolumic relaxation period between the outflow tract and apex (Fig. 10–16). During this phase, the apical pressure waveform is noted to cross over the outflow tract pressure waveform at the start of rapid pressure decline. Apical pressure then continued to fall rapidly, preceding the fall in outflow tract pressure. This pressure difference remained until apical and outflow tract pressures crossed again at approximately the time of tricuspid valve opening. These data suggest that, in some animals, the right ventricular outflow tract may function as a separate chamber, having relaxation characteristics that differ from those of the remainder of the ventricular cavity (40–42). Although we have not, at this time, conclusively documented similar pressure gradients between apex and base, or between apex and outflow tract

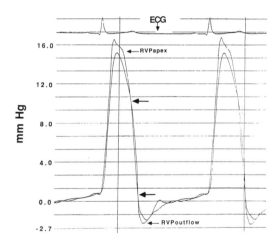

Fig. 10–16. Record in one dog of simultaneous RV apex and outflow tract pressures obtained with micromanometric pressure sensors. During the isovolumic relaxation phase, the apical pressure crosses over outflow tract pressure at the start of rapid pressure decline (upper large arrow). Apical pressure then continues to fall rapidly, preceding the fall in outflow tract pressure. This pressure difference remains until apical and outflow tract pressures cross again at approximately the time of tricuspid valve opening (lower large arrow). Reproduced with permission from Courtois M, Barzilai B, Gutierrez F, Ludbrook PA: Characterization of regional diastolic pressure gradients in the right ventricle. Circulation 82:1413, 1990.

during isovolumic relaxation in the LV, the extensive evidence for changes in LV conformation and for the movement of blood between adjacent regions suggests that intrachamber pressure gradients probably exist in the LV during the isovolumic relaxation phase.

Although we have not recorded a convincing LV intraventricular isovolumic relaxation phase pressure gradient that appears purely related to the movement of blood between adjacent ventricular regions, it is not uncommon to record an artifact in the pressure decay signal during this period (Fig. 10–17), probably because of the above mentioned conformational change in ventricular geometry and/or vibrations related to the closure of the aortic and pulmonary valves. Such pressure signal artifacts, which often occur to varying degrees, affect the calculation of pressure-derived parameters during the isovolumic relaxation phase, and must be minimized by careful, standardized placement of the micromanometer in the LV.

It has been suggested by Rousseau et al. that isovolumic pressure decay rate should be assessed in the first 40 msec after peak −dP/dt (43–44). Data from our laboratory supports this view (45). As shown in Fig. 10–18, the rate of pressure decay following a postextrasystolic contraction (PESC) is delayed by several milliseconds throughout the early portion of the isovolumic relaxation period compared to a normal sinus

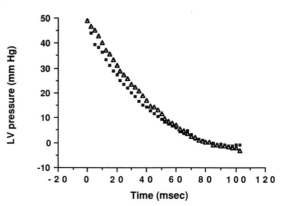

Fig. 10–18. Plot of pressure decay over a matched range in isovolumic relaxation phases after a normal sinus beat (NSR) (squares), and after a postextrasystolic contraction (PESC) (triangles). Rate of pressure decay after the PESC is delayed throughout the early portion of the isovolumic relaxation period. Near the midway point of the isovolumic relaxation period, PESC pressure decay rate catches up with, and subsequently exceeds, that of the NSR beat, eventually falling to an early diastolic pressure level lower than that of NSR. Reproduced with permission from Courtois M, Barzilai B, Fischer AE, Ludbrook PA: Left ventricular isovolumic relaxation rate is slowed, then augmented following extrasystolic potentiation. Coronary Artery Disease 2:501, 1991.

beat. Near the midpoint of this period, PESC pressure decay rate catches up with, and subsequently exceeds, that of the control beat, eventually falling to an early diastolic pressure level lower than that of control. This pattern supports the idea that, under conditions of calcium overload engendered by short-coupled extrasystolic potentiation, the isovolumic relaxation period can appear as two phases. Although the value of 40 msec suggested by Rousseau et al. is not a magic number, in our laboratory we have yet to record an isovolumic relaxation phase that loses its exponential character earlier than 40 msec following peak −dP/dt.

SUMMARY

As the study of the relationship of diastolic function to heart disease advances, a thorough description and understanding of the subtle complexities inherent in the heart during the various phases of diastole are needed. In this chapter, we have endea-

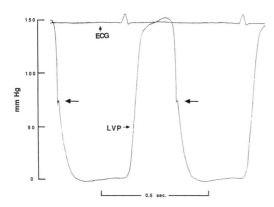

Fig. 10–17. LV pressure recorded with a micromanometer, demonstrating an artifactual "bump" during the isovolumic relaxation period. This artifact is probably related to abrupt changes in LV geometry known to occur during this phase.

vored to describe the salient features of the pressure transients that exist in the ventricles and atria during the different phases of diastole, and to outline the major factors influencing their measurement. Knowledge and control of these potential sources of variability are important for any complete delineation of the process of filling in both the normal and abnormal heart.

REFERENCES

1. Ling D, Rankin JS, Edwards CH, McHale PA, Anderson RW: Regional diastolic mechanics of the left ventricle in the conscious dog. Am J Physiol 236(Heart Circ Physiol 5):H323–H330, 1979.
2. Van de Werf, Minten J, Carmeliet P, De Geest H, Kesteloot H: The genesis of the third and fourth heart sounds: A pressure-flow study in dogs. J Clin Invest 73:1400, 1984.
3. Spencer RF, Greiss FC: Dynamics of ventricular ejection. Circ Res 10:274, 1962.
4. Noble IM: The contribution of blood momentum to left ventricular ejection in the dog. Circ Res 23:663, 1968.
5. Courtois M, Barzilai B, Gutierrez F, Ludbrook PA: Characterization of regional diastolic pressure gradients in the right ventricle. Circulation 82:1413, 1990.
6. Courtois M, Kovács SJ Jr, Ludbrook PA: The transmitral pressure-flow velocity relationship: The importance of regional pressure gradients in the left ventricle. Circulation 78:661, 1988.
7. Ishida Y, Meisner JS, Tsujioka K, et al.: Left ventricular filling dynamics: Influence of left ventricular relaxation and left atrial pressure. Circulation 74:187, 1986.
8. Sabbah HN, Stein PD: Pressure-diameter relations during early diastole in dogs: Incompatibility with the concept of passive left ventricular filling. Circ Res 48:357, 1981.
9. Hori M, Yellin EL, Sonnenblick EH: Left ventricular suction as a mechanism of ventricular filling. Jpn Circ J 46:124, 1982.
10. Yellin EL, Hori M, Yoran C, et al.: Left ventricular filling in the filling and non-filling intact canine heart. Am J Physiol 250:H620, 1986.
11. Nikolic S, Yellin EL, Tamura K, et al.: Passive properties of canine left ventricle: Diastolic stiffness and restoring forces. Circ Res 62:1210, 1988.
12. Patterson SW, Piper H, Starling EH: The regulation of the heart beat. J Physiol 48:465, 1914.
13. Katz LN: The role played by the ventricular relaxation process in filling the ventricle. Am J Physiol 95:542, 1930.
14. Brecher GA: Experimental evidence of ventricular diastolic suction. Circ Res 4:513, 1956.
15. Tyberg JV, Keon WJ, Sonnenblick EH, Urschel CW: Mechanics of ventricular diastole. Cardiovasc Res 4:423, 1970.
16. Caillet D, Crozatier B: Role of myocardial restoring forces in the determination of early diastolic peak velocity of fibre lengthening in the conscious dog. Cardiovasc Res 16:107, 1982.
17. Bahler RC, Martin P: Effects of loading conditions and inotropic state on rapid filling phase of left ventricle. Am J Physiol 248(Heart Circ Physiol 17):H523, 1985.
18. Courtois M, Mechem CJ, Barzilai B, Ludbrook PA: Factors related to end-systolic volume are important determinants of peak early diastolic transmitral flow velocity. Circulation 85:1132, 1992.
19. Courtois M, Vered Z, Barzilai B, et al.: The transmitral pressure-flow velocity relationship: Effect of abrupt preload reduction. Circulation 78:1495, 1988.
20. Choong CY, Hermann HC, Weyman AE, Fifer MA: Preload dependence of Doppler-derived indexes of left ventricular diastolic filling in humans. J Am Coll Cardiol 10:800, 1987.
21. Takagi S, Yokota M, Iwase M, et al.: The important role of left ventricular relaxation and left atrial pressure in the left ventricular filling velocity profile. Am Heart J 118:954, 1989.
22. Ward JM, McGrath RL, Weil JV: Effects of morphine on the peripheral vascular response to sympathetic stimulation. Am J Cardiol 29:659, 1972.
23. Hirota Y: A clinical study of left ventricular relaxation. Circulation 62:756, 1980.
24. Cheng C, Igarashi Y, Little WC: Effect of heart failure on the mechanism of exercise induced augmentation of mitral valve flow (abstract). Circulation 82(suppl III):III-205, 1990.
25. Delemarre BJ, Bot H, Visser CA, Dunning AJ: Pulsed Doppler echocardiographic description of a circular flow pattern in spontaneous left ventricular contrast. J Am Soc Echo 1:114, 1988.
26. Maze SS, Kotler MN, Parry WR: Left ventricular flow characteristics in dilated cardiomyopathy with thrombi: Doppler evaluation (abstract). Circulation 76(suppl IV):IV-126, 1987.
27. Delemarre BJ, Visser CA, Bot H, Dunning AJ: Apical flow pattern and thrombus formation after acute myocardial infarction

(abstract). Circulation 76(suppl IV):IV-227, 1987.

28. Beppu S, Izumi S, Miyatake K, et al.: Abnormal blood pathways in left ventricular cavity in acute myocardial infarction. Circulation 78:157, 1988.

29. Schad N, Romeo F, Fesl H, Nickel O: Noninvasive assessment of regional diastolic left ventricular function with first pass radionuclide functional imaging in ischaemic heart disease. Eur Heart J 7:609, 1986.

30. Courtois M, Kovács SJ Jr, Ludbrook PA: The physiologic early diastolic intraventricular pressure gradient is lost during acute myocardial ischemia. Circulation 81:1688, 1990.

31. Nikolic SD, Feneley M, Octavio PE, et al.: Effect of recoil forces on regional pressure gradients in the left ventricle during diastole. Circulation 82(suppl III):III-605, 1990.

32. Courtois M, Mechem CJ, Barzilai B, Ludbrook PA: The early diastolic pressure-flow relationship is dependent on pressure sampling sites and timing factors. Coronary Artery Disease 3:331, 1992.

33. Courtois M, Barzilai B, Fischer AE, Ludbrook PA: Left ventricular postextrasystolic contraction augments early diastolic filling. Coronary Artery Disease 1:257, 1990.

34. Cassidy SS, Ramanathan M: Dimensional analysis of the left ventricle during PEEP: Relative septal and lateral wall displacements. Am J Physiol 246(Heart Circ Physiol 15):H729, 1984.

35. Robotham JL, Bell RC, Badke FR, Kindred MK: Left ventricular geometry during positive end-expiratory pressure in dogs. Crit Care Med 13:617, 1985.

36. Altieri PI, Wilt SM, Leighton RF: Left ventricular wall motion during the isovolumic relaxation period. Circulation 48:499, 1973.

37. Rademakers FE, Buchalter MB, Weiss JL, et al.: Dissociation between untwisting and filling: An important factor in ventricular suction? Circulation 80(suppl II):II-179, 1989.

38. McInerney JJ, Aronoff RD, Blasko SH, Copenhaver GL, Herr MD: Diastolic collapse: Isovolumic relaxation and early rapid filling. Evidence for diastolic suction? Circulation 82(Suppl III):III-606, 1990.

39. Sasson Z, Hatle L, Appleton CP, et al.: Intraventricular flow during isovolumic relaxation: Description and characterization by Doppler echocardiography. J Am Coll Cardiol 10:539, 1987.

40. Amour JA, Randall WC: Structural basis for cardiac function. Am J Physiol 218:1517, 1970.

41. Pace JB, Keefe JA, Armour JA, Randall WC: Influence of sympathetic nerve stimulation on right ventricular outflow-tract pressures in anesthetized dogs. Circulation Res 24:399, 1969.

42. Raines RA, LeWinter MM, Covell JW: Regional shortening patterns in the canine right ventricle. Am J Physiol 231:1395, 1976.

43. Rousseau MF, Veriter C, Detry JMR, et al.: Impaired early left ventricular relaxation in coronary artery disease: Effects of intracoronary nifedipine. Circulation 62:764, 1980.

44. Rousseau MF, Pouleur H, Detry JMR, Brasseur LA: Relationship between changes in left ventricular inotropic state and relaxation in normal subjects and in patients with coronary artery disease. Circulation 64:736, 1981.

45. Courtois M, Barzilai B, Fischer AE, Ludbrook PA: Left ventricular isovolumic relaxation rate is slowed, then augmented following extrasystolic potentiation. Coronary Artery Disease 2:501, 1991.

Chapter 11

RADIONUCLIDE ANGIOGRAPHIC EVALUATION OF LEFT VENTRICULAR DIASTOLIC FUNCTION

James E. Udelson and Robert O. Bonow

In patients with coronary artery disease, indices of global and regional left ventricular systolic function at rest and during exercise may be obtained by radionuclide ventriculography, and such data provide valuable diagnostic and prognostic information (1–4). Resting left ventricular systolic function is also one of the most important, if not the most important, determinants of prognosis in patients with valvular heart disease (5, 6) and in patients with congestive heart failure (7, 8). Although the most important quantitative variable derived from radionuclide angiographic evaluation of left ventricular function in the majority of cardiac diseases is the ejection fraction, whether measured at rest or during exercise, numerous other quantitative variables, including indexes describing left ventricular diastolic performance, may also be derived. Although these variables have not been demonstrated to have the diagnostic or prognostic power of the ejection fraction, in selected patients they may nonetheless provide clinically relevant information regarding left ventricular function, as well as providing insight into underlying pathophysiology of various cardiac diseases.

LEFT VENTRICULAR DIASTOLIC FILLING

Radionuclide angiographic assessment of left ventricular filling properties is based on analysis of the left ventricular time-activity curve. The time-activity curve represents relative volume changes throughout the cardiac cycle (Fig. 11–1). Such curves are required for deriving all quantitative indexes of ventricular function, including the ejection fraction. With appropriate data acquisition methods and attention to

technical considerations, as outlined below, these volume data may also be used to study left ventricular filling. Several parameters of diastolic function may be computed from the time-activity curve, including the peak rate of rapid diastolic filling, the time to peak filling rate, and the relative contributions of the rapid filling period and of atrial systole to total left ventricular stroke volume (9, 10). In addition, the duration of the isovolumic relaxation period may be computed in approximately 80% of patients (11).

The dynamics of left ventricular filling during rapid filling and atrial systole can also be evaluated using Doppler echocardiography. (See Chap. 12.) Several studies have shown excellent correlations between many radionuclide angiographic and Doppler echocardiographic measurements (12–14), as both techniques assess similar physiologic events. Indices describing the timing of diastolic events, such as the duration of the isovolumic relaxation or the rapid filling period, correlate particularly well with these two techniques. Similarly, agreement is good regarding the relative contributions of rapid filling and atrial systole to total left ventricular stroke volume. Peak filling rate and time to peak filling rate assessed by radionuclide angiography do not correlate well with the magnitude or timing of peak early flow velocity by Doppler echocardiography (12, 13). The events measured by these techniques, the peak volumetric flow and the peak velocity of flow, respectively, occur at different times after the onset of mitral valve opening. However, it has been shown that the radionuclide peak filling rate correlates well with the descent of the Doppler early

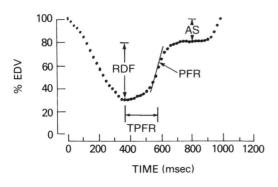

Fig. 11–1. High temporal resolution time-activity curve obtained from radionuclide angiography. Each point represents 20 msec. Variables used to assess left ventricular filling include peak filling rate (PFR), measured as the peak instantaneous slope of a third-order polynomial fit to the rapid filling phase; time to peak filling rate (TPFR), measured from end systole; and the contributions of rapid diastolic filling (RDF) and atrial systole (AS), expressed as a percentage of stroke volume. EDV = end-diastolic volume. Reproduced with permission of Kluwer-Nijhoff Publishing from Bonow RO: Left ventricular filling in ischemic and hypertrophic heart disease. *In* Diastolic Relaxation of the Heart. Edited by W Grossman and BH Lorell. Boston, Martinus Nijhoff Publishers, 1987.

diastolic flow velocity peak (12). Normalization of the radionuclide peak filling rate in terms of stroke volume rather than end-diastolic volume improves the correlation with early peak flow velocity (14). One potential advantage of radionuclide angiography compared to Doppler techniques is the ability to assess the temporal and spatial heterogeneity of left ventricular systolic and diastolic function (16–19), both of which affect global diastolic function in many forms of cardiac disease (19–23). The recent description of pressure gradients within the left ventricle during diastolic filling (15), which may importantly influence local measurement of flow velocity, emphasize the concept that radionuclide angiography and Doppler echocardiography are measuring distinct aspects of left ventricular filling.

Determinants of Left Ventricular Filling

Interpretation of the results of noninvasive data describing ventricular filling, whether obtained using radionuclide an-

giographic or Doppler echocardiographic techniques, is complex. Diastolic filling of the left ventricle represents the simultaneous interaction of multiple factors, including the passive properties determining left ventricular distensibility (or compliance) (24–26), active left ventricular relaxation (27–29), regional ventricular asynchrony (19–23), pericardial constraint and ventricular interaction (30–32), and the prevailing loading conditions, such as afterload (20, 33, 34) and wall tension at the onset of mitral valve opening (20, 33). These factors together combine to influence left ventricular pressure throughout the filling period and interact with left atrial pressure (itself influenced by volume status and venous tone) to create the instantaneous left atrial to left ventricular pressure gradient, the motive force for ventricular filling (35). These many factors must be considered when interpreting diastolic filling measurements and, in many cases, may preclude the complete interpretation of purely noninvasive data. For example, peak filling rate is a noninvasive reflection of the early diastolic pressure difference at mitral valve opening between the left atrium and left ventricle (35), and peak filling rate may be increased merely by increases in the left atrial driving pressure, or decreased by maneuvers that diminish left atrial pressure, such as postural changes (36), in the absence of any change in ventricular properties. (See Chap. 13.)

TECHNICAL CONSIDERATIONS

Data Acquisition

Following labeling of a small volume of the patient's red blood cells with technetium 99m, the tagged red cells are allowed to come into equilibrium with the total blood pool, and a gamma camera is placed over the left thorax for acquisition of the scintigraphic data. For resting studies, up to 800 cardiac cycles of gated-equilibrium information are acquired. From the resultant cardiac image sequence, count activity data within an operator-defined left ventricular region of interest are calculated to create the time-activity curve.

By fitting a third-order polynomial function to the rapid filling period, the peak rate of filling and the time interval from end systole to occurrence of the peak filling rate may be determined (37). In patients with a discernible diastasis interval separating rapid diastolic filling from atrial systole, the relative contribution of atrial systole to total left ventricular stroke volume may be calculated (38). By determining the PR interval from the electrocardiogram and adding 40 msec for electromechanical delay, the duration of atrial mechanical systole can be approximated. The increase in counts over this time period occurring at the final portion of the time-activity curve determines the atrial contribution to total filling (38) (Fig. 11–2).

Appropriate attention must be given to technical details of data acquisition and analysis for evaluation of diastolic events using radionuclide angiography. In particular, the effects of cycle length variability

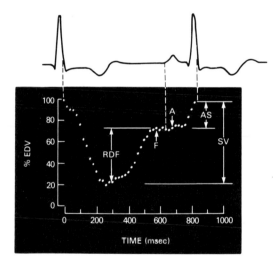

Fig. 11–2. Left ventricular time-activity curve in a patient with hypertrophic cardiomyopathy. Termination of rapid diastolic filling (arrow F) is determined visually. Onset of atrial systole (arrow A) is determined automatically by subtracting the PR interval (140 msec) and the interval from the onset of the QRS to the point of R-wave gating (60 msec) from the cardiac cycle length and then adding 40 msec for assumed atrial electrical mechanical delay. Left ventricular filling volume during rapid diastolic filling (RDF) and atrial systole (AS) are expressed relative to total stroke volume (SV). EDV = end-diastolic volume. Reproduced with permission from Bonow RO, et al.: Atrial systole and left ventricular filling in patients with hypertrophic cardiomyopathy: Effect of verapamil. Am J Cardiol 51:1386, 1983.

(in gated studies), temporal resolution, temporal smoothing, and normalization parameters must be considered.

Effect of Cycle Length Fluctuations and Gating Mode

The diastolic portion of the time-activity curves may be uninterpretable if extrasystolic and post-extrasystolic cycles are included in the data analysis. Such cycles not only distort the diastolic shape of the curve, but also provide misleading information, because these cycles have inherently different contraction and relaxation properties compared with normal sinus beats. Thus, it is general practice to use "beat-length windowing" to exclude cycles that fall out of prespecified cycle length variations around the mean cycle length (usually ± 10%) before data storage.

In normal individuals, an inherent degree of cycle length variability exists during sinus rhythm. This normal degree of sinus arrhythmia may distort the shape of the late diastolic portion of the volume curve because of the loss of counts toward end-diastole, because the frames late in the cardiac cycle contain information from slightly different parts of the late cardiac cycle. Using "frame-mode" acquisition, data from individual cardiac cycles are placed into the series of frames once they have passed through the beat-length window, and the ability to retrieve individual cardiac cycles for post-acquisition processing is lost. The ability to reprocess a study in which excessive cycle length variation has occurred is not possible using frame-mode acquisition. For this reason, "list-mode" acquisition methods may be preferable, in which data from each individual cardiac cycle are stored sequentially in a computer buffer zone and can be retrieved for reprocessing after the acquisition is complete (37). Although this provides the opportunity to more accurately represent late diastolic events, it requires a great deal more computer storage space, which may limit its application in all laboratories. Using list-mode acquisition, one may employ both forward and reverse gating from the R wave to create a time-activity curve

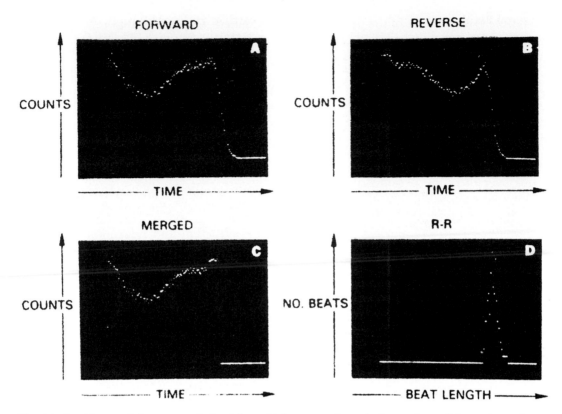

Fig. 11–3. Time-activity curves derived from high temporal resolution radionuclide angiography. In panel A, the data are gated forward from the R-wave; counts drop off toward the end of the cyle because of variations in cycle length and number of courts in the final frames. In panel B, the data are reverse-gated backward from the R-wave. Information regarding rapid filling and atrial systole are completely maintained. In panel C, forward and reverse-gated data are merged to form a complete time-activity curve to reflect accurately systolic as well as early and late diastolic events. Panel D demonstrates the beat length distribution function. Note that the total filling volume caused atrial systole may be underestimated if only the forward gated curve is examined. Reproduced with permission from Bacharach SL, et al.: ECG-gated scintillation probe measurement of left ventricular function. J Nucl Med 18:1176, 1977.

representing the average events in a large number of cardiac cycles, and preserve late diastolic events for analysis (Fig. 11–3) (39). This acquisition mode is particularly important for assessing left ventricular filling, whereas quantifying systolic parameters such as ejection fraction is not as strongly dependent on cycle length variability. It is possible to accurately derive diastolic data from frame-mode acquisitions, but satisfactory results are achieved only if attention is directed to accepting only a narrow range of cardiac cycle lengths for analysis. This may entail prolonging data acquisition to achieve satisfactory count rates, because many more cycles

will be excluded "up front" from storage and analysis. Other approaches include collecting data during atrial pacing at constant heart rate (an intervention which itself may alter filling properties, however), analyzing only single cycles by using first pass methods (40), or using high temporal resolution nonimaging scintillation probes (39, 41).

Alternative gating schemes have been proposed for acquisition of radionuclide data to optimize the quantitative analysis of diastolic parameters (42). However, these modalities have not been widely applied to clinical analysis of diastolic performance in relevant patient subgroups.

Temporal Resolution

The temporal resolution of a radionuclide acquisition is related to the number of frames of information into which the average cardiac cycle is divided. The higher the temporal resolution of the study (that is, the more frames into which the cycle is divided), the more likely that the resultant time-activity curve will accurately reflect the true left ventricular time-volume curve. However, increased temporal resolution reduces the count statistics within each frame. This leads to potentially important counting inaccuracies for each individual data point as lower count statistics lead to greater imprecision of the data, which is then reflected in the global time-activity curve. In contrast, low temporal resolution studies do not accurately reflect subtle inflections in the time-activity curve, and thus do not accurately reflect instantaneous observations such as peak filling rate or peak ejection rate. Previous studies have determined that, when these acquisition methods are used, accurate determination of peak filling rate requires a high temporal resolution left ventricular volume curve using framing rates higher than 25 frames per second, that is, less than 40 msec per frame (43, 44). Lower frame rates are inadequate and result in significant underestimation of peak filling rate. In contrast, lower temporal resolution studies are adequate for evaluation of systolic parameters such as ejection fraction. These concepts have important general implications for assessing ventricular performance because they apply to imaging modalities other than radionuclide angiography, such as magnetic resonance imaging and ultrafast cinecomputed tomography, both of which have inherently low temporal resolution.

Most radionuclide angiographic systems employ an acquisition mode using a fixed time period for each acquisition frame. As noted, this can lead to "drop-off" of counts in the latter frames of a study because of inherent sinus arrhythmia, necessitating reverse-gating to accurately represent late diastolic events (Fig. 11–3). Some systems offer an optional acquisition mode in which the number of frames per cardiac cycle is fixed; thus the temporal duration of analogous frames may vary from cardiac cycle to cardiac cycle. Although this approach theoretically obviates the late cycle fall-off in counts, it makes the assumption that cycle length variability affects all phases of the cardiac cycle equally. This assumption is not necessarily true because cycle length changes predominantly affect late cycle events; earlier events in the cardiac cycle do not "know" that the cycle will be shortened or prolonged on a beat-by-beat basis. Recent data have shown that using the fixed number of frames method may importantly underestimate peak filling rate, and does so to a greater degree with increasing degrees of sinus arrhythmia (45). Thus, an acquisition mode with a fixed temporal duration per frame, using both forward and reverse R-wave gating, appears to most optimally and reproducibly represent diastolic events at rest (45).

Temporal Smoothing

All radionuclide angiographic volume curves have an inherent degree of statistical imprecision. The magnitude of this imprecision is a function of the total number of counts accumulated in the study, the number of counts in each individual frame, and the underlying state of left ventricular function. Studies acquired in patients with depressed left ventricular function (resulting in a flat volume curve) have relatively greater statistical noise as compared to curves from patients with normal left ventricular function, as do studies comprising a relatively low number of total left ventricular counts. To surmount these statistical imprecisions, to reduce noise in the ventricular time-activity curve, and to improve the visual interpretation of radionuclide angiograms, many laboratories routinely employ temporal smoothing techniques to assist in deriving quantitative indexes of systolic and diastolic function. However, such smoothing may introduce important errors into the analysis by changing the shape of the time-activity curve, and may introduce systematic errors into the analysis of diastolic performance (44, 46). Recent data have assessed this potential effect using high resolution time-activity curves from normal subjects, from patients with coronary artery disease, and from patients with hypertrophic cardiomyopathy (46). The time-activity curves were subjected to increasing degrees of temporal smoothing. In each group, increased smoothing progressively and consistently underestimated ejection fraction by up to 5%. A more significant effect was seen on diastolic parameters, as increasing degrees of curve smoothing reduced peak filling rate by up to 23% in normal subjects and by 10% and 15% in patients with coronary artery disease and hypertrophic cardiomyopathy respectively (Fig. 11–4) (46). These errors were increased even further when the same data were reformatted at lower temporal resolution and then subjected to increasing degrees of smoothing: peak filling rate was underestimated by over 30% in all patient groups. Importantly, the underestimation was not uniform, and its magnitude varied considerably among individuals in each of the three groups. Thus, application of temporal smoothing processes may importantly underestimate indices of left ventricular systolic and particularly diastolic

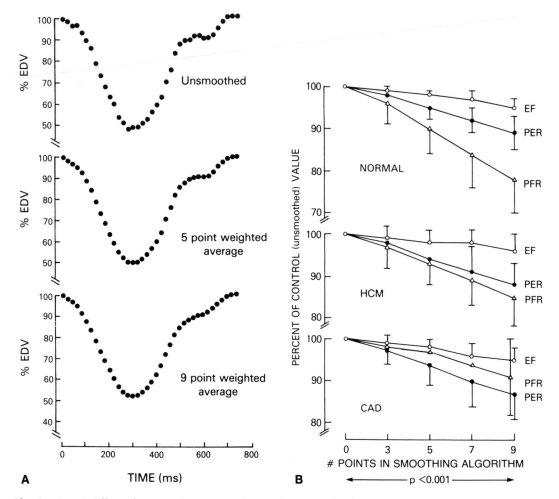

Fig. 11–4. *A,* Effect of progressive temporal smoothing on a background-corrected time-activity curve. The raw curve (unsmoothed) at the top is subjected to 5-point (middle) and then 9-point (bottom) smoothing algorithms. EDV = end diastolic volume. *B,* Effect of progressive temporal smoothing on quantitative measures of left ventricular function in normal subjects and in patients with hypertrophic cardiomyopathy (HC) and coronary artery disease (CAD). Increasing degrees of smoothing are associated with progressive underestimation of ejection fraction (EF), peak ejection rate (PER), and peak filling rate (PFR). Progressive levels of smoothing significantly reduced all three variables in each patient group. Reproduced with permission from Bonow RO, et al.: Influence of temporal smoothing on quantitation of left ventricular function by gated blood pool scintigraphy. Am J Cardiol 64:921, 1989.

function. Application of smoothing algorithms to data obtained at low framing rates increases the error. Again, it should be noted that these concepts are not unique to radionuclide angiography, but also apply to other methods with inherently lower framing rates (and thus lower temporal resolution) such as magnetic resonance imaging or ultrafast cinecomputed tomography.

Normalization Parameters

Because of variations in red cell tagging efficiency and varying attenuation among different patients, the percentage of counts reaching the gamma camera from the left ventricular region of interest as a function of tracer dose is not uniform among patients. Therefore, quantitative variables derived from changes in counts, such as peak filling rate (which is computed in counts/second), must be normalized to a physiologic variable contained within the time-activity curve. Peak filling rate is usually normalized to end-diastolic volume, and expressed as end-diastolic volumes per second. Although normalized peak filling rate has been shown to be a useful index of left ventricular filling for studying diastolic abnormalities in ischemic and hypertrophic heart disease (10), it is influenced not only by the "true" filling rate (in milliliters/second), but also by the normalization parameter itself. In addition, peak filling rate normalized to end-diastolic volume is highly ejection fraction-dependent (9, 47); the higher the ejection fraction, the steeper will be the resulting diastolic filling curve and the higher the normalized peak filling rate. This factor, and others, must be taken into account when studying the effect of interventions on left ventricular filling. An intervention that both increases ejection fraction and increases peak filling normalized to end-diastolic volume may not necessarily be interpreted to indicate a salutary change in ventricular diastolic properties. In contrast, when an intervention increases peak filling rate normalized to end-diastolic volume while at the same time causing no change (or a decrease) in ejection fraction or heart rate, it may be presumed that a change in left ventricular filling has taken

place independent of a change in systolic function.

Peak filling rate may be normalized by other parameters derived from the time-activity curve, such as stroke volume. Stroke volume normalization has the advantage of being ejection fraction independent. It is advisable, when comparing peak filling rates among patient groups or studying the effects of an intervention on peak filling rate, to normalize the data to both end-diastolic volume and stroke volume. Similar findings using both normalization parameters strengthens the contention that true changes in LV filling have occurred. Data from our laboratory have shown that when peak filling rate is normalized to several different variables (such as end-diastolic volume, stroke volume, end-systolic volume, or the instantaneous volume at the time of peak filling rate) in the same patient population, the prevalence of diastolic abnormalities may vary considerably when compared to a normal population (Fig. 11–5) (48). However, the direction and magnitude of a change in peak filling rate during interventions (such as following angioplasty or following oral treatment with verapamil) is generally maintained as long as the normalization pa-

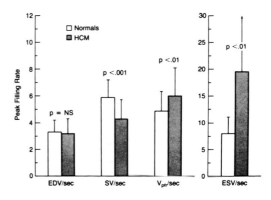

Fig. 11–5. Effect of normalization parameters on peak filling rate derived from the radionuclide time-activity curve in hypertrophic cardiomyopathy (HCM) compared to normal subjects (NL). The count-based values were normalized to end-diastolic volume (EDV), stroke volume (SV), instantaneous volume at the time of peak filling rate (V_{pfr}), and end-systolic volume (ESV). Different normalization parameters may yield distinct results in comparing HCM patients to normal patients. See text for details.

rameter itself does not change significantly (48).

It has been argued that, because normalized peak filling rate does not necessarily represent absolute left ventricular filling velocity, its usefulness as an index of LV filling may be diminished (49). Although the peak rate of left ventricular filling during the rapid filling period does have some relation to left ventricular end-diastolic volume in normal subjects (50), and thus normalization to a parameter such as end-diastolic volume has some degree of physiologic basis, normalized peak filling rate is in itself a diastolic filling "index" whose utility has been demonstrated in studying clinical abnormalities of left ventricular filling in patients with coronary artery disease, hypertrophic cardiomyopathy, and hypertensive heart disease. Although the relationship between normalized peak filling rate (or true filling rate) to more primary factors determining diastolic performance, such as left ventricular relaxation and stiffness, is complex, normalized peak filling rate has been found in many studies to offer clinically useful insights into left ventricular filling abnormalities. In much the same way, the ejection fraction has been found to have important diagnostic and prognostic utility as an index of systolic performance, despite the fact that it is a normalized parameter (stroke volume normalized by end-diastolic volume), and has a complex, nonlinear relationship to primary indexes of left ventricular contractility.

Thus, attention to normalization methods, particularly changes in the normalization parameter itself following intervention, are important factors when assessing left ventricular filling using radionuclide angiography. Normalization methods are likewise problematic in the assessment of passive stiffness and the diastolic pressure-volume relationships. (See Chap. 9.)

Use of First-pass Methodology

Although the analytic techniques described above lend themselves well to gated equilibrium blood pool studies, important inherent methodologic limitations exist in evaluating diastolic filling with first pass methods. Although first-pass techniques have been used to assess diastolic filling

(51), these results should be interpreted cautiously. To equate the rate of change in left ventricular counts during the cardiac cycle with the relative rate of change of left ventricular volume, there is the implicit assumption that a constant proportion exists between counts and volume. This assumption is valid in the case of the equilibrium method, but will usually be invalid with the first-pass method, as the proportionality between counts and volume in the left ventricle is constantly changing (first increasing, then decreasing) as the radioactive bolus traverses the cardiac blood pool (52). This is particularly true during diastole because the new bolus of blood crossing the mitral valve contains a constantly changing radiotracer concentration. Hence, the rate of change of diastolic counts is affected by intrinsic ventricular diastolic properties, by the rapidity with which the radioactive bolus enters and then clears from the left ventricle, and by potentially different count-volume ratios with each transmitral filling bolus. Of note, the more perfect the bolus, with a sudden appearance and sudden clearance from the cardiac chambers, the greater the likelihood of inaccuracy in determining filling rates. Determination of systolic parameters such as ejection fraction is not importantly affected by these concepts. During each systole, the count proportionality to volume within the left ventricular chamber is constant because no new blood is entering the ventricle.

PHYSIOLOGIC CONSIDERATIONS

Effect of Aging

Experimental and clinical data demonstrate an apparent deterioration in left ventricular diastolic function as part of the normal aging process. Aging is associated with increased left ventricular stiffness in experimental animals, representing the effects both of changes in passive myocardial properties (53–55) (related to increased interstitial collagen content) (53, 56, 57) and in active relaxation (related to prolonged contraction duration and impaired calcium sequestration by the sarcoplasmic reticulum) (54, 55, 58–60). This evidence of altered diastolic properties in senescent animals has been supported by noninvasive studies in normal humans demonstrating a reduction in the rate and magnitude of left ventricular rapid diastolic filling as a function of age (Fig. 11–6) (61–65). As the rate

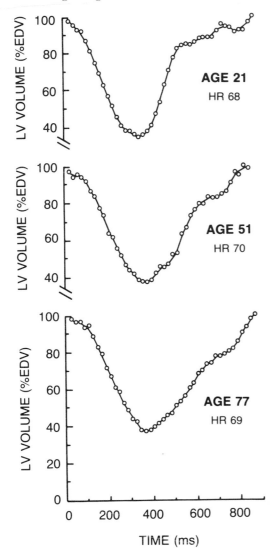

Fig. 11–6. Time-activity curves demonstrating the effect of age on rapid diastolic filling. Global left ventricular (LV) volume curves are shown for three normal volunteers, matched for heart rate and ejection fraction. With increasing age, there is a reduction in the rate as well as the extent of the rapid filling phase of diastole. This is associated with an age-related increase in the contribution of atrial systole to left ventricular stroke volume. Reproduced with permission from Bonow RO, et al.: Effects of aging on asynchronous left ventricular regional function and global ventricular filling in normal human subjects. J Am Coll Cardiol 11:50, 1988.

and extent of rapid diastolic filling decline as a function of age in normal subjects, appropriate age correction is essential before describing left ventricular filling properties in any particular patient or population of patients as "abnormal." (See Chap. 25.)

Effects of Heart Rate and Ejection Fraction

Heart rate and the extent of systolic shortening significantly influence the rate and timing of left ventricular diastolic filling, and differences in heart rate and ejection fraction among subjects (or changes in these variables after an intervention in the same subject) must be considered in interpreting apparent changes in diastolic filling properties. An increase in the rate of diastolic filling is meaningful (insofar as reflecting a favorable change in ventricular filling properties) only in the absence of a simultaneous increase of heart rate or ejection fraction (9, 10).

Ejection fraction is a determinant of filling rate not only in a methodologic sense (as noted previously, end-diastolic volume normalized filling rate is ejection fraction-dependent) but also in the physiologic sense because contractile performance is a determinant of left ventricular relaxation, and would be expected to affect the subsequent filling period. Thus, patients with depressed left ventricular ejection fraction are likely to manifest impaired left ventricular filling (47).

The influence of heart rate on diastolic filling indexes is complex. Although heart rate is directly related to peak filling rate and inversely related to time-to-peak filling rate, these effects are minimized under resting conditions because fluctuations in cardiac cycle length are buffered by variation in the duration of the diastasis interval. However, during exercise to higher heart rates, and loss of the diastasis interval (usually occurring at heart rates above 90 to 95 beats/minute), the buffering effect of the diastasis interval is lost, so that measurements of peak filling rate and time-to-peak filling rate become exquisitely sensitive to fluctuations in cardiac cycle length (66). Furthermore, with disappearance of the diastasis interval at higher heart rates, there is a loss of definition of the different phases of diastole, so that the volume curve attains a symmetric U or V shape. In this setting, decrease in the breadth of the volume curve at increasing heart rate affects the slope of the filling phase, and hence profoundly affects the peak filling rate and time-to-peak filling rate. Very small changes in heart rate and cycle length may result in dramatic changes in peak filling rate. Disappearance of the diastasis interval at higher heart rates creates an additional problem in interpretation of filling data: the rapid diastolic filling period, an interval of ventricular filling influenced by active relaxation and by passive ventricular properties, overlaps with atrial systole, during which the ventricle fills almost entirely passively during atrial contraction. Thus, the ability to study the rapid diastolic filling period, as a reflection of active relaxation and filling, is lost during higher heart rates because of the compounding effect of superimposed atrial systole. These effects are illustrated in Figure 11–7 (67).

These considerations indicate that changes in diastolic filling measurements after an intervention, or differences in these parameters among patient subgroups, should not be analyzed independently and must be interpreted in light of possible differences in ejection fraction and heart rate. For example, the finding that verapamil enhances peak filling rate at rest in patients with coronary artery disease (68) and in hypertrophic cardiomyopathy (69) despite no change (or a reduction) in ejection fraction and a decrease in heart rate may be interpreted as representing a true change in ventricular filing properties independent of heart rate and ejection fraction. A similar change in filling parameters after administration of another agent such as nifedipine, for instance, might not be interpreted in the same way because nifedipine would be expected to increase heart rate and in many patients also increase ejection fraction. Thus, changes in filling parameters may be a nonspecific effect related to changing heart rate and ejec-

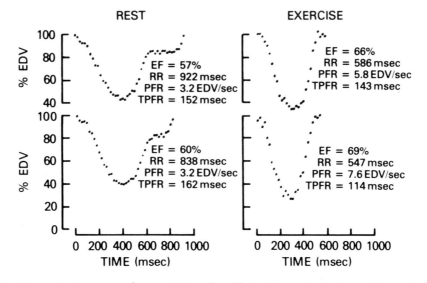

Fig. 11–7. Time-activity curves demonstrating the effect of exercise tachycardia on indexes of left ventricular diastolic filling in a normal volunteer. Two time-activity curves obtained under resting conditions are shown (left panel) at two different resting cycle lengths (PR intervals). Differences in resting cycle length are buffered by changes in the diastasis interval, with little change in the characteristics of the rapid filling phase as assessed by peak filling rate (PFR) and time to peak filling rate (TPFR). During submaximal and then maximal exercise (right panel), with reduction of cycle length and disappearance of the diastasis period, diastolic indexes become highly sensitive to heart rate fluctuations. Peak filling rate and time to peak filling rate change substantially between cycle lengths of 586 msec (heart rate, 102) and 547 msec (heart rate, 110). EDV = end-diastolic volume, EF = ejection fraction. Reproduced with permission from Bonow RO: Radionuclide angiographic evaluation of left ventricular diastolic function. Circulation 84:I-208, 1991.

tion fraction, rather than implying a change in ventricular diastolic properties.

EVALUATION OF LEFT VENTRICULAR FILLING DURING EXERCISE

It has been demonstrated that patients with coronary disease have reduced peak filling rate during exercise compared to normal subjects (51, 70, 71). (See Chap. 15.) Although this has been suggested as a sensitive diagnostic tool to detect coronary disease, this finding must undoubtedly reflect both the different ejection fraction response as well as the different heart rate response to exercise in CAD patients compared to normal, and, in addition, the more symmetric volume curves obtained during exercise will be very sensitive to the differences in heart rate between patients and normal subjects.

Other methodologic aspects of the radionuclide technique limit the assessment of left ventricular filling parameters during exercise. In general, acquisition protocols for radionuclide data during exercise, often with supine or semisupine bicycle exercise, involve acquiring data for 2 or 3 minutes during each 3- to 4-minute exercise stage. Given these relatively short acquisition times (resting studies are acquired for 8 to 10 minutes), there are significantly less favorable count statistics within each exercise acquisition. The resulting time-activity curves tend to be noisier, resulting in potentially greater error in quantitative analysis of the curves. Furthermore, the requirement of normalization of filling rates make interpretation of the exercise data more difficult because the usual normalization parameters (end-diastolic volume and stroke volume) are also changing during exercise.

These methodologic and physiologic considerations have led investigators to explore other methods for evaluating left ventricular diastolic function during exercise using radionuclide techniques. Several groups of investigators have used the end-diastolic volume response to exercise as an index of the extent of total left ventricular filling during exercise, and a test of the ability of the left ventricle to recruit preload reserve. In normal subjects, radionuclide angiographic studies have demon-

strated that, with increasing degrees of supine or upright exercise, end-diastolic volume increases, and this mechanism contributes importantly to enhanced stroke volume seen at increasing levels of exercise (72–74). This is especially the case in elderly subjects (75). Inability to augment end-diastolic volume with exercise has been demonstrated in patients with aortic (76, 77) and mitral stenosis (78) and hypertrophic cardiomyopathy (79), and in patients with heart failure with either preserved (80) or impaired (81) left ventricular systolic performance. In patients with systemic hypertension, the inability to augment end-diastolic volume during exercise in patients with left ventricular hypertrophy is associated with impaired systolic performance (an abnormal ejection fraction response) (82). This provides evidence of a diastolic mechanism for systolic dysfunction.

Assessing the end-diastolic volume response to exercise is not subject to many of the methodologic limitations that plague the analysis of the rate and timing of left ventricular filling during exercise with indexes such as peak filling rate and time-to-peak filling rate. End-diastolic volume or end-diastolic counts can be determined at the beginning of the cardiac cycle by gating to the R wave, and thus is not subject to the influence of the variations in cardiac cycle length. This method of evaluating diastolic performance during exercise can provide important physiologic insight into the ventricular response to exercise in many cardiac disease states.

ASSESSING REGIONAL LEFT VENTRICULAR NONUNIFORMITY

Abnormal ventricular diastolic properties, including reduced rate and extent of left ventricular pressure decline during isovolumic relaxation, reduced rate and extent of left ventricular rapid filling, and altered diastolic pressure-volume relations, are manifestations of impaired left ventricular relaxation, decreased ventricular distensibility, altered loading, or a combination of these effects. These disturbances of global left ventricular diastolic performance are influenced by (and may be causally related to) regional heterogeneity or nonuniformity in the timing and extent of contraction and relaxation (20–23, 83–91). For example, prolonged tension development in one or more regions of the left ventricle that persists beyond aortic valve closure and into early diastole will affect the rate and completeness of left ventricular pressure decline and will alter the intracavitary pressure at any level of diastolic volume, thereby affecting the distensibility characteristics of the left ventricular chamber. Using radionuclide angiography, it is possible to study the presence of regional nonuniformity of systolic and diastolic performance in different disease states, as well as to investigate the relation of regional abnormalities to global indexes of ventricular performance. (See Chaps. 2, 13, and 19.)

Several methods have been developed to quantify regional ventricular function using radionuclide angiography. Vitale et al. originally described the method of sector analysis of gated blood pool scans, in which the total left ventricular region of interest was divided into over 20 sectors, and individual sector time-activity curves were derived (92). For evaluation of regional abnormalities, a first harmonic Fourier expansion may be fitted to these regional time-activity curves, and the phase angle of the Fourier expansion determined. Variation in phase angle among sectors can be used as a measure of relative regional asynchrony. Further analysis of the mathematically modeled sector curves may be performed to derive other regional indices (92).

Instantaneous temporal indexes used for analysis of global ventricular performance (such as time-to-peak ejection rate or time-to-peak filling rate) are not accurate when the left ventricle region of interest is divided into 20 sectors, as the error in such measurements is high given the limited count statistics inherent in each sector. The regional variation in temporal events can be evaluated, however, by combining the 20 sectors into four quadrants of five sectors each to improve count statistics for

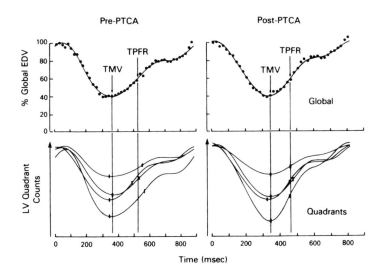

Fig. 11–8. Global and regional time-activity curves in a patient before and after PTCA. Global time-activity curves are presented in the top panels and the four regional quadrant curves (after 3-harmonic filtering) are presented in the bottom panels. Long vertical lines indicate global time to minimum volume (TMV) and time to peak filling rate (TPFR), and heavy short vertical bars indicate individual quadrant TMV and TPFR. Homogeneous values of TMV around the global value indicate relative regional systolic synchrony. However, the variation among quadrants in TPFR before PTCA indicates diastolic dyssynchrony, which is reduced after PTCA. This is associated with a decrease in global time to peak filling rate after PTCA (from 174 to 132 msec) and an increase in global peak filling rate (from 1.5 to 2.7 EDV/sec). There was no change in heart rate or ejection fraction. Reproduced with permission from Bonow RO, et al.: Asynchronous left ventricular regional function and impaired diastolic filling in patients with coronary artery disease: Reversal after coronary angioplasty. Circulation 1:295, 1985.

each region. The quadrant curves can then be fit to Fourier expansions, and from each curve, the time-to-peak ejection rate, time-to-minimum volume, and time-to-peak filling rate may be computed (Fig. 11–8) (18). To assess the regional variation in time-to-peak filling rate as an index of diastolic synchrony, the difference between the global value and the value for each of the four quadrants is calculated and the four differences are averaged. Indexes of regional systolic and diastolic performance derived by this method are highly reproducible (18).

ASSESSMENT OF ISOVOLUMIC RELAXATION PERIOD

The method for assessing the isovolumic relaxation period by radionuclide angiography is based on the observation that most time-activity curves have a visually apparent isovolumic relaxation period, characterized by an interval after the minimal left ventricular volume with a horizontal or slightly positive slope. This period is terminated by the onset of rapid diastolic filling, represented by an inflection point followed by an abrupt increase in slope. This inflection point ending the isovolumic period may be identified by filtering the time-activity curve using Fourier expansions with four harmonics and evaluating the second derivative of this filtered curve (11). The first maximum on this second derivative curve occurring between end systole and the time of the peak filling rate identifies the inflection point marking the onset of rapid filling. The results of this method correlate well with the onset of mitral valve opening by echocardiography (11). The time from end-systole to the time of this inflection point can be defined as the isovolumic relaxation period (Fig. 11–9). Based on previous studies, this computation may be accomplished in up to 90% of normal subjects and a similar proportion of patients with hypertrophic cardiomyopathy. In others, a maximum on the second derivative curve may not occur between end-systole and the peak filling rate, and thus the isovolumic relaxation period may not be identified.

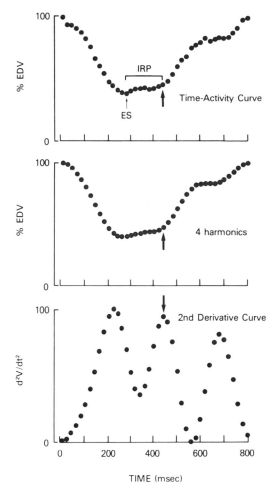

Fig. 11–9. Top panel, raw time-activity curve of a patient with hypertrophic cardiomyopathy. The isovolumic relaxation period (IRP) is visually apparent. Center panel, time-activity curve of the same patient after Fourier filtering using four harmonics. Bottom panel, second derivative curve derived from the filtered curve in center panel. A maximum after end-systole (ES) is present on the derivative curve (arrow), and this time point corresponds to the termination of the isovolumic period in top and center panels. Each point represents 20 msec. EDV = end-diastolic volume. Reproduced with permission from Betocchi S, et al.: Isovolumic relaxation period in hypertrophic cardiomyopathy: Assessment by radionuclide angiography. J Am Coll Cardiol 7:74, 1986.

FIRST THIRD DIASTOLIC FILLING ANALYSIS

Several investigators have used the first-third diastolic filling fraction and first-third filling rate as additional measure-

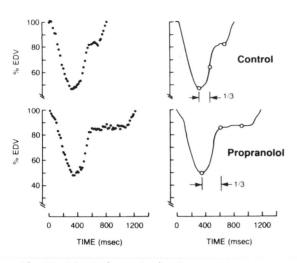

Fig. 11–10. Left ventricular time-activity curves obtained in a patient with coronary artery disease before (Control) and after oral propranolol. The diastolic phase of each cycle is divided into thirds to assess the first third filling fraction and the first-third filling rate. Propranolol did not alter the rapid diastolic filling period or the shape of the rapid filling curve. However, propranolol did increase the cycle length (decreased heart rate), and thereby the diastasis interval has been prolonged. The first-third filling fraction and filling rate are "improved" merely because of the change in cycle length without change in filling characteristics. EDV = end-diastolic volume. Reproduced with permission from Bonow RO, Bacharach SL: Left ventricular diastolic function: Evaluation by radionuclide ventriculography. *In* New Concepts in Cardiac Imaging 1987. Edited by GM Pohost. Chicago, Year Book Medical Publishers, 1987.

ments to assess diastolic filling (51, 70, 93, 94). Unlike measurements of the rate, timing, and extent of rapid diastolic filling, the first-third filling rate or filling fraction does not measure a physiologic event, is exquisitely heart rate-sensitive, and is determined predominantly by the duration of the diastasis interval. For instance, as noted in Figure 11–10, administration of propranolol to a patient with coronary artery disease may have little effect on the rapid diastolic filling phase of diastole. However, by increasing the cardiac cycle length (decreased heart rate), and thereby prolonging the period of diastasis, propranolol will result in a substantial increase in the first-third filling rate and first-third filling frac-

tion. Because the first-third variables are not physiologic markers, and are strongly influenced by heart rate, their use should be discouraged.

COMBINED PRESSURE-VOLUME ANALYSIS OF LEFT VENTRICULAR FUNCTION

To identify potential mechanisms responsible for abnormalities of left ventricular filling identified by noninvasive techniques, it is necessary to examine the factors affecting diastolic filling, including left ventricular relaxation and distensibility. The influence of relaxation and distensibility on the rate, magnitude, and timing of diastolic filling may be studied in the context of the instantaneous relation between left ventricular pressure and volume throughout diastole. It is possible with radionuclide angiography to obtain ventricular volume data in the catheterization laboratory along with simultaneous acquisition of ventricular pressure measurements using micromanometer-tipped catheters, to study the interplay between left ventricular relaxation, filling, and pressure-volume relations (95–101). Simultaneous left ventricular pressure versus time, and volume versus time curves during the cardiac cycle, and the resulting instantaneous left ventricular pressure-volume relations (i.e., the pressure-volume loop) are demonstrated in Figure 11–11. Left ventricular distensibility or compliance may be studied by the contour, location, and slope of the pressure-volume relation during the filling phases of diastole encompassing rapid diastolic filling, diastasis, and atrial systole. Evaluation of left ventricular diastolic function using purely noninvasive techniques is inherently limited because of the inability to obtain instantaneous pressure-volume and pressure-time coordinates. As a result, hemodynamic measurements remain the standard in the evaluation of diastolic function. Combined radionuclide-hemodynamic studies have demonstrated that the noninvasive measures describing rapid diastolic filling correlate significantly with indexes of left ventricular relaxation (such as maximum negative dp/dt and the time constant of relaxation) (97), but that these measurements are also influenced

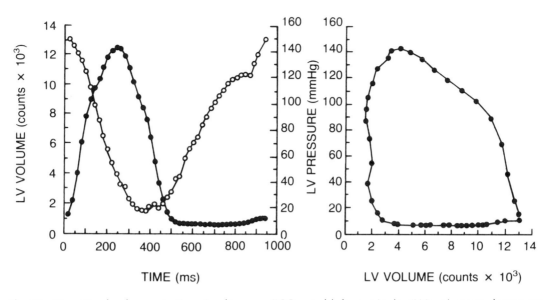

Fig. 11–11. Graphs demonstrating simultaneous ECG-gated left ventricular (LV) volume and pressure curves as a function of time, and the resultant pressure-volume loop obtained in a patient with hypertrophic cardiomyopathy. Data were obtained using radionuclide angiography with a portable gamma camera and a micromanometer-tipped catheter. Reproduced with permission from Bonow RO: Left ventricular filling in ischemic and hypertrophic heart disease. *In* Diastolic Relaxation of the Heart. Edited by W. Grossman and BH Lorell. Boston, Martinus Nijhoff Publishers, 1987.

importantly by left ventricular loading conditions and systolic performance, as noted previously. The combination of invasive and noninvasive radionuclide methodology not only permits correlation of the noninvasive indexes of left ventricular filling with the more accepted hemodynamic indexes, but also provides great versatility in the study of diastolic function. This occurs, in part, because a large number of interventions can be investigated after a single radioisotope dose allowing the construction of multiple high temporal resolution pressure-volume loops, without the limitations of multiple angiographic contrast injections which may alter the hemodynamic milieu. Furthermore, the time-activity curve represents the average of all cardiac cycles that have been acquired. This minimizes the influence of respiratory variation that may importantly affect beat-to-beat parameters of left ventricular volume. Similar methods can also be used to study right ventricular pressure-volume relations (102).

In our laboratory, we have used a system in which the left ventricular pressure signal is digitized and collected in ECG-gated list

mode similar to the radionuclide data, so that the same cycles used to construct the radionuclide time-activity (time-volume) curve are used to construct an average left ventricular pressure versus time curve at a very high temporal resolution (96, 100, 101). The pressure and volume data are then combined to construct the instantaneous pressure-volume relation during the average cardiac cycle (Fig. 11–12).

CLINICAL EVALUATION OF LEFT VENTRICULAR DIASTOLIC FILLING BY RADIONUCLIDE ANGIOGRAPHY

With the appropriate attention to technical detail and with awareness of the methodologic and physiologic considerations inherent in the radionuclide technique, it has been possible to gain numerous insights into left ventricular filling properties in diseases characterized by ischemia or hypertrophy. Many studies have identified abnormal left ventricular diastolic filling properties in the setting of normal ventricular systolic function in patients with coronary artery disease, hypertrophic cardiomyopathy, and hypertensive heart disease.

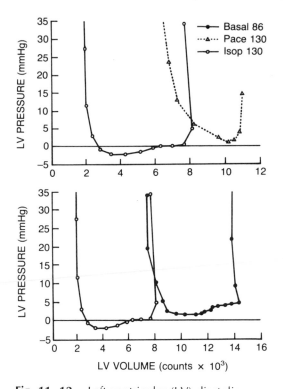

Fig. 11–12. Left ventricular (LV) diastolic pressure-volume relations in a patient without significant cardiovascular disease. In the upper panel, diastolic pressure-volume relations are shown during atrial pacing (Pace) and during isoproterenol (Isop) at similar heart rates (130 beats/minute). With pacing, LV pressure declines throughout most of the filling period. With isoproterenol, pressure fall is complete early in diastole with the subsequent development of negative diastolic pressure. In the lower panel, baseline (basal) and isoproterenol data are compared. The contours of the filling portion of the curves are similar, but the extent of pressure fall during isoproterenol (from a smaller end-systolic volume) is greater, resulting in negative diastolic pressure. The pressure-volume loops were obtained with simultaneous radionuclide angiography and a micromanometer-tipped LV catheter. Reproduced with permission from Udelson JE, et al.: Minimum left ventricular pressure during beta-adrenergic stimulation in human subjects: Evidence for elastic recoil and diastolic "suction" in the normal heart. Circulation 82:1174, 1990.

Coronary Artery Disease

Impaired Diastolic Filling at Rest

The prevalence of impaired diastolic filling at rest in patients with coronary artery disease reported from several centers has varied, reflecting differences in techniques and in patient selection (16, 17, 47, 51, 70, 71, 103, 104). (See Chap. 19.) As in any variable describing left ventricular function, the frequency of abnormal results will depend strongly upon the patient population referred to a given institution for evaluation. Nonetheless, most investigators agree that, in many coronary disease patients with normal regional and global left ventricular systolic function, diastolic filling is impaired under resting conditions, even when there is no evidence of previous myocardial infarction or myocardial ischemia at rest (16, 17, 47, 51, 70, 103, 104).

These findings of impaired filling characteristics at rest in patients with coronary artery disease are of physiologic interest, but the clinical importance of abnormal left ventricular filling at rest is uncertain. Reversible alteration in diastolic performance during exercise, as markers of the presence and severity of inducible ischemia, would be more valuable clinically. Recent data have shown that, in patients with coronary disease and normal resting left ventricular function, impaired left ventricular filling at rest is associated with an abnormal ejection fraction response during exercise (105), an index of the extent of myocardial ischemia. Thus, resting abnormalities of left ventricular filling have important consequences for systolic function during exercise, suggesting that evidence of impaired filling at rest may identify a subset of patients who also have a greater extent of jeopardized myocardium, as reflected by the deterioration in systolic function during exercise, a potential target for therapeutic intervention.

Reversal of Impaired Diastolic Filing

Although it is not possible to perform a definitive noninvasive study to determine mechanisms for impaired LV filling in patients with CAD or other disease states, it is possible to determine the prevalence of abnormal diastolic filling patterns at rest compared with those of a normal control population, and to determine the potential for reversal of these abnormalities after appropriate interventions. For example, improved diastolic filling, with no change in heart rate or systolic function, after an intervention to reduce ischemia and improve coronary flow, would suggest that the impairment in diastolic filling under basal conditions was related to potentially reversible alterations in left ventricular relaxation as a manifestation of subclinical ischemia or reduced coronary flow, rather than to irreversible alterations in compliance stemming from fibrosis or hypertrophy.

In a series of patients with single-vessel coronary disease undergoing percutaneous transluminal coronary angioplasty, radionuclide angiography was performed 1 day before and repeated 2 days after PTCA for assessment of left ventricular filling (106). To exclude patients with clinically overt myocardial fibrosis, selection criteria included a normal resting electrocardiogram with the absence of Q waves, normal global and regional left ventricular systolic function by both contrast and radionuclide angiography, and the absence of a history of myocardial infarction. All studies were performed free from cardiac medications. Although all patients manifested normal regional and global systolic function at rest, global diastolic filling was impaired in over two thirds of patients before PTCA, with either a decreased peak filling rate, prolonged time-to-peak filling rate, or both. After PTCA, heart rate, ejection fraction, and the peak ejection rate were unchanged; rapid diastolic filling improved at rest, however, with an increase in peak fill-

ing rate and a decrease in time-to-peak filling rate (Fig. 11–13) (106).

There are several possible explanations for these findings. If reduced left ventricular filling under resting conditions is a manifestation of subclinical ischemia resulting in impaired relaxation, this might be reversed after angioplasty. Alternatively, improved filling after PTCA could represent enhanced left ventricular relaxation stemming from the mechanical, load-dependent effect of an increased rate of early diastolic coronary flow in a newly patent vessel (33).

Additionally, improved left ventricular filling may result from a favorable effect of the intervention on regional left ventricular diastolic performance, reducing a baseline state of diastolic asynchrony (16–18). In CAD patients without apparent regional wall motion abnormalities at rest, regional systolic events are synchronous, whereas there is significant diastolic asynchrony. The improvement in global left ventricular filling at rest after successful PTCA is associated with a significant reduction in the degree of diastolic asynchrony (See Fig. 11–8) (17, 18, 107). Thus, regional diastolic asynchrony may itself be a reversible manifestation of regional myocardial ischemia or regional reduction in coronary flow and may contribute importantly to impaired global left ventricular diastolic filling.

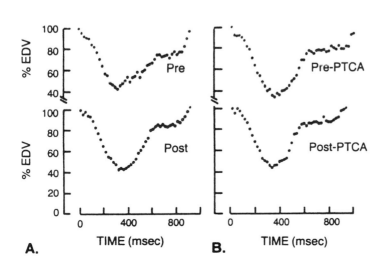

A. TIME (msec)   **B.** TIME (msec)

Fig 11–13. Left ventricular time-activity curves obtained at rest in two patients (panels A and B) with single-vessel coronary artery disease before (Pre) and after (Post) successful coronary angioplasty (PTCA). Ejection fraction and heart rate were not altered by PTCA, but the rate and timing of diastolic filling improved after PTCA. EDV = end-diastolic volume. Reproduced with permission from Bonow RO, et al.: Asynchronous left ventricular regional function and impaired diastolic filling in patients with coronary artery disease: Reversal after coronary angioplasty. Circulation 1:295, 1985.

Impaired left ventricular diastolic filling in patients with CAD may also be modified by pharmacologic interventions. It has been demonstrated that depressed peak filling rate and prolonged time-to-peak filling rate improve after short-term oral verapamil therapy, both at rest and during exercise induced ischemia (108). In contrast, propranolol does not alter diastolic filling properties (108). Verapamil improved indexes of left ventricular diastolic filling despite a significant reduction in the ejection fraction at rest and a decrease in heart rate both at rest and with exercise. These results are analogous to the combined hemodynamic and contrast angiographic data of Lorell et al. which indicate improvement in left ventricular relaxation and diastolic pressure volume relations during pacing-induced ischemia in CAD patients treated acutely with sublingual nifedipine (109).

Hypertrophic Cardiomyopathy

In patients with hypertrophic cardiomyopathy (HCM), abnormal diastolic properties of the hypertrophied ventricle are characteristic features (11, 38, 69, 110, 111) which contribute importantly to clinical manifestations of the disease process. (See Chaps. 22 and 28.) Studies using radionuclide angiography have demonstrated that the rate and extent of rapid filling is reduced in hypertrophic cardiomyopathy, that the time-to-peak filling rate is prolonged, and that the contribution of atrial systole to total left ventricular stroke volume is increased (38, 69). Betocchi et al. demonstrated that the isovolumic relaxation period is prolonged in HCM compared to controls, and is longer in patients with nonobstructive HCM than those with an outflow tract gradient (11). These studies also demonstrated that the prolongation of time-to-peak filling in HCM patients was primarily a result of the prolonged isovolumic relaxation period, as the interval from the onset of rapid filling to the peak filling rate was similar in patients with HCM and controls (11). These data suggest that impaired relaxation is an important determinant of decreased left ventricular filling in patients with HCM. As in patients with CAD, these global abnormalities of diastolic relaxation and filling in

HCM are related to significant systolic and diastolic regional left ventricular asynchrony, as demonstrated by regional analysis of radionuclide angiograms (100, 110).

Verapamil, which is effective in relieving symptoms in many patients with HCM, improves these indexes of global and regional left ventricular relaxation and filling, both on a short-term and a long-term basis (11, 38, 69, 96, 110, 112, 113). Combined radionuclide and hemodynamic measurements indicate that enhanced LV filling after verapamil is associated with improved indexes of left ventricular relaxation and a favorable shift in diastolic pressure-volume relations (96). In contrast, the beta-adrenergic blocker propranolol has not demonstrated favorable effects on left ventricular filling characteristics in patients with HCM (69, 113). Radionuclide angiographic studies have also demonstrated that enhanced left ventricular filling after verapamil correlates with objective symptomatic improvement as measured by exercise treadmill time, suggesting that reversal of left ventricular relaxation and filling abnormalities is an important mechanism by which many patients experience amelioration of symptoms during treatment with verapamil (114). Although the mechanisms of verapamil-mediated improvement in left ventricular filling and in symptoms are multifactorial, we have demonstrated that the magnitude of improvement in peak filling rate following short-term oral verapamil therapy significantly correlates with the extent of reversal of exercise-induced myocardial ischemia in patients with HCM as assessed by tomographic thallium scintigraphy (115).

Essential Hypertension

Abnormal indexes of left ventricular diastolic filling are also identified in many patients with systemic hypertension (82, 93, 116–118). (See Chap. 21.) Although left ventricular hypertrophy is an important predisposing factor leading to impaired ventricular filling in such patients (82, 117, 118), and improvement in filling indexes has been associated with regression of hypertrophy with antihypertensive therapy (119, 120), impaired ventricular filling may be seen in patients without demonstrable left ventricular hypertrophy (118, 121). This may be explained by the effects of heightened afterload with secondary reduction in the rate and extent of left ventricular relaxation and rapid filling (20, 33, 34). Indexes of filling may be normal in the presence of left ventricular hypertrophy, however, particularly in the physiologic hypertrophy of elite athletes (122). Hypertensive patients with ventricular hypertrophy and impaired diastolic filling at rest also manifest a reduction in the exercise-induced augmentation in end-diastolic volume, leading to reduced stroke volume and impaired ejection fraction response to exercise (82). These findings provide clinical evidence of a diastolic mechanism for systolic dysfunction in the hypertrophied left ventricle.

The clinical relevance of impaired filling at rest in patients with hypertension in the absence of symptoms is uncertain. Although it has been demonstrated that such abnormalities are reversible with medical therapy (119, 120), it is not clear whether improvement in filling indexes will have a favorable long-term therapeutic or preventive effect.

There may be clinical relevance in patients with symptoms of congestive heart failure despite preserved left ventricular systolic function. In many such patients, congestive and low-output symptoms arise purely from diastolic mechanisms. A majority of patients with "diastolic heart failure" have underlying essential hypertension as a likely cause (123–125). Radionuclide studies have provided evidence of an abnormal end-diastolic volume response to exercise in these patients as well, associated with an impaired stroke volume response coupled with an increased pulmonary capillary wedge pressure during exercise (80). Thus, abnormal diastolic performance, manifested by an impaired ability to recruit end-diastolic volume, results in physiologic abnormalities of heart failure in these patients with normal systolic function. Although definitive treatment studies are lacking, distinguishing predominant systolic from diastolic dysfunction as the cause of clinical heart failure appears to be important because the management of symptoms arising from each of these syndromes is distinct (126).

Assessment of LV Filling in Left Ventricular Dysfunction

The use of radionuclide angiography to evaluate left ventricular filling parameters in the presence of significant left ventricular systolic dysfunction is complex. The methodologic and physiologic considerations noted previously have an important effect on the derivation of filling parameters by radionuclide angiography in such patients. In evaluating groups of patients with heart failure and left ventricular dysfunction, there is likely to be a wide range of end-diastolic volumes, ejection fractions, and heart rates. Furthermore, the relative flatness of the time-activity curve in patients with poor systolic performance may be associated with statistical imprecisions of the curve, so that even a small fluctuation in one or two data points may importantly affect the calculations of peak filling rate and time-to-peak filling rate. Thus, evaluation of filling parameters in this context should be approached with great caution.

It is expected that evidence of impaired systolic performance will often coexist with abnormalities of diastolic function. (See Chap. 26.) As symptoms of dyspnea in such patients often occur during exertion, the analysis of the diastolic response to exercise may provide insight into physiologic mechanisms. In this regard, recently reported data have shown that patients with asymptomatic left ventricular dysfunction have a distinct end-diastolic volume response to exercise compared to patients with symptomatic heart failure and left ventricular dysfunction (81). Asymptomatic patients augment end-diastolic volume with exercise, associated with an increase in stroke volume. In contrast, symptomatic patients with left ventricular dysfunction are unable to recruit preload, with no change or a decrease in end-diastolic volume during exercise, whereas stroke volume remains constant. Symptomatic patients thus rely totally on the heart rate response during exercise to raise cardiac output, with the attendant potential deleterious effects on myocardial energetics that such a response would impose. Acute administration of the angiotensin-converting enzyme inhibitor enalaprilat improves the end-diastolic volume response to exercise in symptomatic patients with left ventricular dysfunction (81). These data suggest that radionuclide angiographic evaluation of the end-diastolic volume response to exercise may be a useful tool in patients with heart failure and left ventricular dysfunction for assessing the presence of diastolic abnormalities as well as the response to interventions.

SUMMARY

Radionuclide angiographic analysis of left ventricular diastolic filling has provided important information regarding underlying pathophysiologic abnormalities in many cardiac disease states, particularly those characterized by myocardial ischemia or left ventricular hypertrophy. As technical and methodologic considerations involving data acquisition and processing, as well as physiologic factors such as age, heart rate, and systolic function, may all affect variables of left ventricular filling as derived from the radionuclide time-activity curve, these factors must be considered when interpreting filling data. It is also important to emphasize that, in the absence of simultaneous measurement of left ventricular diastolic pressures or wall tension, noninvasive measurement of left ventricular filling parameters (and especially changes in filling indexes after interventions) provides incomplete information regarding ventricular or myocardial diastolic performance. In many patients, and particularly for individual patients, exercise testing evaluating effort tolerance and a symptomatic response to therapeutic maneuvers may be of equal or greater value than serial measurements of left ventricular filling parameters by radionuclide angiographic or Doppler echocardiographic techniques. With appropriate attention to technical and methodologic details, however, analysis of left ventricular diastolic filling by radionuclide angiography can provide pathophysiologically relevant and clinically useful insights into ventricular diastolic performance.

REFERENCES

1. Borer JS, Kent KM, Bacharach SL, et al.: Sensitivity, specificity and predictive accuracy of radionuclide cineangiography during exercise in patients with coronary artery disease: Comparison with exercise electrocardiography. Circulation 60:572, 1979.
2. Jones RH, McEwan P, Newman GE, et al.: Accuracy of diagnosis of coronary artery disease by radionuclide measurement of left ventricular function during rest and exercise. Circulation 64:586, 1981.
3. Pryor DP, Harrell FE, Lee KL, et al.: Prognostic indicators from radionuclide angiography in medically treated patients with coronary artery disease. Am J Cardiol 53: 18, 1984.
4. Bonow RO, Kent KM, Rosing DR, et al.: Exercise-induced ischemia in mildly symptomatic patients with coronary artery disease and preserved left ventricular function: Identification of subgroups at risk of death during medical therapy. N Engl J Med 311:1339, 1984.
5. Philips HR, Levine FH, Carter JE, et al.: Mitral valve replacement for isolated mitral regurgitation: Analysis of clinical course and late postoperative left ventricular ejection fraction. Am J Cardiol 48: 647, 1981.
6. Bonow RO, Picone AL, McIntosh CL, et al.: Survival and functional results after valve replacement for aortic regurgitation from 1976 to 1983: Impact of preoperative left ventricular function. Circulation 72:1244, 1985.
7. Archibald DG, Cohn JN, and VA Cooperative Study Group: A treatment-associated increase in ejection fraction predicts long-term survival in congestive heart failure: the V-HeFT study (abstr). Circulation 74(suppl II):II-309, 1986.
8. Gradman A, Deedwania P, Cody R, et al.: Predictors of total mortality and sudden death in mild to moderate heart failure. J Am Coll Cardiol 14:564, 1989.
9. Bonow RO, Bacharach SL: Left ventricular diastolic function: evaluation by radionuclide ventriculography. *In* New Concepts in Cardiac Imaging 1987. Edited by Pohost GM. Chicago, Year Book Medical Publishers 1987, pp 107–138.
10. Bonow RO: Left ventricular filling in ischemic and hypertrophic heart disease. *In* Diastolic Relaxation of the Heart. Edited by Grossman W and Lorell BH. Boston, Martinus Nijhoff Publishers 1987, pp 231–243.
11. Betocchi S, Bonow RO, Bacharach SL, et al.: Isovolumic relaxation period in hypertrophic cardiomyopathy: Assessment by radionuclide angiography. J Am Coll Cardiol 7:74, 1986.
12. Spirito P, Maron BJ, Bonow RO: Nonin-

vasive assessment of left ventricular diastolic function: Comparative analysis of Doppler echocardiographic and radionuclide angiographic techniques. J Am Coll Cardiol 7:518, 1986.

13. Friedman BJ, Drinkovic N, Miles H, et al.: Assessment of left ventricular diastolic function: Comparison of Doppler echocardiography and gated blood pool scintigraphy. J Am Coll Cardiol 8:1348, 1986.

14. Bowman LK, Lee FA, Jaffe CC, Mattera J, Wackers FJ, Zaret BL: Peak filling rate normalized to mitral stroke volume: a new Doppler echocardiographic filling index validated by radionuclide angiographic techniques. J Am Coll Cardiol 12:937, 1988.

15. Courtois M, Kovacs SJ, Ludbrook PA: The transmitral pressure-flow velocity relationship: the importance of regional pressure gradients in the left ventricle. Circulation 78:661, 1988.

16. Miller TR, Goldman KJ, Sampathkumaran KS, et al.: Analysis of cardiac diastolic function: Application in coronary artery disease. J Nucl Med 24:2, 1983.

17. Yamagishi T, Ozaki M, Kumada T, et al.: Asynchronous left ventricular diastolic filling in patients with isolated disease of the left anterior descending coronary artery: Assessment with radionuclide ventriculography. Circulation 69:933, 1984.

18. Bonow RO, Vitale DF, Bacharach SL, et al.: Asynchronous left ventricular regional function and impaired diastolic filling in patients with coronary artery disease: Reversal after coronary angioplasty. Circulation 71:297, 1985.

19. Bonow RO: Regional left ventricular nonuniformity: Effects on left ventricular diastolic function in ischemic heart disease, in hypertrophic cardiomyopathy, and in the normal heart. Circulation 81(suppl III):III-54, 1990.

20. Brutsaert DL, Rademakers FE, Sys US: Triple control of relaxation: Implications in cardiac disease. Circulation 69:190, 1983.

21. Blaustein AS, Gaasch WH: Myocardial relaxation. VI. Effects of beta-adrenergic tone and asynchrony on left ventricular relaxation rate. Am J Physiol 244:H417, 1983.

22. Brutsaert DL: Nonuniformity: A physiologic modulator of contraction and relaxation of the normal heart. J Am Coll Cardiol 9:341, 1987.

23. Lew YW, Rasmussen CM: Influence of nonuniformity on rate of left ventricular pressure fall in the dog. Am J Physiol 256: H222, 1989.

24. Mirsky I, Cohen PF, Levine JA, et al.: Assessment of left ventricular stiffness in primary myocardial disease and coronary artery disease. Circulation 50:128, 1974.

25. Gaasch WH, Levine HJ, Quinones MA, Alexander JK: Left ventricular compliance: Mechanisms and clinical implications. Am J Cardiol 38:645, 1976.

26. Grossman W, Barry WH: Diastolic pressure-volume relations in the diseased heart. Fed Proc 39:148, 1980.

27. McLaurin LP, Rolett EL, Grossman W: Impaired left ventricular relaxation during pacing-induced ischemia. Am J Cardiol 32:751, 1973.

28. Gaasch WH, Cole JS, Quinones MA, Alexander JK: Dynamic determinants of left ventricular pressure-volume relations in man. Circulation 51:317, 1975.

29. Carroll JD, Hess OM, Hirzel HO, Krayenbuehl HP: Exercise-induced ischemia: The influence of altered relaxation on early diastolic pressures. Circulation 67: 521, 1983.

30. Taylor RR, Covell JW, Sonnenblick EH, Ross J Jr: Dependence of ventricular distensibility on filling of the opposite ventricle. Am J Physiol 213:711, 1967.

31. Ross J Jr: Acute displacement of the diastolic pressure-volume curve of the left ventricle: Role of the pericardium and the right ventricle. Circulation 59:32, 1979.

32. Carroll JD, Lang RM, Neumann A, et al.: The differential effects of positive inotropic and vasodilation therapy on diastolic properties in patients with congestive cardiomyopathy. Circulation 74:815, 1986.

33. Brutsaert DL, Housmans PR, Goethals MA: Dual control of relaxation: Its role in the ventricular function in the mammalian heart. Circ Res 47:637, 1980.

34. Zile MR, Blaustein AS, Gaasch WH: The effect of acute alterations in left ventricular afterload and beta-adrenergic tone on indices of early diastolic filling rate. Circ Res 65:406, 1989.

35. Ishida Y, Meisner JS, Tsujioka K, et al.: Left ventricular filling dynamics: Influence of left ventricular relaxation and left atrial pressure. Circulation 74:187, 1986.

36. Plotnick GD, Kahn B, Rogers WJ, et al.: Effect of postural changes, nitroglycerin, and verapamil on diastolic ventricular function as determined by radionuclide angiography in normal subjects. J Am Coll Cardiol 12:121, 1988.

37. Bacharach SL, Green MV, Borer JS: Instrumentation and data processing in cardiovascular nuclear medicine: Evaluation of ventricular function. Semin Nucl Med 257, 1979.

38. Bonow RO, Frederick TM, Bacharach SL, et al.: Atrial systole and left ventricular filling in patients with hypertrophic cardiomyopathy: Effect of verapamil. Am J Cardiol 51:1386, 1983.

39. Bacharach SL, Green MV, Borer JS, et al.: ECG-gated scintillation probe measurement of left ventricular function. J Nucl Med 18:1176, 1977.

40. Austin EH, Jones RH: Radionuclide left ventricular volume curves in angiographically proven normal subjects and in patients with three vessel coronary disease. Am Heart J 106:1357, 1983.

41. Bacharach SL, Green MV, Borer JS, et al.: Validity of ECG gating: Calculation of parameters describing left ventricular function. J Nucl Med 21:307, 1980.

42. Juni JE, Chen CC: Effects of gating modes on the analysis of left ventricular function in the presence of heart rate variation. J Nucl Med 29:1272, 1988.

43. Bacharach SL, Green MV, Borer JS: Left ventricular peak ejection rate, peak filling rate, and ejection fraction: Frame rate requirements at rest and during exercise. J Nucl Med 20:189, 1980.

44. Bonow RO, Bacharach SL, Crawford-Green C, Green MV: Influence of temporal smoothing on quantitation of left ventricular function by gated blood pool scintigraphy. Am J Cardiol 64:921, 1989.

45. Bacharach SL, Bonow RO, Green MV: Comparison of fixed and variable temporal resolution methods for creating gated cardiac blood-pool image sequences. J Nucl Med 31:38, 1990.

46. Bacharach SL, Green MV, Vitale D, et al.: Fourier filtering cardiac time activity curves: Sharp cutoff filters. *In* Information Processing in Medical Imaging. Edited by Deconinck F. Boston, Martinus Nijhoff Publishers, 1984, pp 266–281.

47. Bonow RO, Bacharach SL, Green MV, et al.: Impaired left ventricular diastolic filling in patients with coronary artery disease: Assessment with radionuclide angiography. Circulation 64:315, 1981.

48. Udelson JE, Bonow RO, Bacharach SL: Peak filling rate by radionuclide angiography: Effect of normalization parameters (abstr). J Am Coll Cardiol 9:4A, 1987.

49. Shaffer P, Bashore T, Magorien D: Do normalized filling rates measured by radionuclide ventriculography actually represent ventricular filling rates (abstr)? J Nucl Med 24:P89, 1983.

50. Hammermeister KE, Warbasse JR: The rate of change of left ventricular volume in man. II. Diastolic events in health and disease. Circulation 49:739, 1974.

51. Reduto LA, Wickemeyer WJ, Young JB, et al.: Left ventricular diastolic performance at rest and during exercise in patients with coronary artery disease: Assessment with first-pass radionuclide angiography. Circulation 63:1228, 1981.

52. Bonow RO, Bacharach SL, Green MV: First pass technique and diastolic phenomena (letter). Circulation 65:640, 1982.

53. Weisfeldt ML, Loeven MH, Shock NW: Resting and active mechanical properties of trabeculae carnae from age male rats. Am J Physiol 220:1921, 1971.

54. Lakatta EG, Yin FCP: Myocardial aging: Function alterations and related cellular mechanisms. Am J Physiol 242:H927, 1982.

55. Capasso JM, Malhotra A, Remily RM, et al.: Effects of age on mechanical and electrical performance of rat myocardium. Am J Physiol 245:H72, 1983.

56. Wilens SL, Sproul EE: Spontaneous cardiovascular disease in the rat. Am J Pathol 14:177, 1938.

57. Schaub MC: The aging of collagen in the heart muscle. Gerontologia 10:38, 1964.

58. Lakatta EG, Gerstenblith G, Angell CS, et al.: Prolonged contraction duration in aged myocardium. J Clin Invest 55:61, 1975.

59. Froelich JP, Lakatta EG, Beard E, et al.: Studies of sarcoplasmic reticulum function and contraction duration in young and aged rat myocardium. J Mol Cell Cardiol 10:427, 1978.

60. Narayanan N: Differential alterations in ATP-supported calcium transport activities of sarcoplasmic reticulum and sarcolemma of aging myocardium. Biochim Biophys Acta 678:442, 1981.

61. Gerstenblith G, Fredericksen J, Yin FCP, et al.: Echocardiographic assessment of a normal aging population. Circulation 56:273, 1977.

62. Miyatake K, Okamoto M, Kinoshita N, et al.: Augmentation of atrial contribution to left ventricular inflow with aging as assessed by intracardiac Doppler flowmetry. Am J Cardiol 53:586, 1984.

63. Miller TR, Grossman SJ, Schechtman KB, et al.: Left ventricular diastolic filling and its association with age. Am J Cardiol 58:531, 1986.

64. Arora RR, Machac J, Goldman HE, et al.: Atrial kinetics and left ventricular diastolic filling in the healthy elderly. J Am Coll Cardiol 9:1255, 1987.

65. Bonow RO, Vitale DF, Bacharach SL, et al.: Effects of aging on asynchronous left ventricular regional function and global

ventricular filling in normal human subjects. J Am Coll Cardiol 11:50, 1988.

66. Bacharach SL, Green MV, Bonow RO, Larson SM: Maximal filling rate during exercise: RR interval normalization. *In* Computers in Cardiology. Long Beach, IEEE Computer Society, 1984, pp 207–210.

67. Bonow RO: Radionuclide angiographic evaluation of left ventricular diastolic function. Circulation 84:I-208, 1991.

68. Bonow RO, Leon MB, Rosing DR, et al.: Effects of verapamil and propranolol on left ventricular systolic function and diastolic filling in patients with coronary artery disease: Radionuclide angiographic studies at rest and during exercise. Circulation 65:1337, 1981.

69. Bonow RO, Rosing DR, Bacharach SL, et al.: Effect of verapamil on left ventricular systolic function and diastolic filling in patients with hypertrophic cardiomyopathy. Circulation 64:787, 1981.

70. Mancini GBJ, Slutsky RA, Norris SL, et al.: Radionuclide analysis of peak filling rate, filling fraction, and time to peak filling rate: Response to supine bicycle exercise in normal subjects and patients with coronary disease. Am J Cardiol 51:43, 1983.

71. Poliner LR, Farber SH, Glaeser DH, et al.: Alteration of diastolic filling rate during exercise radionuclide angiography: A highly sensitive technique for detection of coronary artery disease. Circulation 70: 942, 1984.

72. Poliner LR, Dehmer GJ, Lewis SE, et al.: Left ventricular performance in normal subjects: A comparison of the responses to exercise in the upright and supine positions. Circulation 62:528, 1980.

73. Sorensen SG, Ritchie JL, Caldwell JH, et al.: Serial exercise radionuclide angiography: Validation of count-derived changes in cardiac output and quantitation of maximal exercise ventricular volume change after nitroglycerin and propranolol in normal men. Circulation 61:600, 1980.

74. Higginbotham MB, Morris KG, Williams RS, et al.: Regulation of stroke volume during submaximal and maximal upright exercise in normal man. Circ Res 58:281, 1986.

75. Rodeheffer RJ, Gerstenblith G, Becker LC, et al.: Exercise cardiac output is maintained with advancing age in healthy human subjects: cardiac dilatation and increased stroke volume compensate for a diminished heart rate. Circulation 69:203, 1984.

76. Clyne CA, Arrighi JA, Maron BJ, et al.: Systemic and left ventricular responses to exercise stress in asymptomatic patients with valvular aortic stenosis. Am J Cardiol 68:1469, 1991.

77. Choi BW, Barbour D, Leon MB, et al.: Left ventricular end diastolic volume response to exercise in patients with aortic stenosis (abstr). J Am Coll Cardiol 15:7A, 1990.

78. Choi BW, Barbour DJ, Leon MB, et al.: Left ventricular systolic function and diastolic filling characteristics in patients with severe mitral stenosis (abstr). J Am Coll Cardiol 11:90A, 1988.

79. Choi BW, McCarthy KE, Bacharach SL: Left ventricular end diastolic volume response to exercise in hypertrophic cardiomyopathy (abstr). Circulation 80:II-664, 1989.

80. Kitzman DW, Higginbotham MB, Cobb FR, et al.: Exercise intolerance in patients with heart failure and preserved left ventricular systolic function: Failure of the Frank-Starling mechanism. J Am Coll Cardiol 17:1065, 1991.

81. Konstam MA, Kronenberg MW, Udelson JE, et al.: Preload reserve: A determinant of clinical status in patients with left ventricular systolic dysfunction. Am J Cardiol 69:1591, 1992.

82. Cuocolo A, Sax FL, Brush JE, et al.: Left ventricular hypertrophy and impaired diastolic filling in essential hypertension: Diastolic mechanisms for systolic dysfunction during exercise. Circulation 81:978, 1990.

83. Kumada T, Karliner JS, Pouleur H, et al.: Effects of coronary occlusion on early ventricular diastolic events in conscious dogs. Am J Physiol 237:H542, 1979.

84. Gibson DG, Prewitt TA, Brown DJ: Analysis of left ventricular wall movement during isovolumic relaxation and its relation to coronary artery disease. Br Heart J 38: 1010, 1976.

85. Ludbrook PA, Byrne JD, Tiefenbrunn AJ: Association of asynchronous protodiastolic segmental wall motion with impaired left ventricular relaxation. Circulation 64:1201, 1981.

86. Pouleur H, Rousseau MF, van Eyll C, et al.: Assessment of regional left ventricular relaxation in patients with coronary artery disease: Importance of geometric factors and changes in wall thickness. Circulation 69:696, 1984.

87. Green MV, Jones-Collins BA, Bacharach SL, et al.: Scintigraphic quantitation of asynchronous myocardial motion during

the left ventricular isovolumic relaxation period: A study in the dog during acute ischemia. J Am Coll Cardiol 4:72, 1984.

88. Gaasch WH, Blaustein AS, Bing OHL: Asynchronous (early segmental) relaxation of the left ventricle. J Am Coll Cardiol 5:891, 1985.

89. Sasayama S, Nonogi H, Miyazaki S, et al.: Changes in diastolic properties of the regional myocardium during pacing-induced ischemia in human subjects. J Am Coll Cardiol 5:599, 1985.

90. Grossman W: Why is left ventricular diastolic pressure increased during angina pectoris? J Am Coll Cardiol 5:607, 1985.

91. Takeuchi M, Fujitani K, Kurogane K, et al.: Effects of left ventricular asynchrony on time constant and extrapolated pressure of left ventricular pressure decay in coronary artery disease. J Am Coll Cardiol 6:597, 1985.

92. Vitale DF, Green MV, Bacharach SL, et al.: Assessment of regional left ventricular function by sector analysis: A method for objective evaluation of radionuclide blood pool studies. Am J Cardiol 52:1112, 1983.

93. Inouye I, Massie B, Loge D, et al.: Abnormal left ventricular filling: An early finding in mild to moderate systemic hypertension. Am J Cardiol 53:120, 1985.

94. Inouye IK, Hirsch AT, Loge D, et al.: Left ventricular filling is usually normal in uncomplicated coronary disease. Am Heart J 110:326, 1985.

95. Magorien DJ, Shaffer P, Bush CA, et al.: Assessment of left ventricular pressure-volume relations using gated radionuclide angiography, echocardiography, and micromanometer pressure recordings. Circulation 67:844, 1983.

96. Bonow RO, Ostrow HG, Rosing DR, et al.: Effects of verapamil on left ventricular systolic and diastolic function in patients with hypertrophic cardiomyopathy: Pressure-volume analysis with a nonimaging scintillation probe. Circulation 68:1062, 1983.

97. Magorien DJ, Shaffer P, Bush CA, et al.: Hemodynamic correlates of timing intervals, ejection rate, and filling rate derived from the radionuclide angiographic volume curve. Am J Cardiol 53:567, 1984.

98. McKay RG, Aroesty JM, Heller GV, et al.: Left ventricular pressure-volume diagrams and end-systolic pressure-volume relations in human beings. J Am Coll Cardiol 3:301, 1984.

99. McKay RG, Aroesty JM, Heller GV, et al.: Assessment of the end-systolic pressure-volume relationship in human beings with the use of a time-varying elastance model. Circulation 74:97, 1986.

100. Udelson JE, Cannon RO, Bacharach SL, et al.: Beta-adrenergic stimulation with isoproterenol enhances left ventricular diastolic performance in hypertrophic cardiomyopathy despite potentiation of myocardial ischemia: Comparison to rapid atrial pacing. Circulation 79:371, 1989.

101. Udelson JE, Bacharach SL, Cannon RO, Bonow RO: Minimum left ventricular pressure during beta-adrenergic stimulation in human subjects: Evidence for elastic recoil and diastolic "suction" in the normal heart. Circulation 82:1174, 1990.

102. Brown KA, Ditchey RV: Human right ventricular end-systolic pressure-volume relation defined by maximal elastance. Circulation 78:81, 1988.

103. Polak JF, Kemper AJ, Bianco JA, et al.: Resting early peak diastolic filling rate: A sensitive index of myocardial dysfunction in patients with coronary artery disease. J Nucl Med. 23:471, 1982.

104. Bryhn M: Abnormal left ventricular filling in patients with sustained myocardial relaxation: Assessment of diastolic parameters using radionuclide angiography and echocardiography. Clin Cardiol 7:639, 1984.

105. Perrone-Filardi P, Bacharach SL, Dilsizian V, Bonow RO: Impaired left ventricular filling and regional diastolic asynchrony at rest in coronary artery disease and relation to exercise-induced myocardial ischemia. Am J Cardiol 67:356, 1991.

106. Bonow RO, Kent KM, Rosing DR, et al.: Improved left ventricular diastolic filling in patients with coronary artery disease after percutaneous transluminal coronary angioplasty. Circulation 66:1159, 1982.

107. Melchior JP, Doriot PA, Chatelain P, et al.: Improvement of left ventricular contraction and relaxation synchronism after recanalization of chronic total coronary occlusion by angioplasty. J Am Coll Cardiol 9:763, 1987.

108. Bonow RO, Leon MB, Rosing DR, et al.: Effects of verapamil and propranolol in left ventricular systolic function and diastolic filling in patients with coronary artery disease: Radionuclide angiography studies at rest and during exercise. Circulation 65:1337, 1982.

109. Lorell BH, Turi Z, Grossman W: Modification of left ventricular response to pacing tachycardia by nifedipine in patients with coronary artery disease. Am J Med 71:667, 1981.

110. Bonow RO, Vitale DF, Maron BJ, et al.: Regional left ventricular asynchrony and impaired global ventricular filling in hypertrophic cardiomyopathy: Effect of verapamil. J Am Coll Cardiol 9:1108, 1987.

111. Alvares RF, Shaver JA, Gamble WH, Goodwin JF: Isovolumic relaxation period in hypertrophic cardiomyopathy. J Am Coll Cardiol 3:71, 1984.

112. Hanrath P, Schluter M, Sonntag F, et al.: Influence of verapamil therapy on left ventricular performance at rest and during exercise in hypertrophic cardiomyopathy. Am J Cardiol 52:544, 1983.

113. Speiser KW, Krayenbuehl HP: Reappraisal of the effect of beta blockade on left ventricular filling dynamics in hypertrophic obstructive cardiomyopathy. Eur Heart J 2:21, 1981.

114. Bonow RO, Dilsizian V, Rosing DR, et al.: Verapamil-induced improvement in left ventricular diastolic filling and increased exercise tolerance in patients with hypertrophic cardiomyopathy: Short- and long-term effects. Circulation 72:853, 1985.

115. Udelson JE, Maron BJ, O'Gara PT, Bonow RO: Relation between left ventricular hypertrophy, filling, and perfusion in asymptomatic hypertrophic cardiomyopathy (abstr). J Am Coll Cardiol 13:80A, 1989.

116. Fouad FM, Tarazi RC, Gallagher JH, et al.: Abnormal left ventricular relaxation in hypertensive patients. Clin Sci 59:411s, 1980.

117. Fouad F, Slominiski M, Tarazi RC: Left ventricular diastolic function in hypertension: Relation to left ventricular mass and systolic function. J Am Coll Cardiol 3:1500, 1984.

118. Smith VE, Schulman P, Karimeddini MK, et al.: Rapid ventricular filling in left ventricular hypertrophy. II. Pathologic hypertrophy. J Am Coll Cardiol 5:869, 1985.

119. Smith VE, White WB, Meeran MK, Karimeddini MK: Improved left ventricular filling accompanies reduced left ventricular mass during therapy of essential hypertension. J Am Coll Cardiol 8:1449, 1986.

120. Schulman SP, Weiss JL, Becker LC, et al.: The effects of antihypertensive therapy on left ventricular mass in elderly patients. N Engl J Med 322:1350, 1990.

121. Cuocolo A, Sax FL, Brush JE, et al.: Impaired diastolic function in hypertensive patients without left ventricular hypertrophy (abstr). J Nucl Med 30:780, 1989.

122. Granger CB, Karimeddini MK, Smith VE, et al.: Rapid ventricular filling in left ventricular hypertrophy. I. Physiologic hypertrophy. J Am Coll Cardiol 5:862, 1985.

123. Dougherty AH, Naccarelli GV, Gray EL, et al.: Congestive heart failure with normal systolic function. Am J Cardiol 54:778, 1984.

124. Soufer R, Wohlgelernter D, Vita NA, et al.: Intact systolic left ventricular function in clinical congestive heart failure. Am J Cardiol 55:1032, 1985.

125. Aquirre FV, Pearson AC, Lewen MK, et al.: Usefulness of Doppler echocardiography in the diagnosis of congestive heart failure. Am J Cardiol 63:1098, 1989.

126. Topol EJ, Traill TA, Fortuin NJ: Hypertensive hypertrophic cardiomyopathy of the elderly. N Engl J Med 312:277, 1985.

Chapter 12

DOPPLER ECHOCARDIOGRAPHY AND LEFT VENTRICULAR DIASTOLIC FUNCTION

James D. Thomas

Left ventricular diastolic dysfunction is an important cause of cardiac morbidity and appears to be one of the earliest detectable abnormalities in several disorders (1–6). As previous chapters have indicated, diastolic dysfunction may be considered operationally to be a condition in which *filling* of the left ventricle is impeded, resulting in unacceptable symptoms of either low cardiac output, elevated pulmonary venous pressures, or both. Diastolic performance can be described conceptually by two distinct and occasionally discordant parameters, relaxation and compliance (7–9). To date, the only definitive methods for assessing these parameters have required direct measurement of intracardiac pressures, which can only be obtained by cardiac catheterization. To avoid the risk, expense, and inconvenience of catheterization, many have sought noninvasive methods for assessing diastolic function. These methods generally measure ventricular filling and use these data to infer the true diastolic parameters of the heart. In this chapter, we shall review some of the physical and physiologic principles that connect diastolic function with ventricular filling, concentrating particularly on the use of Doppler echocardiography to assess ventricular diastolic function.

NONINVASIVE ASSESSMENT OF DIASTOLIC FUNCTION

Of the two principal aspects of diastolic function, ventricular stiffness may be re-lated to the local slope of the ventricular pressure-volume curve, whereas relaxation is generally characterized by the exponential time constant for pressure decay during isovolumic relaxation. (See Chap. 4.) Note that both stiffness and relaxation include ventricular pressure in their formal definitions. It is because no noninvasive method is currently capable of directly measuring intracavitary pressure that methods have been developed which use the time course of ventricular *filling* to infer information about ventricular relaxation and compliance.

The ventricular filling pattern was initially obtained from ventricular volumes obtained from radionuclide ventriculograms (10, 11) and M-mode and two-dimensional echocardiograms (12, 13). These sequential volumes were time-differentiated to yield filling rate throughout diastole.

Because of its ease of use and superior temporal and velocity resolution, pulsed Doppler echocardiography has emerged as the preferred method to assess patterns of left ventricular filling (14, 15). In this technique, a pulsed Doppler sample is placed within the mitral inflow tract between the tips of the mitral leaflets, and the temporal pattern of transmitral velocity recorded throughout diastole (Fig. 12–1). The inflow pattern is composed of two principal deflections. The *E-wave* arises from the rapid filling, which occurs just after mitral valve opening with active ventricular relaxation. Thereafter follows a period of diastasis with relatively low velocity flow. A small secondary wave may be seen, caused by inflow from the pulmonary veins. Finally comes the *A-wave*, arising from atrial contraction.

Dr. Thomas is supported in part by a grant from the Bayer Fund for Cardiovascular Research, New York, NY.

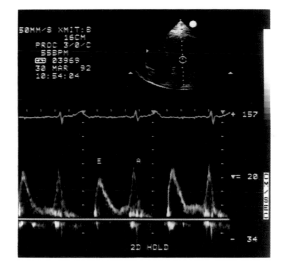

Fig. 12–1. Technique of recording the mitral inflow velocity by pulsed Doppler echocardiography. The sample volume is typically placed between the tips of the mitral leaflets and the velocity recorded with a low wall filter setting.

Numerous empiric indices have been derived from this pattern and proposed as markers for ventricular diastolic function, including the peak and integrated velocities of the E- and A-waves, their ratios, and the acceleration and deceleration times of the early filling wave. It must be recalled that these indices are fundamentally measures of diastolic *filling*, not function. Although ventricular filling is certainly affected by changes in diastolic function, it is similarly influenced by other parameters such as atrial pressure, ventricular systolic function, and atrial compliance.

To appreciate better how the mitral filling pattern relates to ventricular diastolic function, it is important to understand first, the fundamental *physical* determinants of transmitral velocity and second, how these physical determinants relate to parameters of *physiologic* importance such as ventricular relaxation and the end-diastolic pressure-volume curve.

PHYSICAL AND PHYSIOLOGIC DETERMINANTS OF THE MITRAL VELOCITY PATTERN

As a general observation, we note that, at the time of mitral valve opening, the blood within the mitral valve apparatus is stationary. This mass of blood is then accelerated by the growth in the atrioventricular pressure gradient as the ventricle relaxes. Thus, we see that velocity *acceleration* is strongly influenced by ventricular *relaxation*. As the velocity of blood within the mitral valve rises, volume is transferred from the atrium to the ventricle, causing the atrioventricular pressure gradient to fall, which in turn leads to deceleration of blood velocity. Because a change in chamber pressure with changing volume is fundamentally related to chamber compliance, we observe that velocity *deceleration* must be closely tied to ventricular and *compliance*. From these general observations, we will explore in more detail the causes of mitral acceleration and deceleration. (See Chap. 5.)

Velocity Acceleration

Physical Determinants

As a schematic aid to help understand the forces which govern ventricular filling, consider Figure 12–2, which shows a column of blood passing through the mitral valve. This column has a mass given by the product of the density of blood (ρ), the area of the mitral valve (A), and the effective length (L) over which blood accelerates in entering and leaving the valve (16, 17) and shown in in vitro experiments to be approximately proportional to the diameter of the mitral valve (18). This mass is subjected to a force (F) given by the atrioventricular pressure difference (Δp) multiplied by the mitral valve area. By Newton's second law, the acceleration of the blood column dv/dt is equal to the force divided by this mitral mass:

$$\text{acceleration} = dv/dt = \frac{F}{m} = \frac{A\Delta p}{\rho A L} = \frac{\Delta p}{\rho L}$$

(1)

We see by this that mitral valve area per se cancels out, and what remains as the principle mitral inertial term (which we term the mitral *inertance*) is the effective length of the blood column within the mitral valve, identified previously by Yellin and others as a key parameter determining the acceleration of blood through the mitral valve

(19). It is evident from this equation that the larger the transmitral gradient, the greater the acceleration.

If a transmitral pressure difference (Δp_o) were instantaneously applied across the mitral valve, then the velocity within the blood column would rise linearly with time (Fig. 12–3A). In the physiologic situation, the pressure gradient is not applied instantaneously with mitral valve opening, but rather increases gradually as ventricular pressure falls with active relaxation. For a linearly rising gradient, the initial part of the mitral velocity curve would be roughly parabolic, as shown in Figure 12–3B and demonstrated in vivo (20). Acceleration is faster for more rapidly falling ventricular pressure.

Physiologic Determinants

Thus the key determinant of mitral acceleration is the rate of growth in the atrioventricular pressure difference immediately after mitral valve opening (dΔp/dt). Because atrial pressure is roughly constant during isovolumic ventricular relaxation, it is the rate of fall in ventricular pressure at mitral valve opening that primarily determines dΔp/dt. As noted in previous chapters, ventricular pressure fall during isovolumic relaxation may be described by a monoexponential function decaying to a zero asymptote: $p_v(t) = p_{vo}e^{-t/\tau}$, where τ is the isovolumic relaxation time constant, and p_{vo} is ventricular pressure at peak negative dp_v/dt (21). By differentiating this function, we see that the rate of ventricular pressure decline ($-dp_v$/dt) is given by

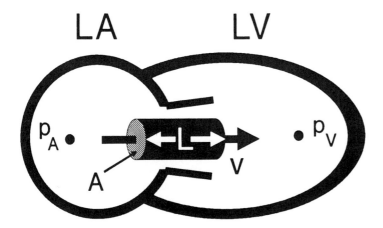

Fig. 12–2. Schematic representation of mitral velocity. A blood column with area A, effective acceleration length L and density ρ is accelerated by the pressure difference between p_A and p_V. Reproduced with permission from Thomas JD, et al.: Physical and Physiologic Determinants of Transmitral Velocity: Numerical Analysis. Am J Physiol 260 (Heart Circ Physiol 29): H1718, 1991. Reprinted with permission from the American Journal of Physiology.

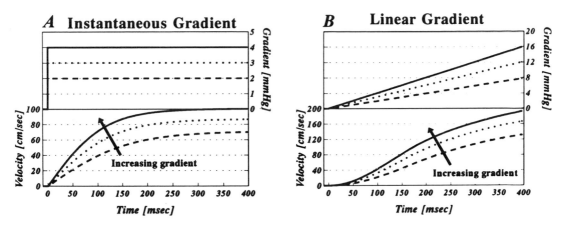

Fig. 12–3. Impact of transmitral gradient on initial acceleration. *A,* sudden application of pressure differentials of 2, 3, and 4 mm Hg leading to a linear rise in velocity with acceleration proportional to the applied gradient and final velocities proportional to the square root of the gradient (by the Bernoulli equation). *B,* gradual application of transmitral gradient leading to initial parabolic acceleration with slope related to rate of pressure rise. Reproduced with permission from Thomas JD, Weyman AE: Echocardiographic Doppler evaluation of left ventricular diastolic function: Physics and physiology. Circulation 84:977, 1991. Reprinted with permission of the American Heart Association.

$p_{vo}e^{-t/\tau}/\tau = p_v(t)/\tau$. At the time of mitral valve opening, ventricular pressure $p_v(t)$ is equal to left atrial pressure (p_{LA}), and therefore the initial rate of growth of the atrioventricular pressure difference ($d\Delta p/dt$) is given by p_{LA}/τ. As shown in Figure 12–4, the initial rate of rise of the atrioventricular pressure gradient is inversely related to τ and directly related to initial atrial pressure.

These competing effects of atrial pressure and ventricular relaxation on mitral acceleration were demonstrated in a canine model in which left atrial pressure and τ could be independently adjusted (22). As shown in Figure 12–5, when left atrial pressure was raised with τ held constant, acceleration increased with a concomitant rise in peak mitral velocity. Conversely (Fig. 12–6), when atrial pressure was held constant and relaxation delayed (by raising ventricular afterload), acceleration was slowed and peak velocity lowered. Other clinical and experimental studies have shown similar results (23–26).

Velocity Deceleration

Now consider the physical and physiologic determinants of velocity deceleration of transmitral flow.

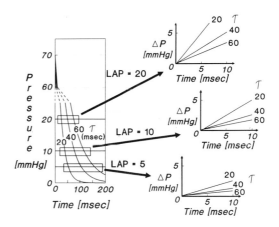

Fig. 12–4. Physiologic determinants of the rate of rise in atrioventricular pressure difference at the onset of ventricular filling. For an isovolumic pressure decay with an overall exponential shape and a time constant of τ, the rate of pressure fall is directly proportional to ventricular pressure (equal to left atrial pressure at mitral valve opening) and inversely related to τ. This is shown in the three inset graphs of pressure difference rise immediately after mitral opening for $\tau = 20$, 40, and 60 msec and left atrial pressure of 5, 10, and 20 mm Hg. Reproduced with permission from Thomas JD, Weyman AE: Echocardiographic Doppler evaluation of left ventricular diastolic function: Physics and physiology. Circulation 84:977, 1991. Reprinted with permission of the American Heart Association.

Physical Determinants

The downslope of the mitral velocity profile is commonly used to assess the severity of mitral stenosis (27–31), with the mitral pressure half-time demonstrated empirically to be roughly inversely proportional to mitral valve area. Theoretical, in vitro, and clinical analyses have demonstrated that the pressure half-time is also directly proportional to the net compliance of the atrium and the ventricle (32). Indeed, it has recently been shown in vitro (33) that there is a very simple relationship between mitral deceleration and the net stiffness of the atrium and ventricle: $-dv/dt = \rho A S_n$, where ρ is blood density (1.05 g/cm^3), A is effective mitral valve area, and S_n is the sum of atrial and ventricular stiffness, the reciprocal of compliance.

This simple analytic expression for deceleration rate can be derived easily. Recall that chamber stiffness (S) is the change in chamber pressure caused by a small change in volume: $S = dp/dV$, defined similarly for the atrium and the ventricle. For mitral valve flow, the critical stiffness parameter combines the atrial and ventricular stiffness and represents the change in atrioventricular gradient for an amount of volume passing through the mitral valve; this *net stiffness* is the sum of the atrial and ventricular stiffness, $S_n = S_A + S_V$, and is defined as $S_n = d\Delta p/dV$. Equivalently, we may consider S_n as the *rate of change* in gradient $(d\Delta p/dt)$ divided by the rate of change of volume (dV/dt). But dV/dt is simply the flow rate (Q) through the mitral valve, given by the mitral velocity multiplied by the effective valve area, $-vA$ (negative because *forward* flow through the valve *reduces* the gradient). If we make one other substitution, replacing Δp with the simplified

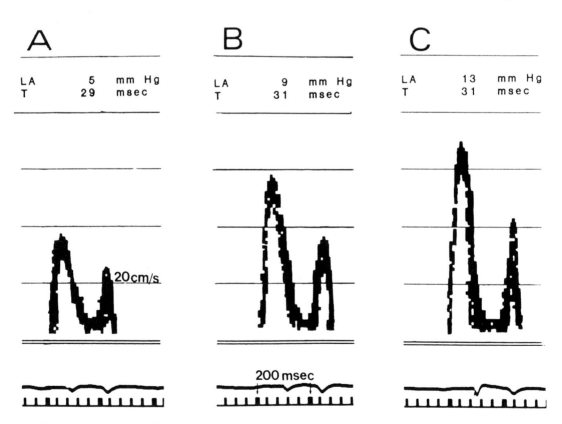

Fig. 12–5. Independent effect of left atrial pressure on the mitral velocity pattern. As LA pressure is increased (with τ held constant), E-wave acceleration and peak velocity increase. Reproduced with permission from Choong CY, et al.: Combined influence of ventricular loading and relaxation on the transmitral flow velocity profile in dogs measured by Doppler echocardiography. Circulation 78:672, 1988. Reprinted with permission of the American Heart Association.

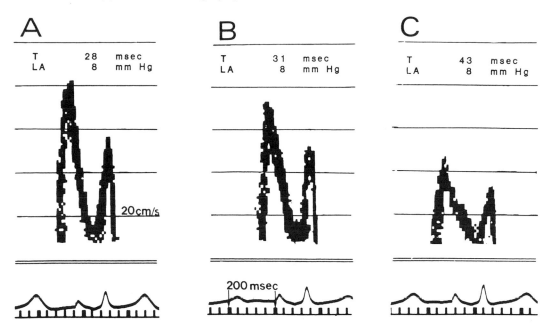

Fig. 12–6. Independent effect of left ventricular relaxation on the mitral velocity pattern. With LA pressure held constant, τ was increased by raising ventricular afterload. This delay in relaxation slowed acceleration and reduced the peak E-wave velocity. Reproduced with permission from Choong CY, et al.: Combined influence of ventricular loading and relaxation on the transmitral flow velocity profile in dogs measured by Doppler echocardiography. Circulation 78:672, 1988. Reprinted with permission of the American Heart Association.

Bernoulli equivalent, $\frac{1}{2}\rho v^2$, then, by the laws of differentiation, $d\Delta p/dt = d(\frac{1}{2}\rho v^2)/dt = \rho v(dv/dt)$. Taken together, these substitutions yield

$$S_n = \frac{d\Delta p/dt}{dV/dt} = \frac{d(\frac{1}{2}\rho v^2)/dt}{-vA}$$
$$= \frac{\rho v(dv/dt)}{vA} = \frac{\rho(dv/dt)}{A}.$$

Rearranging to solve for the deceleration rate $(-dv/dt)$ yields

$$-dv/dt = AS_n/\rho. \qquad (2)$$

Thus, the rate of fall in velocity is directly proportional to the mitral valve area and the net atrial and ventricular stiffness, and *independent* of the pressure difference across the valve. Note that this formulation could have been made in terms of chamber compliance, dV/dp, (i.e., C_A, C_V, and C_n), which is reciprocal to stiffness: $-dv/dt = A/(\rho C_n)$. However, although the stiffness of

two connected chambers is the sum of the component stiffnesses, when atrial and ventricular compliance are combined into net compliance, the relationship is $C_n = (1/C_A + 1/C_V)^{-1} = C_A C_V/(C_A + C_V)$, smaller than either C_A or C_V. The quantitative predictions of Equation 2 have been verified in vitro (33) and in canine experiments with mitral stenosis (34). Figure 12–7 shows Doppler tracings from an in vitro left heart model demonstrating a doubling of the rate of deceleration when net chamber compliance is cut in half.

Two important facts emerge from this analysis. One is that, when the net stiffness (or compliance) is constant during diastolic filling, the mitral velocity decay has a constant slope; that is, the decay is a *straight line*. Such linear decay is commonly observed in mitral stenosis, implying that whatever changes in atrial and ventricular stiffness may occur during diastole, they must be roughly equal and opposite to keep net stiffness constant. The second observation is that the mitral velocity curve can give

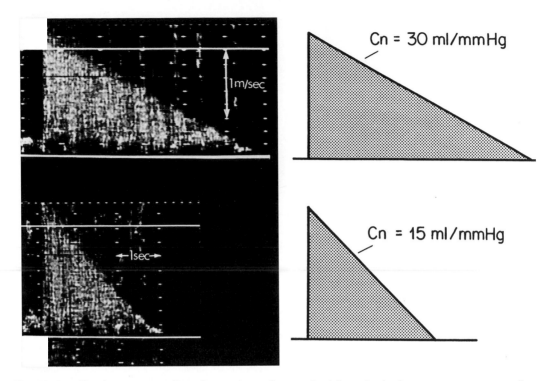

Fig. 12–7. Continuous-wave Doppler tracings of transmitral flow. In the lower curve, net compliance is reduced from 30 to 15 ml/mm Hg by insertion of a rectangular slab in the ventricular chamber. With this reduction in compliance, the slope of the velocity decay is doubled but still linear. Reproduced with permission from Flachskampf FA, et al.: Calculation of atrioventricular compliance from the mitral flow profile: Analytical and *in vitro* study. J Am Coll Cardiol 19:998, 1992. Reprinted with permission of the Journal of the American College of Cardiology.

no unique information about individual chamber pressures or compliance, only the pressure *difference* and the *net* compliance.

Physiologic Determinants

Thus, when the atrial or ventricular compliance is reduced, mitral deceleration is expected to be steeper. These are the *physical determinants* of velocity deceleration. But what are the physiologic determinants of chamber compliance? Compliance is generally equal to the instantaneous slope of the appropriate pressure-volume curve. But as shown in Figure 12–8, compliance can be reduced, either because of a material change in chamber properties (a shift from A to B) or by a shift along a single pressure-volume curve (A to C). Indeed, in some situations diastolic function is clearly impaired (A to D, raising ventricular pressures at all volumes), but without an in-

crease in the steepness in the pressure volume curve.

It should also be recognized that this simplified formula relates specifically to situations where the mitral orifice is restrictive (i.e., mitral stenosis) and relaxation is complete. The latter point is important because, if relaxation is ongoing, the pressure-volume curve gets flatter with time, and ventricular compliance appears higher than it really is. Indeed, early in filling, compliance actually appears to be negative because ventricular pressure falls despite an increase in ventricular volume. We can thus separate the change (dp) in ventricular pressure, which occurs in a time increment dt, into two components:

$$dp = \frac{\partial p}{\partial V}\, dV + \frac{\partial p}{\partial t}\, dt = \frac{\partial p}{\partial V}\, Qdt + \frac{\partial p}{\partial t}\, dt,$$

$$(3)$$

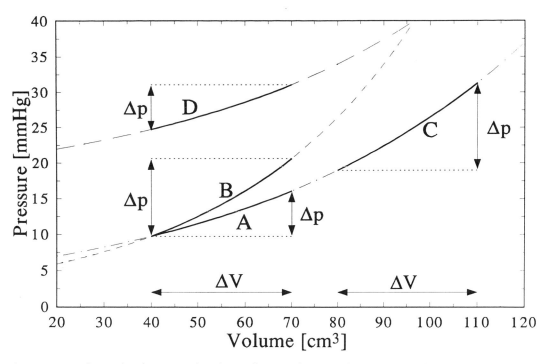

Fig. 12–8. Relationship between chamber stiffness and ventricular pressure-volume curve. Stiffness is the local slope of the p-V curve, which may be increased by an actual steepening of the p-V curve (A→B) or by a shift along the same p-V curve (A→C). Conversely, ventricular pressure may be raised at all volumes without increasing the actual stiffness (A→D). Reproduced with permission from Thomas JD: Assessment of diastolic heart failure by echocardiography. Heart Failure 7:195, 1991. Reprinted with permission of Le Jacq Communications, 47 Arch Street, Greenwich CT.

where $\partial p/\partial V$ is instantaneous chamber stiffness (approximately proportional to chamber pressure) (35, 36) and $\partial p/\partial t$ is the instantaneous rate of relaxation, and we have used the identity $Q = dV/dt$.

These competing effects of relaxation and stiffness are illustrated in Figure 12–9. Here the net rate of change in ventricular pressure (center arrow) is broken into its two components, that related to ongoing relaxation (lower arrow) and that related to filling along the current pressure volume curve (upper arrow). It is evident that relaxation continues to have an effect well into the E-wave so that simply measuring the change in ventricular pressure for a given change in volume will underestimate the actual stiffness of the current ventricular pressure volume curve.

Despite these caveats, it should be appreciated qualitatively that mitral deceleration steepens in situations of reduced ventricular compliance, such as constrictive pericar-

ditis (37), restrictive cardiomyopathy (38), and acute severe aortic insufficiency (39). (See Chap. 23.)

OVERALL DETERMINANTS OF THE EARLY FILLING WAVE

The preceding analysis has demonstrated that velocity acceleration is primarily determined by the ratio of atrial pressure to the ventricular relaxation constant τ, whereas deceleration rate is approximately proportional to the product of mitral valve area and chamber stiffness. However, such a conceptualization cannot tell the whole story because the effects of relaxation carry over into the deceleration period; furthermore, peak velocity, the principal Doppler measurement of early filling, depends in a complex manner on the competing effects of acceleration and deceleration. Therefore, we have developed a mathematical model of ventricular filling that allows the independent effects of many physiologic variables on mitral velocity to be assessed. The details of this model have been described previously (40) and its

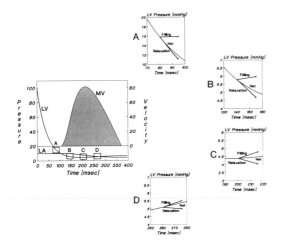

Fig. 12–9. Combined influence of active relaxation and filling on the rate of ventricular pressure change. *A, B, C,* and *D* show ventricular pressure at 80, 140, 200, and 260 msec, respectively, after aortic valve closure, corresponding to the boxed regions in the left-hand graph (mitral valve opening occurs at 103 msec). In each inset, the "filling" (upper) vector shows the rate of change of ventricular pressure if relaxation stopped at that instant and filling continued at the same rate along the current pressure-volume curve. Conversely, the "relaxation" (lower) vector shows the rate of pressure change if filling suddenly ceased but relaxation continued in an isovolumic fashion. The actual pressure change is the sum of these two vectors. Thus, in *A*, the mitral valve has not yet opened, and so the filling vector is horizontal (no filling is occurring) and the relaxation vector completely determines the pressure change. In *B*, filling is occurring but relaxation is still the main determinant of pressure change, causing ventricular pressure to fall even as its volume is rising. In *C*, the filling and relaxation vectors are equal and opposite in magnitude, and the ventricular pressure is constant (and at its minimum). Finally, in *D*, relaxation is almost complete and the rate of ventricular rise is mainly determined by the filling curve. Note, however, that even in *D* relaxation is not negligible even though, at 260 msec from aortic closure, 6.5 time constants have elapsed meaning that relaxation is 99.85% complete. Reproduced with permission from Thomas JD, Weyman AE: Echocardiographic Doppler evaluation of left ventricular diastolic function: Physics and physiology. Circulation 84:977, 1991. Reprinted with permission of the American Heart Association.

predictions summarized in a recent review (41) and are described subsequently. Such a simulation is termed a lumped parameter model because it lumps distributed quantities such as pressure throughout the atrium and ventricle into single numbers. Similar lumped parameter modelling approaches have been described (42–48), as have two-dimensional (49–52) and preliminary three-dimensional (53, 54) approximations to ventricular filling.

Lumped Parameter Mathematical Model

We begin with the schematic anatomy in Figure 12–2, assuming that a cylinder of blood of length (L), area (A) (the effective area of the mitral valve), and density (ρ) is accelerated by the atrioventricular pressure gradient and opposed by the resistance of the mitral valve and the inertance of the blood itself. The left atrium in this model includes the pulmonary veins in a common chamber that receives the full stroke volume from the right ventricle in systole and discharges it by elastic recoil during diastole (pulmonary venous filling can be included separately in the model but were not in this initial work). Left atrial and ventricular compliance are described by functions of chamber pressure that dictate how chamber pressure changes as the volume within that chamber changes.

Governing Equations

One may predict the time course of atrial pressure (p_A), ventricular pressure (p_V), and transmitral velocity (v) by integrating three coupled differential equations:

$$dv/dt = (p_A - p_V - \tfrac{1}{2}\rho v^2 - R)/M, \quad (4)$$

$$dp_A/dt = -Av/C_A \text{ and} \quad (5)$$

$$dp_V/dt = Av/C_V. \quad (6)$$

Equation 1 is in essence Newton's second law:

$$\text{FORCE } [A(p_A - p_V - \tfrac{1}{2}\rho v^2 - R)]$$
$$= \text{MASS } (\rho AL)$$
$$\times \text{ ACCELERATION (dv/dt).}$$

Here $\tfrac{1}{2}\rho v^2$, R, and M are three components of mitral valve impedance. $\tfrac{1}{2}\rho v^2$ is convective mitral valve resistance, related to the conversion of pressure energy within the atrium into kinetic energy as the blood passes through the mitral valve and is most commonly encountered in the Bernoulli equation; R is viscous resistance; and M is an inertial term because of the mass of blood passing through the mitral appara- tus. Note that mitral valve area occurs on both sides of the Newton equation and therefore can be factored out, leaving M represented in this model by (blood den- sity) × (length of the blood column), ρL, with units g/cm^2.

As noted previously, we term M the mi- tral *inertance*. Because blood obviously does not move through the valve as a solid body, our notion of a literal blood column of length (L) is simplistic. A more sophisti- cated analysis has recently related L to the *effective* length over which blood accelerates and decelerates when passing through the mitral valve (55). In this approach, shown schematically in Figure 12–10, we analyze a streamline of blood passing through the mitral valve from atrium to ventricle. The distance along the streamline is given by s, so velocity at any point in space and time is given by v(s,t). As shown in Figure 12–10, v(s,t) can be separated into distinct func- tions of space and time; L can then be ap- proximated by the spatial integral of blood velocity along the streamline divided by the peak velocity along the streamline at that

instant in time, which typically occurs within the mitral valve:

$$L = \int_A^v \frac{v(s)}{v_{MV}}\, ds. \qquad (7)$$

For relatively constant geometry through- out early filling, the profile $v(s)/v_{MV}$ is in- variant, as is L, a fact recently demon- strated by analysis of color Doppler flow maps through the mitral valve (56). Thus, the use of a fixed constant (M) to represent inertance appears justified as a first-order approximation.

Equations 5 and 6 relate the change in chamber pressure (dp/dt) with flow (given by the product of effective valve area and mitral velocity, Av) into or out of that chamber. C_A is instantaneous left atrial compliance, whereas C_V is ventricular com- pliance, each reflective of the chamber pressure-volume curve because compli- ance is by definition [change in chamber volume]/[change in chamber pressure], or dV/dp. Equation 6 may also include a time- dependent term describing left ventricular relaxation, similar to Equation 3.

When the parameters R, M, and A are specified, along with the characteristics of the atrial and ventricular pressure-volume curves and the initial chamber pressures, Equations 4 through 6 can be integrated directly to yield the time course of atrial and ventricular pressure and mitral veloc-

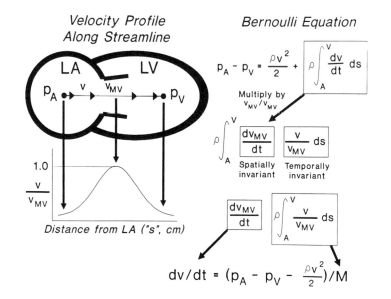

Fig. 12–10. Schematic repre- sentation of mitral inertance. By assuming that flow geome- try is relatively constant through diastole, we may ex- press the velocity (v) anywhere along the central streamline from the LA to the LV as the product of a spatially invariant term v_{MV} (the same as v in Fig- ure 12–1) and a temporally in- variant term v/v_{MV}. This simpli- fies the Bernoulli equation to Equation 4 as discussed in the text. Reproduced with permis- sion from Thomas JD, Weyman AE: Numerical modeling of ventricular filling. Ann Biomed Engineering 20:19, 1992. Re- produced with permission of Pergamon Press.

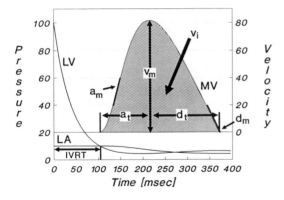

Fig. 12–11. Chamber pressures and mitral velocity from the baseline calculation (V_{vk} = 60 cm^3; s = 40 msec; ESV = 60 cm^3; V_{Ak} = 60 cm^3; A = 4 cm^2; p_{AO} = 10 mm Hg) defining the Doppler indices and isovolumic relaxation time used in the analysis. LA = left atrial pressure; LV = left ventricular pressure; MV = transmittal velocity. Other symbols are defined in Table 12–1. v_t (duration of the early filling wave) is given by $a_t + d_t$. Reproduced with permission from Thomas JD et al.: Analysis of the early transmitral Doppler velocity curve: Effect of primary physiologic changes and compensatory preload adjustment. J Am Coll Cardiol 16:644, 1990. Reprinted with permission of American College of Cardiology.

ity throughout the early filling wave (atrial contraction has also been modelled (47, 52), but are not discussed here). Figure 12–11 shows an example set of curves produced by integrating these equations, demonstrating how Doppler indices in common clinical use can be derived.

Changes in Mitral Velocity Caused by Isolated Parameter Manipulation

Figure 12–12 shows a series of numerical solutions of our mathematical model, displaying left ventricular diastolic pressure-volume curves along with the Doppler velocity pattern resulting from alterations in

left atrial pressure (Fig. 12–12A and 12–12B), τ (Fig. 12–12C and 12–12D), ventricular compliance (Fig. 12–12E and 12–12F), and ventricular end-systolic volume (Fig. 12–12G and 12–12H). Also shown are several commonly measured noninvasive indices calculated from these curves: the peak velocity (E, cm/sec), the maximal acceleration (A) and deceleration rates (D, both in m/sec^2), and the velocity time integral of the E-wave (VTI, cm). Isovolumic relaxation time (IVRT), the time from aortic valve closure to mitral valve opening, is shown by the short vertical line at the start of mitral velocity curve. For each pair of graphs, the middle curve displays identical baseline data (LA pressure = 10 mm Hg, τ = 40 msec, exponential ventricular volume constant = 60 cm^3, and ventricular end-systolic volume = 60 cm^3, the same parameters as in Fig. 12–11); the other two curves in each graph show a decrease and increase in the parameter of interest.

Influence of Atrial Pressure

In Figure 12–12A and B, increasing atrial pressure leads to a shortening of the isovolumic relaxation time, increased acceleration rate, and a significantly increased peak velocity and time velocity integral, results predicted from the preceding physical analysis. On the pressure-volume relationship, this increased filling is manifest as a larger end-diastolic volume.

Influence of Ventricular Relaxation

Figure 12–12C and D display changes in the τ. The most striking effect of slow relaxation is a delay in filling with little actual imitation in total filling. The peak velocity is slightly depressed with reduced acceleration as expected from the inverse re-

Fig. 12–12. Mathematical modeling of early ventricular filling showing the influence of atrial pressure (*A* and *B*), ventricular relaxation time constant (*C* and *D*), ventricular stiffness (*E* and *F*), and ventricular end-systolic volume (*G* and *H*) on diastolic pressure-volume loops (left graphs) and early filling velocity pattern (right graphs). In all cases, the center curve represents the same data (a "baseline" condition) with the other two curves showing an increase and a decrease in the parameter of interest. Reproduced with permission from Thomas JD, Weyman AE: Echocardiographic Doppler evaluation of left ventricular diastolic function: Physics and physiology. Circulation 84:977, 1991. Reprinted with permission of the American Heart Association.

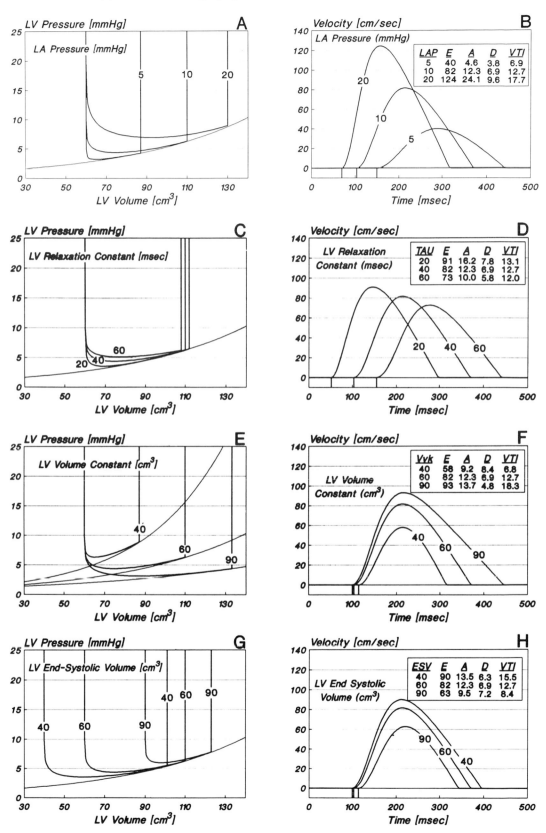

lationship between τ and deceleration; the isovolumic relaxation time is markedly prolonged. Interestingly, the pressure-volume loops themselves do not differ greatly because relaxation is merely delayed, not incomplete. Even when $\tau = 60$ msec, the ventricle reaches the fully relaxed curve by the end of the E-wave; however, with further prolongation in τ, relaxation may remain incomplete throughout early filling, the ventricle would never reach its fully relaxed pressure-volume curve, and stroke volume would be more markedly reduced.

Influence of Intrinsic Myocardial Stiffness

Figure 12–12E shows three different ventricular pressure-volume curves in which the fundamental chamber elasticity is varied. The numbers shown (left ventricular volume constant V_{vk}) represent the volume that must be added to the ventricle to raise its pressure by a factor of e, 2.71828 . . . The instantaneous stiffness of these pressure-volume curves, dp/dV, is represented by their local slope; for an exponential function this slope is given by chamber pressure divided by the volume constant. Thus, the 40 cm^3 curve is the stiffest at all pressures, and this leads to a markedly stunted E-wave in Figure 12–12F.

Influence of Ventricular Systolic Function

The curves in Figure 12–12G and 12–H demonstrate the effect that systolic performance has on diastolic filling. Each curve is based on the same diastolic ventricular pressure-volume curve and relaxation rate. All that is varied is the end-systolic ventricular volume (produced for example by changes in inotropic state or variation in afterload with the same end-systolic pressure-volume relation). As predicted by the observations in Figure 12–8, the overall effect on the E-wave is similar to those seen in Figure 12–12E and F because higher end-systolic volume causes the ventricle to fill at a steeper portion of its pressure-volume curve.

Variation in Doppler Indices with Isolated Changes in Physiologic Parameters

Figure 12–13 displays the proportional change in several Doppler indices caused by small proportional changes in each of the physiologic parameters. To use this figure to define the changes in peak velocity with atrial pressure, for instance, one finds a value of 0.74 associated with the p_{Ao}-v_m bar. Thus a 10% increase in p_{Ao} should lead to a 0.74·10% or 7.4% increase in v_m.

DETERMINANTS OF THE ATRIAL FILLING WAVE

Physical and Physiologic Determinants

Our analysis to date has neglected the causes of the atrial filling wave. In the simplest analysis, the *physical* determinants of the A-wave are essentially the same as those for the E-wave: velocity acceleration is determined by the growing atrioventricular pressure difference with atrial contraction, whereas deceleration reflects equilibration of this gradient because of either the transfer of blood from atrium to ventricle or the end of atrial contraction. The *physiology* of atrial contraction, however, is less studied and less well understood than the "passive" phase of ventricular filling. In general, however, we may observe that the magnitude of the A-wave is a function of atrial preload, afterload, and atrial systolic function.

Atrial Preload

Firstly, analogous to the Starling law connecting myofibril stretch and contractile force in the ventricle, it has been shown that the strength of atrial contraction is directly affected by its preload (57, 58), that is, the atrial volume (and pressure) at the time of atrial activation. Thus, a high left atrial pressure at the time of atrial contraction (caused, for instance, by delayed relaxation in the ventricle, tachycardia, or first-degree atrioventricular block) would cause a larger A-wave.

Atrial Afterload

The second determinant of A-wave magnitude is atrial afterload, specifically the stiffness of the ventricle at the time of atrial contraction. Thus, if the ventricle is extremely stiff (e.g., constrictive pericarditis), little atrial volume is transported across the mitral valve regardless of the strength of contraction, and the A-wave is blunted.

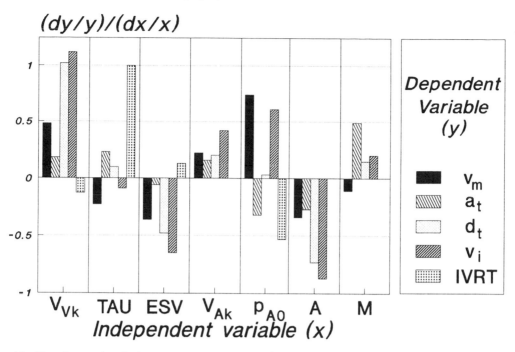

Fig. 12–13. Proportional change in noninvasive indices for small, isolated proportional changes in physiologic parameters. For instance, a 10% increase in the ventricular volume constant (far left-hand set of bars) would lead to a 0.48·10% or 4.8% increase in peak velocity, a 1.8% increase in acceleration time, a 10.2% increase in deceleration time, an 11.2% increase in the E-wave velocity time integral, and a 1.3% decrease in the isovolumic relaxation time. Reproduced with permission from Thomas JD, et al.: Analysis of the early transmitral Doppler velocity curve affect of primary physiologic changes and compensatory pre-load adjustment. J Am Coll Cardiol 16:644, 1990. Reprinted with permission of the American College of Cardiology.

This issue is compounded by the fact that an alternative exit for blood from the atrium exists, retrograde up the pulmonary veins, which might be expected to present a more favorable egress than a very stiff ventricle.

Atrial Systolic Function

The final determinant of A-wave magnitude may be the most important and least understood factor: the systolic performance of the atrium per se. It has been shown (59) that, after cardioversion from atrial fibrillation, atrial mechanical function may take several weeks to return to normal. In the wide spectrum of disease encountered in evaluating ventricular diastolic function, atrial mechanical function is likely to range from severely depressed to hyperdynamic. Unfortunately, atrial systolic function is difficult to measure and

is often is not considered in interpreting mitral velocity patterns.

CHARACTERISTIC MITRAL VELOCITY PATTERNS

Figure 12–14 demonstrates three common patterns of ventricular filling that have been described in various physiologic and pathologic conditions. The first of these (Fig. 12–13A) is commonly observed in healthy young patients without other evidence for ventricular diastolic dysfunction, and may be considered the "normal" filling pattern. It is characterized by brisk E-wave acceleration with slower deceleration and E-wave that exceeds the A-wave both in peak velocity and integrated velocity. From this normal pattern, two very different patterns have been described for situations with ventricular diastolic dysfunction.

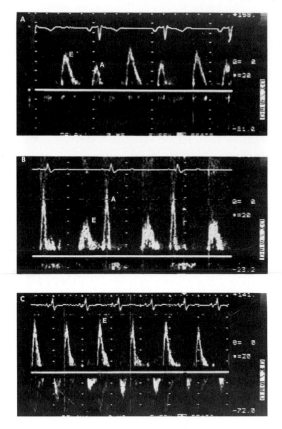

Fig. 12–14. Typical Doppler mitral inflow patterns. The normal pattern in *A* is characterized by an early or E-wave, which is larger than the A-wave in both maximal velocity and in integrated area. Shown in *B* is the filling pattern most commonly associated with diastolic dysfunction: a low amplitude E-wave indicating delayed and reduced early filling, followed by a much larger A-wave. *C* demonstrates an entirely different filing pattern associated most commonly with restrictive situations. In this pattern, the E-wave has an abnormally high peak velocity, but with very rapid deceleration, leading to a brief filling wave. The A-wave is very small (in this case so small that it does not rise above the Doppler wall filter.) Reproduced with permission from Thomas JD, Weyman AE: Echocardiographic Doppler evaluation of left ventricular diastolic function: Physics and physiology. Circulation 84:977, 1991. Reprinted with permission of the American Heart Association.

Pattern of Delayed Relaxation

The first of these "pathologic" patterns is shown in Figure 12–14 and is characterized by a prolonged isovolumic relaxation time, slowed acceleration and deceleration, low peak velocity, and a reduced ratio of E to A wave velocity, typically less than 1. This type of pattern was the first one suggested as indicating diastolic dysfunction, and has been observed in situations such as hypertrophic cardiomyopathy (60–63), secondary hypertrophy (64), morbid obesity (65), myocardial infarction (66, 67), acute ischemia caused by increased myocardial oxygen demand (68) and transient coronary occlusion (69–73), and dilated cardiomyopathy (74), as well as immediately after coronary artery bypass grafting (75). Reversal of this pattern has even been used to assess the benefit of pharmacologic therapy (76–78), coronary angioplasty (79), and septal myomectomy (80). Unfortunately, although group means of the Doppler indices differed from normal in these studies, a great deal of overlap occurred, so that in individual patients, the patterns were less predictable. Furthermore, reduction in the E/A wave ratio has been described as a consequence of normal aging (81–83), tachycardia (83), decreased left atrial pressure (25, 84–86), and head-up positional change with a tilt-table (87).

Causes of Delayed Relaxation Pattern

By examining Figure 12–12, we see possible explanations for the etiology of this pattern. First, if relaxation were delayed, IVRT would be prolonged and E-wave velocity and acceleration would be reduced. The increase in A-wave velocity might be caused by relatively high atrial pressure at the time of atrial activation with the ventricle becoming progressively more compliant with ongoing relaxation. Indeed, the pattern in Figure 12–14B is often referred to as the pattern of delayed relaxation. On the other hand, we see from Figure 12–12B that simple reduction in atrial pressure will reproduce most of the features of this pattern with prolonged IVRT and reduced E-wave acceleration and peak velocity. Peak A velocity typically is reduced in this situation but not as markedly as the E-wave velocity so that the E/A ratio falls.

Pattern of Increased Stiffness

In recent years, a second general pathologic pattern has been described (Fig. 12–14C), generally associated with more advanced diastolic dysfunction than that of Figure 12–14B. In distinction with the pattern of delayed relaxation, this pattern is associated with *shortened* IVRT, *increased* peak E-velocity and acceleration with extremely steep deceleration, and a small (or even absent) A-wave leading to an *increase* in the E/A-wave ratio. This pattern has been reported in patients with heart transplant rejection (88, 89), in constrictive (35) and restrictive (36, 90, 91) processes, and in acute severe aortic regurgitation (37). It has even been shown that patients may shift from the pattern in Figure 12–14B to that in Figure 12–14C as the severity of amyloid cardiomyopathy progresses, often with a period in between when the mitral filling pattern resembles Figure 12–13A, termed pseudonormalization (Fig. 12–15) (92).

Causes of Restrictive Pattern

How can this pattern be explained pathophysiologically? Examination of Figure 12–12 shows that neither reduced compliance nor delayed relaxation alone produces such an E-wave as that in Figure 12–14C. The key observation is that Figure 12–12 shows the changes anticipated from *isolated* changes in these parameters, with the other physiologic parameters held constant. In the clinical situation, however, compensatory mechanisms are often invoked to reduce the impact of diastolic dysfunction (93). For instance, the reduced early filling observed with diminished ventricular compliance may be offset partly by an increase in heart rate, inotropic state (if possible), and perhaps most commonly a rise in left atrial pressure.

Importance of Preload Compensation

For example, Figure 12–16 shows the effect of reduced ventricular compliance with and without preload compensation. When the ventricular volume constant is reduced in isolation (increasing chamber stiffness by 50%), peak E-wave velocity and acceleration are diminished, with an appearance similar to that of Figure 12–14B. By contrast, when left atrial pressure is allowed to rise to return the E-wave time velocity integral to baseline (in this case from 10 to 29.6 mm Hg), the result is a very tall narrow E-wave with very short IVRT, simi-

lar to Figure 12–14C. This complex interplay of ventricular relaxation, stiffness and preload has been examined in patients with varying degrees of systolic dysfunction (94). In patients with normal systolic function, the E-wave deceleration time was closely related to ventricular τ (the E-waves became flatter with delayed relaxation), whereas in patients with systolic dysfunction, E-waves were tall and narrow, with deceleration time inversely related to left atrial pressure and myocardial stiffness. The restrictive pattern of filling has been reported to be accentuated during mental arithmetic in patients with impaired systolic function, with a close relationship between deceleration rate and pulmonary capillary wedge pressure (95).

Proportional Changes in Doppler Indices with Preload Compensation

Figure 12–17 demonstrates proportional changes in each of the Doppler indices for proportional changes in the physiologic indices, but now adjusting atrial pressure to keep stroke volume constant. Note that atrial pressure has become a dependent variable, with bars showing the proportional change in ρ_{Ao} needed to offset the proportional change in the specified physiologic parameter.

CLINICAL INTERPRETATION OF MITRAL FILLING PATTERNS

The conclusions that we can apply to mitral velocity patterns observed clinically are discussed in the following paragraphs. (See Chaps. 23 and 24.)

"Restrictive" Pattern

The most straightforward of these is that of Figure 12–14C, with the tall, narrow E-wave and absent A-wave. Such a pattern appears to be fairly specific for the combination of reduced ventricular compliance (either primary or caused by ventricular systolic dysfunction) in combination with elevated left atrial pressure. The observation of this pattern has important prognostic implications. In amyloidosis patients, the worst one-year survival was observed in those with the highest E- to A-wave ratio and the shortest deceleration times (96).

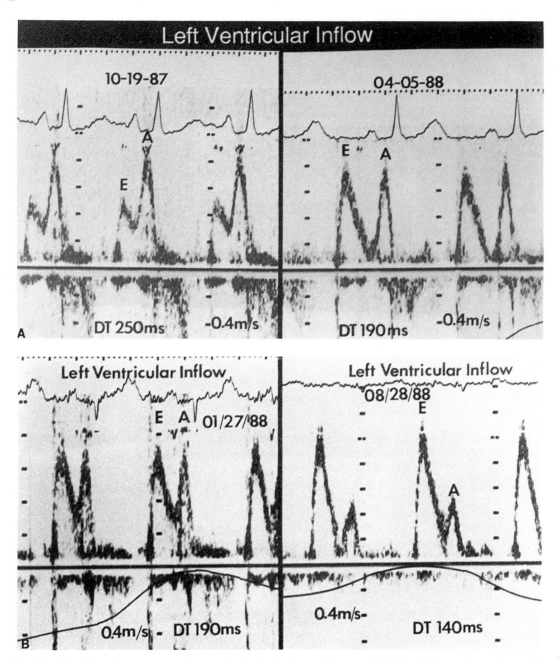

Fig. 12–15. Changing patterns of transmitral velocity in cardiac amyloidosis. *A*, Over a 6-month period, ventricular inflow pattern changed from a pattern of delayed relaxation to a pseudonormalized one. *B*, In another patient, filling changed from a pseudonormalized one to one characteristic of restriction. Reproduced with permission from Klein AL, et al.: Serial Doppler echocardiographic follow-up of left ventricular diastolic function in cardiac amyloidosis. J Am Coll Cardiol 16:1135, 1990. Reprinted with permission of the American College of Cardiology.

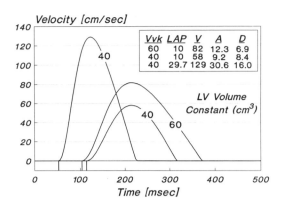

Vvk	LAP	V	A	D
60	10	82	12.3	6.9
40	10	58	9.2	8.4
40	29.7	129	30.6	16.0

Fig. 12–16. Effect of preload compensation on the early filing wave. When the ventricular volume constant is reduced from 60 to 40 cm³ while holding atrial pressure constant at 10 mm Hg the E-wave is reduced in magnitude similarly to that seen in 6B. However, if LA pressure is instead allowed to rise to 29.3 mm Hg to maintain the diastolic stroke volume, the resultant E-wave has a very short IVRT, high velocity, and steep deceleration, similar to the pattern of 6C. Reproduced with permission from Thomas JD: Assessment of diastolic heart failure by echocardiography. Heart Failure 7:195, 1991. Reprinted with permission of Le Jacq Communications, 47 Arch Street, Greenwich CT.

Similarly, in patients with dilated cardiomyopathy, presence of a restrictive pattern of filling was more predictive of severe symptoms than indices of systolic function (97). It has also been associated with the presence of mitral regurgitation in patients with systolic dysfunction (98).

"Delayed Relaxation" Pattern

The pattern in Figure 12–14B is more difficult to interpret. In situations in which left atrial pressure is known to be elevated (for instance, by hemodynamic monitoring or the presence of rales on examination), we may be fairly confident that ventricular relaxation is delayed. However, such a pattern may also be seen with reduced atrial pressure or as a consequence of normal aging (presumably caused by an age-related decrease in relaxation). The observation of this pattern in isolation must therefore be interpreted with caution.

"Normal" Pattern

Likewise, the "normal" pattern in Figure 12–14A is also problematic. For the vast majority of the time, it represents true normality in a young person. In some situations, it is seen in persons with significant diastolic dysfunction and just enough preload compensation to move them halfway from the pattern in Figure 12–14B to that in Figure 12–14C.

NEW APPROACHES TO DOPPLER ASSESSMENT OF DIASTOLIC FUNCTION

It should be evident from the foregoing discussion that a given set of physiologic parameters (atrial and ventricular compliance, mitral valve impedance, ventricular relaxation, etc.) will predict a unique pattern of transmitral velocity. Unfortunately, in the clinical situation, our desire is to reverse the process, i.e., to use an observed mitral pattern to predict the constituent physiologic parameters. Unfortunately, consideration of the "normal" and "pseudonormal" patterns demonstrates that a single filling pattern may result from a multitude of physiologic parameters. It is the fundamental insolvability of this *inverse problem* (attempting to work backwards from an observable pattern to the underlying determinants of that pattern) that causes confusion in the Doppler assessment of diastolic function.

General Approach to the "Inverse Problem"

When a single observable set of data (transmitral velocity pattern) may result from a multitude of underlying determinants, the general approach is to gather additional data that relate to the same physiologic determinants but in a *different manner* from the mitral pattern. Fortunately, numerous other types of data may be recorded noninvasively to define better the true parameters of diastolic function.

Pulmonary Venous Velocity Patterns

For example, how might one distinguish the "normal" pattern in Figure 12–14A from the "pseudonormal" patterns in Figure 12–15? One possible approach is to analyze the pulmonary venous (PV) velocity pattern along with the transmitral pattern, a technique described recently for transesophageal (99) and transthoracic echocardiography (100).

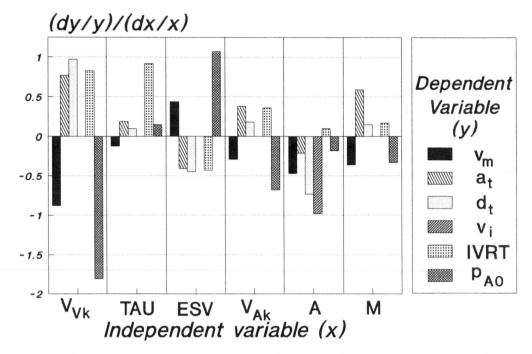

Fig. 12–17. Proportional change in noninvasive indices for small proportional changes in physiologic parameters with compensation in atrial pressure to keep stroke volume constant. Thus, a 10% increase in the ventricular volume constant can be compensated by a 1.8·10% or 18% decrease in atrial pressure. This combination causes an 8.8% decrease in peak velocity, a 7.7% increase in acceleration time, a 9.7% increase in deceleration time, an 8.3% increase in the isovolumic relaxation time, and no change in the E-wave time velocity integral (by definition of the constraining condition). (From Klein, et al.: Analysis of the early transmitral Doppler velocity curve affect of primary physiologic changes and compensatory preload adjustment. Reproduced with permission from Thomas JD, et al.: Analysis of the early transmitral Doppler velocity curve affect of primary physiologic changes and compensatory pre-load adjustment. J Am Coll Cardiol 16:644, 1990. Reprinted with permission of the American College of Cardiology.

Characteristics of Pulmonary Venous Velocities

Figure 12–18 demonstrates the technique for recording pulmonary venous velocities by transesophageal echocardiography. Using color Doppler to guide placement of the pulsed Doppler sample volume within the distal pulmonary vein, one may observe three distinct velocity waves. During ventricular systole (S), there is prominent forward flow into the atrium. At the time of mitral valve opening, the atrium empties rapidly into the ventricle; the associated fall in atrial pressure allows blood to flow from the pulmonary vein as a diastolic wave (D). Finally, with atrial contraction, pressure in the atrium may exceed that in the pulmonary vein, causing a reversal of flow up the vein (A).

Association of PV A-wave Reversal with Atrial Systolic Function and Ventricular Stiffness

It appears that analysis of the reversal of velocity with atrial systole may help in assessing both intrinsic atrial function and ventricular stiffness. For instance, with normal atrial function and ventricular compliance, one would expect the mitral A-wave to be large relative to the pulmonary venous A-wave reversal. In contrast, if ventricular compliance is reduced, the pulmonary reversal would be enhanced relative to the mitral A-wave. Finally, if atrial systolic dysfunction is present, both waves should be diminished in magnitude. Thus the *sum* of the forward transmitral A-wave and the reversed PV A-wave is an indicator of atrial systolic function, whereas the *ratio* of the

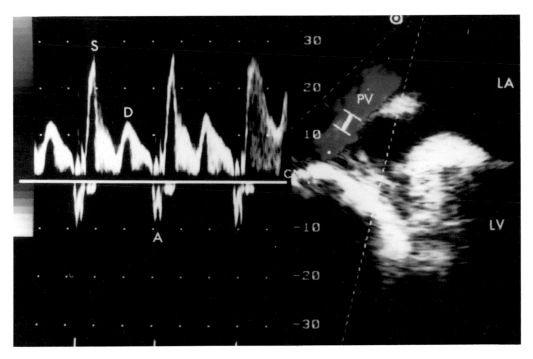

Fig. 12–18. Recording of pulmonary venous velocity by transesophageal echocardiography. Using color Doppler as a guide, the pulsed Doppler sample volume is placed in the pulmonary vein to record forward flow in systole (S), diastole (D), and reversal of flow with atrial contraction (A).

PV A-wave to the mitral A-wave should be related to ventricular compliance.

For instance, Figure 12–19 displays the changes in mitral and pulmonary venous velocity when fluids are infused (99). Note that both mitral and PV A-waves are increased, but their ratio remains approximately the same, indicating that the predominant impact is an increase in atrial stroke volume without significant change in ventricular compliance. In contrast, Figure 12–20 shows the effect of nitroglycerin infusion, showing a reduction in PV A-wave with preserved mitral A-wave, indicating an improvement in ventricular compliance with relatively constant atrial stroke volume.

Use of the Color Doppler M-mode Display

The preceding discussion on the simultaneous analysis of mitral and pulmonary venous velocities illustrates the utility of examining velocity at multiple points within the heart. A natural extension of this is the use of Doppler flow mapping, which displays velocity throughout a two-dimensional sector in the heart. Unfortunately, the frame rate for such a sector scan is only about 20 Hz, too slow to resolve the fine temporal events of mitral acceleration and deceleration. An alternative display is the *color Doppler M-mode*, which shows velocity along a single scan line (at about 1 mm resolution) and updated every 5 or 10 msec (Fig. 12–21). (See Chap. 19.) This technique has been used to show delayed propagation of flow to the LV apex (101). Particularly attractive is the analysis of a scan line passing from the left atrium to the left ventricle through the middle of the mitral annulus. Such a scan line approximates closely the actual course of blood passing from the atrium to the ventricle and thus represents flow along a *streamline*. For inviscid flow along a streamline, the enormously complex Navier-Stokes equations reduce to the much simpler *Euler equation* (102):

$$\rho\left[\frac{\partial v}{\partial t} + v\,\frac{\partial v}{\partial s}\right] = -\frac{\partial p}{\partial s}, \qquad (8)$$

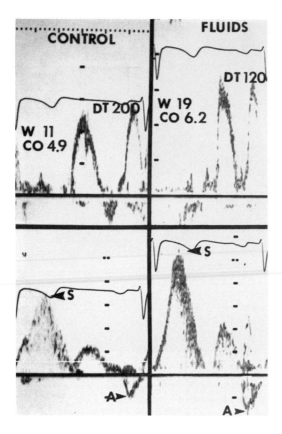

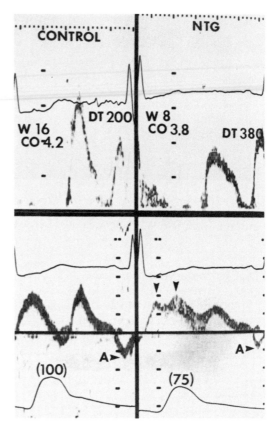

presence of ventricular restoring forces in early diastole (i.e., the E-wave is "pulled," the A-wave is "pushed"). Furthermore, we observed that the E-wave was particularly displaced in patients with hypertrophied, hyperdynamic ventricles. It is hoped that analysis of the actual Doppler velocities, output in digital fashion, may allow quantification of intraventricular pressure

Fig. 12–19. Impact of fluid infusion on mitral (top) and pulmonary venous (bottom) velocity patterns. With fluids, pulmonary capillary wedge pressure (W, mm Hg) increased along with cardiac output (CO, l/min) associated with an increase in the magnitude of both mitral and pulmonary venous A-wave (A), indicating an increase in atrial stroke volume with little change in ventricular compliance. Reproduced with permission from Nishimura RA, et al.: Relation of pulmonary vein to mitral flow velocities by transesophageal Doppler Echocardiography: Effect of different loading condition. Circulation 81:1488, 1990. Reprinted with permission of the American Heart Association.

Fig. 12–20. Impact of nitroglycerin infusion (NTG) on mitral (top) and pulmonary venous (bottom) velocity patterns. With NTG, pulmonary capillary wedge pressure (W, mm Hg) decreased along with cardiac output (CO, l/min) associated with a decrease in the magnitude of pulmonary venous A-wave (A) but preservation of mitral A-wave, suggesting an improvement in ventricular compliance with relatively little change in atrial stroke volume. Reproduced with permission from Nishimura RA, et al.: Relation of pulmonary vein to mitral flow velocities by transesophageal Doppler echocardiography: Effect of different loading condition. Circulation 81:1488, 1990. Reprinted with permission of the American Heart Association.

where v is the local velocity, p is local pressure, s is distance along the streamline, t is time, and ρ is blood density. Thus, when velocity is stationary in space and time ($\partial v/\partial t = \partial v/\partial s = 0$), this should identify a local minimum in pressure ($\partial p/\partial s = 0$). We have shown in a preliminary report (103) that this stationary point of the E-wave is displaced apically relative to the A-wave, which appears to be consistent with the

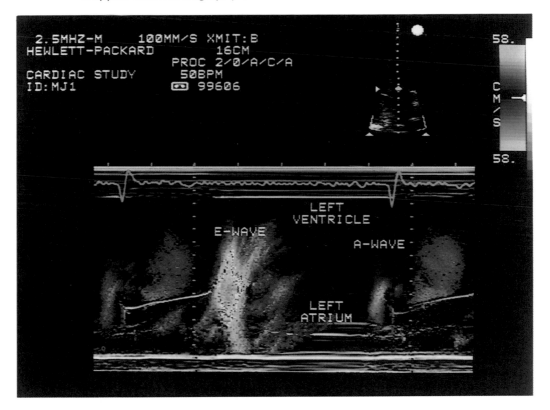

Fig. 12–21. Color Doppler M-mode recording of transmitral velocity. With the cursor line directed through the mitral valve, the spatiotemporal pattern of velocity is shown along a streamline from the mid-atrium to the ventricular apex.

gradients, whose existence have been demonstrated by direct recording (20). (See Chap. 10.)

Reports have outlined two possible clinical uses for this color Doppler M-mode display of mitral inflow. The first application is the calculation of mitral inertance as outlined in Equation 7 and Figure 12–10, integrating velocity along a streamline, normalized to peak instantaneous mitral velocity. Derivation of inertance in this way allows the calculation of transmitral pressure gradient by applying the complete Bernoulli equation:

$$\Delta p = \frac{1}{2}\rho(\Delta v^2) + M\frac{dv}{dt}. \qquad (9)$$

In a canine experiment (104), inclusion of the inertial term allowed the time course of the transmitral gradient to be estimated with much higher accuracy than previously. Such an analysis might allow $-dp_{LV}/dt$ at mitral valve opening to be calculated, a term closely related to ventricular relaxation.

An approach even more closely tied to ventricular relaxation is characterization of the propagation speed of the early filling wave into the ventricle. One study used the leading edge of the mitral E-wave, measuring its propagation speed as slope on the color Doppler M-mode (105). These authors demonstrated a strong negative correlation between propagation speed and LV τ. A more robust approach is to determine the position within the LV inflow tract of the velocity centroid, v_c:

$$v_c(t) = \frac{\int_A^V s\, v(s,t)\, ds}{\int_A^V v(s,t)\, ds}$$

where s is the distance along the scan-line

from the left atrium and v(s,t) is the spatio-temporal map of velocity from the color M-mode (106). Centroid velocity was consistently less than the actual velocities within the filling wave and correlated inversely to changes in LV τ under conditions of β-adrenergic stimulation and blockade (104).

CONCLUSIONS

A tremendous amount of physiologic information is contained in the left filling pattern, and the high temporal, spatial, and velocity resolution of Doppler echocardiography makes it the optimal modality for assessing ventricular filling. Even a qualitative analytical approach allows important clinical observations about ventricular diastolic function to be made about several Doppler filling patterns. However, it is critical to remember that diastolic *filling* is not equivalent to diastolic *function*: the mitral valve and left atrium play important roles in determining transmitral flow, and compensatory mechanisms may yield radically different patterns for the same ventricular compliance and relaxation. To sort out this complex interplay of factors requires more sophisticated analysis of Doppler filling patterns, and a great deal of fundamental research must be done to achieve this goal. An improved understanding of the physical and physiologic basis for Doppler filling curves should allow their more intelligent interpretation and improve the noninvasive assessment of ventricular diastolic function.

REFERENCES

1. Hirota Y: A clinical study of left ventricular relaxation. Circulation 62:756, 1980.
2. Rousseau MF, Pouleur H, Detry JMR, Brasseur LA: Relaxation between changes in left ventricular inotropic state and relaxation in normal subjects and patients with coronary artery disease. Circulation 64:736, 1981.
3. Dougherty AH, et al.: Congestive heart failure with normal systolic function. Am J Cardiol 54:778, 1984.
4. Topol EJ, Traill TA, Fortuin NJ: Hypertensive hypertrophic cardiomyopathy in the elderly. N Engl J Med 312:277, 1985.
5. Soufer R, et al.: Intact systolic left ventricular function in clinical congestive heart failure. Am J Cardiol 53:567, 1984.
6. Aroesty JM, et al.: Simultaneous assessment of left ventricular systolic and diastolic dysfunction during pacing-induced ischemia. Circulation 71:889, 1985.
7. Gilbert JC, Glantz SA: Determinants of left ventricular filling and the diastolic pressure-volume relation. Circ Res 64:827, 1989.
8. Yellin EL, Nikolic S, Frater RW: Left ventricular filling dynamics and diastolic function. Prog Cardiovasc Dis 32:242, 1990.
9. Mirsky I, Pasipoularides A: Clinical assessment of diastolic function. Prog Cardiovasc Dis 32:391, 1990.
10. Bonow RO, et al.: Impaired diastolic filling in patients with coronary artery disease: Assessment with radionuclide angiography. Circulation 64:315, 1981.
11. Magorien DJ, et al.: Hemodynamic correlates for timing intervals, ejection rate and filling rate derived from the radionuclide angiographic volume curve. Am J Cardiol 53:567, 1984.
12. Sanderson JE, et al.: Left ventricular relaxation and filling in hypertrophic cardiomyopathy: An echocardiographic study. Br Heart J 40:596, 1978.
13. Upton MI, Gibson DG: The study of left ventricular filling from digitized echocardiograms. Prog Cardiovasc Dis 20:359, 1978.
14. Rokey R, et al.: Determiniation of parameters of left ventricular diastolic filling with pulsed Doppler echocardiography: Comparison with cineangiography. Circulation 71:543, 1985.
15. Spirito P, Maron BJ, Bonow RO: Noninvasive assessment of left ventricular diastolic function: Comparative analysis of Doppler echocardiographic and radionuclide angiographic techniques. J Am Coll Cardiol 7:518, 1986.
16. Bakalyar DM, Hauser AM, Timmis GC: Theoretical description of blood flow through the mitral orifice. J Biomech Eng 111:141, 1989.
17. Pasipoularides A: Clinical assessment of ventricular ejection dynamics with and without outflow obstruction. J Am Coll Cardiol 15:859, 1990.
18. Flachskampf FA, et al.: Calculation of mitral inertial mass: A factor critical to extracting relaxation from Doppler filling profiles; an *in vitro* study (abstract). Circulation 80:II-567, 1989.
19. Yellin EL: Mitral valve motion, intracardiac dynamics and flow pattern modelling: Physiology and pathophysiology. *In* Ghista's Advances in Cardiovascular Phys-

ics, Vol 5. Basel, S. Karger, 1983, pp. 137–161.

20. Courtois M, Kovács SJ, Jr, Judbrook PA: Transmitral pressure-flow velocity relation: Importance of regional pressure gradients in the left ventricle during diastole. Circulation 78:661, 1988.

21. Weiss JL, Frederikson JW, Weisfeldt JL: Hemodynamic determinants of the time-course of fall in canine left ventricular pressure. J Clin Invest 58:751, 1976.

22. Choong CY, et al.: Combined influence of ventricular loading and relaxation in the transmitral flow velocity profile in dogs measured by Doppler echocardiography. Circulation 78:672, 1988.

23. Takahashi T, et al.: Significance of left atrial pressure and left ventricular relaxation as determinants of left ventricular early diastolic filling in man. Jpn Heart J 31:319, 1990.

24. Stoddard ME, et al.: Influence of alteration in preload on the pattern of left ventricular diastolic filling as assessed by Doppler echocardiography in humans. Circulation 79:1226, 1989.

25. Appleton CA, Hatle LK, Popp RL: Relation of transmitral flow velocity patterns to left ventricular diastolic function: New insights from a combined hemodynamic and Doppler echocardiographic study. J Am Coll Cardiol 12:426, 1988.

26. Davidson WR, Pasquale MJ, Aronoff RD: Doppler left ventricular filling pattern is closely related to ventricular relaxation abnormalities (abstract). J Am Coll Cardiol 13:197A, 1989.

27. Hatle L, Angelsen B, Tromsdal A: Noninvasive assessment of atrioventricular pressure half-time by Doppler ultrasound. Circulation 60:1096, 1979.

28. Smith MD, et al.: Comparative accuracy of two-dimensional echocardiography and Doppler pressure half-time methods in assessing severity of mitral stenosis in patients with and without prior commissurotomy. Circulation 73:100, 1986.

29. Bryg RJ, et al.: Effect of atrial fibrillation and mitral regurgitation on calculated mitral valve area in mitral stenosis. Am J Cardiol 57:634, 1986.

30. Williams GA, Labovitz AJ: Doppler hemodynamic evaluation of prosthetic (Starr-Edwards and Bjork-Shiley) and bioprosthetic (Hancock and Carpentier-Edwards) cardiac valves. Am J Cardiol 56:325, 1985.

31. Ryan T, Armstrong WF, Dillon JC, Feigenbaum H: Doppler echocardiographic evaluation of patients with porcine mitral valves. Am Heart J 111:237, 1986.

32. Thomas JD, et al.: Inaccuracy of the mitral pressure half-time immediately following percutaneous mitral valvotomy: Dependence on transmitral gradient and left atrial and ventricular compliance. Circulation 78:980, 1988.

33. Flachskampf FA, Weyman AE, Guererro JL, Thomas JD: Calculation of atrioventricular compliance from the mitral flow profile: Analytical and in vitro study. J Am Coll Cardiol 19:998, 1992.

34. Flachskampf FA, et al.: *In vivo* determination of net left atrioventricular compliance from mitral Doppler profiles (abstr). Circulation 82(Supplement III):III-127, 1990.

35. Templeton GH, Donald TC, III, Mitchell JH, Hefner LL: Dynamic stiffness of papillary muscle during contraction and relaxation. Am J Physiol 224:692, 1973.

36. Templeton GH, Ecker RR, Mitchell JH: Left ventricular stiffness during diastole and systole: The influence of changes in volume and inotropic state. Cardiovasc Res 6:95, 1972.

37. Hatle LK, Appleton CP, Popp RL: Differentiation of constrictive pericarditis and restrictive cardiomyopathy by Doppler echocardiography. Circulation 79:357, 1989.

38. Appleton C, Hatle L, Popp R: Demonstration of restrictive ventricular physiology by Doppler echocardiography. J Am Coll Cardiol 11:757, 1987.

39. Oh JK, et al.: Characteristic Doppler echocardiographic pattern of mitral inflow velocity in severe aortic regurgitation. J Am Coll Cardiol 14:1712, 1989.

40. Thomas JD, Newell JB, Choong CYP, Weyman AE: Physical and physiological determinants of transmitral velocity: Numerical analysis. Am J Physiol (in press).

41. Thomas JD, Weyman AE: Echocardiographic Doppler evaluation of left ventricular diastolic function: Physics and physiology. Circulation 84:977, 1991.

42. Meissner JS, Pajaro OE, Yellin EL: Investigation of left ventricular filling dynamics: Development of a model. Einstein Quart J Biol Med 4:47, 1986.

43. Keren G, et al.: Interrelationship of mid-diastolic mitral valve motion, pulmonary venous flow, and transmitral flow. Circulation 74:36, 1986.

44. Kovács SJ, Barzilai B, Perez JE: Evaluation of diastolic function with Doppler echocardiography: The PDF formalism. Am J Physiol 252(Heart Circ Physiol 21):H178, 1987.

45. Bakalyar DM, Hauser AM, Timmis GC:

Theoretical description of blood flow through the mitral orifice. J Biomech Eng 111:141, 1989.

46. Beyar R, Sideman S: Atrioventricular interactions: A theoretical simulation study. Am J Physiol 252:H653, 1987.

47. Lau VK, Sagawa K: Model analysis of the contribution of atrial contraction to ventricular filling. Ann Biomed Eng 7:167, 1979.

48. Chadwick RS, Brun P: A theoretical model of left ventricular filling and interpretation of echographic waveforms. *In* Cardiovascular Dynamics and Models. Proceedings of the NIH-Inserm Workshops, Colloque Inserm. *183*, Inserm, Paris, 1988, pp. 339–348.

49. Peskin CS: Numerical analysis of blood flow in the heart J Comput Phys 25:220, 1977.

50. McQueen DM, Peskin CS, Yellin EL: Fluid dynamics of the mitral valve: Physiologic aspects of a mathematical model. Am J Physiol 242(Heart Circ Physiol 11): H1095, 1982.

51. McQueen DM, Peskin CS: Computer-assisted design of pivoting disc prosthetic mitral valves. J Thorac Cardiovasc Surg 86:126, 1983.

52. Meissner JS, et al.: Effects of timing of atrial systole on ventricular filling and mitral valve closure: Computer and dog studies. Am J Physiol 249(Heart Circ Physiol 18):H604, 1985.

53. Peskin CS, McQueen DM: A three-dimensional computational method for blood flow in the heart. I. Immersed elastic fibers in a viscous incompressible fluid. J Comput Phys 81:372, 1989.

54. McQueen DM, Peskin CS: A three-dimensional computational method for blood flow in the heart: II. Contractile fibers. J Comput Phys 82:289, 1989.

55. Thomas JD: Numerical modelling of ventricular filling. Ann Biomed Engineering 20:19, 1992.

56. Aghassi D, Vandervoort PM, Thomas JD: Calculating mitral inertial mass in patients: A critical parameter in the assessment of diastolic function. J Am Coll Cardiol 19(Suppl A):214A, 1992.

57. Alexander J, Jr, Sunagawa K, Chang N, Sagawa K: Instantaneous pressure-volume relation of the ejecting left atrium. Circ Res 61:209, 1987.

58. Lau VK, Sagawa K, Suga H: Instantaneous pressure volume relationship of right atrium during isovolumic contraction in the canine heart. Am J Physiol 236(Heart Circ Physiol 5):H672, 1979.

59. Manning WJ, Leeman DE, Gotch PJ, Come PC: Pulsed Doppler evaluation of atrial mechanical function after electrical cardioversion of atrial fibrillation. J Am Coll Cardiol 13:617, 1989.

60. Takenaka K, et al.: Left ventricular filling in hypertrophic cardiomyopathy: A pulsed Doppler echocardiographic study. J Am Coll Cardiol 7:1263, 1986.

61. Bryg RJ, Pearson AC, Williams GA, Labovitz AJ: Left ventricular systolic and diastolic flow abnormalities determined by Doppler echocardiography in obstructive hypertrophic cardiomyopathy. Am J Cardiol 59:925, 1987.

62. Maron BJ, et al.: Noninvasive assessment of left ventricular diastolic function by pulsed Doppler echocardiography in patients with hypertrophic cardiomyopathy. J Am Coll Cardiol 10:733, 1987.

63. Pearson AC, Gudipati CV, Labovitz AJ: Systolic and diastolic flow abnormalities in elderly patients with hypertensive hypertrophic cardiomyopathy. J Am Coll Cardiol 12:989, 1988.

64. Otto CM, Pearlman AS, Amsler LC: Doppler echocardiographic evaluation of left ventricular diastolic filling in isolated valvular aortic stenosis. Am J Cardiol 63: 313, 1989.

65. Zarich SW, et al.: Left ventricular filling abnormalities in asymptomatic morbid obesity. Am J Cardiol 68:377, 1991.

66. Fujii J, et al.: Noninvasive assessment of left and right ventricular filling in myocardial infarction with a two-dimensional Doppler echocardiographic method. J Am Coll Cardiol 56:921, 1985.

67. Visser CA, et al.: Pulsed Doppler-derived mitral inflow velocity in acute myocardial infarction: an early prognostic indicator (abstract). J Am Coll Cardiol 7:136A, 1986.

68. Ilecito S, et al.: Doppler echocardiographic evaluation of the effect of atrial pacing-induced ischemia on left ventricular filling in patients with coronary artery disease. J Am Coll Cardiol 11:953, 1988.

69. Wind BE, et al.: Pulsed Doppler assessment of left ventricular diastolic filling in coronary artery disease before and immediately after coronary angioplasty. Am J Cardiol 59:1041, 1987.

70. Labovitz AJ, et al.: Evaluation of left ventricular systolic and diastolic dysfunction during transient myocardial ischaemia produced by angioplasty. J Am Col Cardiol 10:748, 1987.

71. Raisaro A, et al.: Doppler evaluation of left ventricular diastolic filling function

during angioplasty (abstract). J Am Coll Cardiol 9:213A, 1987.

72. de Bruyne B, et al.: Doppler assessment of left ventricular diastolic filling during brief coronary occlusion. Am Heart J 117: 629, 1989.

73. Doria E, Agostini P, Loaldi A, Fiorentini C: Doppler assessment of left ventricular filling pattern in silent ischemia in patients with Prinzmetal's angina. Am J Cardiol 66:1055, 1990.

74. Takenaka K, et al.: Pulsed Doppler echocardiographic study of left ventricular filling in dilated cardiomyopathy. Am J Cardiol 58:143, 1986.

75. Wehlage DR, Bohrer H, Ruffmann K: Impairment of left ventricular diastolic function during coronary artery bypass grafting. Anesthesia 45:549, 1990.

76. Iwase M, et al.: Effects of diltiazem on left ventricular diastolic behavior in patients with hypertrophic cardiomyopathy: Evaluation with exercise pulsed Doppler echocardiography. J Am Coll Cardiol 9:1099, 1987.

77. Phillips RA, et al.: Doppler echocardiographic analysis of left ventricular filling in treated hypertensive patients. J Am Coll Cardiol 9:317, 1987.

78. Lee RT, Lord CP, Plappert T, St. John Sutton M: Effects of nifedipine on transmitral Doppler blood flow velocity profile in patients with concentric left ventricular hypertrophy. Am Heart J 119:1130, 1990.

79. Snow FR, et al.: Doppler echocardiographic evaluation of left ventricular diastolic function after percutaneous transluminal coronary angioplasty for unstable angina pectoris or acute myocardial infarction. Am J Cardiol 65:840, 1990.

80. Masuyama T, Nellessen U, Stinson EB, Popp RL: Improvement in left ventricular diastolic filling by septal myectomy in hypertrophic cardiomyopathy. J Am Soc Echo 3:196, 1990.

81. Bryg RJ, Williams GA, Labovitz AJ: Effect of aging on left ventricular diastolic filling in normal subjects. Am J Cardiol 59:971, 1987.

82. Gardin JM, et al.: Doppler transmitral flow velocity parameters: Relationship between age, body surface area, blood pressure and gender in normal subjects. Am J Noninvas Cardiol 1:3, 1987.

83. Appleton CA, Carucci MJ, Henry CP: Influence of incremental changes in heart rate on mitral flow velocity in lightly sedated conscious dogs. J Am Coll Cardiol 17:227, 1991.

84. Choong CYC, Herrmann HC, Weyman AE, Fifer MA: Preload dependence of Doppler-derived indices of left ventricular diastolic function in humans. J Am Coll Cardiol 10:800, 1987.

85. Ishida Y, et al.: Left ventricular filling dynamics: Influence of left ventricular relaxation and left atrial pressure. Circulation 74:187, 1986.

86. Stoddard MF, et al.; Influence of alteration in preload on the pattern of left ventricular diastolic filling as assessed by Doppler echocardiography in humans. Circulation 79:1226, 1989.

87. Downes TR, et al.: Effect of alteration in loading conditions on both normal and abnormal patterns of left ventricular filling in healthy individuals. Am J Cardiol 65: 377, 1990.

88. Desruennes M, et al.: Doppler echocardiography from the diagnosis of acute cardiac allograft rejection. J Am Coll Cardiol 12:63, 1988.

89. Valantine HA, et al.: A hemodynamic and Doppler echocardiographic study of ventricular function in long-term cardiac allograft recipients. Circulation 79:66, 1989.

90. Klein AL, et al.: Doppler characterization of left ventricular diastolic function in cardiac amyloidosis. J Am Coll Cardiol 13: 1017, 1989.

91. Spirito P, Lupi G, Melevendi C, Vecchio C: Restrictive diastolic abnormalities identified by Doppler echocardiography in patients with thalassemia major. Circulation 82:88, 1990.

92. Klein AL, et al.: Serial Doppler echocardiographic follow-up of left ventricular diastolic function in cardiac amyloidosis. J Am Coll Cardiol 16:1135, 1990.

93. Thomas JD, Choong CYP, Flachskampf FA, Weyman AE: Analysis of the early transmitral Doppler velocity curve: Effect of primary physiologic changes and compensatory preload adjustment. J Am Coll Cardiol 16:644, 1990.

94. Himura Y, et al.: Importance of left ventricular systolic function in the assessment of left ventricular diastolic function with Doppler transmitral flow velocity recording. J Am Coll Cardiol 18:753, 1991.

95. Giannuzzi P, et al.: Effects of mental exercise in patients with dilated cardiomyopathy and congestive heart failure: An echocardiographic Doppler study. Circulation 83[suppl II]:95.II-155, 1991.

96. Klein AL, et al.: Prognostic significance of Doppler measures of diastolic function in cardiac amyloidosis: A Doppler echocardiography study. Circulation 83:808, 1991.

97. Vanoverschelde J-LJ, Raphael DA, Robert

AR, Cosyns JR: Left ventricular filing in dilated cardiomyopathy: Relation to functional class and hemodynamics. J Am Col Cardiol 15:1288, 1990.

98. Ng KSK, Gibson DG: Relation of filling pattern to diastolic function in severe left ventricular disease. Br Heart J 63:209, 1990.

99. Nishimura RA, Abel MD, Hatle LK, Tajik AJ: Relation of pulmonary vein to mitral flow velocities by transesophageal Doppler echocardiogarphy: Effect of different loading conditions. Circulation 81:1488, 1990.

100. Masuyama T, et al.: Pulmonary venous flow velocity pattern as assessed with transthoracic pulsed Doppler echocardiography in subjects without cardiac disease. Am J Cardiol 67:1396, 1991.

101. Jacobs LE, Kotler MN, Parry WR: Flow patterns in dilated cardiomyopathy: A pulsed-wave and color flow Doppler study. J Am Soc Echo 3:294, 1990.

102. Tritton DF: Physical Fluid Dynamics. Oxford, Clarendon Press, 1988, pp. 48–72.

103. Thomas JD, et al.: Spatiotemporal distribution of mitral inflow velocity: Use of the color Doppler M-mode echocardiogram to investigate intracardiac pressure gradients (abstract). Medical & Biological Engineering & Computing 29(Suppl I):130, 1991.

104. Greenberg NL, Vandervoort PM, Powell KA, Thomas JD: Computation of transmitral pressure gradients from color Doppler M-mode images. Submitted to ASME Proceedings 6/92.

105. Brun P, Tribouilloy C, Duval A-M, et al.: Left ventricular flow propagation during early filling is related to wall relaxation: A color M-mode Doppler analysis. J Am Coll Cardiol 20:420, 1992.

106. Thomas JD, Greenberg NA, Vandervoort PM, Aghassi DS, Hunt BF: Digital analysis of transmitral color Doppler M-mode data: A potential new approach to the noninvasive assessment of diastolic function. Computers in Cardiology 1992, pp 631–635.

Chapter 13

HEMODYNAMIC LOADS AND LEFT VENTRICULAR DIASTOLIC FUNCTION: FACTORS AFFECTING THE INDICES OF ISOVOLUMETRIC AND AUXOTONIC RELAXATION

Michael R. Zile, Rick A. Nishimura, and William H. Gaasch

The clinical assessment of left ventricular (LV) diastolic function is important for at least two reasons. First, as many as one third of all patients who develop signs and symptoms of congestive heart failure have normal systolic function (1–10). In such patients, congestive heart failure is often related to an abnormality of LV diastolic function. Because the therapeutic approach to diastolic failure is distinctly different from that used in systolic failure (3, 4, 7, 11, 12), successful treatment of patients with congestive heart failure depends on accurate clinical assessment of LV systolic and diastolic function. Second, diastolic dysfunction may be present before discernible abnormalities of systolic function; thus, some disease processes can present with isolated abnormalities of diastolic function. The assessment of diastolic function in such patients may allow early detection of the disease process before symptoms develop; selected indices of diastolic function may be used to follow the natural history of the disease process and to assess the effects of treatment (11–22). Incorrect interpretation of the indices of diastolic function may lead the clinician to suspect the presence of diastolic dysfunction when it is not present or to conclude that a pharmacologic intervention successfully corrected an abnormality in diastolic function when it merely changed LV loading conditions. These potential errors in the assessment of diastolic function can be caused by a failure to appreciate and assess the mechanical and hemodynamic determinants of the indices used to evaluate diastolic function (22–31).

All of the clinical parameters of diastolic function can be affected not only by alterations in the intrinsic process of myocardial relaxation, but also by ventricular heterogeneity and changes in loading conditions. Therefore, an accurate assessment of diastolic function depends on a clear understanding of the hemodynamic determinants of the relaxation parameters and an ability to integrate such information into the interpretation of the data.

The purpose of this chapter is to describe the clinical parameters used to assess LV diastolic function and define the mechanical and hemodynamic factors that affect these parameters. An understanding of the effects of changes in homogeneity and especially load is essential if we are to interpret accurately the indices of LV relaxation.

METHODS OF EVALUATING RELAXATION

Relaxation refers to the process by which the myocardium returns to its initial or resting length and tension (i.e., sarcomeres relengthen in part as a consequence of calcium reuptake by the sarcoplasmic reticulum); in clinical terms, relaxation generally refers to all of the processes by which the left ventricle returns to its presystolic or end-diastolic pressure and volume. It should be recognized, however, that the process of active myocardial relaxation is essentially complete by mid diastole (at least in the normal heart) and that late diastolic filling is primarily related to the passive properties of the ventricle and atrial contraction. Attempts to evaluate relaxation in the intact left ventricle are based on measurements made during two periods: the isovolumic relaxation period and the diastolic filling period.

Isovolumic Relaxation

Noninvasive methods used to quantify the rate of isovolumic relaxation include the echocardiographic and phonocardiographic measurement of isovolumic relaxation time. Cardiac catheterization is necessary to assess the rate of LV pressure decline (peak negative dP/dt and the isovolumic relaxation time constant).

Isovolumic relaxation time (IVRT) is calculated as the time period from aortic valve closure to mitral valve opening. In general, when the rate of LV isovolumic pressure decline is slow, IVRT is prolonged. However, this parameter is influenced by factors other than the rate of relaxation (i.e., the timing of aortic valve closure and mitral valve opening); it should, therefore, be interpreted with caution (32). For example, an elevated left atrial pressure can cause earlier opening of the mitral valve and a decrease in the IVRT. Recognizing such hemodynamic determinants, this parameter remains a useful non-invasive index of LV relaxation.

Peak negative dP/dt reflects events that occur very early during LV pressure decline, near the instant of aortic valve closure. During acute hemodynamic interventions, peak negative dP/dt is directly related to LV systolic pressure. For these reasons, this parameter is not widely used in the assessment of LV relaxation. However, when systolic loads are constant, a lower dP/dt generally indicates a slower relaxation.

The time constant of LV isovolumic pressure decline (τ) reflects the entire course of LV pressure decline. The time constant is equal to the time required for LV pressure to fall to approximately one third of its initial value. Because LV pressure decline generally follows a monoexponential course, a plot of the natural log of pressure versus time forms a linear relation; the time constant is equal to the inverse slope of this linear relation. When isovolumic relaxation is impaired, pressure decline is slowed, the slope of the log pressure versus time relation declines, and τ in-

creases. This definition of the time constant is based on the work of Weiss et al. (33):

$$P = P_0 e^{-t/\tau} \qquad (1)$$

To apply these methods to the clinical assessment of LV relaxation, it should be noted that Weiss used transmural LV pressure, assumed that LV pressure decline was isovolumic and monoexponential, and that the baseline pressure toward which this exponential decayed was zero. However, τ is generally calculated using LV cavity pressure, not transmural pressure. The experiments of Frais et al. (34) indicate that τ, calculated from LV intracavitary pressure using the Weiss equation, is altered by changes in pericardial pressure when myocardial relaxation itself was unchanged. This is important in the clinical assessment of diastolic function because some acute hemodynamic and pharmacologic intervention and some chronic disease processes may cause significant changes in pericardial pressure. Fortunately, however, Frais et al. (34) also demonstrated that two alternate methods to calculate τ, using LV cavitary pressure, were not affected by changes in pericardial pressure. First, the "derivative" method of Craig et al. (35) calculates the isovolumic time constant τ as the inverse slope of the linear relation between dP/dt and P using the equation:

$$dP/dt = -1/\tau(P - P_B) \qquad (2)$$

τ calculated using these methods is not affected by changes in pericardial pressure, but because it is based on the time derivative of pressure, it may be inaccurate when the derivative signal becomes noisy. In the second method, LV intracavitary pressure and time are analyzed using the equation:

$$P = P_0 e^{-t/\tau} + P_B \qquad (3)$$

Using this formula, P_B (the baseline pressure toward which the exponential decays) is calculated and the resultant value of τ is unaffected by changes in pericardial pressure.

Other studies (36, 37) indicate that LV pressure decline does not always follow a perfectly monoexponential decay. This may be especially important in the presence of aortic stenosis. Therefore, it is important to examine the linearity of the log P versus time relation and calculate the time constant using equations 1 through 3 only when the relation between log P and time has a high linear correlation coefficient. Alternatively, data can be analyzed using a biexponential approach or a three-constant nonlinear regression analysis (29). (See Chaps. 4 and 5.)

Because of the limitations just described, it is prudent to calculate the time constant of isovolumic pressure decline using more than one method. When agreement exists between methods, it is likely that τ accurately reflects the time course of pressure decline. In disease processes such as coronary heart disease, mitral regurgitation and aortic regurgitation, LV pressure decline may not be isovolumic. Therefore, a truly isovolumic time constant cannot be calculated.

Diastolic Filling

Ventricular filling normally occurs in three phases: the rapid early diastolic filling period, slow filling (diastasis), and late diastolic filling produced by atrial contraction. Approximately two thirds of the normal end diastolic volume enters the ventricle during the rapid filling period. Early diastolic filling can be assessed by measuring the maximum filling rate, the time to peak filling rate (i.e., the time from end systolic to peak positive dV/dt), the extent of filling (i.e., the fractional filling that occurs during the rapid filling period) and the acceleration and deceleration rate of the rapid filling wave. Atrial contraction contributes up to 20% of end diastolic volume in the normal heart. This phase of filling can be evaluated by examining the extent and velocity of filling that occurs during atrial contraction or the ratio of early to late filling rates.

Cardiac Catheterization and Angiography

Simultaneous measurements of LV pressure, volume, and geometry can be made throughout diastolic filling. Such measurements allow an assessment of filling dynamics; in addition catheterization has the advantage that isovolumic relaxation, chamber compliance, and loading conditions can also be assessed. However, this invasive technique cannot be repeated frequently, nor is it suitable for serial measurements during the course of the disease or its treatment.

Echocardiography

This method allows assessment of beat-to-beat changes in diastolic filling and is well suited for serial measurements over time in a single patient. (See Chap. 12.) The M-mode echocardiogram has the advantage of providing information about dimension and wall thickness throughout the cardiac cycle at a very rapid sampling rate. These data can be used to calculate the peak rate of increase in LV dimension (peak positive dD/dt), and peak wall thinning rate (peak negative dTh/dt). Because these parameters do not provide direct measurements of the rate of change of LV volume, they must be considered indices of filling. In the absence of segmental wall motion abnormalities, however, they have an excellent correlation with catheterization-derived measures of the rate of change of volume (38).

Echo-Doppler Techniques

This method provides transmitral flow velocity (meters/sec) data during rapid early diastolic filling (E wave velocity) and during late filling produced by atrial contraction (A wave velocity). There are two methods of interpreting Doppler-derived transmitral flow velocities. One interprets velocities when the sample volume is placed at the level of the mitral annulus. The integral of the flow velocity can be used to derive volumetric flow (mL/sec) if the area of the annulus can be determined. Thus, measurements of peak filling rates and the temporal occurrence of the peak rates can be obtained from the peak velocities. These measurements assume a circular constant orifice and laminar flow, neither of which is present in humans. Nonetheless, under steady-state conditions, most studies indicate that Doppler-derived measurements of peak and late filling rates correlate well with those derived from other methods (23, 24, 39, 40). A second method interprets velocities from the sample volume placed at the highest velocity of transmitral flow; this occurs at the tip of the mitral leaflets as they open into the left ventricle in early diastole. This second method is most commonly used in clinical studies of diseased hearts and research involving changes in left ventricular loading conditions. Altered hemodynamic loads can cause substantial changes in these Doppler velocity patterns, independent of changes in the diastolic properties of the ventricle.

Radionuclide Ventriculography

This method provides a time-activity curve that is not dependent on LV geometry and is produced by averaging many cardiac cycles. (See Chap. 11.) Indices of filling rate such as peak filling rate, time to peak filling rate, and filling fractions can be derived from this curve. However, because the results represent average volume transients, beat-to-beat changes in diastolic function cannot be assessed using this technique.

DETERMINANTS OF RELAXATION RATE

Relaxation is controlled by a complex interaction between deactivation (the time-dependent decay of active force generating capacity), homogeneity (temporal and functional uniformity) and loading conditions (forces affecting myocardial length and tension); this process is then modulated by neurohumoral, metabolic, and pharmacologic influences (25). Thus, relaxation indices reflect intensity of the "intrinsic" myocardial relaxing system only if loading conditions, homogeneity, and neurohumoral influences are constant. (See Chap. 2.) In the discussion below, we focus on how changes in homogeneity and loading conditions affect clinical indices of LV relaxation rate.

The discussion that follows does not include late ventricular filling that results from atrial contraction. The extent and velocity of late filling are determined by interactions between atrial function and ventricular compliance. A discussion of these factors is beyond the scope of this chapter.

Heterogeneity

Heterogeneity is present when regional variations occur in the onset, rate, or extent of segmental muscle shortening and/or lengthening. (See Chap. 19.) Asynchrony can be defined as a temporal dispersion of contraction-relaxation sequences. Some fibers or segments are activated late in the cardiac cycle, causing continued shortening in one area while relaxation and lengthening are beginning in another area. Asynergy is a functional dispersion of contraction-relaxation sequences, causing marked differences in the extent of shortening among segments, with increased muscle shortening in one area (hyperkinesis) and decreased shortening in an another area (hypokinesis or akinesis). Asynchrony and asynergy prolong the contraction-relaxation sequence; this causes the time course of isovolumic pressure decline to be slowed, mitral valve opening to be delayed, and the rate of rapid filling to be decreased (41).

Experiments in the Intact Dog Heart. Several studies indicate that an acute increase in heterogeneity (independent of changes in loading conditions and myocardial deactivation) can slow the rate of LV isovolumic pressure decline and early diastolic filling (41–44). For example, sequential atrial-ventricular pacing has been shown to produce asynchrony, no measurable change in ventricular load, a significant increase in the relaxation time constant, and a significant fall in filling rate (42). Similar studies in patients with dual-chamber pacemakers indicate that sequential atrial-ventricular pacing induced asynchrony results in slower LV relaxation and decreased early filling rate (45, 46).

Clinical Implications. One of the mechanisms underlying abnormal relaxation and filling rate in patients with chronic heart disease is heterogeneity within the wall. For example, asynergy is produced when a myocardial infarction results in hypokinesis in the infarcted segment with normal motion or even hyperkinesis in the noninfarcted segments. Even when a disease process does not significantly alter load or deactivation, the presence of heterogeneity can prolong pressure decline and slow filling. Various studies have shown that principal mechanisms causing abnormal filling in coronary artery disease, hypertrophic cardiomyopathy, and aging are asynchrony, asynergy, or both (47–58). In addition, a change in heterogeneity caused by mechanical or pharmacologic treatment of coronary artery disease or hypertrophic cardiomyopathy may contribute to improvement in these measures of diastolic function. Pharmacologic and mechanical treatment of coronary disease and hypertrophic cardiomyopathy have been shown to lessen heterogeneity and improve LV relaxation and filling (48–51).

Ventricular Loading Conditions

Ventricular loading conditions are best described by calculating the forces or stresses within the LV wall. Ventricular load can be divided into preload (end diastolic force), afterload (wall forces generated during systole), and lengthening load (force applied during diastole).

Preload

There is a remarkable yet unnecessary confusion regarding the effect of acute changes in preload (end diastolic force) on the rate of LV relaxation and filling (28, 59–74). This confusion exists because: (1) some investigators define and use the term preload incorrectly; (2) some of the methods used to alter preload also caused changes in afterload and lengthening load, each of which has independent effects on relaxation and filling; and (3) some of the studies examining the effects of changes in preload did not include measurements of pressure and, therefore, did not directly assess either preload or lengthening load (66–73). Preload represents the force applied to the myocardium at *end* diastole. Preload should clearly be distinguished from forces present during *early* diastole (during the periods of isovolumic pressure decline and early diastolic filling). These early diastolic forces will be discussed as "lengthening load" (see below). This distinction is of signal importance because recent studies have shown that an isolated increase in end diastolic stress (preload) does effect a change in relaxation or filling, whereas an increase in the left atrial to LV pressure gradient (lengthening load) does alter relaxation and filling (59–64, 74–79).

Left atrial pressure at end diastole may reflect preload; however, mean left atrial pressure and left atrial pressure in early diastole certainly do not represent LV preload. Only those hemodynamic parameters that influence end diastolic fiber stretch or sarcomere length (such as end-diastolic pressure or volume) represent measures of preload. Inferior vena cava occlusion, intravenous nitroglycerin, and lower body negative pressure effect changes in left atrial and LV pressure and volume throughout diastole. In addition, these interventions may change systolic pressure and volume. Therefore, these interventions alter preload, afterload, and lengthening load, the latter two of which clearly affect the rate of relaxation and filling. Therefore, in the discussion that follows, we will examine the effects of an isolated change in preload (end diastolic force) on relaxation and filling and contrast these effects with those caused by isolated changes in afterload and lengthening load.

Experiments in the Intact Dog Heart. The effects of an abrupt increase in LV preload were studied by inserting a large bore catheter into the LV apex of an anesthetized dog and rapidly infusing blood into the LV during a single diastole (60). Using a second catheter in the central aorta, LV systolic pressure could be held constant by withdrawing aortic blood during systole (Fig. 13–1). Thus, these single beat interventions allowed an assessment of LV isovolumic relaxation rate during an LV infusion with simultaneous withdrawal of aortic blood (preload increased with unchanged afterload). This method allowed a comparison of data from the control beat with data from the preloaded beat, but it did not allow sufficient time for neurohumoral or reflex changes to influence the results. In 23 paired beats (control versus LV infusion), systolic pressure was held constant and no change occurred in the isovolumic relaxation time constant (60). Thus, an isolated increase in LV preload was not associated with a change in the isovolumic relaxation rate. This result is consonant with data from a study by Hori et al. (65) in which an isolated change in preload did not influence the rate of LV pressure decline.

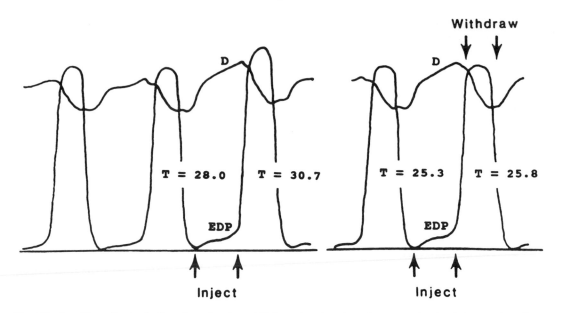

Fig. 13–1. The effect of altered preload on LV isovolumic relaxation rate. In the left panel, volume was infused into the ventricle during a single diastole (inject); end-diastolic pressure (P) and dimension (D) increased, as did left ventricular systolic pressure. As a result, the isovolumic relaxation time constant (T) fell. In the right panel, a similar diastolic infusion is made, but in this case a rapid withdrawal of blood from an aortic cannula provided constant systolic pressure (despite the increment in preload); under these circumstances, there was no change in the isovolumic relaxation rate. Adapted with permission from Gaasch WH, et al.: Myocardial relaxation: Effects of preload on the time course of isovolumetric relaxation. Circulation 73:1037, 1986.

The effect of an isolated change in LV preload on early diastolic filling of the next diastole has not been studied in the intact heart. However, studies in isolated cardiac muscles, discussed below, indicate that an isolated change in myocardial preload does not affect the subsequent lengthening rate. Moreover, using multivariate analysis, studies in an open chest, right heart bypass model indicate that LV preload (end diastolic pressure) is not a primary determinants of early diastolic filling rate (64).

Experiments in Isolated Cardiac Muscle. The independent effect of a change in preload on relaxation can best be studied in physiologically sequenced isolated muscle preparations in which the loading sequence of the intact heart is simulated; isometric contraction is followed by shortening of the muscle and isometric relaxation precedes lengthening. In such studies, either the length or the tension is controlled by an electronic servosystem and a digital computer; thus, total load (the sum

of preload and afterload) can be held constant over a wide range of preloads (59). Isometric relaxation (tension decline at constant muscle length) is analogous to isovolumic pressure decline in the intact left ventricle; isotonic lengthening (muscle lengthening at constant tension) is analogous to filling in the intact left ventricle.

The effect of an isolated change in preload on isometric relaxation was studied by varying preload from 30% to 100% of resting tension at L_{max}; all comparisons were made at a constant total load and constant lengthening load. An example of a typical experiment is shown in Figure 13–2. The time course of isometric force decline (shown in the lower left panel of Figure 13–2) did not change over a wide range of preloads; the time course of isometric relaxation was superimposable at the five different preloads. This was a consistent finding in all muscles studied. These experiments indicated that the maximum rate of isometric tension decline is independent of preload (59). Thus, isometric relaxation (in the isolated muscle) and isovolumic relaxation (in the intact heart) are independent of preload. The time course of isotonic lengthening (shown in the upper left panel of Fig. 13–2) did not change despite variations in preload. As shown in the right panel of Figure 13–2, the average values for maximum isotonic relaxation (lengthening) rate were independent of preload (59). Note that the load on the muscle during isotonic relaxation (i.e., during lengthening) was equal in all five experiments; if lengthening load is not held constant, lengthening rate may vary (see subsequent text). Similar results have been obtained in hypoxic and hypertrophic myocardium (62).

Clinical Implications. Varma et al. (63) used inferior vena caval occlusion in pa-

tients undergoing cardiac catheterization to study the effect of changes in preload on the rate of isovolumic pressure decline. These investigators limited their analysis to beats that occurred early after the start of interior vena caval occlusion in which LV end-diastolic pressure was falling (decrease preload) but there were as yet no changes in LV systolic pressure (constant afterload). In these beats, LV end-diastolic pressure fell from 18 ± 6 to 9 ± 6 mmHg; there were no changes in LV systolic pressure, heart rate or the relaxation time constant. These results confirm the preload independence of isovolumic relaxation rate in man. Other investigators have examined echo-Doppler and radionuclide indices of LV early diastolic filling rate during interventions, which alter left atrial pressure and LV preload (66–73). Unfortunately,

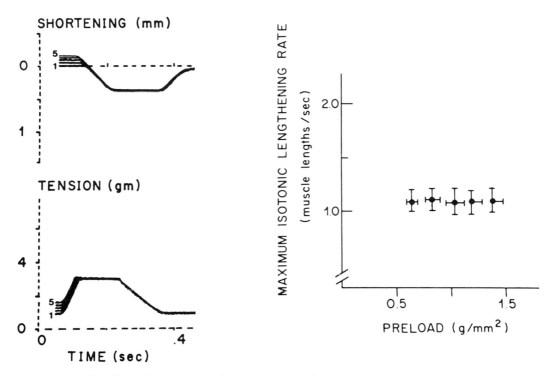

Fig. 13–2. Isolated muscle preload studies. Five levels of preload were set before contraction. Neither isometric nor isotonic relaxation rates were affected by changes in preload, as shown by the superimposed force and length tracings (left panels). In the panel on the right, the average results from six papillary muscle experiments are shown. When preload was increased from 0.65 to 1.37 g/mm², maximum isotonic relaxation (lengthening) rate remained constant. Reproduced with permission of the American Heart Association from Zile MR, et al.: Mechanical determinants of the rate of isotonic lengthening in rat left ventricular myocardium. Circ Res 60:815, 1987.

LV afterload, left atrial pressure, and lengthening loads were allowed to vary; for this reason, it was not possible to assess the independent effect of preload. This is discussed further in the section on lengthening load (see subsequent text).

Afterload

The effect of changes in afterload, measured as LV systolic wall stress, on LV relaxation and filling depends on the magnitude of the change in load, on the time during contraction that load is changed, and on the method used to change load. Loads applied early in the contraction (within the first two thirds of ejection), generally prolong the rate of myocardial relaxation and slow the rate of early filling (25, 80–85). During contraction, activating calcium is available to the contractile proteins, more crossbridges are recruited, systole is prolonged, myocardial relaxation and filling occur later and at a slower rate. In this chapter, these afterloads are termed early systolic (contraction) loads. By contrast, loads applied late in contraction (during the last one third of ejection) generally cause relaxation to be premature and more rapid (25, 80–85). These afterloads are termed late systolic (relaxation) loads. During this period, the available calcium is below the threshold necessary for activating new crossbridges, existing crossbridges cannot support an additional load, the muscle yields, and relaxation is premature.

Relaxation and filling also depend on the method used to alter afterload. Different experimental techniques can cause variable activation of reflexes and variations in the time course of change in LV pressure and volume during ejection (65, 86, 88–90). Afterload, when altered by steady state infusions of vasopressor agents, may affect baroreceptor and other mechanical and neurohumoral reflex activity, each of which may independently affect relaxation. This limitation requires studies performed with such pharmacologic agents to be done after sympathetic and parasympathetic blockade which in turn adds to the complexity of the experimental design. Afterload can also be altered by brief mechanical occlusion of the aorta using an aortic crossclamp in open-chest dogs or an intra-aortic balloon in the conscious intact state (see subsequent text). These mechanical occlusions produce variably afterloaded or single isovolumic beats and provide data that are not contaminated by neurohumoral or reflex mechanisms. Despite differences in methodology, most published data indicate that an increase in LV afterload results in an increase in the isovolumic relaxation time constant and a decrease in LV early filling rate. However, the degree to which afterload affects relaxation may vary, partly because of differences in the time course of changes in LV pressure and volume during contraction. For example, Hori et al. have demonstrated that relaxation is variably affected by the timing of peak LV pressure and the timing of end ejection (see subsequent text) (65, 71, 87).

Early Systolic (Contraction) Load

Experiments in the Intact Dog Heart. To determine the effects of an isolated increase in afterload, a large vascular clamp placed around the descending aorta was used to produce variably afterloaded beats by clamping the descending aorta for three cardiac cycles (43, 91, 92). An example of such an experiment is shown in Figure 13–3. The average results from a series of aortic crossclamp experiments are shown in Figure 13–4. These experiments indicate that there was a direct relation between LV afterload and the isovolumic relaxation time constant. Systolic pressure increased from 124 ± 6 mmHg in the control beat to 176 ± 11 mmHg in the third crossclamp beat; T increased from 20 ± 2 to 30 ± 4 msec. It should be noted that the crossclamp experiment does not cause a pure increase in afterload; end diastolic pressure shows a progressive rise after the first crossclamp beat. However, because preload does not affect the rate of isovolumic pressure decline, these results indicate a direct relationship between systolic load and the relaxation time constant.

The effect of afterload on LV peak filling rate was also studied in the anesthetized dog model using the aortic crossclamp technique (92). Segment length and minor axis dimension were measured with sonomicrometers and the peak rate of in-

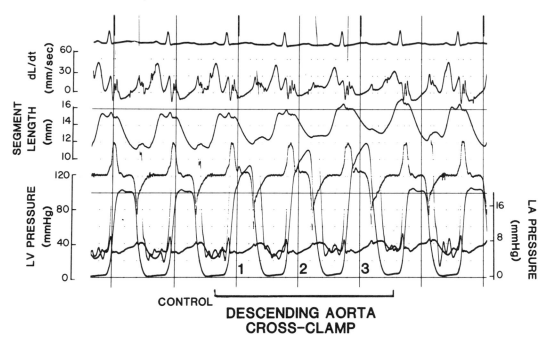

CONTROL

DESCENDING AORTA CROSS-CLAMP

Fig. 13–3. Example of the effects of a mechanically induced (descending aorta cross-clamp) change in afterload. LV pressure (micromanometer), the first derivative of pressure (dP/dt), LV midwall segment length (ultrasonic crystals), and the first derivative of length (dL/dt) are shown. Left atrial (LA) pressure and LV diastolic pressure are shown at high gain. With application of the descending aorta clamp, the LV systolic pressure and length progressively increased while fractional shortening and peak lengthening rate progressively decreased. Reproduced with permission of the American Heart Association from Zile et al.: The effect of acute alterations in left ventricular afterload and β-adrenergic tone on indices of early diastolic filling rate. Circ Res 65:406, 1989.

crease of these parameters (during the rapid filling period) was taken as an index of LV peak filling rate. The average results from a series of aortic crossclamp experi- ments are shown in Figure 13–5. In these studies, both of the indices of peak filling rate (peak positive dL/dt and dD/dt) were found to be inversely related to LV af-

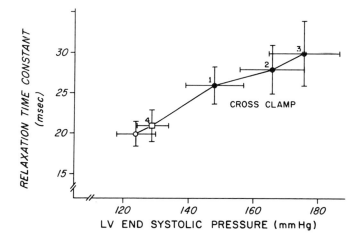

Fig. 13–4. Relationship between the relaxation time constant and LV end-systolic pressure. After abrupt occlusion of the descending thoracic aorta, both LV systolic pressure and relaxation time constant increased progressively (closed circles labeled 1, 2, and 3). Release of the occlusion resulted in prompt return (open square) toward control value (open circle). Reproduced with permission of the American Physiological Society from Blaustein AS, Gaasch WH: Myocardial relaxation. VI. Effects of β-adrenergic tone and asynchrony on LV relaxation rate. Am J Physiol 244:H417, 1983.

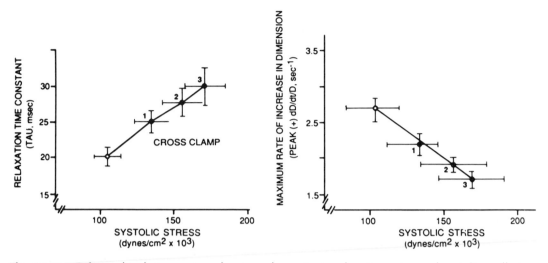

Fig. 13–5. Relationship between isovolumic and auxotonic relaxation rates and systolic wall stress. Data were obtained by abrupt occlusion (cross-clamp) of the descending aorta. Open circle = control; closed circles (1, 2, 3) = aortic occlusion. Abrupt occlusion of the descending aorta produced an increase in LV systolic wall stress, an increase in the relaxation time constant (slowed isovolumic relaxation), and a decreased myocardial lengthening rate (slowed auxotonic relaxation).

terload (92). These data and those published by Bahler and Martin (86); Caillet et al. (93), and Karliner et al. (87) indicate that during acute hemodynamic interventions, isovolumic relaxation rate and early diastolic filling rate are inversely related to LV afterload. This inverse relation is, at least partly, based on the changes in elastic restoring forces produced by changes in afterload. When afterload is increased, stroke volume falls, end-systolic volume increases, and the effect on restoring forces is attenuated. In addition, because end systolic volume is increased, length-dependent deactivation is decreased. These factors cause a slowed and delayed left ventricular pressure decline, an increased minimum left ventricular pressure, a decreased transmitral pressure gradient, and slowed left ventricular early filling.

The role of systolic pressure or afterload as a determinant of isovolumic relaxation was examined further by Hori et al. (65, 88, 89). They produced variable afterload beats by clamping the ascending or descending aorta; the ascending aortic clamps manifested an earlier peaking pressure while the descending clamps produced a late peaking pressure (the peak systolic pressure was similar, but the time course of pressure differed in the two in-

terventions). These experiments in the anesthetized open-chest dog clearly demonstrated that a late peaking systolic pressure (descending aorta clamp) resulted in a substantial increase in T (75 ± 3 to 122 ± 10 msec); an ascending aortic clamp with an early peaking pressure (of the same magnitude) was associated with a smaller increase in T (67 ± 3 to 86 ± 8 msec). These data are consonant with the experiments of Bahler et al. (86) and Gaasch et al. (90), who performed ascending and descending aortic crossclamps in anesthetized dogs. Based on these differences in relaxation rate between early and late peaking pressure, Hori et al. (88, 89) concluded that the "loading sequence is a major determinant of afterload-dependent relaxation in the intact canine heart." Hori et al. (65) also suggested that the history of ejection affects the rate of LV relaxation. Thus, when LV pressure, end systolic volume, and ejection rate were held constant, a delay in end ejection time (i.e., shortening persists longer and the onset of isovolumic pressure decline is delayed) caused LV pressure decline to fall more rapidly. They hypothesized that a delay in end-ejection allowed shortening to persist into a period when intracellular calcium concentration is low, shortening deactivation is pronounced, crossbridge cycling is reduced and relaxation can proceed more rapidly.

It should be recognized that the ascending and descending clamp interventions produced by Hori et al. (65, 88, 89) and others (86, 90) are not the same as the abrupt changes in load studied by Brutsaert (25) and others (80–85). The loads applied by Hori were applied early and maintained throughout contraction; the time course of pressure varied according to whether the clamp was applied to the ascending or descending aorta. By contrast, Brutsaert emphasized the effects of an abrupt load increment late in the cardiac cycle. The changes in LV relaxation produced by Brutsaert's abrupt late load clamps are manifestations of load-dependent relaxation, and are discussed below as "late systolic (relaxation) load."

Clinical Implications. On the basis of the experimental data, it might be expected that abnormal LV systolic loading conditions might contribute to the relaxation abnormalities seen in patients with systemic arterial hypertension. Unfortunately, no studies have been published on the subject of LV relaxation in patients with hypertensive crisis, but it is likely that an acute increase in systolic pressure (an early systolic contraction load) could cause prolonged relaxation, elevated LV diastolic pressures, decreased LV filling rate and, especially if the heart rate is rapid, pulmonary venous hypertension, dyspnea, and even congestive heart failure. On the other hand, an acute reduction in arterial pressure might contribute to improved LV relaxation and a decrease in LV diastolic pressures in such patients.

In contrast to a large body of experimental data, two studies in human beings (94, 95) indicate no change in the rate of LV isovolumic pressure decline or early filling when afterload was increased by methoxamine infusions. The reason for the disparity is unknown, but it is possible that the effect of altered load is less pronounced in normal than in abnormal hearts (or anesthetized animals).

Patients with chronically elevated arterial pressure also exhibit abnormalities of LV relaxation and filling. Some studies indicate that these abnormalities of relaxation are related to increased LV mass (96–99), whereas others implicate abnormal loading (97, 100–102) or other processes (21). Fouad et al. (97) and Smith et al. (101) and others (103, 104) have shown that hypertensive patients with or without hypertrophy have decreased early diastolic rates and have noted an inverse relation between filling rate and systolic wall stress. Others have failed to demonstrate a relationship between peak filling rate and arterial pressure (100, 102), but these investigators did not assess changes in LV wall stress, which is a more appropriate index of myocardial load than is systolic pressure. Unfortunately, it has not been possible to separate or dissect out the effects of autonomic tone, antihypertensive drugs, ischemia, LV asynergy, or even the extent of LV hypertrophy as independent determinants of relaxation in patients with heart disease. This is clearly an important area for future research.

The observation that an acute change in systolic load affects LV relaxation and filling have important implications for understanding the mechanism(s) by which pharmacologic agents influence relaxation in patients with heart disease. For example, calcium channel blocking agents tend to normalize the prolonged relaxation that is so typical of hypertrophic cardiomyopathy (105–109). Paulus et al. (105), however, have shown that nitroprusside also increases relaxation rate in this disorder; these authors conclude that the increase in relaxation rate produced by calcium channel blockers was at least partly caused by a systolic unloading effect. Indeed, if we are to understand completely the effects of any drug on LV relaxation, all loading and other determinants of relaxation rate must be considered; this is true for mitral and pulmonary venous flow velocities (110).

Late Systolic (Relaxation) Loads

Late systolic loads can be defined as those applied during the latter portion of ejection and during the isovolumic relaxation period (i.e., approximately within 50 to 100 msec of aortic valve closure). These late systolic (relaxation) loads are therefore present before the onset of filling; they should be distinguished from loads applied during the filling period (such loads are termed "lengthening" or "filling" loads.

Experiments in Isolated Cardiac Muscle. Late in the cardiac cycle, during deactivation when cytosolic calcium is below the threshold necessary for activating new crossbridges, a load increment results in the premature onset of myocardial relaxation; because existing crossbridges cannot support the additional load, the muscle yields, and relaxation is premature and more rapid. In studying this phenomenon, Brutsaert (25) referred to observations made in isolated cat papillary muscle experiments in which he and his associates observed that isotonic contractions with progressively lighter afterloads manifest progressively shorter overall duration; this appeared to be due to an abbreviation of the relaxation phase rather than to changes in the earlier phases of the contractile cycle. He further noted that an abrupt load increment applied during the relaxation phase resulted in a premature onset of relaxation. This "load-dependent relaxation" was demonstrated in mammalian ventricular muscle, but it did not appear to be a property of muscle from frog ventricles (in which there is only a sparse sarcoplasmic reticulum), nor was it present in mammalian myocardium that was hypoxic or treated with caffeine. Brutsaert used this and other evidence to propose that calcium-sequestering membranes are required for the process that gives rise to the load dependence of relaxation (25). (See Chap. 2.)

In a series of elegant experiments, Brutsaert and associates clearly demonstrated that a load increment that is established early in the contraction phase (i.e., an early systolic or contraction load), produces a result that is opposite to those that occur when changes in load are imposed during relaxation (i.e., late systolic or relaxation load). Thus, in distinct contrast to the effects of an early systolic load, a late systolic load caused a premature onset of relaxation and a reduction in the duration of mechanical activity (25). Moreover, an increase in the magnitude of a late load (with timing held constant) caused more rapid relaxation. Brutsaert has emphasized the existence of a transition zone where the effects of a contraction load change into those of a relaxation load. Furthermore, differences in the timing of the transition

zone would modulate the effects of a given load increment; the transition zone occurs later and is eventually abolished (mammalian myocardium becomes load independent) when the myocardium is made hypoxic or ischemic (25). The existence and recognition of the transition zone is important in studies of load-dependent relaxation in the intact heart (81, 83) (discussed below). Differences between studies in the intact left ventricle may be explained partly by differences in the precise timing of this transition zone. Thus, the magnitude of timing of the load and the inherent load dependency of the myocardium interact to control relaxation.

Experiments in the Intact Dog Heart. Similar to the isolated muscle studies, myocardial relaxation in the intact left ventricle also manifests a load dependency (80–89, 111); an example is shown in Figure 13–6. Load-dependent relaxation was studied in the intact heart by using a computer-controlled servo-pump that was programmed to produce a rapid volume increment (i.e., a quick stretch) at a specified time in the cardiac cycle (81). In anesthetized dogs, the servo-pump was attached to the LV apex and the effects of volume increments on LV relaxation were studied; each volume increment or quick stretch was produced by infusing 6 mL into the LV within a 15 msec interval. Volume increments were given throughout systole so that the effects of an early (contraction) load could be contrasted with the effects of a late (relaxation) load. To prevent reflex or other feedback mechanisms from influencing the results, each intervention was performed in a single beat and the intervention beats were separated by 20 stabilization beats. In both ejecting and nonejecting beats, a quick stretch in the latter half of systole caused a premature onset of relaxation and a more rapid rate of pressure decline. The duration of the relaxation phase was typically reduced by 10 to 15%.

Similar results were obtained when an intra-aortic balloon was inflated during late systole, immediately before aortic valve closure (Fig. 13–7). This intervention produced a small, late systolic pressure increment and resulted in an earlier, more rapid relaxation (83). Thus, the onset of pressure decline was premature, the initial rate of

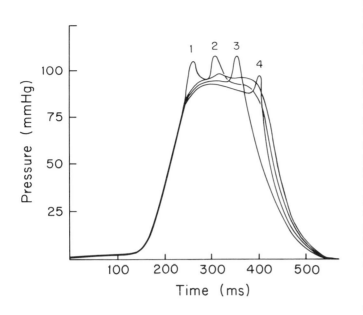

Fig. 13–6. The effect of quick volume infusions on the time course of LV pressure. Six milliliters of blood were injected into the ventricle within a 15-msec interval. An early systolic volume infusion, given in the first quarter of the ejection period, caused an increase in the duration of systole; the control beat (not shown for clarity) was nearly coincident with the second intervention beat. By contrast, late systolic volume infusions, during the third and fourth quarters of ejection, caused an abbreviation of systole. Such an effect on late systolic loads can be attributed to the load dependency of mammalian heart muscle. Note that the transition from a prolongation effect to an abbreviation effect occurred in the second quarter of the ejection period. Reproduced with permission of the American Heart Association from Ariel Y, et al.: Load-dependent relaxation with late systolic volume steps: Servo-pump studies in the intact canine heart. Circulation 75:1287, 1987.

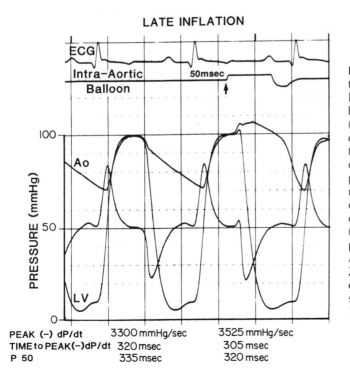

Fig. 13–7. The effect of a late systolic (relaxation) load on left ventricular pressure transients. An intra-aortic balloon, inflated at the end of ejection (50 msec before aortic notch) produced a small increment in late systolic pressure. This "relaxation" load caused LV pressure decline to occur prematurely (decreased time to peak negative dP/dt) and more rapidly (decreased peak negative dP/dt); a decrease in the duration of contraction (decreased P50) was also seen. Reproduced with permission of the American Physiological Society from Zile MR, Gaasch WH: Load-dependent left ventricular relaxation in conscious dogs. Am J Physiol 261:H691, 1991.

LV pressure decline was accelerated, and the duration of contraction was abbreviated. However, when animals were treated with caffeine (a drug known to depress calcium uptake by the sarcoplasmic reticulum), late systolic balloon inflations did not alter the onset or rate of LV pressure decline. These data indicate that myocardial relaxation is load-dependent in the intact conscious dog and that load-dependent relaxation is attenuated by interventions which depress sarcoplasmic reticulum function.

These data are consonant with the studies of Noble et al. (84), and Zatko et al. (85) but appear to be at odds with the studies of Gillebert et al. (82). The apparent differences in the latter study can probably be explained on the basis of the exact timing of the systolic load increments. It appears that the late systolic balloon inflations were performed during the middle one third of ejection (82), just before the transition zone and not during the last one third of ejection. The importance of this transition zone has been discussed by Brutsaert (25), Ariel (81), and Zile (83). It is likely that changes in the timing of the mechanical transition zone reflect changes in calcium uptake (reuptake) by the sarcoplasmic reticulum. Thus, the presence of load-dependent relaxation and its timing can be used as a mechanical probe to assess the functional state of the sarcoplasmic reticulum.

Clinical Implications. Short-term hemodynamic or other interventions may be associated with abrupt changes in late systolic loading conditions. For example, during the Valsalva maneuver there are marked changes in central aortic pulse morphology. These changes in aortic pressure are caused partly by changes in reflected pressure waves (112) which are likely to influence LV relaxation through an effect on early and late load alterations. Depending on which load predominates, LV relaxation may be slower or more rapid. Abrupt changes in coronary blood flow immediately after aortic valve closure might also provide a "late" stretch to myocardial fibers adjacent to the coronary arteries. In this manner, a coronary erectile effect might promote relaxation (113). It is possible, therefore, that the increased LV

filling rate seen after successful coronary angioplasty could, at least partly, be caused by the mechanical effects of increased coronary filling (51). These and other late systolic events deserve further study if we are to understand completely the hemodynamic determinants of relaxation in the intact heart.

The load dependency of LV relaxation makes it likely that even small pressure or volume increments could influence the end-systolic indices of LV contractility (i.e., indices based on end-systolic pressure-volume relations). Note that the pressure coordinates in late systole are markedly different (despite unchanged contractile state) in the four beats shown in Figure 13–6. Reflected pressure waves or other late systolic events might contribute to similar changes in patients with or without heart disease. Thus, under some circumstances, the load dependency of relaxation might limit the use of late systolic pressure-volume data in the assessment of LV contractility.

Lengthening Load

Relaxation throughout the period of rapid ventricular filling (auxotonic relaxation) is especially difficult to assess because of the interdependencies of pressure and volume, neither of which is constant during this interval. Because the changes in ventricular volume greatly exceed the changes in pressure during this period, most attempts to characterize auxotonic relaxation utilize measurements of the rate of change of LV volume or dimension. As will be seen, factors independent of the intrinsic process of myocardial relaxation may influence filling rate. In particular, the transmitral pressure gradient (the difference between left atrial and LV pressure) is the primary determinant of transmitral flow and LV filling rate (30). In addition, however, alterations in myocardial load or wall stress after the onset of filling may also influence LV filling or myocardial lengthening rate (25). In this section, we present data from isolated cardiac muscle and intact dog experiments which indicate that myocardial lengthening and LV filling rates are determined in part by the lengthening load present during the rapid filling period. In contrast to preload, which represents end-diastolic load, lengthening loads refer to the myocardial loads that are present during early diastole, during the rapid filling period.

Experiments in the Intact Dog Heart. It is well established that a primary determinant of LV early diastolic filling rate is the left atrial to left ventricular (transmitral) pressure gradient. Ishida et al. made precise measurements of transmitral pressure and flow and isovolumic relaxation rate during acute alterations in LV preload and afterload (75). Their experiments demonstrated that an increased transmitral pressure gradient resulted in an increased peak filling rate (more rapid auxotonic relaxation) despite an increase in the time constant of isovolumic relaxation (indicating slower isovolumic relaxation). These investigators also studied the effects of a graded increase in afterload (angiotensin infusion) on filling and found that filling rate could

be maintained in the presence of slowed isovolumic relaxation if the transmitral pressure gradient was sufficiently high. Their observations provide a basis for the interpretation of altered filling rates in clinical and experimental studies of LV relaxation and filling.

An example of the effect of changes in venous return on transmitral flow velocity is shown in Figure 13–8 (114). Reduced venous return (produced by inferior vena cava occlusion) causes a decline in the early diastolic transmitral pressure gradient and a fall in the early diastolic velocity. By contrast, an increase in venous return (produced by intravenous saline infusion) causes an increase in the early diastolic pressure gradient and an increase in the early diastolic velocity. As was discussed previously, these changes in transmitral velocity are associated with changes in LV preload, but they are caused by changes in

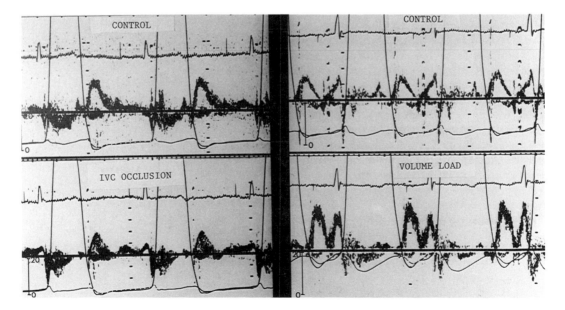

Fig. 13–8. The effect of alterations in venous return on transmitral flow velocities. Inferior vena caval (IVC) occlusion decreased the venous return and the transmitral pressure gradient fell (panels on the left). These changes caused a decrease in early and late transmitral flow velocities. By contrast, a volume load increased venous return, and the transmitral pressure gradient and the transmitral flow velocities increased. Adapted with permission from Nishimura RA, et al.: Significance of Doppler indices of diastolic filling of the left ventricle: Comparison with invasive hemodynamics in a canine model. Am Heart J 118:1248, 1989.

in the left atrial pressure and the trans-mitral pressure gradient.

A number of other studies in conscious dogs (64, 74, 76, 78, 115) and in man (61, 77) have also demonstrated the direct relation between the transmitral pressure gradient and peak early diastolic filling rate. In addition, these studies indicate that, whether the transmitral pressure gradient changes because of a primary change in left atrial pressure or a primary change in LV diastolic pressure, it is the transmitral pressure gradient itself and not its individual determinants that primarily influence peak early diastolic filling rate. By contrast, the rate of acceleration and deceleration of the early filling wave are affected by the absolute left atrial pressure during filling and the rate of isovolumic relaxation (64, 74, 78). In addition to the transmitral pressure gradient, changes in the intraventricular pressure gradients during early filling also affect peak early diastolic filling (79). However, none of these studies directly address the issue of myocardial loading conditions and the effect of load or wall stress on myocardial fiber lengthening during the diastolic filling period. These loads, which were studied in isolated cardiac muscles, are discussed below.

Experiments in Isolated Cardiac Muscle. Isotonic relaxation (lengthening) in the isolated muscle preparation is analogous to auxotonic relaxation (filling) in the intact left ventricle. Because the magnitude and timing of isolated muscle loads can be precisely controlled, the independent effect of load on isotonic lengthening can be assessed in a quantitative fashion. It should be recognized, however, that lengthening load in the isolated muscle is not strictly equivalent to the transmitral pressure gradient or to left atrial pressure. Thus, lengthening load experiments provide insight into the effects of variations in LV wall stress during rapid filling (the load which promotes fiber lengthening). As will be seen, a load increment during this period promotes relaxation and re-extension in such a way that LV filling promotes filling.

The effects of changes in lengthening load were studied in isolated physiologically sequenced rat papillary muscles; an

example is shown in Figure 13–9. After isometric tension declined for a predetermined period of time, a series of force clamps (with progressively larger loads) was applied, thus raising the level of load on the muscle during isotonic lengthening. In this manner, the magnitude of the lengthening load could be changed while holding the time of application constant. Alternately, the timing of the load could be varied with a load of constant magnitude. As shown in Figure 13–9, a progressive increase in lengthening load (from one to four) resulted in a progressive increase in muscle lengthening rate (59). The average data from all six muscles are shown in the right panel of Figure 13–9. This figure also indicates that the rate of isotonic lengthening is greater as the load is applied later in the course of tension decline; this is presumably due to greater muscle deactivation near the end of isometric tension decline. These results, if extrapolated to the intact heart, indicate that loading the LV during the rapid filling period should enhance filling by promoting myocardial lengthening; in effect, chamber filling promotes myocardial lengthening.

Clinical Implications. In the two clinical studies which measured LV pressure and left atrial pressure, multivariate analysis demonstrated that changes in peak filling rate correlated strongly with changes in the transmitral pressure gradient (61, 73). This association between peak filling rate and transmitral pressure gradient has at least three important clinical implications. It explains the mechanism by which: (1) mitral regurgitation increases peak filling rate, (2) changes in load produced by changes in lower body negative suction and nitroglycerin alter peak filling rate, and (3) normal peak filling rate may be present in a disease process normally associated with abnormal relaxation.

Mitral regurgitation, like volume loading, causes an increase in left atrial pressure and an increase in the transmitral pressure gradient during early diastole; this can result in an unusually rapid filling rates (116). In addition to the hemodynamic effect of a high transmitral pressure gradient, explosive filling of the LV chamber produces a sharp increment in wall stress that can promote myocardial length-

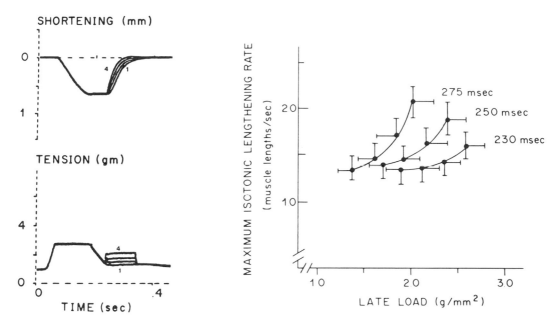

Fig. 13–9. Effects of a change in the magnitude of lengthening load on isotonic lengthening rate. As shown in the panel on the left, isometric tension was allowed to fall for a predetermined period of time and a series of force clamps at progressively larger loads (labeled 1 to 4) were applied, thus raising the level of load on the muscle during isotonic lengthening. As the magnitude of the load increased (from 1 to 4), isotonic lengthening rate increased. In the panel on the right, average data from six muscles indicate the effects of load clamps applied at three points in time during isometric relaxation (230, 250, and 275 milliseconds after muscle stimulation). At any given time, isotonic lengthening rate increased as the magnitude of load increased. The slope of the curvilinear relationship between isotonic lengthening rate and the magnitude of late load became steeper at later times during isometric relaxation. Thus, isotonic lengthening rate (at a common load) increased as the load was applied later in the course of tension decline. Reproduced with permission of the American Heart Association from Zile MR, et al.: Mechanical determinants of the rate of isotonic lengthening in rat left ventricular myocardium. Circ Res 60:815, 1987.

ening (an abrupt load increment during relaxation promotes lengthening); this second mechanism underlying rapid filling in mitral regurgitation is based on the Laplace relation between pressure, radius and wall thickness (25). Finally, restoring forces that are prominent when end systolic volume is small (especially in acute mitral regurgitation) might decrease early LV pressure, increase transmitral pressure gradient, and also contribute to the rapid early diastolic filling rates (102, 117, 118). In mitral regurgitation, therefore, several mechanical factors acting in concert can contribute to an increase in LV early diastolic filling rate.

When an increase in the transmitral pressure gradient is superimposed on pathologic conditions that ordinarily cause impaired relaxation, the filling rate may be more rapid than otherwise expected. (See Chap. 12.) For example, in dilated cardiomyopathy, relaxation rates are generally reduced; however, when mitral regurgitation is superimposed, filling rates can be relatively rapid (119). Likewise, patients with hypertrophic cardiomyopathy may exhibit unexpectedly normal or rapid filling rates in the presence of mitral regurgitation (120–122). Thus, the presence of mitral regurgitation or the presence of other factors that alter the transmitral pressure gradient might act as dynamic determinants of peak early diastolic filling rate in patients with a variety of cardiac disorders. In this regard, Murakami et al. (123) made the important observation that patients with aortic stenosis and normal LV wall stress at the instant of mitral valve opening had a normal filling rate, whereas patients with aortic stenosis and an increased LV wall stress at the instant of mitral valve opening had increased early filling rates. After corrective surgery, this latter group had a decline in wall stress at the instant of mitral valve opening, a decline in left atrial pressure, a decline in the transmitral pressure gradient, and a reduction in filling rate. These data highlight the clinical importance of the transmitral pressure gradient and early diastolic lengthening loads as determinants of LV filling rate.

As is discussed elsewhere in this text, the mitral flow velocity curves obtained by Doppler echocardiography provide a noninvasive method for examining this period of early, rapid filling. When the highest velocity at the tip of the mitral valve leaflets as they open during diastole is determined, a relative measure of the transmitral pressure gradient is obtained. The initial peak velocity, termed "E-velocity," provides information concerning early, rapid filing. (See Chaps. 12, 23, and 24.)

A low E-velocity can be seen in two clinical situations. The first is when there is abnormally slow or prolonged ventricular relaxation, caused by abnormal inactivation, nonuniformity, or a high early systolic load. The second instance, in which a low E-velocity may be present, is when there is a low left atrial pressure despite normal relaxation. These two instances can be distinguished by interrogation of the pulmonary veins. The retrograde velocity at atrial contraction into the pulmonary veins provides adjunctive information to the mitral flow velocities. At this instant, the mitral valve is widely opened, forming a conduit between the pulmonary veins, left atrium, and left ventricle. Atrial contraction causes retrograde flow into the pulmonary vein and antegrade flow across the mitral valve, the degree of which depends on the pressure and compliance in the left ventricle and the left atrium. In the first instance (i.e., abnormal relaxation), a relatively high velocity is seen at atrial contraction in both the mitral and pulmonary vein velocities. This is because of the impaired filling that has occurred in early diastole with a relatively large atrial volume before atrial contraction, with a resultant high atrial stroke volume. In the second instance (i.e., iso-

lated low left atrial pressure) there is a low velocity at atrial contraction back into the pulmonary vein because of the low atrial preload.

A normal E-velocity may also be seen in patients with LV hypertrophy (and abnormal relaxation) who are beginning to demonstrate hemodynamic deterioration. In this "pseudonormalization" pattern, increased left atrial pressures cause a higher driving pressure across the mitral valve, resulting in an increase of the E-velocity to normal levels. Differentiation of the normal pattern from "pseudonormalization" may be made by assessing the pulmonary vein velocities. A high initial E-velocity can be seen in any circumstance when the left atrial pressure and mitral valve opening pressure are high. Thus, it is seen in patients with decompensated, dilated cardiomyopathy or ischemic cardiomyopathy in the end stage. It is also seen when severe mitral regurgitation is present.

The LV pressure and echo Doppler data shown in Figure 13–10 illustrate several of the loading issues discussed above; this example also illustrates the potential for misinterpretation of the Doppler data if hemodynamic and loading changes are not considered. The administration of Verapamil to a patient with restrictive cardiomyopathy caused an increase in the isovolumic relaxation time constant, an increase in the early diastolic transmitral velocity, and an increase in end diastolic pressure. Thus, transmitral flow velocity increased in the presence of a slower isovolumic relaxation and higher LV diastolic pressures; the velocity "pseudnormalized" in the presence of impaired diastolic function, presumably because of an increase in left atrial pressure.

CONCLUSIONS

Left ventricular diastolic function can be assessed using invasive and noninvasive techniques to measure the rate of LV isovolumic pressure decline (isovolumic relaxation rate) and the rate of ventricular filling (auxotonic relaxation rate). Changes in these indices of diastolic function can reflect alterations in the intrinsic relaxation process; however, they may also reflect changes in hemodynamic loading condi-

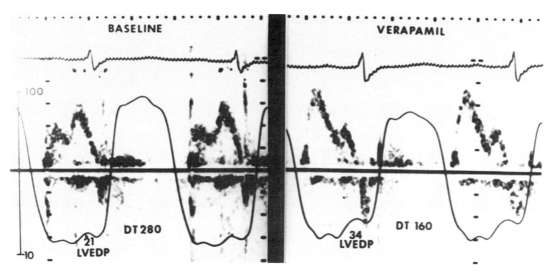

Fig. 13–10. The effect of verapamil on LV diastolic pressure and LV inflow (Doppler) velocities. DT = deceleration time, LVEDP = left ventricular end diastolic pressure. The administration of verapamil was associated with a slower isovolumic pressure decline and an increased end diastolic pressure. However, the Doppler signal indicates that the deceleration time decreased and the early diastolic velocity increased. See text for details.

tions. For example, an increase in early systolic pressure (a contraction load) can cause a reduction in the isovolumic relaxation rate, whereas a decrease in systolic pressure generally results in a more rapid isovolumic relaxation rate. These effects are modulated by the timing and magnitude of the load alteration and by the functional state of the myocardium and its relaxing system. Auxotonic relaxation (filling) rate is primarily affected by changes in the transmitral pressure gradient. Thus, left atrial pressure and left ventricular lengthening loads and pressures affect the filling rate. Abnormally slow filling rates may be "pseudonormalized" if left atrial pressure increases. An accurate assessment of LV diastolic function depends on a clear understanding of the hemodynamic and other factors that influence the indices of relaxation. Under most circumstances, hemodynamic loading conditions have a relatively small effect on isovolumic relaxation and a substantial effect on auxotonic relaxation.

REFERENCES

1. Dougherty AH, et al.: Congestive heart failure with normal systolic function. Am J Cardiol 54:778, 1984.
2. Soufer R, et al.: Intact systolic left ventricular function in clinical congestive heart failure. Am J Cardiol 55:1032, 1985.
3. Given BD, Lee TH, Stone PH, Dzau VJ: Nifedipine in severely hypertensive patients with congestive heart failure and preserved ventricular systolic function. Arch Intern Med 145:281, 1985.
4. Topol EJ, Traill TA, Fortuin NJ: Hypertensive hypertrophic cardiomyopathy of the elderly. N Engl J Med 312:277, 1985.
5. Wong WF, Gold S, Fukuyama O, Blanchette PL: Diastolic dysfunction in elderly patients with congestive heart failure. Am J Cardiol 63:1526, 1989.
6. Aguirre FV, et al.: Usefulness of Doppler echocardiography in the diagnosis of congestive heart failure. Am J Cardiol 63:1098, 1989.
7. Setaro JF, et al.: Usefulness of verapamil for congestive heart failure associated with abnormal left ventricular diastolic filling and normal left ventricular systolic performance. Am J Cardiol 66:981, 1990.
8. Doria E, Agostoni P, Loaldi A, Fiorentini C: Doppler assessment of left ventricular filling pattern in silent ischemia in patients with Prinzmetal's angina. Am J Cardiol 66:1055, 1990.
9. Kitzman DW, et al.: Exercise intolerance in patients with heart failure and preserved left ventricular systolic function: Failure of the Frank-Starling mechanism. J Am Coll Cardiol 17:1065, 1991.

10. Stauffer JC, Gaasch WH: Recognition and treatment of left ventricular diastolic dysfunction. Prog Cardiovasc Dis 32:319, 1990.

11. Heywood JT: Calcium antagonists and left ventricular function. Am J Cardiol 68: 52C, 1991.

12. Bolognesi R, et al.: Effects of acute K-strophantidin administration on left ventricular relaxation and filling phase in coronary artery disease. Am J Cardiol 69:169, 1992.

13. Dineen E, Brent BN: Aortic valve stenosis: Comparison of patients with to those without chronic congestive heart failure. Am J Cardiol 57:419, 1986.

14. Nicod P, et al.: Influence of prognosis and morbidity of left ventricular ejection fraction with and without signs of left ventricular failure after acute myocardial infarction. Am J Cardiol 61:1165, 1988.

15. Pearson AC, Gudipati CV, Labovitz AJ: Systolic and diastolic flow abnormalities in elderly patients with hypertensive hypertrophic cardiomyopathy. J Am Coll Cardiol 12:989, 1988.

16. Aronow WS, Ahn C, Kronzon I: Prognosis of congestive heart failure in elderly patients with normal versus abnormal left ventricular systolic function associated with coronary artery disease. Am J Cardiol 66:1257, 1990.

17. Cohn JN, Johnson G: Heart failure with normal ejection fraction. The V-heft study. Circulation 81(suppl III):III-48, 1990.

18. Clements IP, Brown ML, Zinsmeister AR, Gibbons RJ: Influence of left ventricular diastolic filling on symptoms and survival in patients with decreased left ventricular systolic function. Am J Cardiol 67:1245, 1991.

19. Judge KW, et al.: Congestive heart failure symptoms in patients with preserved left ventricular systolic function: Analysis of the CASS registry. J Am Coll Cardiol 18: 377, 1991.

20. Packer M: Abnormalities of diastolic function as a potential cause of exercise intolerance in chronic heart failure. Circulation 81(suppl III):III-78, 1990.

21. Lorell BH, Grossman W: Cardiac hypertrophy: The consequence for diastole. J Am Coll Cardiol 9:1189, 1987.

22. Grossman W: Diastolic dysfunction in congestive heart failure. N Engl J Med 325:1557, 1991.

23. Nishimura RA, Housmans PR, Hatle LK, Tajak AJ: Assessment of diastolic function of the heart: Background and current applications of Doppler echocardiography. Part 1: Physiologic and pathophysiologic features. Mayo Clin Proc 64:71, 1989.

24. Nishimura RA, Abel MD, Hatle LK, Tajik AJ: Assessment of diastolic function of the heart: Background and current applications of Doppler echocardiography. Part II: Clinical studies. Mayo Clin Proc 64: 181, 1989.

25. Brutsaert DL, Sys SU: Relaxation and diastole of the heart. Physiol Rev 69:1228, 1989.

26. Gilbert JC, Glantz SA: Determinants of left ventricular filing and of the diastolic pressure-volume relation. Circ Res 64: 827, 1989.

27. Little WC, Downes TR: Clinical evaluation of left ventricular diastolic performance. Prog Cardiovasc Dis 32:273, 1990.

28. Zile MR, Gaasch WH: Mechanical loads and the isovolumic and filling indices of left ventricular relaxation. Prog Cardiovasc Dis 32:333, 1990.

29. Mirsky I, Pasipoularides A: Clinical assessment of diastolic function. Prog Cardiovasc Dis 32:291, 1990.

30. Yellin EL, Nikolic S, Frater RWM: Left ventricular filling dynamics and diastolic function. Prog Cardiovasc Dis 32:247, 1990.

31. Lew WYW: Evaluation of left ventricular diastolic function. Circulation 79:1393, 1989.

32. Myreng Y, Smiseth OA: Assessment of left ventricular relaxation by Doppler echocardiography. Circulation 81:260, 1990.

33. Weiss JL, Frederiksen JW, Weisfeldt ML: Hemodynamic determinants of the time course of fall in canine left ventricular pressure. J Clin Invest 58:751, 1976.

34. Frais MA, et al.: The dependence of the time constant of left ventricular isovolumic relaxation (τ) on pericardial pressure. Circulation 81:1071, 1990.

35. Craig WE, Murgo JP, Pasipoularides A: Evaluation of the time course of LV isovolumic relaxation in humans. *In* Diastolic Relaxation of the Heart. Edited by W Grossman and BH Lorell. Boston, Martinus Nijhoff, 1985.

36. Katayama K, et al.: Studies on the mono-exponential nature of the LV pressure fall during isovolumic relaxation period in the diseased heart. Jpn Circ J 51:1273, 1987.

37. Yellin EL, et al.: Left ventricular relaxation in the filling and nonfilling intact canine heart. Am J Physiol 250:H620, 1986.

38. Feigenbaum H: Echocardiography. 4th Ed. Philadelphia, Lea & Febiger, 1986.

39. Rokey R, et al.: Determination of parameters of left ventricular diastolic filling with pulsed Doppler echocardiography: Comparison with cineangiography. Circulation 71:543, 1985.

40. Spirito P, Maron BJ, Bonow RO: Noninvasive assessment of left ventricular diastolic function: Comparative analysis of Doppler echocardiographic and radionuclide angiographic techniques. J Am Coll Cardiol 7:518, 1986.

41. Brutsaert DL: Nonuniformity: A physiologic modulator of contraction and relaxation of the normal heart. J Am Coll Cardiol 9:341, 1987.

42. Zile MR, Blaustein AS, Shimizu G, Gaasch WH: Right ventricular pacing reduces the rate of left ventricular relaxation and filling. J Am Coll Cardiol 10:702, 1987.

43. Blaustein AS, Gaasch WH: Myocardial relaxation. VI. Effects of β-adrenergic tone and asynchrony on LV relaxation rate. Am J Physiol 244:H417, 1983.

44. Heyndricks GR, Paulus WJ: Effect of asynchrony on left ventricular relaxation. Circulation 81(suppl):III-41, 1990.

45. Pearson AC, et al.: Doppler echocardiographic assessment of the effect of varying atrioventricular delay and pacemaker mode on left ventricular filling. Am Heart J 115:611, 1988.

46. Bedotto JB, et al.: Alterations in left ventricular relaxation during atrioventricular pacing in humans. J Am Coll Cardiol 15:658, 1990.

47. Bonow RO: Left ventricular filling in ischemic and hypertrophied heart disease. *In* Diastolic Relaxation of the Heart. Edited by W Grossman and BH Lorell. Boston, Martinus Nijhoff, 1985.

48. Bonow RO, et al.: Effects of verapamil and propranolol on left ventricular systolic function and diastolic fulling in patients with coronary artery disease: radionuclide angiographic studies at rest and during exercise. Circulation 65:1337, 1981.

49. Carroll JD, et al.: Left ventricular systolic and diastolic function in coronary artery disease: effects of revascularization on exercise-induced ischemia. Circulation 72:119, 1985.

50. Mizuno K, et al.: Improved regional and global diastolic performance in patients with coronary artery disease after percutaneous transluminal coronary angioplasty. Am Heart J 115:302, 1988.

51. Bonow RO, et al.: Asynchronous left ventricular regional function and impaired global filling in patients with coronary artery disease after coronary angioplasty. Circulation 71:297, 1985.

52. Bonow RO: Regional left ventricular nonuniformity. Effects on left ventricular diastolic function in ischemic heart disease, hypertrophic cardiomyopathy, and the normal heart. Circulation 81(suppl III):III-54, 1990.

53. Bareiss P, et al.: Alterations in left ventricular diastolic function in chronic ischemic heart failure. Assessment by radionuclide angiography. Circulation 81(suppl III):III-71, 1990.

54. Perrone-Filardi P, Bacharach SL, Dilsizian V, Bonow RO: Impaired left ventricular filling and regional diastolic asynchrony at rest in coronary artery disease and relation to exercise-induced myocardial ischemia. Am J Cardiol 67:356, 1991.

55. Hayashida W, et al.: Left ventricular regional relaxation and its nonuniformtiy in hypertrophic nonobstructive cardiomyopathy. Circulation 84:1496, 1991.

56. Vanoverschelde JJ, et al.: Asynchronous (segmental early) relaxation impairs left ventricular filling in patients with coronary artery disease and normal systolic function. J Am Coll Cardiol 18:1251, 1991.

57. Bonow RO, et al.: Effects of aging on asynchronous left ventricular regional function and global ventricular filling in normal human subjects. J Am Coll Cardiol 11:50, 1988.

58. Ludbrook PA, Byrne JD, Tiefenbrunn AJ: Association of asynchronous protodiastolic segmental wall motion with impaired left ventricular relaxation. Circulation 64:1201, 1981.

59. Zile MR, et al.: Mechanical determinants of the rate of isotonic lengthening in rat left ventricular myocardium. Circ Res 60:815, 1987.

60. Gaasch WH, Carroll JD, Blaustein AS, Bing OHL: Myocardial relaxation: Effects of preload on the time course of isovolumetric relaxation. Circulation 73:1037, 1986.

61. Choong CY, et al.: Preload dependence of Doppler-derived indexes of left ventricular diastolic function in humans. J Am Coll Cardiol 10:800, 1987.

62. Zile MR, et al.: The effect of preload on relaxation rate in normal, hypoxic and hypertrophic myocardium. Am J Physiol 258:H191, 1989.

63. Varma SK, Owen RM, Smucker ML, Feldman MD: Is τ a preload-independent measure of isovolumetric relaxation? Circulation 80:1757, 1989.

64. Choong CY, et al.: Combined influence of ventricular loading and relaxation on the

transmitral flow velocity profile in dogs measured by Doppler echocardiography. Circulation 78:672, 1988.

65. Hori M, et al.: Delayed end ejection increases isovolumic ventricular relaxation rate in isolated perfused canine hearts. Circ Res 68:300, 1991.

66. Fitzovich DE, Hamaguchi M, Tull WB, Young DB: Chronic hypokalemia and the left ventricular responses to epinephrine and preload. J Am Coll Cardiol 18:1105, 1991.

67. Downes TR, et al.: Effect of alteration in loading conditions on both normal and abnormal patterns of left ventricular filling in healthy individuals. Am J Cardiol 65: 377, 1990.

68. Hayashi K, et al.: Evaluation of preload reserve during isometric exercise testing in patients wtih old myocardial infarction: Doppler echocardiographic study. J Am Coll Cardiol 17:106, 1991.

69. Plotnick GD, et al.: Effect of postural changes, nitroglycerin and verapamil on diastolic ventricular function as determined by radionuclide angiography in normal subjects. J Am Coll Cardiol 12: 121, 1988.

70. Triulzi MO, Castini D, Ornaghi M, Vitolo E: Effects of preload reduction on mitral flow velocity pattern in normal subjects. Am J Cardiol 66:995, 1990.

71. Takahashi T, et al.: Doppler echocardiographic-determined changes in left ventricular diastolic filling flow velocity during the lower body positive and negative pressure method. Am J Cardiol 65:237, 1990.

72. Stoddard MF, et al.: Influence of alteration in preload on the pattern of left ventricular diastolic filling as assessed by Doppler echocardiography in humans. Circulation 79:1226, 1989.

73. Lavine SJ, Campbell CA, Held C, Johnson V: Effect of nitroglycerin-induced reduction of left ventricular filling pressure on diastolic filling in acute dilated heart failure. J Am Coll Cardiol 14:233, 1989.

74. Courtois M, et al.: The transmitral pressure-flow velocity relation. Effect of abrupt preload reduction. Circulation 78: 1459, 1988.

75. Ishida Y, et al.: Left ventricular filling dynamics: influence of left ventricular relaxation and left atrial pressure. Circulation 74:187, 1986.

76. Cheng C, Igarashi Y, Little WC: Mechanism of augmented rate of left ventricular filling during exercise. Circ Res 70:9, 1992.

77. Masuyama T, Goar FG, Alderman EL, Popp RL: Effects of nitroprusside on transmitral flow velocity patterns in extreme heart failure: a combined hemodynamic and doppler echocardiographic study of varying loading conditions. J Am Coll Cardiol 16:1175, 1990.

78. Thomas JD, Choong CY, Flaschskampf FA, Weyman AE: Analysis of the early transmitral doppler velocity curve: Effect of primary physiologic changes and compensatory preload adjustment. J Am Coll Cardiol 16:644, 1990.

79. Courtois M, Kovacs S, Ludbrook PA: Transmitral pressure-flow velocity relation. Importance of regional pressure gradients in the left ventricle during diastole. Circulation 78:661, 1988.

80. Kil PJM, Schiereck P: Influence of the velocity of changes in end-diastolic volume on the Starling Mechanism of isolated left ventricles. Eur J Physiol 396:243, 1983.

81. Ariel Y, Gaasch WH, Bogen DK, McMahon TA: Load-dependent relaxation with late systolic volume steps: servo-pump studies in the intact canine heart. Circulation 75:1287, 1987.

82. Gillebert TC, Lew WYW: Influence of systolic pressure profile on rate of left ventricular pressure fall. Am J Physiol 261: H805, 1991.

83. Zile MR, Gaasch WH: Load-dependent left ventricular relaxation in conscious dogs. Am J Physiol 261:H691, 1991.

84. Noble MIM: The contribution of blood momentum to left ventricular ejection in the dog. Circ Res 32:663, 1968.

85. Zatko FJ, Martin P, Bahler PC: Time course of systolic loading is an important determinant of ventricular relaxation. Am J Physiol 21:H461, 1987.

86. Bahler RC, Martin P: Effects of loading conditions and inotropic state on rapid filling phase of left ventricle. Am J Physiol 248:H523, 1985.

87. Karliner JS, et al.: Pharmacologic and hemodynamic influences on the rate of isovolumic left ventricular relaxation in the normal conscious dog. J Clin Invest 60: 511, 1977.

88. Hori M, et al.: Ejection timing as a major determinant of left ventricular relaxation rate in isolated perfused canine heart. Circ Res 55:31, 1984.

89. Hori M, et al.: Loading sequence is a major determinant of afterload-dependent relaxation in intact canine heart. Am J Physiol 249:H747, 1985.

90. Gaasch WH, Blaustein AS, Adam D: Myocardial relaxation IV: mechanical deter-

minants of the time course of left ventricular pressure decline during isovolumic relaxation. Eur Heart J 1:111, 1980.

91. Gaasch WH, et al.: Myocardial relaxation II. Hemodynamic determinants of the rate of left ventricular isovolumic pressure decline. Am J Physiol 239:H1, 1980.

92. Zile MR, Blaustein AS, Gaasch WH: The effects of acute alterations in left ventricular afterload and B-adrenergic tone on indices of early diastolic filling rate. Circ Res 65:406, 1989.

93. Caillet D, Crozatier B: Role of myocardial restoring forces in the determination of early diastolic peak velocity of fibre lengthening in the conscious dog. Cardiovasc Res 16:107, 1982.

94. Starling MR, Montgomery DG, Mancini J, Walsh RA: Load independence of the rate of isovolumic relaxation in man. Circulation 76:1274, 1987.

95. Colan SD, Borow KM, Neumann A: Effects of loading conditions and contractile state (methoxamine and dobutamine) on left ventricular early diastolic function in normal subjects. Am J Cardiol 55:790, 1985.

96. Shimizu G, Zile MR, Blaustein AS, Gaasch WH: Left ventricular chamber filling and midwall fiber lengthening in patients with left ventricular hypertrophy: Overestimation of fiber velocities by conventional midwall measurements. Circulation 71:266, 1985.

97. Fouad FM, Slominski JM, Tarazi RC: Left ventricular diastolic function in hypertension: Relation to left ventricular mass and systolic function. J Am Coll Cardiol 3:1500, 1984.

98. Fouad FM, Slominski MJ, Tarazi RC, Gallagher JH: Alterations in left ventricular filling with beta-adrenergic blockade. Am J Cardiol 51:161, 1983.

99. Inouye I, et al.: Failure of antihypertensive therapy with diuretic, beta-blocking and calcium channel-blocking drugs to consistently reverse left ventricular diastolic filling abnormalities. Am J Cardiol 53:1583, 1984.

100. Inouye I, et al.: Abnormal left ventricular filling: An early finding in mild to moderate systemic hypertension. Am J Cardiol 53:120, 1984.

101. Smith VE, et al.: Rapid ventricular filling in left ventricular hypertrophy. II. Pathologic hypertrophy. J Am Coll Cardiol 5:869, 1985.

102. Papademetriou V, Gottdiener JS, Fletcher RD, Freis ED: Echocardiographic assessment by computer-assisted analysis of diastolic left ventricular function and hypertrophy in borderline or mild systemic hypertension. Am J Cardiol 56:546, 1985.

103. Phillips RA, et al.: Determinants of abnormal left ventricular filling in early hypertension. J Am Coll Cardiol 14:979, 1989.

104. White WB, Schulman P, Dey HM, Katz AM: Effects of age and 24-hour ambulatory blood pressure on rapid left ventricular filling. Am J Cardiol 63:1343, 1989.

105. Paulus WJ, et al.: Comparison of the effects of nitroprusside and nifedipine on diastolic properties in patients with hypertrophic cardiomyopathy: altered left ventricular loading or improved muscle inactivation? J Am Coll Cardiol 2:879, 1983.

106. Hanrath P, et al.: Effect of verapamil on left ventricular filling in hypertrophic cardiomyopathy. Am J Cardiol 45:1258, 1980.

107. Bonow RO, et al.: Effects of verapamil on left ventricular systolic function and diastolic filling in patients with hypertrophic cardiomyopathy. Circulation 64:787, 1981.

108. TenCate FJ, Serruys PW, Mey S, Roelandt J: Effects of short-term administration of verapamil on left ventricular relaxation and filling dynamics measured by a combined hemodynamic-ultrasonic technique in patients with hypertrophic cardiomyopathy. Circulation 68:1274, 1983.

109. Betocchi S, et al.: Effects of sublingual nifedipine on hemodynamics of systolic and diastolic function in patients with hypertrophic cardiomyopathy. Circulation 72:1001, 1985.

110. Nishimura RA, Abel MD, Hatie LK, Tajik AJ: Relation of pulmonary vein to mitral flow velocities by transesophageal Doppler echocardiography. Circulation 81:1488, 1990.

111. Goethals MA, et al.: Influence of abrupt pressure increments on left ventricular relaxation. Am J Cardiol 45:392, 1980 (abstr).

112. Murgo JP, Westerhof N, Giolma JP, Altobelli SA: Aortic input impedance in normal man: Relationship to pressure wave forms. Circulation 62:105, 1980.

113. Vogel WM, et al.: Acute alterations in left ventricular diastolic chamber stiffness. Role in the erectile effect of coronary artery pressure and flow in normal and damaged hearts. Circ Res 51:465, 1982.

114. Nishimura RA, et al.: Significance of Doppler indices of diastolic filling of the left ventricle: Comparison with invasive hemodynamics in a canine model. Am Heart J 118:1248, 1989.

115. Cheng C, et al.: Effect of loading conditions, contractile state, and heart rate on early diastolic left ventricular filling in conscious dogs. Circ Res 66:814, 1990.
116. Osbakken MD, Bove AA: Use of left ventricular filling and ejection patterns in assessing severity of chronic mitral and aortic regurgitation. Am J Cardiol 53:1054, 1984.
117. Tyberg JV, et al.: Mechanics of ventricular diastole. Cardiovasc Res 4:423, 1970.
118. Sonneblick EH: The structural basis and importance of restoring forces and elastic recoil for the filling of the heart. Eur Heart J 1:107, 1980.
119. Takenaka K, et al.: Pulsed doppler echocardiographic study of left ventricular filling in dilated cardiomyopathy. Am J Cardiol 58:143, 1986.
120. Bryg RJ, Pearson AC, Williams GA, Labovitz AJ: Left ventricular systolic and diastolic flow abnormalities determined by Doppler echocardiography in obstructive hypertrophic cardiomyopathy. Am J Cardiol 59:925, 1987.
121. Maron BJ, et al.: Noninvasive assessment of left ventricular diastolic function by pulsed Doppler echocardiography in patients with hypertrophic cardiomyopathy. J Am Coll Cardiol 10:733, 1987.
122. Shaikh MA, Lavine SJ: Effect of mitral regurgitation on diastolic filling with left ventricular hypertrophy. Am J Cardiol 61:590, 1988.
123. Murakami T, et al.: Diastolic filling dynamics in patients with aortic stenosis. Circulation 73:1162, 1986.

Part Three

*CLINICAL DISORDERS OF
LEFT VENTRICULAR
DIASTOLIC FUNCTION*

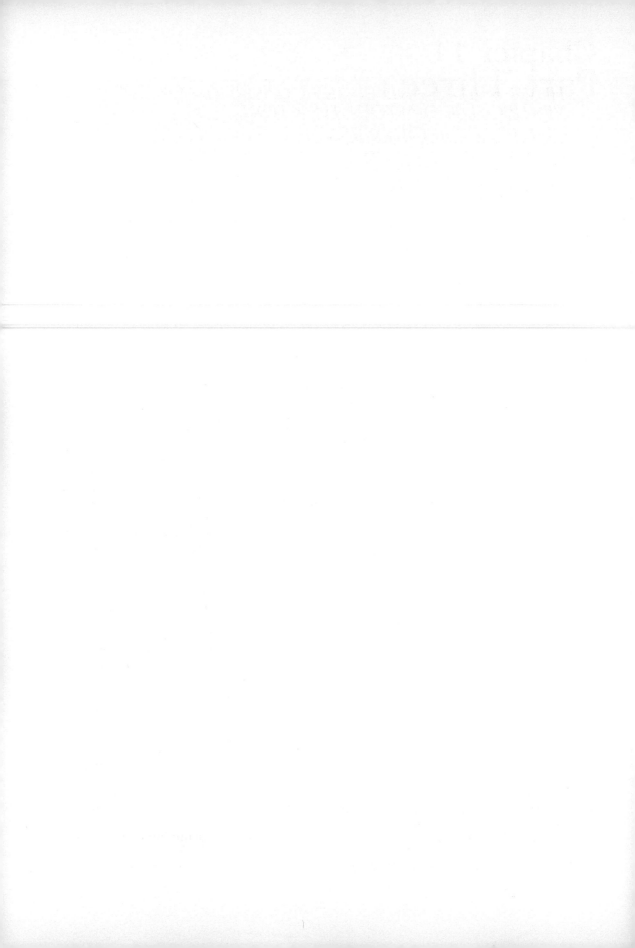

Chapter 14

HEART FAILURE AND CLINICAL DISORDERS OF LEFT VENTRICULAR DIASTOLIC FUNCTION

William H. Gaasch, Alvin S. Blaustein, and Martin M. LeWinter

Congestive heart failure (CHF) is a clinical syndrome that is caused by a wide variety of disorders that include valvular, myocardial, pericardial, and other diseases. The pathophysiology of CHF has been examined and re-examined by clinicians and physiologists. A major focus of their deliberations has been the important distinction between left ventricular (LV) systolic and diastolic dysfunction (Figure 14–1). Simply stated, *systolic dysfunction* can be considered a defect in the ability of the myofibrils to shorten against a load; thus, the left ventricle loses its ability to eject blood into the high-pressure aorta. The term *diastolic dysfunction* implies that the ventricle cannot accept blood at low pressures; ventricular filling is slow, delayed, or incomplete unless atrial pressure increases. Consequently, pulmonary and/or systemic venous congestion develops. Thus, the signs and symptoms of pulmonary and/or systemic venous congestion are not primarily the result of systolic dysfunction; rather, they are related to alterations in the diastolic properties of the LV chamber.

Diastolic dysfunction of the left ventricle is caused by conditions that alter the LV diastolic pressure-volume relation which in turn leads to an impaired capacity to fill; it may exist with little or no systolic dysfunction. In its mildest form, diastolic dysfunction may be manifest only as a slow or delayed pattern of relaxation and filling, and normal or only minor elevations of LV diastolic pressure. Thus, in patients with LV hypertrophy or coronary disease, an alteration in diastolic filling can be an early indicator of disease. In other patients, LV filling may be sufficiently impaired to cause a substantial rise in left atrial pressure. Under these circumstances, diastolic dys-

function may be manifest as overt congestive heart failure (even in the presence of normal or near-normal systolic function). In some ways, therefore, diastolic dysfunction is similar to mitral stenosis, in which impaired filling is caused by a reduced effective mitral orifice area. Thus, the concept of diastolic dysfunction as a mechanism underlying heart failure is analogous to the notion of "backward failure."

In this chapter, some of the factors influencing the LV diastolic pressure-volume relations and the mechanisms underlying diastolic dysfunction are summarized. Our purpose is to provide a general overview of pathophysiology, diagnosis, and therapy in patients with CHF that is caused by LV diastolic dysfunction; in such patients, the cause is most commonly hypertrophy and/ or ischemic heart disease. For a more complete and detailed review of these topics including definitions of terms, the reader is referred to the subsequent chapters and other sources (1–16).

PATHOPHYSIOLOGY

An appreciation of the determinants of the curvilinear diastolic pressure-volume relation is essential to an understanding of diastolic dysfunction. It has long been recognized that the pressure within a ventricular chamber is directly related to the distending volume, and that during steady-state conditions, the LV diastolic pressure is determined by the chamber volume, the wall volume (i.e., myocardial mass), and the physical properties (i.e., stiffness) of the wall. (See Chap. 9.) This relationship is, however, not fixed. During abrupt hemodynamic or other acute interventions, the influence of several other factors can be superimposed on the passive diastolic pres-

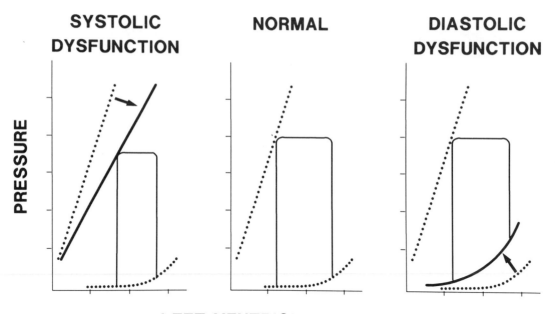

Fig. 14–1. Diagram of left ventricle (LV) pressure-volume loops in systolic and diastolic dysfunction. In systolic dysfunction (left panel), the end-systolic pressure-volume line is displaced downward and to the right; there is diminished capacity to eject blood into a high pressure aorta. In diastolic dysfunction (right panel), the diastolic pressure-volume relation is displaced upward and to the left; there is diminished capacity to fill at low diastolic pressures. Adapted with permission from Katz AM: Influence of altered inotropy and lusitropy on ventricular pressure-volume loops. J Am Coll Cardiol 11:438, 1988.

sure-volume curve (Fig. 14–2). These include variations in the rate and extent of myocardial relaxation, changes in LV elastic recoil, the effect of the pericardium and right ventricle, the coronary erectile effect, and others. As will be seen, these factors alone or in concert may contribute to acute or chronic alterations in the diastolic pressure-volume curve and/or the isovolumic and filling indexes of LV relaxation.

Acute Changes in Diastolic Properties

The mechanisms underlying most acute alterations in the diastolic pressure-volume curve are generally classified as to whether they occur as a consequence of (1) a preload or strain depending change in compliance, (2) a shift to a different pressure volume curve, or (3) a combination of the two. All three can result in elevated left atrial pressure, pulmonary venous hypertension and the signs or symptoms of congestive failure. Several illustrative examples will be used to describe such changes.

Pericardial Effect

The pericardium surrounds and constrains the entire heart; at volumes above its reserve volume it is less distensible than the ventricle, and therefore limits the distensibility of the heart and increases the mechanical interaction among the four chambers (17–20). In the absence of a pericardium, the static diastolic pressure-volume relation is affected by the geometry and elasticity of the left ventricle (i.e., chamber volume, wall mass, and the composition of the wall); it is not substantially affected by pharmacologic or other hemodynamic interventions (21). This is analogous to the resting length-tension relation of isolated cardiac muscle that, for example, is not affected by positive inotropic interventions (22). When the pericardium is intact, however, volume loading and even pharmacologic interventions may contribute to significant changes in the diastolic pressure-volume relation. (See Chap. 6.)

An example of the pericardial effect is shown in Figure 14–3. In this dog experi-

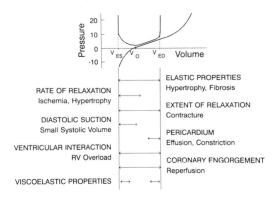

Fig. 14–2. Diastolic pressure-volume relations (upper panel) and the factors that influence these relations. The effects of each of these factors depend on the time at which they occur; some factors exert their influence in early diastole (i.e., relaxation rate and diastolic suction), others in late diastole (i.e., pericardium), and still others throughout diastole (i.e., elastic properties). V_{ES} = end-systolic volume; V_O = equilibrium volume, V_{ED} = end-diastolic volume; RV = right ventricle. Adapted with permission from Gilbert JC, Glantz SA: Determinants of left ventricular filling and of the diastolic pressure-volume relationship. Circ Res 64:827, 1989.

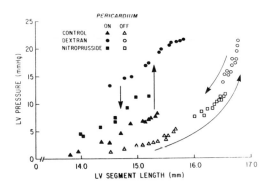

Fig. 14–3. Left ventricular (LV) diastolic pressure segment length relations before and after removal of the pericardium. In the absence of the pericardium (open symbols), dextran infusion followed by the administration of nitroprusside produced shifts that appear to be on the same pressure-length line; this represents a preload-dependent change in chamber compliance. When the pericardium is intact, similar interventions cause vertical ("parallel") displacements of the pressure-length curves. Adapted with permission from Ross J Jr: Acute displacement of the diastolic pressure-volume curve of the left ventricle: Role of the pericardium and the right ventricle. Circulation 59: 32, 1979.

ment, an acute increase in preload (dextran infusion) was followed by unloading (nitroprusside); these interventions were performed before and after pericardiectomy (5). With an open pericardium, the diastolic pressure-length coordinates are not displaced from the baseline curvilinear pressure-length relation during the loading and unloading interventions; they merely move up or down the same curve and there is no change in the chamber stiffness constant. This has been called a preload-dependent change in compliance (1). By contrast, when the pericardium is intact, a similar volume infusion results in a substantial upward displacement of the pressure-length relation. As the cardiac chamber volumes increase (and total intrapericardial volume increases), the pericardium becomes relatively inelastic and resists further stretch. Consequently, pressure in the pericardial space rises, and the pericardium exerts a restraining force that limits a further increase in LV volume. As a result, the LV diastolic pressures are much higher and the chamber is less distensible. The administration of nitroprusside, a venous and arteriolar dilator, causes a decrease in the total intrapericardial volume so that pericardial pressures fall and the pressure-length coordinates approach those obtained during the control state. This example highlights the importance of the pericardium as a determinant of LV diastolic pressure, and it illustrates the mechanism underlying a preload dependent change in compliance.

Similar shifts in the diastolic pressure-volume relation have been observed in normal and diseased human hearts. These effects are especially important in assessing and interpreting changes in right and left heart filling pressures during the treatment of patients with heart failure (23). The influence of the pericardium and ventricular interaction on LV diastolic function is discussed in more detail in Chapter 6.

Angina Pectoris

Myocardial ischemia can depress cellular concentrations of high-energy phosphates. As a result, the energy requiring process of calcium uptake (reuptake) by the sarco-

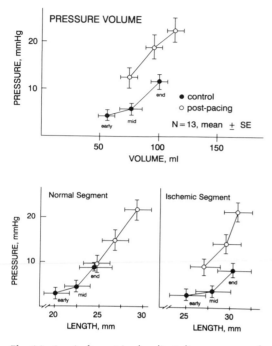

Fig. 14–4. Left ventricular diastolic pressure-volume and pressure-length relations before and after pacing-induced angina pectoris. In the postpacing state (upper panel), the diastolic pressure-volume coordinates are shifted upwards. The pressure-length analysis (lower panels) reveals that the nonischemic myocardial fibers lengthen along the same pressure-length curve; by contrast, there is a marked stiffening of the myocardium in the ischemic segment. Adapted with permission from Sasayama et al.: Changes in diastolic properties of the regional myocardium during pacing-induced ischemia in human subjects. J Am Coll Cardiol 5: 599, 1985.

plasmic reticulum is impaired and relaxation may be slowed, incomplete, and inhomogeneous; the ischemic myocardium becomes less distensible and the LV filling pressure rises (24). As is shown in Figure 14–4, there may be little or no length change in the ischemic region, but the nonischemic fibers lengthen, move to a steeper portion of their diastolic pressure-length curve, and utilize the Frank-Starling mechanism to maintain stroke volume (25). Thus, the increase in LV filling pressure that occurs during angina pectoris is caused at least partly by regionally impaired myocardial relaxation and a complex interaction between the ischemic and nonischemic segments. Such changes in the

diastolic properties of the human LV have been observed during vasospastic (Prinzmetal's) angina, during pacing or exercise-induced angina, and even with transient coronary occlusion during catheter-balloon angioplasty (12, 14). The pathophysiology of myocardial ischemia and hypoxia is discussed further in Chapters 15, 16, and 17.

Chronic Changes in Diastolic Properties

Myocardial Hypertrophy

Aortic stenosis, systemic arterial hypertension, and hypertrophic cardiomyopathy may lead to elevated LV diastolic pressures through several passive and active mechanisms. Increased myocardial mass (i.e., a low volume-mass ratio) can influence chamber stiffness through geometric mechanisms alone (4); a ventricle with a thick wall may exhibit reduced distensibility even though the intrinsic myocardial stiffness is normal. Myocardial fibrosis, commonly present in the subendocardium of hypertrophied hearts, may also affect chamber distensibility through its influence on intrinsic myocardial stiffness (26). Thus, fibrosis increases the stiffness of each unit of the LV wall and contributes to a reduced chamber distensibility that is independent of wall thickness. In addition to these altered "passive" properties, the active process of myocardial relaxation may be abnormal in hypertrophic hearts (27). In such hearts, the ability of the sarcoplasmic reticulum to sequester calcium is depressed. As a result, cytosolic calcium transients are prolonged, myocardial relaxation is slow, the decay of tension in the wall is delayed and prolonged, and LV diastolic pressure is higher than that predicted from passive pressure-volume relations (28–30). Thus, a combination of passive and active abnormalities leads to a reduced LV chamber distensibility in LV hypertrophy. (See Chaps. 20 and 21.)

Chronic Coronary Heart Disease

Myocardial fibrosis that develops after infarction can influence the diastolic properties of the left ventricle directly or may have secondary effects on noninfarcted regions. Infarcted ventricles, especially aneu-

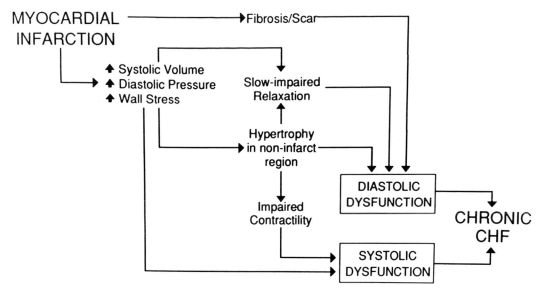

Fig. 14–5. Diagram of the mechanisms leading to left ventricular remodeling and chronic congestive heart failure (CHF) after myocardial infarction. The earliest events (increased systolic volume, increased diastolic pressure, increased wall stress) occur as a result of decreased myocardial fiber shortening in the ischemic region. Later, scar formation, myocardial hypertrophy, and their interactions contribute to systolic and diastolic dysfunction, and to the development of CHF. Adapted with permission from Grossman W: Diastolic dysfunction and congestive heart failure. Circulation 81 (Suppl III):1, 1990.

rysmal segments, exhibit fixed irreversible alterations in stiffness (31, 32). The noninfarcted segment may be stretched to a steeper (stiffer) portion of the diastolic pressure-length relation. In addition, compensatory hypertrophy of the noninfarcted segment develops, and as a result, passive stiffness and active relaxation of these regions may be abnormal. If there is residual ischemia in the noninfarcted region, the relaxation process may be further impaired. Thus, LV diastolic dysfunction after myocardial infarction can be related to fixed alterations in the passive elastic properties of some segments and dynamic changes in the active relaxation of others. Such functional and temporal nonuniformities have a significant effect on diastolic function (33, 34). (See Chap. 18.)

These and other mechanisms that underlie the development of CHF in chronic coronary heart disease are illustrated in Figure 14–5. (See Chap. 18.) Some forms of medical therapy may reduce cardiac dilation, interrupt the development of fibrosis or hypertrophy, and hopefully prevent the development of systolic and diastolic dysfunction, and CHF (see section on treatment, in subsequent text).

DIAGNOSIS OF DIASTOLIC DYSFUNCTION

A complete evaluation of the diastolic properties of the LV requires calculation of LV chamber and myocardial stiffness constants as well as operating (end-diastolic) pressure, stress, and stiffness; the more dynamic processes of relaxation and filling require measurement of LV pressure and volume transients during diastole (12, 14, 16). These parameters and indices of diastolic function can provide meaningful information only if the hemodynamic, metabolic, and neuropharmacologic factors that influence them are considered. For example, left atrial pressure is a major determinant of the LV filling rate; for this reason, changes in filling rate are difficult to interpret unless simultaneous measurements of left atrial pressure are made. This is a formidable task requiring extensive invasive techniques. Because such detailed measurements are complex and time-consuming, a complete assessment of cardiac diastolic is rarely made in clinical practice. However, a practical clinical assessment of diastole is possible using less invasive methods and tests that are tailored to answer specific questions (35, 36).

One third of the patients with signs and symptoms of CHF are found to have a normal LV systolic ejection fraction and the diagnosis of diastolic dysfunction is therefore considered (37, 38). Although many, if not most, of these patients have at least a component of diastolic dysfunction, the diagnosis requires exclusion of pulmonary disorders and mitral valve disease as well as other rare mechanical causes of impaired LV filling (e.g., cor triatriatum, pulmonary venous occlusive disease). In clinical practice, the presence of pulmonary rales and radiographic evidence of pulmonary venous hypertension in combination with a normal ejection fraction is usually sufficient to suggest the diagnosis of diastolic dysfunction. In this fashion, Dougherty et al. (37) and Soufer et al. (38) used echocardiographic and radionuclide techniques to assess the frequency of diastolic dysfunction in patients with signs and symptoms of congestive heart failure. Dougherty et al. reported that 36% of their patients had normal or near-normal LV systolic function (ejection fraction >45%); Soufer et al. reported that 42% of their patients had intact systolic function of the LV. Both groups emphasized a high incidence of diastolic dysfunction in such patients. These and other reports certainly indicate that dyspnea and other signs or symptoms of congestive heart failure do not necessarily indicate systolic dysfunction; therefore, signs and symptoms alone should not be used as a indication for therapy directed toward systolic dysfunction.

Having made the diagnosis of diastolic dysfunction, it may be possible to dissect out the cause by considering the LV end-diastolic volume to mass or radius to thickness ratio (9); this is especially true if fixed abnormalities of the passive pressure-volume relation are present. Thus, if the LV wall thickness is increased, myocardial hypertrophy or infiltrative disease are likely culprits; if not, stiff (fibrotic) myocardium or intermittent myocardial ischemia is probably responsible for the diastolic dysfunction. Although hypertrophy and ischemia are certainly the most common causes of LV diastolic dysfunction, restrictive myocardial disease such as cardiac amyloidosis or constrictive pericarditis should always be considered in the differential diagnosis. Pulmonary hypertension in patients with pulmonary vascular or parenchymal disease, or even intracardiac shunts may cause enlargement of the right heart which can contribute to increased LV chamber stiffness. On occasion, cardiac catheterization, myocardial biopsy, or special radiographic studies (i.e., computed tomography) or magnetic resonance imaging may be necessary to clarify the diagnosis of myocardial or pericardial disease. Atrial pacing (24, 25) or exercise (39, 40) studies may also provide diagnostic information by uncovering an ischemic response or by revealing a limitation of filling or other abnormality not present in the basal state.

Some patients who are admitted to an intensive care unit with acute pulmonary edema exhibit a normal ejection fraction (37, 38, 41–44); many of these cases may be related to hypertension and/or LV ischemia, whereas others may be caused by excessive volume administration. When the diagnosis is in doubt, it can be appropriate to proceed with a "diagnostic-therapeutic trial." (See Chap. 26.) However, recognizing the difficulties of evaluating LV function at the bedside, it may be necessary to confirm the presence of elevated pulmonary venous pressure with right heart catheterization.

TREATMENT OF HEART FAILURE AND DIASTOLIC DYSFUNCTION

Traditional therapy directed at improving systolic performance has little place in the management of heart failure caused by diastolic dysfunction. In the absence of systolic dysfunction, there is no reason to administer digitalis. Arterial vasodilators may produce hypotension. In patients with hypertrophic or coronary heart disease, diastolic dysfunction is best managed with beta adrenergic receptor blocking agents, calcium channel blocking drugs, or both. These drugs slow the heart rate and improve the balance between myocardial oxygen supply and demand; indirectly, they may increase myocardial relaxation rate.

With these principles in mind, a general approach to therapy will be outlined and treatment of specific types of diastolic dysfunction will be presented.

A major goal of therapy should be to reduce pulmonary and systemic venous pressures, and in this way lessen the congestive symptoms. Although diuretics and salt restriction are effective, special care must be taken to avoid excessive volume depletion and reduced cardiac output. Because of the steep (stiff) diastolic pressure-volume curve, large changes in diastolic pressure can be achieved with only modest changes in volume. Venodilators, such as nitrates, are useful preloading-reducing agents, because they are short-acting and rapidly reversible, and have the additional benefits of providing an anti-ischemic effect. As with diuretics, however, special care must be taken to avoid excessive preload reduction.

Maintenance of a properly timed atrial contraction is important in preserving LV filling in late diastole. Thus, efforts should be made to preserve normal sinus rhythm and to employ cardioversion when atrial arrhythmia is present; when a pacemaker is indicated for heart block, an atrioventricular sequential pacemaker should be utilized.

Prevention of LV hypertrophy by treating the hypertensive patient is an obvious and desirable goal. Once hypertrophy is established, medications that reduce both arterial pressure and LV mass should probably be used; methyldopa, beta-blocking agents, calcium channel blockers, and converting enzyme inhibitors can accomplish these aims, whereas hydralazine and minoxidil do not. Whether regression of LV hypertrophy is associated with improved diastolic function is a question that remains largely unanswered. (See Chap. 21.) Hypertensive patients who present with CHF caused by diastolic dysfunction may respond well to sublingual nifedipine (43).

Beneficial slowing of the heart rate can be achieved with the use of beta-adrenergic receptor blockers or calcium channel blockers, or other bradycardiac drugs. Although a reduction in heart rate may promote LV filling by increasing the filling time, a most important effect of these drugs is energy sparing (improved balance of myocardial oxygen supply and demand)

and, in some instances, a decrease in myocardial ischemia. By slowing the rate and prolonging diastole, the myocardium is provided with additional time to re-establish a normal cytosolic calcium level which can contribute to a reduction in diastolic tone and lower LV diastolic pressures. Thus, a slower rate may be associated with an improvement in the "function-frequency relationship." The optimal heart rate in patients with diastolic dysfunction is not known, but theoretical arguments support the notion that a relative bradycardia is desirable in hypertrophic hearts (45).

If a beta-adrenergic receptor blocking agent is administered, consideration should be given to the use of one with intrinsic sympathomimetic activity, especially in patients with CHF. Such agents can blunt an exercise induced increase in heart rate (and MVO_2) with little potential to depress myocardial relaxation at rest. This approach, although theoretically appealing, has not been tested in controlled studies.

The acute increase in LV diastolic pressure that occurs during myocardial ischemia can be treated with nitroglycerin, but a more rational goal is to prevent myocardial ischemia and its diastolic consequences, both acute (impaired LV relaxation) and chronic (fibrosis and scar). Thus, beta-adrenergic receptor blockers, calcium channel blocking drugs, and nitroglycerin are essential ingredients in the treatment and prevention of diastolic dysfunction.

Positive inotropic drugs and arterial dilators appear to have no place in the management of congestive heart failure that is caused by diastolic dysfunction. Indeed, some vasodilators may cause substantial hypotension (42), especially if used with diuretics and nitrates; therefore, this class of drugs should generally be avoided in the treatment of patients with diastolic dysfunction. However, in acute hypertension, especially when heart failure is present, the systolic unloading effects of nifedipine, ACE inhibitors, and nitrates may provide a dramatic hemodynamic and symptomatic improvement.

Coronary Heart Disease

Diastolic dysfunction has been reported to be present in as many as 90% of patients with coronary artery disease (46). Its manifestations vary in different subsets of patients, and the treatment depends partly on symptomatic status and clinical subset (14, 47). These include (1) generally asymptomatic patients with or without a history of myocardial infarction, (2) patients with myocardial ischemia and/or acutely evolving myocardial infarction, and (3) patients with chronic coronary heart disease, especially those with old anterior myocardial infarction; many, if not most, patients in this category eventually develop CHF.

Experimental data indicate that it may be possible to improve or protect diastolic function with pharmacologic agents (48, 49), but it has not yet been possible to confirm a direct relaxing effect of such agents in patients with coronary disease. Most attempts to treat abnormal LV relaxation and filling involve interventions that improve the balance between myocardial oxygen supply and demand (39, 50–56). Thus, the clinical benefits of beta-blocking drugs and calcium channel blocking drugs are likely to be caused by their negative inotropic and chronotropic effects and their coronary vasodilator properties. Like medical treatments, coronary angioplasty and bypass surgery can be effective in the treatment of diastolic dysfunction (51, 52, 54–56).

During or immediately after myocardial infarction, elevated LV diastolic pressures and pulmonary (or systemic) venous congestion are treated with diuretics, nitrates, and converting enzyme inhibitors. Over the long term, ventricular unloading with nitrates or converting enzyme inhibitors may prevent or attenuate the deleterious LV remodeling (Figure 14–5) that eventually contributes to chronic heart failure (57–60). If chronic failure develops, emphasis is placed on cautious administration of diuretics, nitrates, and converting enzyme inhibitors. Coexisting systolic dysfunction may require additional treatment with vasodilators and positive inotropic agents.

Hypertensive Heart Disease

It is well established that abnormal LV relaxation is common in patients with hypertensive heart disease, even before substantial hypertrophy is present (61–67). However, it is not at all clear that antihypertensive therapy has a beneficial effect on the diastolic properties of the LV. Some data indicate that short-term therapy with hydrochlorothiazide, beta-blockers, or diltiazem does not result in improved LV relaxation (68). Others have found that the administration of beta blockers improves filling in hypertensive patients, but only if they experience a decrease in arterial pressure (69, 70). These and other published studies indicate that beta-blocking agents can cause a decrease in the rate of relaxation and filling unless ischemia is lessened and/or arterial pressure is reduced. Calcium channel blockers may likewise contribute to improved diastolic function in hypertrophy secondary to hypertension (71–73). Unfortunately, it is not known whether or not a regression of hypertensive LV hypertrophy is associated with improved diastolic filling, symptoms, or prognosis. At present, therefore, it would seem prudent to emphasize the treatment of arterial hypertension and approach the problem of LV diastolic dysfunction only if symptoms dictate the need for treatment. Thus the patient with hypertensive heart disease and CHF caused by diastolic dysfunction is managed according to the general scheme presented previously; sublingual nifedipine or other vasodilator therapy can provide short-term benefits in hypertensive patients with CHF (43).

Some elderly patients with marked LV hypertrophy and only modest hypertension experience disabling symptoms of dyspnea and angina. Systolic function of the left ventricle is normal in many of these patients, and there is little rationale for the use of digitalis or arterial dilators. Indeed, some vasodilators may cause hypotension, dizziness, and even syncope in some patients. By contrast, therapy directed at diastolic dysfunction can result in substantial symptomatic improvement (30, 42).

Hypertrophic Cardiomyopathy

In a sense, hypertrophic cardiomyopathy is the prototype for diastolic dysfunction. (See Chap. 22.) LV systolic function is generally supernormal, yet dyspnea and pulmonary congestion are significant clinical features. Thus, diastolic dysfunction of the LV represents a most important functional abnormality in hypertrophic cardiomyopathy (74). These hearts exhibit slow isovolumic relaxation (75, 76), impaired diastolic filling (61, 77–79), and a prominent atrial contribution to LV diastolic pressure and volume (80). Despite a large body of clinical investigation, it remains difficult to sort out the individual factors that affect diastolic events. For this reason, it is difficult to explain the mechanisms underlying various therapeutic interventions. The therapies discussed in this section primarily apply to patients with angina and/or dyspnea.

Beta-adrenergic receptor blocking agents have been used in the symptomatic treatment of patients with hypertrophic cardiomyopathy for over 20 years. Early studies indicated that these agents had a beneficial effect on diastolic function (81–83); it was assumed that improved relaxation and filling were responsible for symptomatic improvement. Currently, some authorities have little enthusiasm for the use of beta blockers in symptomatic patients with nonobstructive hypertrophic cardiomyopathy (74). Indeed, recent studies have not confirmed a direct relaxing effect of beta blockers (84, 85). Beta-adrenergic receptor blocking agents do, however, have potential benefits in this disorder; they blunt the exercise-induced tachycardia and attenuate or prevent myocardial ischemia.

Calcium channel blocking agents have also been used extensively in the treatment of hypertrophic cardiomyopathy. The beneficial effects of these agents may result from regression of the inappropriate hypertrophy (86), a direct effect on abnormal calcium transport (87, 88), a reduction in regional asynchrony (89), a nonspecific effect on relaxation (90), or a beneficial effect on the balance between myocardial oxygen supply and demand. It is well established that the administration of calcium channel blockers can improve or even normalize the indexes of relaxation in hypertrophic cardiomyopathy (85, 87, 91–94). Based on the observation that the relaxing effects of these drugs cannot be explained simply on the basis of altered loading conditions (88), it is reasonable to suggest that abnormal

myocardial calcium metabolism is corrected by calcium channel blockers and that this results in a beneficial effect on diastolic relaxation and filling. Alternatively, these agents may prevent the recurrent effects of myocardial ischemia and thereby cause improved myocardial relaxation and filling. Although these arguments remain speculative, there is a correlation between ventricular asynchrony (89), filling rate, symptoms, and exercise performance. The fact that verapamil can cause an increased filling rate and symptomatic relief without a change in diastolic pressure or volume indicates that symptoms are more closely related to filling dynamics than to passive chamber compliance.

There is probably no reason to select one calcium channel blocker over another if the primary goal is to treat diastolic dysfunction in nonobstructive hypertrophic cardiomyopathy. However, if latent or established outflow obstruction is present, agents that cause a major reduction in systemic vascular resistance should be avoided; under these circumstances, verapamil is probably the preferred calcium channel blocker. (See Chap. 28.) The dosage is adjusted on the basis of symptomatic relief, not on a predetermined dosage schedule.

Left ventricular myotomy or myectomy may provide dramatic relief of symptoms in selected patients with hypertrophic cardiomyopathy. Indeed, some authorities believe that the symptomatic relief that follows successful surgery exceeds that achieved with drug therapy (74). The decline in diastolic pressure that follows these surgical procedures is probably caused by alterations in LV geometry. It is likely that the reduction in diastolic pressure that commonly occurs after mitral valve replacement is also largely the result of an effect on chamber geometry (95, 96); this procedure is infrequently used in hypertrophic cardiomyopathy, and its major goal is to correct mitral regurgitation.

Dual-chamber cardiac pacing may be an alternative to cardiac surgery in patients with hypertrophic obstructive cardiomyopathy who are symptomatic despite medical therapy. Such treatment results in hemodynamic and symptomatic improvement

(97), but the effects of dual-chamber pacing on diastolic function are not known.

The development of overt CHF is especially ominous in these patients. It is initially treated by preload reduction and attempts to maintain arterial pressure; atrial arrhythmias should be converted to sinus rhythm; beta-blockers and calcium channel blockers are used in selected patients.

PROGNOSIS

In broad populations of patients with CHF, mortality is inversely related to the systolic ejection fraction. This notion might therefore lead to the conclusion that survival in patients with CHF caused by diastolic dysfunction is excellent (because systolic function tends to be preserved in such patients). In the Veterans Administration Cooperative Study (V-HeFT), patients with chronic CHF and a normal or near-normal (>45%) ejection fraction exhibited an annual mortality that was less than half of that seen in those with a low ejection fraction (98). Thus, prognosis in those with preserved systolic function (annual mortality = 8%) was better than in those with depressed systolic function (annual mortality = 19%). In another study, patients with CHF and preserved systolic function exhibited 46% mortality over a 7-year period of follow up (99); the mortality was highest in the first and lower thereafter, but these data are not substantially different from the V-HeFT results. Data from the Coronary Artery Surgery Study (CASS) registry indicate a 6-year mortality of 18% in patients with CHF and a preserved ejection fraction (>45%); over the same 6-year period, mortality in a control group without CHF was 9% (100). In this study, the presence of coronary disease had a substantial effect on the survival of patients with CHF and a normal ejection fraction. A 32% mortality was seen 6 years in patients with three-vessel coronary disease; by contrast, the 6-year mortality in patients without coronary disease was only 8%. These CASS data are consonant with the experience of others who have described a similar low mortality in patients with diastolic dysfunction and normal coronary arteriography (101). In this latter study, diastolic dysfunction was defined as elevated filling pressures and a normal LV ejection fraction; morbidity and recurrent hospitalizations for CHF remained a major problem, but the annual mortality was only 1 to 2%.

It appears, therefore, that LV diastolic dysfunction, even in patients with CHF, is associated with a lower mortality than is seen in patients with CHF due to systolic dysfunction; this is especially true if coronary artery disease is not a contributing factor. In patients with coronary disease (and CHF with a normal ejection fraction) the mortality is higher, but the prognosis does not approach the grave outlook of patients with coronary disease and CHF in association with a low ejection fraction.

The pathophysiology, treatment, and prognosis of heart failure caused by diastolic dysfunction differ from those seen in systolic dysfunction. If improved therapies for diastolic dysfunction are to be developed, it will be important to refine our understanding of the natural history of patients with this form of heart disease.

REFERENCES

1. Gaasch WH, Levine HJ, Quinones MA, Alexander JK: Left ventricular compliance: Mechanisms and clinical implications. Am J Cardiol, 38:645, 1976.
2. Grossman W, McLaurin LP: Diastolic properties of the left ventricle. Ann Intern Med, 84:316–326, 1976.
3. Mirsky I: Assessment of passive elastic stiffness of cardiac muscle: Mathematical concepts, physiologic and clinical considerations, directions of future research. Prog Cardiovasc Dis 18:277, 1976.
4. Glantz SA, Parmley WW: Factors which affect the diastolic pressure-volume curve. Circ Res 42:171, 1978.
5. Ross J Jr: Acute displacement of the diastolic pressure-volume curve of the left ventricle: Role of the pericardium and the right ventricle. Circulation 59:32, 1979.
6. Brutsaert DL, Housmans PR, Goethals MA: Dual control of relaxation: Its role in the ventricular function in the mammalian heart. Circ Res 47:637, 1980.
7. Mirsky I: Assessment of diastolic function: Suggested methods and future considerations. Circulation 69:836, 1984.
8. Brutsaert DL, Rademakers FE, Sys SU, et al.: Ventricular relaxation. *In* The Ventricle. Edited by Levine HJ, Gaasch WH. Boston, Martinus Nijhoff, 1985, pp. 123–132.

9. Gaasch WH, Apstein CS, Levine HJ: Diastolic properties of the left ventricle. *In* The Ventricle. Edited by Levine HJ, Gaasch WH. Boston, Martinus Nijhoff, 1985, pp. 143–170.

10. Tyberg JV: Ventricular interaction and the pericardium. *In* The Ventricle. Edited by Levine HJ, Gaasch WH. Boston, Martinus Nijhoff, 1985, pp. 171–184.

11. Katz AM: Influence of altered inotropy and lusitropy on ventricular pressure-volume loops. J Am Coll Cardiol 11:438, 1988.

12. Gilbert JC, Glantz SA: Determinants of left ventricular filling and of the diastolic pressure-volume relationship. Circ Res 64:827, 1989.

13. Brutsaert DL, Sys SU: Relaxation and diastole of the heart. Physiol Rev 69:1228, 1989.

14. Gaasch WH: Diastolic dysfunction of the left ventricle: Importance to the clinician. *In* Advances in Internal Medicine, vol 35. Edited by JJ Leonard. Boston, Yearbook Medical Publishers, Inc., 1990, pp. 311–340.

15. Grossman W: Diastolic dysfunction and congestive heart failure. Circulation 81, suppl III (1990), 1–7.

16. Mirsky I, Pasipoularides A: Clinical assessment of diastolic function. Prog Cardiovasc Dis 32:291, 1990.

17. Glantz SA, Misbach GA, Moores WY, et al.: The pericardium substantially affects the left ventricular diastolic pressure-volume relationship in the dog. Circ Res 42:433, 1978.

18. Shirato K, Shabetai R, Bhargave V, et al.: Alteration of the left ventricular diastolic pressure-segment length relation produced by the pericardium: Effects of cardiac distention and afterload reduction in conscious dogs. Circulation 57:1191, 1978.

19. Mirsky I, Rankin JS: The effects of geometry, elasticity, and external pressures on the diastolic pressure-volume and stiffness-stress relations: How important is the pericardium? Circ Res 44:601, 1979.

20. Smiseth OA, Frais MA, Kingma I, et al.: Assessment of pericardial constraint: measured after pericardiocentesis. J Am Coll Cardiol 7:307, 1986.

21. Wildenthal K, Mullins CB, Harris MD, et al.: Left ventricular end-diastolic distensibility after norepinephrine and propranolol. Am J Physiol 217:812, 1969.

22. Sonnenblick EH, Ross J Jr, Covell JW, et al.: Alterations in resting length-tension relations of cardiac muscle induced by changes in contractile force. Circ Res 19:980, 1966.

23. Carroll JD, Lang RM, Neuman AL, et al.: The differential effects of positive inotropic and vasodilator therapy on diastolic properties in patients with congestive cardiomyopathy. Circulation 74:815, 1986.

24. Grossman W: Why is left ventricular diastolic pressure increased during angina pectoris? J Am Coll Cardiol 5:607, 1985.

25. Sasayama S, Nonogi H, Miyazaki S, et al.: Changes in diastolic properties of the regional myocardium during pacing-induced ischemia in human subjects. J Am Coll Cardiol 5:599, 1985.

26. Gaasch WH, Bing OHL, Mirsky I: Chamber compliance and myocardial stiffness in left ventricular hypertrophy. Eur Heart J 3:139, 1982.

27. Lorell BH, Grossman W: Cardiac hypertrophy: The consequences for diastole. J Am Coll Cardiol 9:1189, 1987.

28. Scheuer J: Alteration in sarcoplasmic reticulum function. *In* Perspectives in Cardiovascular Research, vol 7: Myocardial Hypertrophy and Failure. Edited by Tarezi RC, Dunbar JB. New York, Raven Press, 1983, pp. 111–122.

29. Morgan JP, Morgan KG: Calcium and cardiovascular function: Intracellular calcium levels during contraction and relaxation of mammalian cardiac and vascular smooth muscle as detected by aequorin. Am J Med 77 (Suppl 5A):33, 1984.

30. Lorell BH: Left ventricular diastolic pressure-volume relations: Understanding and managing congestive heart failure. Heart Failure 4:206, 1988.

31. Mirsky I, Cohn PF, Levine JA, et al.: Assessment of left ventricular stiffness in primary myocardial disease and coronary artery disease. Circulation 50:128, 1974.

32. Parmley WW, Chuck L, Kivowitz C, et al.: In vitro length-tension relations of human ventricular aneurysms: Relation of stiffness to mechanical advantage. Am J Cardiol 32:889, 1973.

33. Gaasch WH, Blaustein AS, Bing OHL: Asynchronous (segmental early) relaxation of the left ventricle. J Am Coll Cardiol 5:891, 1985.

34. Brutsaert DL: Nonuniformity: A physiologic modulator of contraction and relaxation of the normal heart. J Am Coll Cardiol 9:341, 1987.

35. Harizi RC, Bianco JA, Alpert JS: Diastolic function of the heart in clinical cardiology. Arch Intern Med 148:99, 1988.

36. Stauffer JC, Gaasch WH: Recognition and treatment of left ventricular diastolic dys-

function. Prog Cardiovasc Dis 32:319, 1990.

37. Dougherty AH, Naccarelli GV, Gray EL, et al.: Congestive heart failure with normal systolic function. Am J Cardiol 54: 778, 1984.

38. Soufer R, Wohlgelernter D, Vita NA, et al.: Intact systolic left ventricular function in clinical congestive heart failure. Am J Cardiol 55:1032, 1985.

39. Bonow RO, Leon MB, Rosing DR, et al.: Effects of verapamil and propranolol on left ventricular function and diastolic filling in patients with coronary artery disease: Radionuclide angiographic studies at rest and during exercise. Circulation 65:1337, 1981.

40. Kitzman DW, Higginbotham MB, Cobb FR, Sheikh KH, Sullivan MJ: Heart failure in patients with heart failure and preserved left ventricular systolic function: failure of the Frank-Starling mechanism. J Am Coll Cardiol 17:1065, 1991.

41. Kunis R, Greenberg H, Yeoh CB, et al.: Coronary revascularization for recurrent pulmonary edema in elderly patients with ischemic heart disease and preserved ventricular function. N Engl J Med 313:1207, 1985.

42. Topol EJ, Traill TA, Fortuin NJ: Hypertensive hypertrophic cardiomyopathy of the elderly. N Engl J Med 312:277, 1985.

43. Given BD, Lee TH, Stone PH, et al.: Nifedipine in severely hypertensive patients with congestive heart failure and preserved ventricular function. Arch Intern Med 145:281, 1985.

44. Parfrey PS, Harnett JD, Griffiths SM, et al.: Congestive heart failure in dialysis patients. Arch Intern Med 148:1519, 1988.

45. Levine HJ: Optimum heart rate of large failing hearts. Am J Cardiol 61:633, 1988.

46. Bonow RO, Bacharach SL, Green MV, et al.: Impaired left ventricular diastolic filling in patients with coronary artery disease: Assessment with radionuclide angiography. Circulation 64:315, 1981.

47. Bonow RO: Left ventricular filling in ischemic and hypertrophic heart disease. *In* Diastolic Relaxation of the Heart. Edited by Grossman W, Lorell BH. Boston, Martinus Nijhoff, 1988, pp. 231–243.

48. Tilton GD, Bush LR, Apprill PG, et al.: Effect of diltiazem and propranolol on left ventricular segmental relaxation during temporary coronary arterial occlusion and one month reperfusion in conscious dogs. Circulation 71:165, 1985.

49. Fujibayashi Y, Yamazaki S, Chang BL, et al.: Comparative echocardiographic study

of recovery of diastolic versus systolic function after brief periods of coronary occlusion: Differential effects of intravenous nifedipine administered before and during occlusion. J Am Coll Cardiol 6: 1289, 1985.

50. Lorell BH, Turi Z, Grossman WH: Modification of left ventricular response to pacing tachycardia by nifedipine in patients with coronary artery disease. Am J Med 71:667, 1981.

51. Bonow RO, Kent KM, Rosing DR, et al.: Improved left ventricular diastolic filling in patients with coronary artery disease after percutaneous transluminal coronary angioplasty. Circulation 66:1159, 1982.

52. Carroll JD, Hess OM, Hirzel HO, et al.: Left ventricular systolic and diastolic function in coronary artery disease: Effects of revascularization on exercise-induced ischemia. Circulation 72:119, 1985.

53. Nakamura Y, Sasayama S, Nonogi H, et al.: Effects of pacing-induced ischemia on early left ventricular filling and regional myocardial dynamics and their modification by nifedipine. Circulation 76:1232, 1987.

54. Mizuno K, Arakawa K, Shibuya T, et al.: Improved regional and global diastolic performance in patients with coronary artery disease after percutaneous transluminal coronary angioplasty. Am Heart J 115: 302, 1988.

55. Lawson WE, Seifert F, Anagnostopoulos C, et al.: Effect of coronary artery bypass grafting on left ventricular diastolic function. Am J Cardiol 61:283, 1988.

56. Humphrey LS, Topol EJ, Rosenfeld GI, et al.: Immediate enhancement of left ventricular relaxation by coronary artery bypass grafting: Intraoperative assessment. Circulation 77:886, 1988.

57. Pfeffer JM, Pfeffer MA, Braunwald E: Influence of chronic captopril therapy on the infarcted left ventricle of the rat. Circ Res 57:84, 1985.

58. Pfeffer MA, Pfeffer JM, Steinberg C, et al.: Survival after an experimental myocardial infarction: Beneficial effects of long-term therapy with captopril. Circulation 72:406, 1985.

59. McKay RG, Pfeffer MA, Pasternak RC, et al.: Left ventricular remodeling after myocardial infarction: A corollary to infarct expansion. Circulation 74:693, 1986.

60. Jugdett BI, Warnica JW: Intravenous nitroglycerine therapy to limit myocardial infarct size, expansion, and complications: Effect of timing, dosage, and infarct location. Circulation 78:906, 1988.

61. Hanrath P, Mathey DG, Seigert R, et al.: Left ventricular relaxation and filling pattern in different forms of left ventricular hypertrophy: An echocardiographic study. Am J Cardiol 45:15, 1980.
62. Inouye I, Massie B, Loge D, et al.: Abnormal left ventricular filling: An early finding in mild to moderate systemic hypertension. Am J Cardiol 53:120, 1984.
63. Fouad FM, Slominski JM, Tarazi RC: Left ventricular diastolic function in hypertension: Relation to left ventricular mass and systolic function. J Am Coll Cardiol 3:1500, 1984.
64. Smith VE, Schulman P, Karimeddini MK, et al.: Rapid ventricular filling in left ventricular hypertrophy: II. Pathologic hypertrophy. J Am Coll Cardiol 5:869, 1985.
65. Shimizu G, Zile MR, Blaustein AS, Gaasch WH: Left ventricular chamber filling and midwall fiber lengthening in patients with left ventricular hypertrophy: Overestimation of fiber velocities by conventional midwall measurements. Circulation 71:266, 1985.
66. Gibson DG, Traill TA, Hall RJC, et al.: Echocardiographic features of secondary left ventricular hypertrophy. Br Heart J 41:54, 1979.
67. Tarazi RC: The heart in hypertension. N Engl J Med 312:308, 1985.
68. Inouye IK, Massie BM, Loge D, et al.: Failure of antihypertensive therapy with diuretic, beta-blocking and calcium channel-blocking drugs to consistently reverse left ventricular diastolic filling abnormalities. Am J Cardiol 53:1583, 1984.
69. Fouad FM, Slominski MJ, Tarazi RC, et al.: Alterations in left ventricular filling with beta-adrenergic blockade. Am J Cardiol 51:161, 1983.
70. Hartford M, Wendelhag I, Berglund G, et al.: Cardiovascular and renal effects of long-term antihypertensive treatment. JAMA 259:2553, 1988.
71. Smith VE, White WB, Meeran MK, et al.: Improved left ventricular filling accompanies reduced left ventricular mass during therapy of essential hypertension. J Am Coll Cardiol 8:1449, 1986.
72. Betocchi S, Cuocolo A, Pace L, et al.: Effects of intravenous verapamil administration on left ventricular diastolic function in systemic hypertension. Am J Cardiol 59:624, 1987.
73. Giles TD, Sander GE, Roffidal LC, et al.: Comparison of nifedipine and hydrochlorothiazide for systemic hypertension. Am J Cardiol 60:103, 1987.
74. Wigle ED, Sasson Z, Henderson MA, et al.: Hypertrophic cardiomyopathy: The importance of the site and the extent of hypertrophy: A review. Prog Cardiovasc Dis 28:1, 1985.
75. Alvares RF, Shaver JA, Gamble WH, et al.: Isovolumic relaxation period in hypertrophic cardiomyopathy. J Am Coll Cardiol 3:71, 1984.
76. Betocchi S, Bonow RO, Bacharach SL, et al.: Isovolumic relaxation period in hypertrophic cardiomyopathy: Assessment by radionuclide angiography. J Am Coll Cardiol 7:74, 1986.
77. Sanderson JE, Gibson DG, Brown DJ, et al.: Left ventricular filling in hypertrophic cardiomyopathy: An angiographic study. Br Heart J 39:661, 1977.
78. Sanderson JE, Traill TA, St. John-Sutton MG, et al.: Left ventricular relaxation and filling in hypertrophic cardiomyopathy: An echocardiographic study. Br Heart J 40:596, 1978.
79. Stewart S, Mason DT, Braunwald E: Impaired rate of left ventricular filling in idiopathic hypertrophic subaortic stenosis and valvular aortic stenosis. Circulation 37:8, 1968.
80. Bonow RO, Frederick TM, Bacharach SL, et al.: Atrial systole and left ventricular filling in hypertrophic cardiomyopathy: Effect of verapamil. Am J Cardiol 51:1386, 1983.
81. Lewis BS, Mitha AS, Bakst A, et al.: Haemodynamic effects of beta blockade in hypertrophic cardiomyopathy using Sectral (acebutolol). Cardiovasc Res 8:249, 1974.
82. Swanton RH, Brooksby IAB, Jenkins BS, et al.: Hemodynamic studies of beta blockade in hypertrophic obstructive cardiomyopathy. Eur J Cardiol 5:327, 1977.
83. Alvares RF, Goodwin JF: Non-invasive assessment of diastolic function in hypertrophic cardiomyopathy on and off beta adrenergic blocking drugs. Br Heart J 48:204, 1982.
84. Hess OM, Grimm J, Krayenbuehl HP: Diastolic function in hypertrophic cardiomyopathy: Effects of propranolol and verapamil on diastolic stiffness. Eur Heart J 4:47, 1983.
85. Suwa M, Hirota Y, Kawamura K: Improvement in left ventricular diastolic function during intravenous and oral diltiazem therapy in patients with hypertrophic cardiomyopathy: An echocardiographic study. Am J Cardiol 54:1047, 1984.
86. Kaltenbach M, Hopf R, Kober G, et al.: Treatment of hypertrophic obstructive

cardiomyopathy with verapamil. Br Heart J 42:35, 1979.

87. Lorell BH, Paulus WJ, Grossman W, et al.: Modification of abnormal left ventricular diastolic properties by nifedipine in patients with hypertrophic cardiomyopathy. Circulation 65:499, 1982.

88. Paulus WJ, Lorell BH, Craig WE, et al.: Comparison of the effects of nitroprusside and nifedipine on diastolic properties in patients with hypertrophic cardiomyopathy: Altered left ventricular loading or improved muscle inactivation? J Am Coll Cardiol 2:879, 1983.

89. Bonow RO, Dilsizian V, Rosing DR, et al.: Verapamil-induced improvement in left ventricular diastolic filling and increased exercise tolerance in patients with hypertrophic cardiomyopathy: Short- and long-term effects. Circulation 72:853, 1985.

90. Hanrath P, Mathey DG, Kremer P, et al.: Effect of verapamil on left ventricular isovolumic relaxation time and regional left ventricular filling in hypertrophic cardiomyopathy. Am J Cardiol 45:1258, 1980.

91. Suwa M, Hirota Y, Kawamura K: Effects of nifedipine on left ventricular systolic and diastolic function in hypertrophic nonobstructive cardiomyopathy: An echocardiographic observation. J Cardiovasc Ultrasonogr 2:9, 1983.

92. Hess OM, Murakami T, Krayenbuehl HP: Does verapamil improve left ventricular relaxation in patients with myocardial hypertrophy? Circulation 74:530, 1986.

93. Iwase M, Sotobata I, Takagi S, et al.: Effects of diltiazem on left ventricular diastolic behavior in patients with hypertrophic cardiomyopathy: Evaluation with exercise pulsed doppler echocardiography. J Am Coll Cardiol 9:1099, 1987.

94. Shaffer EM, Rocchini AP, Spicer RL, et al.: Effects of verapamil on left ventricular diastolic filling in children with hypertrophic cardiomyopathy. Am J Cardiol 61:413, 1988.

95. Fighali S, Krajcer Z, Leachman RD: Septal myomectomy and mitral valve replacement for idiopathic hypertrophic subaortic stenosis: Short and long-term follow-up. J Am Coll Cardiol 3:1127, 1984.

96. Leachman RD, Krajcer Z, Azic T, et al.: Mitral valve replacement in hypertrophic cardiomyopathy: Ten-year follow-up in 54 patients. Am J Cardiol 60:1416, 1987.

97. Fananapazir L, Cannon RO, Tripodi D, Panza JA: Dual chamber pacing is an alternative to cardiac surgery in hypertrophic cardiomyopathy patients with symptoms refractory to medical therapy. Circulation 84 (Suppl IV):326, 1991.

98. Cohn JN, Johnson G: Heart failure with normal ejection fraction: The V-HeFT study. Circulation 81 (Suppl. III):48, 1990.

99. Setaro JF, Remetz M, Zaret BL, Soufer R: Prognosis of patients with congestive heart failure and intact systolic function: a seven year follow up. Circulation 80 (Suppl II):275, 1989.

100. Judge KW, Pawitan Y, Caldwell J, et al.: Congestive heart failure in patients with preserved left ventricular systolic function: Analysis of the CASS registry. J Am Coll Cardiol 18:377, 1991.

101. Brogan WC, Hillis LD, Flores ED, et al.: The natural history of isolated left ventricular diastolic dysfunction. Am J Med 92:627, 1992.

Chapter 15

EXERCISE-INDUCED ANGINA PECTORIS

John D. Carroll and Eugenia P. Carroll

"They who are afflicted with it, are seized while they are walking, (more especially if it be uphill, and soon after eating) with a painful and most disagreeable sensation in the breast, which seems as it would extinguish life, if it were to increase or to continue, but the moment they stand still all this uneasiness vanishes."

> William Heberden, M.D.
> Commentaries on the History
> and Care of Diseases
> London, 1802.

Exercise-induced angina pectoris exemplifies a cause of cardiac symptoms that emerges or worsens with physical activity. The severity of angina or myocardial ischemia is frequently graded by the amount and type of physical activity necessary for induction. Furthermore, controlled degrees of exercise are routinely used in most patients to assess whether angina and laboratory abnormalities indicative of ischemia are present, and further to suggest whether there is anatomically mild or extensive coronary artery disease.

Diastolic and systolic properties of the left ventricle are immediately altered when exercise causes ischemia. Clinically, the induced abnormalities of systolic function (i.e., ejection fraction and regional wall motion abnormalities) are relatively easy to both identify and measure, and are generally used, rather than diastolic abnormalities, to diagnose and quantify coronary artery disease. Yet an understanding of diastole is essential to understanding the pathophysiology of coronary artery disease and multiple diseases in which myocardial ischemia occurs during exercise. Also, many of the symptoms and signs of exercise-induced ischemia can be understood only by studying the diastolic properties of the left ventricle.

The induction of ischemia by exercise in the setting of a coronary artery stenosis involves the interaction of a variety of factors which are outlined in Table 15–1. A discussion of diastolic dysfunction in exercise-induced ischemia is appropriately put in the context of two other topics: the physiology of exercise and myocardial oxygen supply and demand.

Circulatory adjustments during exercise may be divided into chronic and acute. The acute adjustments are most important in understanding exercise-induced ischemia because most patients with significant coronary artery disease are not conditioned athletes. Whereas athletes have chronic adjustments in left ventricular mass, size, and shape from extensive exercise programs, the majority of patients with exercise-induced ischemia are below average in cardiovascular conditioning given their risk factors, and avoidance of activities that provoke angina pectoris.

Important differences exist between the physiology of exercise that is dynamic versus static, upright versus supine, and submaximal versus maximal. For purposes of this discussion, the emphasis is on dynamic, symptom-limited exercise that is generally in a supine position for invasive studies and in an upright position for nuclear studies. (See Chap. 11.)

The major changes in left ventricular diastolic function during exercise are listed in Table 15–2. Exercise-induced changes in diastolic function are key factors in allowing the augmentation in cardiac output to occur without a detrimental increase in filling pressures (1, 2). These acute adjustments are used to understand the disruption in diastolic function due to the superimposition of ischemia. The landmarks in diastole pertinent to a discussion of exer-

Table 15–1. Factors Involved in the Induction of Exercise-Induced Ischemia

Marked increases in myocardial oxygen demand:
- Increased contractile state
- Increased heart rate
- Increased wall stresses

Inability to sufficiently augment coronary flow:
- Coronary artery stenosis
- Exercise-induced coronary vasoconstriction
- Decreased coronary perfusion pressure
- Increased coronary venous pressures
- Limited coronary collateral flow
- Tachycardia-mediated decrease in diastole

cise-induced ischemia are clarified in Figure 15–1.

The diastolic dysfunction caused by exercise-induced ischemia is not only a complex interplay between the physiology of exercise and the mechanical abnormalities of myocardial ischemia, but is also importantly modified by subtle to gross histologic changes in the myocardium. Focal or confluent areas of fibrosis in the wall of the left ventricle alter diastolic function. The superimposition of ischemia-induced mechanical abnormalities further induces changes in filling pressures, filling characteristics, etc. Therefore, the subsequent discussion looks at both the exercise-in-

Table 15–2. Alterations in Left Ventricular Diastolic Function During Normal Exercise

Abbreviation of diastolic filling time:
- Increased heart rate shortens diastole
- Altered left atrial pressure and left ventricular diastolic
- Pressure modify time of mitral valve opening/closing

Augmentation of filling rates:
- Accelerated relaxation
- Enhanced elastic recoil
- Increased left atrial pressure

Enhanced chamber compliance

Accelerated isovolumic pressure decay:
- Sympathetically mediated myocardial effect
- Enhanced elastic recoil
- Decreased end-systolic chamber size

duced abnormalities occurring from ischemia and then turn to the exercise-induced abnormalities of diastolic function from the chronic scar due to previous myocardial infarction.

EXERCISE-INDUCED ABNORMALITIES IN DIASTOLIC FUNCTION DURING ISCHEMIA

Filling Pressures

Much of the early clinical work on diastolic function was directed at understanding the increase in left ventricular filling pressures after myocardial infarction and during angina pectoris. Transient ischemia with or without the pain of angina is associated with a rise in left ventricular filling pressures (2–4). Figure 15–2 illustrates that, in the absence of exercise-induced ischemia, low diastolic pressures are maintained during exercise. During exercise-induced ischemia, however, there is an increase in pulmonary capillary pressure not infrequently above 20 mm Hg, in association with a variety of changes in left ventricular function (Table 15-3). If acute papillary muscle dysfunction is caused by the ischemia or if the quantity of ischemic myocardium is a large, as with left main coronary artery stenosis, frank pulmonary edema may be induced by transient ischemia. At the opposite extreme are episodes of ischemia with a small increase in left ventricular end-diastolic pressure. These episodes are often silent, i.e., asymptomatic (5).

The rise in filling pressures is associated with dilatation of the left atrium and pulmonary vessels which may be as important as the ischemic myocardium in producing symptoms (6, 7). Transient changes in lung compliance which accompany acute elevations of left ventricular filling pressures may also contribute to the sense of dyspnea, often referred to as an anginal equivalent.

Diastolic Pressure-Volume Relation

Shifts in the diastolic pressure-volume relation are seen during angina pectoris and silent ischemia when they are induced by rapid atrial pacing or exercise (8–15). The degree of the shift does show some variability regarding the relative displace-

LANDMARKS IN DIASTOLE

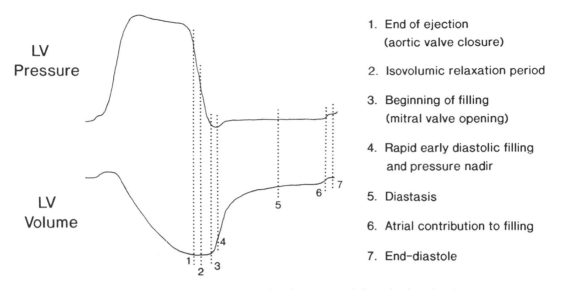

LV
Pressure

LV
Volume

1. End of ejection
   (aortic valve closure)

2. Isovolumic relaxation period

3. Beginning of filling
   (mitral valve opening)

4. Rapid early diastolic filling
   and pressure nadir

5. Diastasis

6. Atrial contribution to filling

7. End-diastole

Fig. 15–1. Landmarks in diastole pertinent to the discussion of diastolic function in coronary artery disease. With permission from Carroll JD, Carroll EP: Diastolic function in coronary artery disease. Herz (Germany) 16:1, 1991.

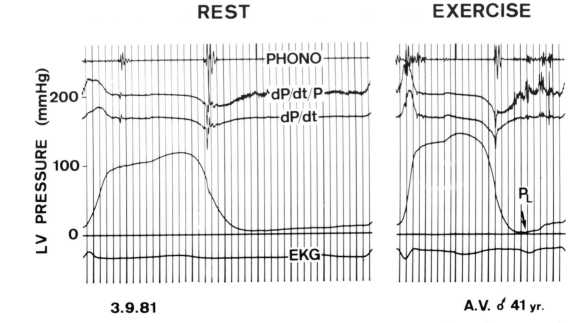

REST   EXERCISE

3.9.81   A.V. ♂ 41 yr.

Fig. 15–2. Left ventricular pressure before and during exercise in a patient with no ischemia. Diastolic pressures remain low with a tendency for a small decrease in early diastolic pressure (P_L) and a small increase in end-diastolic pressure.

Table 15–3.   Hemodynamic Changes During Exercise With and Without Accompanying Ischemia

	Normal Exercise	Exercise-Induced Ischemia
Heart rate	Increased	Variable
Mean arterial pressure	Increased	Blunted increase
Central venous pressure	Unchanged	Increased or unchanged
Pulmonary wedge pressure	Unchanged	Greatly increased
Cardiac output	Greatly increased	Moderately increased
Stroke volume	Increased	Variable
Left Ventricular Pressure		
Systolic	Increased	Variable
End-diastolic	Slightly increased	Greatly increased
Early diastolic	Decreased	Greatly increased
Maximum +Dp/dt	Greatly increased	Variable
Isovolumic relaxation rate	Greatly increased	Slightly increased
Left Ventricular Size		
End-diastolic	Variable	Increased
End-systolic	Decreased	Increased
Ejection fraction	Increased	Decreased
Early diastolic filling rates	Greatly increased	Moderately increased
Late diastolic filling rates	Greatly increased	Variable

ment of diastolic volumes and whether the shift involves early, late, or all of diastole (Fig. 15–3). This heterogeneity suggests that each patient shows a quantitatively variable contribution of the different determinants of the pressure-volume relation, i.e., altered isovolumic relaxation, acute chamber dilation, pericardial/right ventricular interaction and alterations of passive muscle stiffness (Fig. 15–4).

The most common diastolic pressure-volume shift seen in myocardial ischemia is a parallel shift with a rise in diastolic pressures at all volumes (Fig. 15–5). The nearly universal increase in end-systolic volume produces a rightward shift of the early diastolic pressure-volume coordinates. This classical shift in the diastolic pressure-volume relation presents a difficulty in quantifying the shift. Using conventional ap-

DIASTOLIC PRESSURE - VOLUME RELATIONS

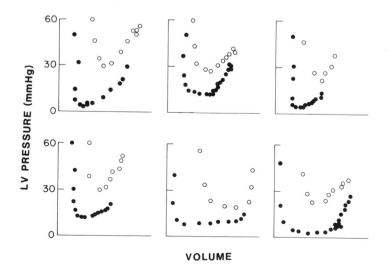

VOLUME

Fig. 15–3. Six left ventricular diastolic-volume plots from different patients with coronary artery disease illustrate some of the heterogeneity seen with ischemia. By end-diastole, some patients, e.g., middle figure, lower row, have no or little shift in their diastolic pressure-volume relation. The open circles are during exercise-induced ischemia and the closed circles are at rest. With permission from Carroll JD, Carroll EP: Diastolic function in coronary artery disease. Herz (Germany) 16:1, 1991.

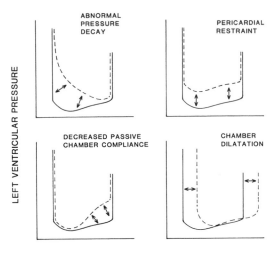

Fig. 15–4. Four mechanisms for shifts in the diastolic pressure-volume relation. During ischemia, each mechanism may contribute to a variable degree in an individual patient, to the upward shift. With permission from Carroll JD, et al.: The differential effects of positive inotropic and vasodilator therapy on diastolic properties in patients with congestive cardiomyopathy. Circulation 74:815, 1986. With permission from the American Heart Association.

proaches of computing an index of chamber compliance is inaccurate because the shift is parallel (16). Although mathematical solutions may quantify the shift, physiologically their use is problematic. The chamber properties are clearly in an

unsteady state, thus making chronic, passive compliance a difficult concept to apply to the left ventricle during angina pectoris. The variable contribution of extrinsic factors influencing left ventricular properties adds another element of complexity. Specifically, acute ischemia may invoke pericardial restraining effects and ventricular interaction which further elevate intracardiac pressures, which no longer represent true distending pressures. Given these limitations in interpreting the nature of shifts in the diastolic pressure-volume relation, we now examine some of the pathophysiologic mechanisms that may cause the shift during ischemia.

The rise in diastolic pressures is clearly not totally caused by simple, acute chamber dilation. Yet, in some patients the increase in end-diastolic volume may be so substantial that the rest and angina diastolic pressure-volume coordinates may minimally overlap.

Abnormal myocardial relaxation may significantly alter the diastolic pressure-volume relationship in some patients (2, 17, 18). This shift would be expected to involve early diastole to a greater extent that late diastole, especially if relaxation is slowed but still an ongoing process in the ischemic myocardium (Fig. 15–4, upper left panel). If the muscle was not able to totally relax, a likely scenario in the brief diastole with tachycardia, the relaxation-related shift could extend to end-diastole.

With the completion of pressure decay,

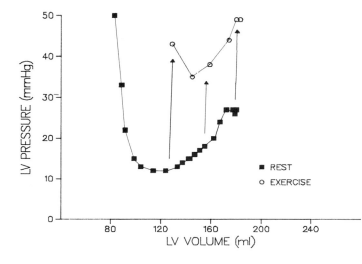

Fig. 15–5. The classical pressure-volume shift of ischemia is illustrated by this patient. At all diastolic volumes pressure is clearly elevated compared to the resting coordinates. With permission from Carroll JD, Carroll EP: Diastolic function in coronary artery disease. Herz (Germany) 16:1, 1991.

diastolic function is primarily determined by the passive chamber properties (18–22). Passive chamber properties are the result of many factors, including myocardial stiffness, wall thickness, the pericardium, and viscous effects (23). During ischemia, the left ventricle may never become totally relaxed, and thus chamber properties are even more complex. Likewise, nonhomogeneous contraction and relaxation during ischemia occur in such a way that myocardial stiffness may be grossly abnormal in one area and normal in another (24–31). The pressure-volume relation represents the net product of these factors. (See Chap. 19.)

There is ample evidence that myocardial stiffness, in addition to chamber stiffness, increases during acute ischemia. The evidence comes from experimental and clinical studies (24, 25, 32–34). The intracellular events leading to altered muscle stiffness are being actively investigated. Calcium sequestration by the sarcoplasmic reticulum appears to be impaired; this is most likely to contribute to impaired relaxation (35).

Viscous factors are important to consider in the pathophysiology of ischemia in the clinical setting (23). The diastolic pressure-volume relation in the isolated heart preparation can be derived by slowing varying intraventricular volume in a fully relaxed chamber, thus minimizing viscous effects. However, in clinical studies, diastolic pressure-volume relations are derived from single diastoles in which volume changes occur at rapid rates; such rapid rates occur in early diastole and with atrial contraction. When the pressure-volume coordinates during rapid volume fluxes significantly deviate from the pressure-volume curve obtained with slow rates, a viscous effect is operative. Therefore, viscous factors may be important in interpreting data from patients with coronary artery disease. Viscous effects are proportional to intrinsic myocardial stiffness. Fibrotic muscle is expected to demonstrate a significant viscous element during rapid length changes with chamber filling.

The normal pericardium resists stretch if there is a significant and acute increase in total intrapericardial volume (36). (See Chap. 6.) The atria and right ventricle may

acutely dilate from the elevation of left ventricular filling pressures during ischemia. If total intrapericardial volume increases so that intrapericardial pressure rises above its normal low values, an acute pericardial effect on left ventricular chamber properties may become manifest (Figure 15–4). This would produce an elevation in pressure for a given volume in the left ventricle as well as in other cardiac chambers. Clinically, this has been a problem to study because both total intrapericardial volume and pressure are difficult to measure by current routine techniques. Therefore, changes in right atrial pressure have been used as an indirect index of pericardial effect. If the pericardium does play a role in left ventricular chamber properties, right atrial pressures should be elevated during angina. Indeed, during exercise-induced ischemia, right atrial pressures have been shown to increase; however, there has been no consistency in the presence of increased right atrial pressures or in the degree of upward shift in the left ventricle's diastolic pressure-volume relation compared with the change in right atrial pressure (37). In addition, other factors may elevate right atrial pressures, for example, right ventricular ischemia. The pericardium, the right ventricle, or both play a significant role in determining left ventricular chamber properties during ischemia in some patients, but these methodologic limitations obscure their overall importance. Studies of right ventricular function during exercise-induced left ventricular suggest that right ventricular ischemia is often not present but that acute increases in pulmonary artery pressure may be important in elevating right ventricular pressures (38, 39). Parallel changes in filling pressures of both chambers have been shown and support the hypothesis that ventricular interaction is a factor in the upward shift of the diastolic pressure-volume relation (38, 39).

Left Ventricular Pressure Decay

The isovolumic relaxation period links the dynamics of ventricular ejection to diastolic events. During this period, pressure falls in the chamber as the muscle relaxes. Pressure decay can be quantitated by various methods (16). Maximum negative dP/

dt was initially used to quantify alterations in pressure decay, but this value has the disadvantage of being influenced by the timing of aortic valve closure and of representing pressure decay at only one moment. Subsequently, several approaches have been used to quantify the isovolumic relaxation period. The duration of the isovolumic relaxation period can be measured accurately using phonocardiographic identification of aortic valve closure and echocardiographic visualization of mitral valve opening. Yet this time is determined not only by the rapidity of pressure fall between these two valve actions, but also by the other determinants of valve opening and closing. More attention has been focused on mathematical models to quantitate the rate of pressure decay in the isovolumic relaxation period. The simplest approach is to calculate a T ½, which is defined as the time it takes pressure to fall to one half of its end-systolic value. Other methods have quantitated the exponential nature of pressure decay during the isovolumic period. A plot of the natural logarithm of pressure versus time is quite linear. The negative reciprocal of the slope of this line is the time constant of relaxation or pressure decay, often called tau. This model mathematically forces pressure decay to zero, which is of concern in the clinical setting, when intrathoracic and intrapericardial pressures may invalidate this assumption. A plot of pressure versus the simultaneous value of dP/dt as seen in Figure 15–6 is also nearly linear for the isovolumic relaxation period and does not inherently assume a zero value (2). The negative reciprocal of the slope of this line is also a time constant of pressure decay, but it cannot be directly compared with the value derived from the natural log method, because the X-axis intercept, P_b, also describes the character of pressure decay (Fig. 15–6). Although small deviations from linearity are seen, both methods give a quantitative assessment of pressure decay that is useful in clinical studies. These parameters of pressure decay quantify global chamber events and do not tell the observer whether one wall of the chamber is relaxing abnormally during ischemia while the other portions of the chamber are functioning normally. The global measurements of pressure decay are useful mainly in understanding acutely altered diastolic chamber properties. Several reviews provide comprehensive reading in the area of myocardial relaxation and techniques of quantifying relaxation (16, 18).

The character of pressure decay is dynamic, determined on a beat-to-beat basis (18). It changes in response to a variety of factors. During normal exercise, pressure decay is greatly accelerated and produces

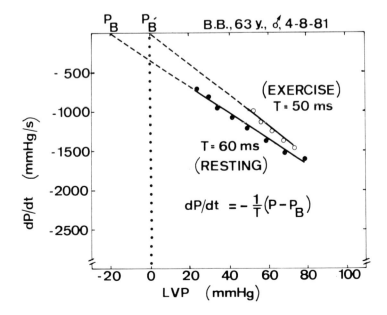

Fig. 15–6. Left ventricular pressure decay is represented as a plot of dP/dt versus pressure coordinates using data from the isovolumic relaxation period. During exercise-induced ischemia, there is a decrease in T, but the pressure axis intercept P_b increases.

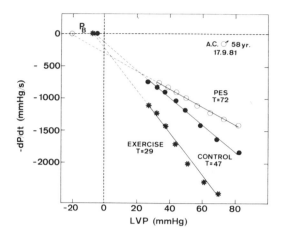

Fig. 15–7. Pressure decay is modified by a variety of factors. Here one subject underwent exercise (*) and then extrasystoles were induced to look at pressure decay in the post-extrasystolic (PES) beat (open circles) having systolic potentiation. Note that exercise greatly accelerates pressure decay but a similar degree of systolic augmentation in the post-extrasystolic beat is paired with a slowed pressure decay. With permission from Carroll JD, et al.: Left ventricular isovolumic pressure decay and diastolic mechanics after post-extrasystolic potentiation and during exercise. Am J Cardiol 51:583, 1983.

a low value of tau, which is important in allowing the ventricle to fill rapidly at low intraventricular pressures. Following an extrasystole may be slowing of relaxation despite augmentation of systolic function in the postextrasystolic beat (Fig. 15–7). During pacing-induced ischemia, tau is prolonged, indicating slower pressure decay (15). During exercise-induced ischemia, tau is reduced (Figure 15–6), but the reduction is significantly less than that which occurs in those exercising without ischemia (2).

Abnormally slow pressure decay has several effects on ventricular function. It delays mitral valve opening and thus shortens the time for filling. It elevates diastolic pressure, particularly in early diastole. It also causes an upward shift in the diastolic pressure-volume relation (Fig. 15–4). This occurs because, at a given diastolic volume, the pressure represents, in part, incompletely decayed pressure from the previous systole. This shift is distinctly abnormal because pressure decay from the previous

systole in the normal ventricle is virtually complete by early diastole; pressures thereafter mainly reflect the passive chamber properties in the normal heart.

Abnormally slow pressure decay during ischemia is the result of many factors (18). Ischemia directly impairs the rapidity and completeness of muscle relaxation. It is possible that the myocardium in the ischemic wall never completely relaxes between systoles. This incomplete relaxation translates, at the ventricular or chamber level, into slow pressure decay that fails to achieve a pressure level expected for a totally relaxed chamber. Other factors also affect the way pressure decays in the left ventricle. Abnormal loads, i.e., high wall stresses, and asynchrony can prolong pressure decay, whereas sympathetic stimulation can accelerate it.

Filling Dynamics

If the left ventricle becomes acutely stiffer during ischemia, filling should be altered. This does occur, but in a complex fashion that depends on how ischemia was induced (see Chap. 17) and how filling is quantitated (see Chaps. 11 and 12). Left ventricular filling is a dynamic process involving the interaction of active and passive properties of the atria and ventricles (40, 41). It cannot be fully understood solely by measuring filling rates. The rate of left ventricular pressure decay and the subsequent atrial-ventricular pressure gradient are major factors determining early filling volume and rates. The preload-dependent change in left ventricular chamber stiffness becomes increasingly more important as filling progresses. That is, as the chamber reaches a steeper portion of the pressure-volume relation, further filling is resisted by the stiffening chamber. (See Chap. 9.) Finally, the strength and timing of atrial systole determine the final portion of filling volume, which in turn determines the end-diastolic preload (40).

By itself, the abnormally slow pressure decay during ischemia should restrict early diastolic filling. Indeed it does, but early filling rates are also dependent on the atrial driving pressure for filling (40, 42). During exercise-induced ischemia, mitral valve opening occurred at an average value of over 40 mm Hg. Thus, the atrial driving pressure for early filling may offset abnormalities of relaxation, which, when unopposed, tends to slow early filling.

An early diastolic intraventricular pressure gradient is normally present in the left ventricle but is lost during acute ischemia (43). Elastic recoil that appears to cause this physiologic early diastolic gradients is normally produced by the elastic potential energy in the small, deformed left ventricle at end-systole (43). Myocardial ischemia, with its disruption of systolic function, may disturb this mechanism that keeps early diastolic pressures low at rest and actually subzero during exercise in subjects free of cardiovascular disease (1).

In the left panel of Figure 15–8, filling curves at rest and during exercise are shown for a patient free of significant cardiovascular disease. Note three periods at rest: rapid early filling, diastasis, and subsequent filling due to atrial contraction. With exercise, the time for filling is brief because of tachycardia, yet the total filling volume, which is equal to stroke volume, increases.

Filling is rapid and monophasic, without the three periods seen at rest. No elevation of atrial driving pressure occurs in young, healthy persons during exercise, although there may be some elevation in older individuals without signs of cardiovascular disease. In the right panel of Figure 15–8, the reduced filling volume of a patient in whom ischemia developed with exercise is shown. In this case, it appears that the filling rate during exercise in the first half of diastole is not as rapid as it was in the control patient. Several studies using nuclear techniques have shown reduced peak filling rates during ischemia (44, 45). This reduction presumably reflects abnormal pressure decay in the left ventricle. Other studies using angiographic techniques have shown peak filling rates that may increase during exercise-induced ischemia (40). This difference may potentially reflect the methods employed in calculating filling rates. In addition, the grossly elevated atrial driving pressures can overcome the pressure decay abnormalities. Filling rates are influenced by many factors; certainly,

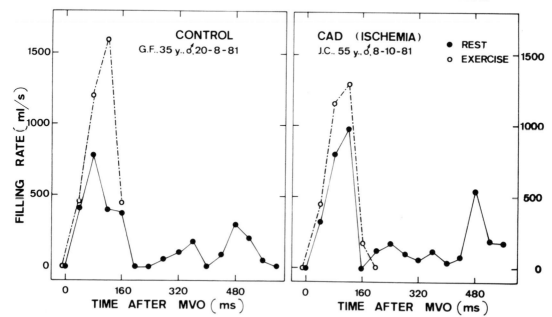

LEFT VENTRICULAR FILLING RATE DURING EXERCISE

Fig. 15–8. Left ventricular filling rates are shown during rest and during exercise in a subject free of significant cardiovascular disease (left panel and one with exercise-induced ischemia (right panel). MVO = mitral valve opening. With permission from Carroll JD, et al.: Dynamics of left ventricular filling at rest and during exercise. Circulation 68:59, 1983. With permission from the American Heart Association.

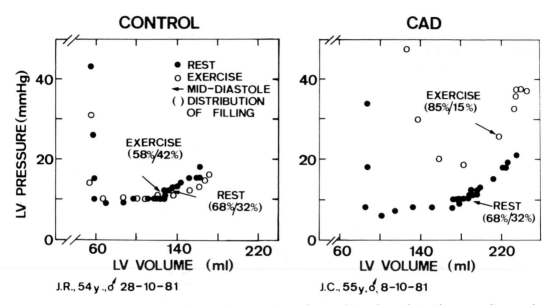

Fig. 15–9. Diastolic pressure-volume plots are shown for a subject free of significant cardiovascular disease (left panel) and one with exercise-induced ischemia (right panel). The time of mid-diastole is noted and the distribution of filling between the first half and second half of diastole is given for both patients at rest and during exercise. In the control subject, filling is augmented throughout diastole. During exercise-induced ischemia, filing is augmented in the first half of diastole but decelerates during the second half.

fast filling should not be thought of in association with qualitative terms such as "good," because the elevated atrial pressures producing these rates are not normal.

During exercise, filling rates are normally increased during both the first and second halves of diastole (Table 15–3). During exercise-induced ischemia, there is often a significant decrease in the amount of filling that occurs in the second half of diastole (40). This is demonstrated in Figure 15–9. Filling virtually stops for the second half of diastole during exercise-induced ischemia. The restriction to late diastolic filling may be due to several other factors, including diminished atrial systole. In conclusion, it is not surprising that multiple techniques have found a diversity of filling patterns in coronary artery disease (46–64).

Duration of Mechanical Abnormalities

Filling pressures, diastolic pressure-volume shifts, abnormalities of pressure decay, and ventricular filling are all disrupted by myocardial ischemia during exercise, as discussed in the previous text.

The duration of these abnormalities after exercise has been terminated is not well studied. Abnormalities in peak filling rates may persist for several days following maximal exercise (65). Abnormalities of diastolic function commonly persist at rest when systolic abnormalities have resolved after exercise. Therefore, it is plausible that many patients with resting abnormal radionucleotide filling patterns and normal systolic performance may be demonstrating the lingering effects of previous episodes of exercise-induced ischemia (66). Particularly high-intensity exercise results in marker and prolonged mechanical abnormalities (67).

MYOCARDIAL FIBROSIS AND EXERCISE-INDUCED ABNORMALITIES IN DIASTOLIC FUNCTION

Filling Pressures

Myocardial fibrosis is frequently associated with a rise in end-diastolic pressures, but the impact on left atrial pressure and pulmonary artery pressures is often blunted, especially if sinus rhythm is maintained. These latter sites of pressure measurement are more commonly elevated when left ventricular diastolic pressures are elevated throughout diastole. Myocardial fibrosis may not do this, especially if, as in coronary artery disease, only focal areas of the myocardium are altered by the presence of excessive fibrotic tissue (68).

The increase in filling pressure in the presence of myocardial fibrosis is highly dependent on the volume status of the patients. An expansion of cardiopulmonary blood volume from salt retention or venoconstriction may unmask the adverse effects of myocardial fibrosis on filling pressures.

Diastolic Pressure-Volume Relations

The importance of intravascular fluid status and filling pressures is better understood by examination of the diastolic pressure-volume relation in the ventricle scarred from past infarction. The resting pressure-volume relation may appear unremarkable in a patient with a large anterior wall scar from a remote infarction. Yet, with the stress of exercise diastolic volumes

increase, presumably caused by the increased central blood volume seen with exercise, and diastolic pressures become grossly elevated (46, 47). No ischemia need be induced to cause a rise in end-diastolic pressure (Fig. 15–10).

Myocardial fibrosis, such as that following myocardial infarction, has a major effect on left ventricular diastolic pressure-volume relation. (See Chap. 8.) Unlike changes in only wall thickness, increased amounts of collagen result in a change in the stiffness of the muscle itself, i.e., an alteration in myocardial stiffness. As shown in Figure 15–11, in a rat model of fibrosis, 6 weeks after microsphere embolization, the end-diastolic stress-strain relation is altered in myocardium containing an excessive amount of fibrosis.

Myocardium is composed of myocytes supported within an extracellular matrix consisting largely of the fibrillar protein collagen (69–74). Remodelling of this fibrosis matrix following experimental infarction increases myocardial stiffness. This can be seen, for example, following coronary artery embolization (74). Al-

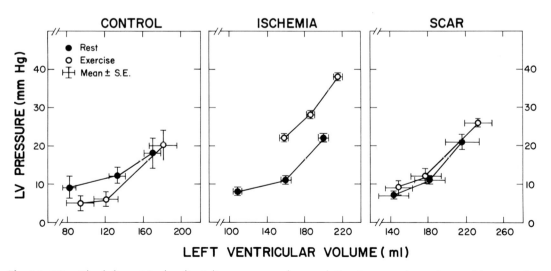

Fig. 15–10. The left ventricular diastolic pressure-volume relation in controls, patients withe exercise-induced ischemia, and in patients with a scar from prior infarction but no exercise-induced ischemia. The coordinates represent averages. See text for details. With permission from Carroll JD, et al.: Dynamics of left ventricular filling at rest and during exercise. Circulation 68:59, 1983. With permission from the American Heart Association.

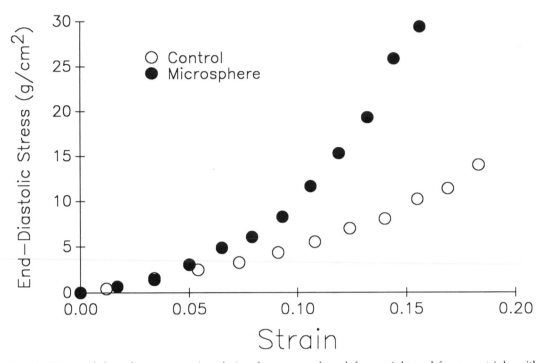

Fig. 15–11. End-diastolic stress-strain relation for a normal rat left ventricle and for a ventricle with extensive myocardial fibrosis from coronary microsphere embolization. Note the shift toward increased muscle stiffness in the fibrotic left ventricle. With permission from Carroll JD, Carroll EP: Diastolic function in coronary artery disease. Herz (Germany) 16:1, 1991.

though the accumulation of collagen serves to maintain the structural integrity and tensile strength of the myocardium after infarction, the altered diastolic properties may increase filling pressures and reduce the efficiency of the Starling mechanism to maintain stroke volume. (See Chap. 16.)

The more exponential diastolic stress-strain relation following infarction may be caused by the addition of inelastic collagen fibers in an inseries arrangement with the myocardium (74). The specific location of collagen along with its alignment with adjacent structures needs to be studied to more completely understand how myocyte loading and myocardial stiffness are altered for infarction.

Filling Dynamics and Pressure Decay

Filling patterns in patients recovered from myocardial infarction show a great deal of variability (40). This is not unexpected because filling dynamics are determined by both left ventricular and left atrium passive and active properties, loading conditions, heart rate, and mitral valve function. Therefore, one factor present in many patients with myocardial fibrosis, such as reduced chamber compliance, may be offset by another, such as atrial hypertrophy with a vigorous atrial contribution to filling. In early diastole, slowed left ventricular pressure decay may not result in reduced early filling because left atrial driving pressure is increased from chronic intravascular volume expansion. Thus, unlike acute ischemia, myocardial fibrosis following infarction is often accompanied by various adaptive changes in structure and function.

In response to exercise, normal filling rates are present in patients with past myocardial infarction (40). This occurred despite a limited acceleration of left ventricular pressure decay during exercise which was apparently balanced by an increase in left atrial driving pressure.

CONCLUSIONS

Exercise has unique effects on diastole, affecting relaxation, pressure-volume relations, and filling dynamics. The ventricle scarred from prior myocardial infarction has new structural characteristics that modify this response to exercise. Yet the distortion of normal diastolic function during exercise becomes the greatest and most complex when exercise induces myocardial ischemia in the ventricle, either with normal structure or scarred from previous events. The pathophysiology of exercise-induced angina, although complex, has been studied extensively and has revealed much about normal and abnormal diastolic properties of the left ventricle.

REFERENCES

1. Nonogi H, Hess OM, Ritter M, Krayenbuehl HP: Diastolic properties of the normal left ventricle during supine exercise. Br Heart J 60:30, 1988.
2. Carroll JD, Hess OM, Hirzel HO, Krayenbuehl HP: Exercise-induced ischemia: The influence of altered relaxation on early diastolic pressures. Circulation 67:521, 1983.
3. Grossman W: Why is left ventricular diastolic pressure increased during angina pectoris? J Am Coll Cardiol 5:607, 1985.
4. Mahmarian JJ, Pratt CM: Silent myocardial ischemia in patients with coronary artery disease. Possible links with diastolic left ventricular dysfunction. Circulation 81 (Suppl 2):III-33, 1990.
5. Maseri A, Chierchia S, Davies G, Glazier J: Mechanisms of ischemic cardiac pain and of silent myocardial ischemia. Am J Med 79:7, 1985.
6. Turino GM: Origins of cardiac dyspnea. Primary Cardiol 7:76, 1981.
7. Mannting F: Pulmonary thallium uptake: Correlation with systolic and diastolic left ventricular function at rest and during exercise. Am Heart J 119:1137, 1990.
8. Tomoike H, et al.: Regional myocardial dysfunction and hemodynamic abnormalities with strenuous exercise in dogs with limited coronary flow. Circ Res 42:487, 1978.
9. Horwitz LD, Peterson DF, Bishop VS: Effect of regional myocardial ischemia on cardiac pump performance during exercise. Am J Physiol 234:H157, 1978.
10. Paulus WJ, Serizawa T, Grossman H: Altered left ventricular diastolic properties during pacing-induced ischemia in dogs with coronary stenoses. Circ Res 50:218, 1982.
11. Dwyer EM: Left ventricular pressure-volume alterations and regional disorders of contraction during myocardial ischemia induced by atrial pacing. Circulation 42:1111, 1970.
12. Barry WH, et al.: Changes in diastolic stiffness and tone of the left ventricle during angina pectoris. Circulation 49:255, 1974.
13. Mann T, et al.: Factors contributing to altered left ventricular diastolic properties during angina pectoris. Circulation 59:14, 1979.
14. Mann T, et al.: Effect of angina on the left ventricular diastolic pressure-volume relationship. Circulation 55:761, 1977.
15. Grossman W, Serizawa T, Carabello BA: Studies of the mechanisms of altered left ventricular diastolic pressure-volume relationship. Eur Heart J 1 (Suppl A):141, 1980.
16. Mirsky I: Assessment of diastolic function: Suggested methods and future considerations. Circulation 69:836, 1984.
17. Glantz SA, Parmley WW: Factors which affect the diastolic pressure-volume curve. Circ Res 42:171, 1978.
18. Brutsaert DL, Rademakers FE, Sys SU: Triple control of relaxation: Implications in cardiac disease. Circulation 69:190, 1984.
19. Grossman W, Barry WH: Diastolic pressure-volume relations in the diseased heart. Fed Proc 39:148, 1980.
20. Sasayama S, Nakamura Y, Kawai C: Effects of nifedipine on left ventricular distensibility, relaxation and filling dynamics during pacing-induced myocardial ischemia. Am J Cardiol 63:102E, 1989.
21. Grossman W, McLaurin LP: Diastolic properties of the left ventricle. Ann Intern Med 84:316, 1976.
22. Gaasch WH, et al.: Left ventricular compliance: Mechanisms and clinical implications. Am J Cardiol 38:645, 1976.
23. Rankin JS, et al.: Diastolic myocardial mechanics and the regulation of cardiac performance. *In* Diastolic Relaxation of the Heart. 1st Ed. Edited by W Grossman, BH Lorell. Boston, Martinus Nijhoff Publishing, 1988.
24. Hess OM, et al.: Diastolic myocardial wall stiffness and ventricular relaxation during partial and complete coronary occlusions in the conscious dog. Circ Res 52:387, 1983.
25. Momomura S, Bradley AB, Grossman W: Left ventricular diastolic pressure-segment length relations and end-diastolic distensibility in dogs with coronary stenosis. Circ Res 55:203, 1984.

26. Sasayama S, et al.: Changes in diastolic properties of the regional myocardium during pacing-induced ischemia in human subjects. J Am Coll Cardiol 5:599, 1985.

27. Carroll JD, et al.: Systolic function during exercise in patients with coronary artery disease. J Am Coll Cardiol 2:206, 1983.

28. Pouleur H, et al.: Impaired regional diastolic distensibility in coronary artery disease: Relations with dynamic left ventricular compliance. Am Heart J 112:721, 1986.

29. Mizuno K, et al.: Improved regional and global diastolic performance in patients with coronary artery disease after percutaneous transluminal coronary angioplasty. Am Heart J 115:302, 1988.

30. Bonow RO, et al.: Asynchronous left ventricular regional function and impaired global diastolic filling in patients with coronary artery disease: reversal after coronary angioplasty. Circulation 71:297, 1985.

31. Smalling RW, Kelley KO, Kirkeeide RL, Gould KL: Comparison of early systolic and early diastolic regional function during regional ischemia in a chronically instrumented canine model. J Am Coll Cardiol 2: 263, 1983.

32. Grossman W: Relaxation and diastolic distensibility of the regionally ischemic left ventricle. In Diastolic Relaxation of the Heart. 1st Ed. Edited by W Grossman, BH Lorell. Boston, Martinus Nijhoff Publishing, 1988.

33. Sasayama S: Altered diastolic distensibility during angina pectoris. In Diastolic Relaxation of the Heart. 1st Ed. Edited by W Grossman, BH Lorell. Boston, Martinus Nijhoff Publishing, 1988.

34. Pouleur H, Rousseau MF: Regional diastolic dysfunction in coronary artery disease: clinical and therapeutic implications. In Diastolic Relaxation of the Heart. 1st Ed. Edited by W Grossman, BH Lorell. Boston, Martinus Nijhoff Publishing, 1988.

35. Hirsch AT, et al.: The effect of caffeine on exercise tolerance and left ventricular function in patients with coronary artery disease. Ann Intern Med 110:593, 1989.

36. Mirsky I, Rankin JS: The effects of geometry, elasticity, and external pressure on the diastolic pressure-volume and stiffness-stress relations: How important is the pericardium? Circ Res 44:601, 1979.

37. Carroll JD, Hess OM, Hirzel HO, Krayenbuehl HP: Inconsistency of changes in right atrial pressure during exercise-induced left ventricular ischemia (abstract). Circulation 68 (Suppl 3):102, 1983.

38. Heywood JT, et al.: Right ventricular systolic function during exercise with and without significant coronary artery disease. Am J Cardiol 67:681, 1991.

39. Heywood JT, et al.: Right ventricular diastolic function during exercise: effect of ischemia. J Am Coll Cardiol 16:611, 1990.

40. Carroll JD, Hess OM, Hirzel HO, Krayenbuehl HP: Dynamics of left ventricular filling at rest and during exercise. Circulation 68:59, 1983.

41. Yellin EL, Sonnenblick EH, Frater RWM: Dynamic determinants of left ventricular filling: An overview. In Cardiac Dynamics. 1st edition. Edited by J Baan, AC Arntzenius, EL Yellin. The Hague, Martinus Nijhoff, 1980.

42. Miyazaki S, et al.: Changes of left ventricular diastolic function in exercising dogs without and with ischemia. Circulation 81: 1058, 1990.

43. Courtois M, Kovacs SJ, Ludbrook PA: Physiological early diastolic intraventricular pressure gradient is lost during acute myocardial ischemia. Circulation 81:1688, 1990.

44. Reduto LA, et al.: Left ventricular diastolic performance at rest and during exercise in patients with coronary artery disease. Circulation 63:1228, 1981.

45. Bonow RO, et al.: Impaired left ventricular diastolic filling in patients with coronary artery disease: Assessment with radionuclide angiography. Circulation 64:315, 1981.

46. Carroll J, et al.: Left ventricular systolic and diastolic function in patients with coronary artery disease: Effects of revascularization on exercise-induced ischemia. Circulation 72:119, 1985.

47. Carroll JD, et al.: Effects of ischemia, bypass surgery and past infarction on myocardial contraction, relaxation and compliance during exercise. Am J Cardiol 63:65E, 1989.

48. Hammermeister KE, Wawrbasse JR: The rate of change of left ventricular volume in man: II. Diastolic events in health and disease. Circulation 49:739, 1974.

49. Ishida Y, et al.: Peak rapid filling rate may not reflect left ventricular relation properties when left atrial pressure compensates for changes in loading conditions (abstract). Circulation 70:349, 1984.

50. Werner GS, et al.: Impaired relationship between Doppler echocardiographic parameters of diastolic function and left ventricular filling pressure during acute ischemia. Am Heart J 120:63, 1990.

51. Downes TR, et al.: Mechanism of altered pattern of left ventricular filling with aging in subjects without cardiac disease. Am J Cardiol 64:523, 1989.

52. Stoddard MF, et al.: Influence of alteration in preload on the pattern of left ventricular diastolic filling as assessed by Doppler echocardiography in humans. Circulation 79: 1226, 1989.

53. Dawson JR, Gibson DG: Left ventricular filling and early diastolic function at rest and during angina in patients with coronary artery disease. Br Heart J 61:248, 1989.

54. Myreng Y, Myhre E: Effects of verapamil on left ventricular relaxation and filling dynamics in coronary artery disease: a study by pulsed Doppler echocardiography. Am Heart J 117:870, 1989.

55. Myreng Y, Ihlen H, NitterHauge S: Effects of beta-adrenergic blockade on left ventricular relaxation and filling dynamics in coronary artery disease: A pulsed Doppler echocardiography study. Eur Heart J 9: 1167, 1988.

56. de-Bruyne B, et al.: Doppler assessment of left ventricular diastolic filling during brief coronary occlusion. Am Heart J 117:629, 1989.

57. Stoddard MF, et al.: Left ventricular diastolic function: Comparison of pulsed Doppler echocardiographic and hemodynamic indexes in subjects with and without coronary artery disease. J Am Coll Cardiol 13:327, 1989.

58. Kuecherer HF, Ruffmann K, Schaefer E, Kuebler W: Doppler echocardiographic assessment of left ventricular filling dynamics in patients with coronary heart disease and normal systolic function. Eur Heart J 9:649, 1989.

59. Appleton CP, Hatle LK, Popp RL: Relation of transmitral flow velocity patterns to left ventricular diastolic function: New insights from a combined hemodynamic and Doppler echocardiographic study. J Am Coll Cardiol 12:426, 1989.

60. Mitchell GD, et al.: Assessment of mitral flow velocity with exercise by an index of stress-induced left ventricular ischemia in coronary artery disease. Am J Cardiol 61: 536, 1988.

61. Arora RR, et al.: Atrial kinetics and left ventricular diastolic filling in the healthy elderly. J Am Coll Cardiol 9:1255, 1987.

62. Miller TR, Fountos A, Biello DR, Ludbrook PA: Detection of coronary artery disease by analysis of coronary filling. J Nucl Med 28:837, 1987.

63. Inouye IK, et al.: Left ventricular filling is usually normal in uncomplicated coronary disease. Am Heart J 110:326, 1985.

64. Bonow RO, et al.: Improved left ventricular diastolic filling in patients with coronary artery disease after percutaneous transluminal coronary angioplasty. Circulation 66: 1159, 1982.

65. Fragasso G, et al.: Symptom-limited exercise testing causes sustained diastolic dysfunction in patients with coronary disease and low effort tolerance. J Am Coll Cardiol 17:1251, 1991.

66. Perrone-Filardi P, Bacharach SL, Dilsizian V, Bonow RO: Impaired left ventricular filling and regional diastolic asynchrony at rest in coronary artery disease and relation to exercise-induced myocardial ischemia. Am J Cardiol 67:356, 1991.

67. Homans D, et al.: Effect of exercise intensity and duration on regional function during and after exercise-induced ischemia. Circulation 83:2029, 1991.

68. Hess OM, et al.: Myocardial structure of LV segments with and without exercise-induced wall motion abnormalities in patients with coronary artery disease (abstract). J Am Coll Cardiol 1:734, 1983.

69. Borg TK, Caulfield JB: The collagen matrix of the heart. Fed Proc 40:2037, 1981.

70. Robinson TF, et al.: Structure and function of connective tissue in cardiac muscle: Collagen types I and III in endomysial struts and pericellular fibers. Scanning Microsc. 2:1005, 1988.

71. Weber KT, et al.: Collagen in the hypertrophied pressure-overloaded myocardium. Circulation 75:40, 1987.

72. Judgitt BI, Amy TBM: Healing after myocardial infarction in the dog: Changes in infarct hydroxyproline and topography. J Am Coll Cardiol 7:91, 1986.

73. Hefner LL, Bowen TE: Elastic components of cat papillary muscle. Am J Physiol 212: 1221, 1987.

74. Carroll EP, Janicki JS, Pick R, Weber KT: Myocardial stiffness and reparative fibrosis following coronary embolisation in the rat. Cardiovasc Res 23:655, 1989.

Chapter 16

DIASTOLIC DYSFUNCTION DURING PACING-INDUCED ANGINA PECTORIS

Yasuyuki Nakamura and Shigetake Sasayama

THE MECHANISM FOR INDUCTION OF ISCHEMIA BY RAPID PACING

Several methods have been used to elucidate potentially ischemic myocardium that functions normally at the resting state but becomes disturbed in function in the stressed state. These include dynamic exercise test (1, 2), isometric exercise test (3), infusion of catecholamines such as dobutamine (4), and chronotropic stress test with pacing tachycardia (5–7). Among these stress tests, pacing tachycardia is the most convenient method because of its easy applicability, good reproducibility, reliability, and safety.

The mechanism for induction of ischemia by rapid pacing has been attributed to an increase in myocardial oxygen consumption secondary to the increased heart rate and to an increase in myocardial contractility related to the Treppe effect (8). Compared with dynamic exercise, however, a rise in rate-pressure product (heart rate × peak systolic pressure), an estimate of myocardial oxygen consumption is minimal (9). (See Chap. 15.) Furthermore, the minute stroke work with rapid pacing does not increase significantly enough to account for ischemia in patients with coronary artery disease because the stroke work per beat during rapid pacing falls substantially because of a drop in the stroke volume which inversely correlates with heart rate, and with no change or even a decrease in the aortic pressure. But ischemia does occur with rapid pacing in patients with coronary artery disease. Parker and co-workers measured arterial and coronary sinus blood lactate concentration before, during, and after rapid pacing, and have demonstrated the shift from lactate extraction to lactate production with pacing (10).

More recently, Heller and co-workers have demonstrated myocardial ischemia on thallium myocardial scan during rapid pacing in patients with coronary artery disease (11). Thallium redistribution was present on the delayed images.

Because ischemia is definitely induced with rapid pacing in patients with coronary artery disease despite a minimal increase in myocardial oxygen demand, a more important mechanism for ischemia with this intervention has to be substantiated. With rapid pacing, the diastolic filling period shortens inversely with the heart rate. Initially, the isovolumic relaxation rate may not change, in contrast to tachycardia induced by exercise or catecholamine infusion, in which case it accelerates. Shortening of the diastole and no change in the relaxation rate during rapid pacing may not have any deleterious effects on coronary circulation in normal subjects, but this condition can limit coronary flow in patients in whom coronary reserve is diminished and hence may result in ischemia. Ischemia causes impaired relaxation and a decrease in left ventricular compliance. These two changes may further limit the coronary circulation in such patients, and thus a vicious circle may be established. Therefore, one of the important mechanisms for ischemia with rapid pacing in patients with diminished coronary reserve appears to be the generation of the vicious circle in coronary circulation.

QUANTITATIVE ANALYSIS OF REGIONAL MYOCARDIAL FUNCTION

Automatic Processing of Cineventriculograms for Analysis of Regional Myocardial Function

Simultaneous left ventricular pressure measurement with high-fidelity micromanometer-tipped catheter and frame-by-frame analysis of left ventricular volume are of fundamental importance for studies of ventricular function utilizing cineventriculograms in humans. To reduce tedious and laborious tasks involved in the frame-by-frame analysis of consecutive cine film and to expedite analysis without observers' variation, we developed an automatic processing system using computers (6, 12, 13). The left ventricular images on each cine film were scanned by a flying spot scanner and stored on magnetic disc. Digitized images consisted of 128×128 pixels with gray levels of 256 values. The spatial derivatives of the gray levels were then obtained and the left ventricular boundaries were automatically determined using a heuristic method to search for the local maximal gradient values. The algorithm of the boundary tracing consists of two major weight coefficients for direction and depth of search. The former enables avoidance of an abrupt change in the direction of edge tracing and the latter is to refer to the sequential information of several remote edge points. In addition, the boundary of the preceding frame is always referred to as a global guidance. This border algorithm closely imitates visual detection of a boundary by the human eye (6, 12, 13).

When the entire edge was detected, the position of the aortic valve was determined at the area where the separation of the segments across the outflow tract of the left ventricle is the shortest. The apex is determined at the point with the longest distance from the midpoint of the aortic valve.

The left ventricular volumes (V) were calculated by a modification of Kennedy's formula (14):

$$V = 0.687 \times C^3 \times A^2/L + 1.9 \text{ mL}$$

where A is the area of the ventricle, calculated from the amount of pixels surrounded by the left ventricular boundary; L is the longest measured length between the midpoint of aortic valve and the apex; C is the linear correction factors for the magnification of a unit of length (one pixel), which was derived from the comparison to the known area of 1 cm² grid filmed in parallel to the tube at the position of the heart.

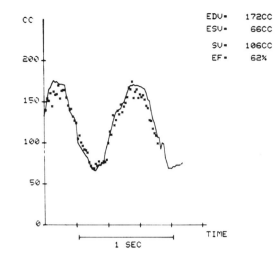

Fig. 16–1. Left ventricular volume calculated manually, (cross) plotted with respect to time of exposure and automated time-volume curve, in the same patient. Reproduced with permission from Sasayama S, et al.: An automated method for left ventricular volume measurement from the cineventriculography with minimal doses of contrast medium. Am J Cardiol 48:746, 1981.

Figure 16–1 shows the conventionally determined left ventricular volumes plotted with respect to time exposure and superimposed on the automated time volume curve of the same patient. Because there was close agreement in these two values, our computerized method of volume calculation proved to be valid (13).

Quantitative Assessment of Regional Wall Motion

Although, in the experimental settings, the development of systolic bulge following ligation of the coronary artery supplying that area has been known since the original description of Tennant and Wiggers (15), it has not been until recent years that an assessment of similar regional myocardial phenomenon became possible in clinical settings.

Fixed External Reference Markers for Regional Wall Motion Analysis. An important consideration in precise identification of localized myocardial dysfunction resulting from coronary artery disease is the reference system used. It is necessary to achieve proper superimposition of sequential ventricular images. We chose a reference system employing fixed external markers, because when it is used, the regional wall motion abnormalities have been shown to be most accurately represented as predicted by the location of myocardial infarction (6, 12, 13).

Radial System for Regional Wall Motion Analysis. When attempting to quantify the extent of the regional wall motion abnormalities, the fixing of a reference point to which the inward wall motion can be related is more controversial. To evaluate regional wall motion, three models have been considered: (1) radial system, (2) chord system, and (3) area system. Karsch and co-workers (16) compared the three quantitative methods in the 30° right anterior oblique and 60° left anterior oblique projections and concluded that the radial method provided the best separation of normal and abnormal regions and best reflected symmetric uniform motion of the ventricular silhouette with intact coronary arteries. On the other hand, Gelberg and co-workers (17) reported that the area method was the most accurate in assessing local wall motion abnormalities. However, in this area system, the ventricular silhouette was divided into five areas in the right anterior oblique view and three areas in the left anterior oblique view. Therefore, although the wall motion disturbance in each area could be represented by the abnormality of systolic reduction for the respective area, such a large grouping of segments is not likely to sufficiently characterize the extent of abnormal wall motion.

It has been widely accepted that the direction of ventricular wall motion is much closer to natural behavior for all areas if it is expressed along radial lines. In our study, the sequential ventricular silhouettes automatically determined were superimposed by using external reference markers. The geometric center of end-diastolic silhouette was chosen as the fixed reference point to which concentric wall motion was related. The position of the center of gravity was examined in each ventricular silhouette in five normal subjects, and its spatial movement proved to be normal. If asynchronous contraction occurs, this point will shift toward that area (6).

ALTERATIONS IN EARLY LEFT VENTRICULAR FILLING WITH ISCHEMIA

Early left ventricular filling is important for ventricular ejection because the predominant filling takes place during this period. Controversy exists as to whether or not ischemia causes reduction in the peak rate of early ventricular filling. The peak rate of early ventricular filling demonstrated by radionuclide angiography in patients with coronary artery disease has been shown to be diminished. Bonow and co-workers reported that the abnormality of the early ventricular filling was independent of left ventricular systolic function and the presence or absence of previous myocardial infarction (18). However, the active relaxation of myocardium has been shown to be heavily influenced by the systolic dynamics. Thus, a substantial amount of elastic energy is stored during the process of systolic shortening; this provides for an elastic recoil to expand the muscle in early diastole (19). Sasayama and co-workers produced experimental heart failure in canine hearts by continuous rapid ventricular pacing. Thereby diastolic pressure-volume curve shifted upward and to the right along with the single relation together with a conspicuous upward shift of the early diastolic portion of the pressure-volume curve (Fig. 16–2). This shift indicates that, in the failing heart, left ventricular relaxation was severely impaired but myocardial distensibility remained unaltered. Inotropic stimulation substantially improved left ventricular relaxation of the failing heart. This improvement of relaxation appears to be mediated partly by increased systolic shortening with enhancement of internal restoring forces within the ventricle (19). A study by Carroll and co-workers, in which left cineventriculography during exercise was analyzed, showed that early left ventricular filling was augmented in patients with ischemia as well as in patients without ischemia (2). This study showed that the increase in peak filling rate during exercise was caused by a higher left atrial pressure in patients in whom ischemia developed. Furthermore, Aroesty and co-workers, who used radionuclide ventriculography during pacing, achieved similar results (20).

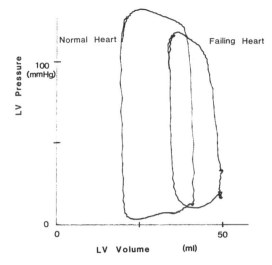

Fig. 16–2. Representative pressure-volume loops obtained in the control state (left) and after pacing (right). In the failing heart, an increase in diastolic volume was accompanied by a comparable rise in diastolic pressure. Therefore, the diagram shifted upward and to the right along with the single diastolic pressure-volume relationship; however, there was a distinct upward shift of the early diastolic portion of the loops. Reproduced with permission from Sasayama S, Asanoi H, Ishizaka S: Mechanics of contraction and relaxation of the ventricle in experimental heart failure produced by rapid ventricular pacing in the conscious dog. Eur Heart J 12 (Suppl. C), 1991.

These studies have paid attention to overall ventricular filling. An ischemic insult, however, is primarily regional in nature; the analysis of regional myocardial function in addition to the determination of global ventricular performance is crucial. (See Chap. 19.) Our study was designed to investigate regional myocardial dynamics in addition to global ventricular filling in patients with coronary artery disease during postpacing ischemic periods.

Analysis of Pacing-Induced Changes in Hemodynamics and Ventricular Function in Coronary Artery Disease

The effect of pacing was studied in 11 patients with coronary artery disease. All of the 11 patients with coronary artery disease developed typical anginal pain during pacing tachycardia, and the hemodynamics and the ventricular functions were examined in the postpacing beat. The heart rate

and the peak left ventricular pressure did not change significantly with pacing stress (Fig. 16–3). The left ventricular end-diastolic pressure rose significantly with ischemic intervention. Impairment of ventricular ejection is indicated by decreases in the ejection fraction and the percent shortening (%L) of the ischemic segment. The relaxation time constant increased significantly, implying impairment of relaxation with ischemia. The %L of the control segment did not change in postpacing beats. The peak rate of early left ventricular filling (LVPF), the LVPF/stroke volume (SV), and the LVPF/end-diastolic volume (EDV) did not change significantly.

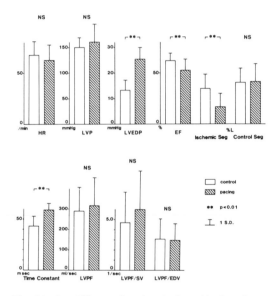

Fig. 16–3. Effects of pacing-induced ischemia on hemodynamics and ventricular function. Control data are shown by open bars and postpacing data by shaded bars. The heart rate (HR) and the peak left ventricular pressure (LVP) did not change significantly. The left ventricular end-diastolic pressure (LVEDP) rose significantly with ischemic intervention. Impairment of ventricular ejection is indicated by decreases in the ejection fraction (EF) and the percent shortening (%L) of the ischemic segment. The relaxation time constant (Time Constant) increased significantly, implying impairment of relaxation with ischemia. The %L of the control segment did not change in postpacing beats. The peak rate of early left ventricular filling (LVPF), the LVPF/stroke volume (SV), and the LVPF/end-diastolic volume (EDF) did not change significantly. ** p < 0.01, NS = not statistically significant. n = 11 except for Time Constant, where n = 7.

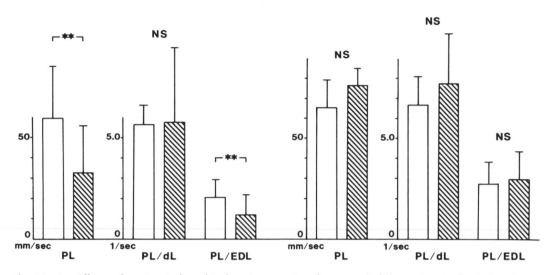

Fig. 16–4. Effects of pacing-induced ischemia on regional myocardial dynamics. In the ischemic segment, the peak rate of lengthening (PL) decreased with pacing-induced ischemia, as did the PL/end-diastolic segment length (EDL). However, the PL/extent of shortening (dL) did not change with ischemic intervention. Analysis of the control segment showed a tendency to increase in these three variables in postpacing beats. Reproduced with permission from Nakamura Y, et al.: Effects of pacing-induced ischemia on early left ventricular filling and regional myocardial dynamics and their modification by nifedipine. Circulation 76:1232, 1987.

Figure 16–4 shows the effects of pacing-induced ischemia on regional myocardial lengthening. In the ischemic segment, the peak rate of lengthening (PL) decreased with pacing-induced ischemia, as did the PL/end-diastolic segment length (EDL). However, the PL/extent of shortening (dL) did not change with ischemic intervention. Analysis of the control segment showed a tendency to increase in these three variables in postpacing beats. In short, substantial deterioration in the global ejection, the segment shortening, and the relaxation occurred during pacing-induced ischemia in the patients with coronary artery disease. Early diastolic global filling rate did not change, probably because of an increase in left atrial pressure with ischemia.

Analyses of Asynchrony Induced by Ischemia

The results of analyses of asynchrony in left ventricular filling induced by ischemia are shown in Figure 16–5. In the study patients, the time from mitral valve opening to the left ventricular peak filling rate (MVO-PF) was slightly but not significantly decreased in postpacing beats. The absolute time difference between peak left ventricular filling and segmental peak lengthening was increased significantly by ischemic intervention in the ischemic segment but not in the control segment. Therefore, the degree of asynchrony in left ventricular filling increased with ischemia in the patients with coronary artery disease.

Alterations in Early Diastolic Function during Ischemia

Ischemia caused reduction in global regional left ventricular contraction, impairment in relaxation, asynchrony in left ventricular filling, and an increase in chamber stiffness. All of these alterations should have caused a reduction in the peak rate of early left ventricular filing (21, 22). However, the peak rate of early left ventricular filling did not decrease in this study. The aforementioned alterations caused by ischemia appear to have resulted in a concomitant increase in left atrial pressure at the time of early left ventricular filling, which was estimated by an increase in left ventricular end-diastolic pressure. Therefore, an increase in left ventricular filling pressure appears to be the mechanism for the unchanged peak rate of early left ventricular filling despite unfavorable alterations in systolic and diastolic factors that affect the rate of early left ventricular filling with ischemia.

Regional analysis in our study revealed an interesting mechanism for determining the peak rate of segmental lengthening (i.e., the peak rate of segmental lengthening decreased in the ischemic segment with ischemia), but the reduction in the rate was in proportion to the reduction in the extent of muscle shortening because the peak rate of segmental lengthening normalized for the extent of shortening did not change with ischemia. Analysis of the control segment showed some increase in the peak

rate of segmental lengthening; the peak rate of segmental lengthening normalized for extent of shortening, however, was not statistically significant.

Using an isolated heart muscle preparation contracting in physiologic sequence with the aid of a servo system, Tamiya and coworkers (23) found that the maximal velocity of isotonic muscle lengthening during diastole depends on the extent of muscle shortening during systole, and that the change in preload, afterload, and inotropic state altar the isotonic lengthening velocity only because these factors affect the extent of shortening, so that the maximal lengthening velocity divided by the extent of muscle shortening remains constant when these factors are altered. Therefore, the process of isotonic muscle lengthening simply resembles the recoiling of a spring. Although Tamiya and coworkers did not test the effect of hypoxia or ischemia on isotonic muscle-lengthening velocity, from

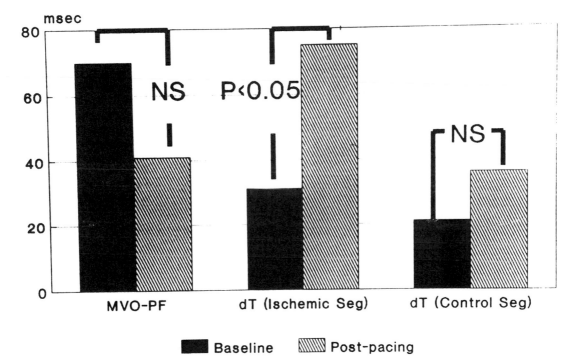

Fig. 16–5. The time from mitral valve opening to left ventricular peak filling rate (MVO-PF) tended to decrease, but the change was not statistically significant in postpacing beats (70 ± 47 to 41 ± 27 ms). The absolute time difference between left ventricular peak filling and segmental peak lengthening (dT) increased significantly in the ischemic segment (31 ± 28 to 75 ± 48 msec, p < 0.05), but not in the control segment (21 ± 16 to 36 ± 26 msec, NS).

the results of this study it can be concluded that the mechanism of reduction in the peak rate of lengthening with ischemia in the ischemic segment is caused by a decrease in the extent of shortening with ischemia because the peak rate of segmental lengthening normalized for the extent of shortening did not change with ischemia.

CHANGES IN PASSIVE ELASTIC PROPERTIES OF THE GLOBAL AND THE REGIONAL MYOCARDIUM DURING PACING-INDUCED ISCHEMIA

Changes in passive elastic properties of the global and the regional myocardium during pacing-induced ischemia were studied in seven patients with coronary artery disease. The pressure-length loops for every fourth grid of 128 radial grids were generated for the purpose of this study. Figure 16–6 showed representative pressure-length loops constructed by relating the length of each radial grid to instantaneous left ventricular pressure throughout the cardiac cycle. To analyze the effect of

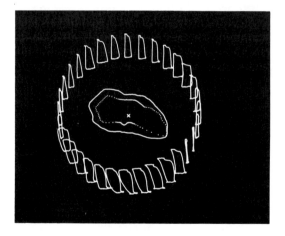

Fig. 16–6. Representative pressure-length loops constructed by relating the length of each radial grid to instantaneous left ventricular pressure throughout the cardiac cycle. The loops were originally generated for 128 radial grids, but were reduced to every fourth grid, resulting in a display of 32 loops over the entire ventricular circumference. The center of gravity of the entire ventricular end-diastolic frame is indicated by the dot. Reproduced with permission from Sasayama S, et al.: Changes in diastolic properties of the regional myocardium during pacing-induced ischemia in human subjects. JACC 5:599, 1985.

pacing stress on the ischemic myocardium, a potentially ischemic section corresponding to the known coronary lesions, in which active shortening was preserved, was compared with that of the normal section perfused with intact coronary arteries (Fig. 16–7). In the patients with overt myocardial infarction, the section that included the central ischemic region was excluded because neither dyskinetic nor akinetic motion of the definite infarction area was modified substantially by pacing stress.

First, diastolic passive properties of the global left ventricle were examined. Figure 16–8 (A and B) shows diastolic pressure-volume curves before and after rapid pacing in all seven patients. The pressure-volume curves shifted upward remarkably in the postpacing beat in four patients (Cases 1 to 4, Fig. 16-8A), whereas the curve shifted more to the right associated with upward shift in three patients (Cases 5 to 7, Fig. 16–8B).

Next, diastolic passive properties of the regional myocardium were examined. Plots of left ventricular pressure against normal and ischemic segment length throughout passive ventricular filling are shown in Figure 16–9 (A and B). In all the cases, the increase in diastolic pressure was accompanied by the comparable increases in end-diastolic length in the normal segment. Thus, the normal segment appeared to be operating at the higher portion on the single pressure-length curve. In the ischemic segment, pressure was higher at any given segment length in the postpacing beat and the pressure-length curves unequivocally shifted upward, indicating regional alteration of the diastolic passive properties of the ischemic myocardium. Accordingly, the observed global shifts of the pressure-volume relation were net results determined by the interaction of regional diastolic properties of the normal and ischemic myocardium.

Impairment of ventricular function in ischemic heart disease depends on the mechanical dysfunction of different regions of the left ventricle, and analysis of a single pressure-volume curve does not adequately define the contractile property of the ventricular myocardium during ischemia (6, 12, 13). This principle holds true in the analysis of diastolic passive

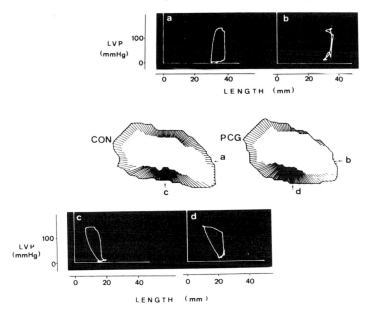

Fig. 16–7. Comparison of pressure-length loops at resting state (control [CON]) (grid a and grid c) and after rapid cardiac pacing (PCG) (grid b and grid d) for the representative two segments in the normal (lower panel) and ischemic (upper panel) areas. Pacing stress caused a remarkable increase in the left ventricular diastolic pressure and striking deformation on the loop configuration. LVP = left ventricular pressure. Reproduced with permission from Sasayama S, et al.: Changes in diastolic properties of the regional myocardium during pacing-induced ischemia in human subjects. JACC 5:599, 1985.

property of the myocardium during ischemia in patients with coronary artery disease. When global left ventricular passive elastic property was analyzed by the diastolic pressure-volume relation in these patients, two different responses were observed. In four cases, left ventricular end-diastolic pressure increased out of proportion to changes in end-diastolic volume, with the left ventricular diastolic pressure-volume curve being shifted upward; in the remaining three patients, the increased end-diastolic pressure during ischemia was accompanied by an increase in left ventricular end-diastolic volume. These observations emphasize again the controversy concerning the factors responsible for the increased end-diastolic pressure during angina. Several possibilities exist: altered left ventricular diastolic properties with reduced compliance, transient left ventricular failure, or factors extrinsic to the left ventricular myocardium, such as loading conditions of the right ventricle (24), effects of the pericardium (25) and coronary perfusion (26). However, increasing clinical and experimental studies have indicated that the factors extrinsic to the left ventricular myocardium do not account for the changes in left ventricular pressure-volume relation during ischemia, and that myocardial stiffness, per se, increases during ischemia (27–31).

When the regional responses were analyzed, the displacement of the segmental diastolic pressure-length relation during pacing-induced ischemia was remarkably consistent, depending on the ischemic status of the respective segment. We observed an upward shift of the segmental pressure-length relation in the ischemic region during angina. However, in the control segment, the elevation of end-diastolic pressure was accompanied by a comparable increase in end-diastolic length, and the segment appeared to have moved up on the single pressure-length curve to the higher and steeper portion (32). Thus, the analysis of regional myocardial function is indispensable because global function only reflects the sum of the changes in regional myocardial segment.

SUMMARY: LEFT VENTRICULAR DIASTOLIC DYSFUNCTION IN PACING-INDUCED ANGINA PECTORIS

We have previously shown that impairment of left ventricular systolic function during angina can only be adequately described when segmental wall motion analyses are performed in addition to global analyses (6, 12, 13). This principle holds true in the analysis of diastolic function of the left ventricle during ischemia in patients with coronary artery disease. That is,

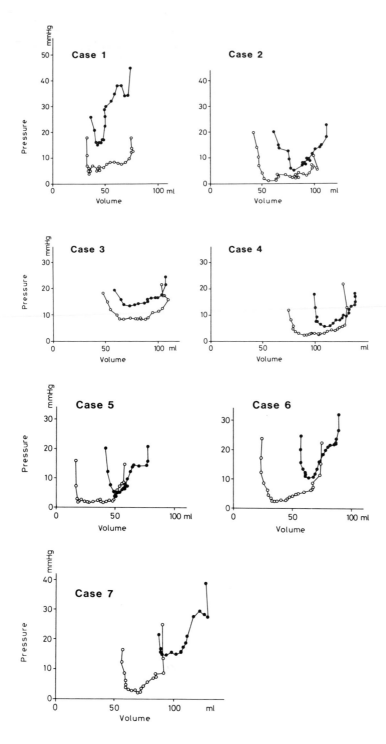

Fig. 16–8. *A* and *B,* left ventricular diastolic pressure-volume relations before (open circle) and after (closed circle) rapid cardiac pacing in seven patients with coronary artery disease. The curve shifted directly upward in four patients (Cases 1 to 4, A) and upward and more to the right in three patients (Cases 5 to 7, B) in the postpacing beat compared with the control. Reproduced with permission from Sasayama S, et al.: Changes in diastolic properties of the regional myocardium during pacing-induced ischemia in human subjects. JACC 5:599, 1985.

although isovolumic relaxation was impaired judging from an increase in isovolumic relaxation time constant, the peak rate of early left ventricular filling obtained from frame-by-frame analysis of left ventriculograms did not change significantly during ischemia. When regional wall motion was analyzed, however, asynchrony in early diastolic filling and a reduction in peak rate of segmental lengthening were

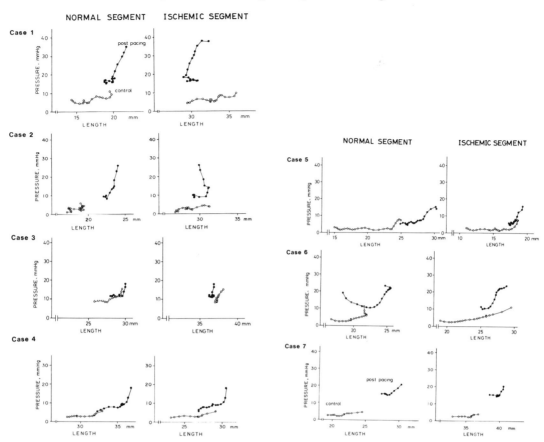

Fig. 16–9. *A* and *B,* Plots of left ventricular pressure against normal (left panels) and ischemic (right panels) segment lengths before (open circle) and after (closed circle) rapid cardiac pacing in all seven patients. Despite variations in response in pressure-volume curves (upward in Cases 1 to 4 [A] and to the right in Cases 5 to 7 [B]), there are uniform changes in the pressure-length relation, the normal segment moving up to the higher portion of the single pressure-length relation and the ischemic segment shifting upward directly. Reproduced with permission from Sasayama S, et al.: Changes in diastolic properties of the regional myocardium during pacing-induced ischemia in human subjects. JACC 5:599, 1985.

demonstrated. Likewise, analysis of global left ventricular passive elastic property by the diastolic pressure-volume relation in these patients resulted in nonuniform responses. On the other hand, when the regional responses were analyzed, the displacement of the segmental diastolic pressure-length relation during pacing-induced ischemia was remarkably consistent. That is, we observed an upward shift of the segmental pressure-length relation in the ischemic region during angina, and in the control segment, the elevation of end-diastolic pressure was accompanied by a comparable increase in end-diastolic length and the segment appeared to have moved up on the single pressure-length curve to

the higher and steeper portion. Impaired isovolumic relaxation and an increase in diastolic stiffness of the ischemic myocardium contribute to pulmonary congestion and dyspnea during ischemia.

REFERENCES

1. Thadani U, West RO, Mathew TM, Parker JO: Hemodynamics at rest and during supine and sitting bicycle exercise in patients with coronary artery disease. Am J Cardiol 39:776, 1977.
2. Carroll JD, Hess OM, Hirzel HO, Krayenbuehl HP: Dynamics of left ventricular filling at rest and during exercise. Circulation 68:59, 1983.
3. Helfant RH, DeVilla MA, Meister SG: Ef-

fect of sustained isometric handgrip exercise on left ventricular performance. Circulation 44:982, 1971.

4. Mannering D, Cripps T, Leech G, et al.: The dobutamine stress test as an alternative to exercise testing after acute myocardial infarction. Br Heart J 59:521, 1988.

5. Sowton GE, Balcon R, Cross D, Frick MH: Measurement of the angina threshold using atrial pacing. Cardiovasc Res 1:301, 1967.

6. Fujita M, Sasayama S, Kawai C, Eiho S, Kuwahara M: Automatic processing of cine-ventriculograms for analysis of regional myocardial function. Circulation 63:1065, 1981.

7. Nakamura Y, Sasayama S, Nonogi H, et al.: Effects of pacing-induced ischemia on early left ventricular filling and regional myocardial dynamics and their modification by nifedipine. Circulation 76:1232, 1987.

8. Ricci D, Orlick A, Alderman E: Role of tachycardia as an inotropic stimulus in man. J Clin Invest 63:695, 1979.

9. McKay RG, Grossman W: Hemodynamic stress testing during pacing tachycardia. *In* Cardiac catheterization and angiography, 3rd edition. Edited by Grossman W. Philadelphia, Lea & Febiger, 1986, pp. 267–281.

10. Parker JO, Chiong MA, West RO, Case RB: Sequential alterations in myocardial lactate metabolism, S-T segments, and left ventricular functions during angina induced by atrial pacing. Circulation 40:113, 1969.

11. Heller GV, Aroesry JM, Parker JA, et al.: The pacing stress test: thallium-201 myocardial imaging after atrial pacing: Diagnostic value in detecting coronary artery disease compared with exercise testing. J Am Coll Cardiol 3:1197, 1984.

12. Sasayama S, Nonogi H, Kawai C: Assessment of left ventricular function using an angiographic method. Jpn Circ J 46:1127, 1982.

13. Sasayama S, Nonogi H, Kawai C, et al.: An automated method for left ventricular volume measurement from the cineventriculography with minimal doses of contrast medium. Am J Cardiol 48:746, 1981.

14. Kennedy JW, Trenholme SE, Kasser IS: Left ventricular volume and mass from single plane angiogram. A comparison of anteroposterior and right anterior oblique methods. Am Heart J 80:343, 1970.

15. Tennant R, Wiggers CJ: The effect of coronary occlusion on myocardial contraction. Am J Physiol 112:351, 1935.

16. Karsch KR, Lamm U, Blanke H, Rentrop KP: Comparison of nineteen quantitative models for assessment of localized left ventricular wall motion abnormalities. Clin Cardiol 3:123, 1980.

17. Gelberg HJ, Brundage BH, Glants S, Parmley WW: Quantitative left ventricular wall motion analysis: A comparison of area, chord and radial methods. Circulation 59:991, 1979.

18. Bonow RD, Bacharach SL, Green MV, et al.: Impaired left ventricular diastolic filling in patients with coronary artery disease: assessment with radionuclide angiography. Circulation 64:315, 1981.

19. Sasayama S, Asanoi H, Ishizaka S: Mechanics of contraction and relaxation of the ventricle in experimental heart failure produced by rapid ventricular pacing in the conscious dog. Eur Heart J 12 (Suppl. C): 35–41, 1991.

20. Aroesty JM, McKay RG, Heller GV, et al.: Simultaneous assessment of left ventricular systolic and diastolic dysfunction during pacing-induced ischemia. Circulation 71: 889, 1985.

21. Kumada T, Karliner JS, Pouler H, et al.: Effects of coronary occlusion on early ventricular diastolic events in conscious dogs. Am J Physiol 237:H542, 1979.

22. Yamagishi T, Ozaki M, Kumada T, et al.: Asynchronous left ventricular diastolic filling in patients with isolated disease of the left anterior descending coronary artery: Assessment with radionuclide ventriculography. Circulation 69:933, 1984.

23. Tamiya K, Sugawara M, Sakurai Y: Maximum lengthening velocity during isotonic relaxation at preload in canine papillary muscle. Am J Physiol 237:H83, 1979.

24. Visner MS, Arentzen CE, Crumbley AJ III, et al.: The effects of pressure-induced right ventricular hypertrophy or left ventricular diastolic properties and dynamic geometry in the conscious dog. Circulation 74:410, 1986.

25. Spotonitz HM, Kaiser GA: The effect of the pericardium on pressure-volume relations in the canine left ventricle. J Surg Res 11: 375, 1971.

26. Salisbury PF, Cross CE, Rieben PA: Influence of coronary artery pressure upon myocardial elasticity. Circ Res 8:794, 1960.

27. Wijns W, Serruys PW, Slager CJ, et al.: Effect of coronary occlusion during percutaneous transluminal angioplasty in humans on left ventricular chamber stiffness and regional diastolic pressure-radius relations. JACC 7:455, 1986.

28. Visner MS, Arentzen CE, Parrish DG, et al.: Effects of global ischemia on diastolic properties of the left ventricle in the conscious dog. Circulation 71:610, 1985.

29. Serizawa T, Carabello BA, Grossman W:

Effect of pacing-induced ischemia on left ventricular diastolic pressure-volume relations in dogs with coronary stenosis. Circ Res 46:430, 1980.

30. Paulus WJ, Serizawa T, Grossman W: Altered left ventricular diastolic properties during pacing-induced ischemia in dogs with coronary stenosis. Potentiation by caffeine. Circ Res 50:218, 1982.

31. Templeton GH, Wildenthal K, Mitchell JH: Influence of coronary blood flow on left ventricular contractility and stiffness. Am J Physiol 223:1216, 1972.

32. Sasayama S, Nonogi H, Miyazaki S, et al.: Changes in diastolic properties of the regional myocardium during pacing-induced ischemia in human subjects. JACC 5:599, 1985.

Chapter 17

DIFFERENT EFFECTS OF "SUPPLY" AND "DEMAND" ISCHEMIA ON LEFT VENTRICULAR DIASTOLIC FUNCTION IN HUMANS

Walter J. Paulus, Jean G.F. Bronzwaer, Bernard de Bruyne, and William Grossman

In the past, duration of ischemia has received more attention as a determinant of mechanical function of ischemic myocardium than the precise nature of the ischemic insult. This led to a classification (1–3) of the myocardial effects of an ischemic episode into reversible dysfunction as occurs after a brief coronary occlusion, myocardial stunning as observed following reperfusion after a longer coronary occlusion, and hibernation characterized by slow recovery of myocardial function on restoration of perfusion after protracted episodes of ischemia.

The precise nature of the ischemic insult has aroused scientific interest as an important modulator of resulting mechanical dysfunction of ischemic myocardium (4). In excised and isovolumic rodent hearts, left ventricular peak-systolic pressure is less depressed after a brief episode of hypoxia than after no-flow ischemia, and a brief episode of hypoxia (but not of ischemia) causes a rise of left ventricular end-diastolic pressure (5). In anesthetized dogs, 3 minutes of pacing tachycardia in the presence of coronary stenoses (demand ischemia) affect ischemic myocardium differently from 3 minutes of coronary occlusion (supply ischemia) (6, 7). Another example of modulation of mechanical dysfunction of ischemic myocardium by the nature of the ischemic insult is preconditioning to a prolonged ischemic insult by brief foregoing ischemic episodes (8).

Since the advent of coronary angioplasty, the myocardial effects of brief ischemic episodes could easily be investigated in humans during angioplasty balloon coronary occlusions. Initial studies assessed the effects of brief ischemic episodes of balloon coronary occlusion in terms of loss of global and regional systolic function (9). These studies were followed by analysis of diastolic myocardial function (10), which appeared to be an earlier and more sensitive marker of myocardial ischemia during balloon coronary occlusion (11). The specific nature of balloon coronary occlusion ischemia was subsequently characterized in man by pharmacologic modulation of the ischemic insult (12), by demonstration of preconditioning during repetitive balloon coronary occlusions (13), and by comparison to regional left ventricular wall motion during pacing angina (14). The studies presented in this chapter make further use of angioplasty balloon coronary occlusion to explore in man diastolic myocardial function (14) and metabolic alterations (15) during coronary occlusion (no-flow ischemia), during pacing-induced angina (low flow-high demand ischemia), and during coronary occlusion with maintained hypoxic perfusion distal to the balloon occlusion (hypoxia) (16). (See Chaps. 15 and 16.)

METHODS

Patient Characteristics

Thirty-four patients were included in the present studies. All had exercise-induced angina. No patient had angina at rest or previous myocardial infarction as evident from the electrocardiogram (ECG) at rest and the normal global and regional left ventricular wall motion on the left ventricular angiogram. Prior diagnostic left heart catheterization and coronary angiography revealed normal left ventricular function at rest, single-vessel coronary disease consisting of a significant (>80%) proximal LAD stenosis, and absence of spontaneously visible collaterals to the distal LAD on contralateral coronary injection. All drugs with inotropic effects were withheld before the study except in two patients, who experienced angina at moderate exercise in the last 48 hours before hospital admission. Premedication consisted of 10 mg diazepam. All patients gave informed consent. There was no complication related to procedure or study protocol.

Study Protocols

A 7 French (F) pigtail Sentron tip-micromanometer catheter and an 8F angioplasty guiding catheter were advanced from the left and right femoral arteries. In 11 patients, a 6F NIH catheter was advanced into the coronary sinus from an antecubital vein or from the right femoral vein. The high-fidelity tip-micromanometer left ventricular pressure signal and a single plane 30 degrees right anterior oblique left ventricular angiogram were recorded simultaneously in the resting state using angiographic markers, an injection marker, and 0.5 mL/kg ioxaglate as contrast agent. Following this baseline left ventricular angiogram, three different study protocols were followed:

Protocol 1: Comparative effects of pacing-induced and balloon coronary occlusion ischemia on left ventricular diastolic function in man (n = 12) (14). Right ventricular pacing was initiated at a rate of 90 beats/min and was increased in a stepwise manner by 30 beats/min every 2 minutes. Pacing was continued until the appearance of angina. A second left ventricular angiogram with simultaneous recording of left ventricular pressure was obtained immediately on cessation of pacing. After the second left ventricular angiogram, end-diastolic left ventricular pressure was allowed to return to baseline value before the angioplasty procedure was started. A third left ventricular angiogram with simultaneous recording of left ventricular pressure was obtained just before balloon deflation

at the end of a fourth angioplasty balloon inflation of 60 seconds' duration.

Protocol 2: Metabolic alterations during pacing-induced and balloon coronary occlusion ischemia in man (n = 11) (15): Right ventricular pacing was initiated at a rate of 90 beats/min and increased in a stepwise manner by 30 beats/min every 2 minutes. Pacing was continued until the appearance of angina. A second left ventricular angiogram with simultaneous recording of left ventricular pressure was obtained immediately on cessation of pacing. Blood samples were drawn from the coronary sinus catheter and from the side-arm of an arterial sheath before pacing, during the last 15 seconds of each pacing step and 10, 30, and 120 seconds after cessation of pacing. After the second left ventricular angiogram, end-diastolic left ventricular pressures were allowed to return to baseline value before the angioplasty procedure was started. A third left ventricular angiogram with simultaneous recording of left ventricular pressure was obtained just before balloon deflation at the end of a second angioplasty balloon inflation of 60 seconds duration. Blood samples were drawn from the coronary sinus catheter and from the side-arm of an arterial sheath before the second balloon inflation, after 30 seconds during the second balloon occlusion and 10, 30, and 120 seconds after deflation of the balloon. Concentrations of H^+, K^+, and lactate were determined on each blood sample.

Protocol 3: Comparative effects of hypoxia and ischemia on left ventricular diastolic function in man (n = 11) (16). A second left ventricular angiogram with simultaneous recording of left ventricular pressure was obtained just before balloon deflation at the end of a second angioplasty balloon inflation of 60 seconds duration. After the second left ventricular angiogram, end-diastolic left ventricular pressure was allowed to return to baseline value before starting a third angioplasty balloon inflation of equal duration to the second balloon inflation (51 ± 12 sec). During the third angioplasty balloon inflation, saline was perfused (1 mL/sec) through the distal lumen of the balloon catheter. At the end of the third angioplasty balloon inflation just before deflation of the balloon, a third left ventricular angiogram with simultaneous recording of left ventricular pressure was obtained.

All patients experienced chest pain and ischemic ST segment changes during the pacing stress test and the balloon occlusions of coronary angioplasty. Coronary angioplasty was successful in all patients with minimal residual coronary stenosis.

Data Acquisition and Analysis

Left ventricular volumes and pressures were matched using cine frame markers. Left ventricular volumes were calculated according to the area-length method and a regression formula. Frame-by-frame analysis was performed on the third to fourth beat after contrast appearance and nonsinus or potentiated beats were excluded from the analysis. Regional wall motion was analyzed using the end-diastolic center of mass as a reference point and 28 sectors emerging from the center of mass. Radial length was calculated for each frame as the distance from the center of mass to the endocardial contour of an ischemic and nonischemic sector (17, 18). Percentage systolic shortening was expressed as the ratio of the difference between the end-diastolic and end-systolic radial lengths divided by the end-diastolic radial length. In each individual, the reported angiographic value is the mean of three measurements (intraobserver variability for left ventricular volume = 1.5%; intraobserver variability for radial length = 1.6%). A monoexponential curve fit with a 0 mm Hg asymptote pressure was used to calculate the time constant of left ventricular pressure decay (19) from the left ventricular tip-micromanometer left ventricular pressure signal, which was digitized from the moment of left ventricular dP/dt min to a left ventricular pressure, which equaled left ventricular end-diastolic pressure plus 5 mm Hg. Diastolic left ventricular pressure-volume plots and diastolic left ventricular pressure-radial length plots of the ischemic segment were constructed by matching corresponding points of left ventricular pressure with respectively left ventricular volume and radial length of the ischemic segment. Shifts of the diastolic left ventricular pressure-radial length plots were quantified to provide an index of dia-

stolic distensibility of the ischemic segment by calculating a mean pressure value (P_m) over which overlapping portions of the diastolic left ventricular pressure-radial length plots had moved upward. P_m was obtained by planimetry of an area enclosed by the two diastolic left ventricular pressure-radial length plots and two lines perpendicular to the radial length axis at the outer borders of the overlap region (14).

Statistical Analysis

Results are given as mean ± standard deviation. Statistical significance was set at $p < 0.05$ and was obtained by Student's test for paired data and Bonferroni's method of multiple comparison.

RESULTS

Comparative Effects of Pacing-Induced and Balloon Coronary Occlusion Ischemia on Left Ventricular Diastolic Function in Humans (n = 12)

Left ventricular (LV) hemodynamic and angiographic data at rest (REST), immediately on cessation of pacing (= Pacing-induced Ischemia; PI) and at the end of balloon coronary occlusion (CO) are shown in Figures 17–1 and 17–2. Ejection Fraction (EF) decreased from 77 ± 7% at rest to 71 ± 9% immediately following pacing tachycardia (NS) and to 47 ± 11% at the end of CO ($p < 0.01$ versus REST and PI) with individual EF data varying from 73% to 30% at the end of CO. Left ventricular end-diastolic pressure (LVEDP) rose from 14 ± 4 mm Hg at rest to 24 ± 7 mm Hg ($p < 0.01$) immediately following pacing and to 21 ± 8 mm Hg ($p < 0.01$) at the end of CO. Left ventricular end-diastolic volume index (LVEDVI) rose from 83 ± 19 mL/m^2 at rest to 88 ± 17 mL/m^2 immediately following pacing (NS) and to 96 ± 16 mL/m^2 at the end of CO ($p < 0.05$ versus R and PI). For the pooled patient data, these findings are consistent with PI causing an upward shift of the end-diastolic LV pressure-volume relation and CO causing an upward and rightward shift of the relation. However, individual patient response was variable, as is evident from Figure 17–3, which shows examples of diastolic LV pressure-volume relations, representing ex-

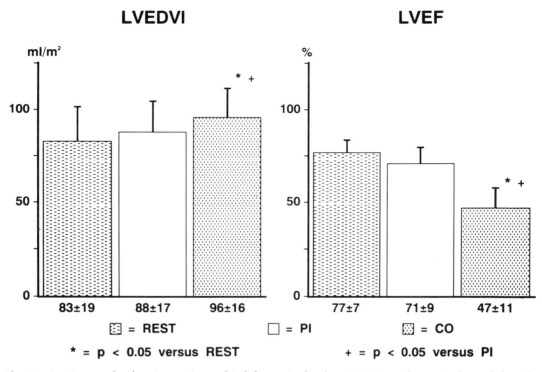

Fig. 17–1. Bar graphs showing angiographic left ventricular data (LVEDVI: Left ventricular end-diastolic volume index; LVEF: Left ventricular ejection fraction) obtained at rest (REST), during pacing-induced ischemia (PI), and at the end of balloon coronary occlusion (CO). Only at the end of CO was there a significant rise of LVEDVI and a significant fall of LVEF with respect to both REST and PI data.

tremes of responses to CO. In the left-hand panel, ejection fraction was preserved at the end of CO and an upward shift of the diastolic LV pressure-volume relation was observed both immediately after pacing and at the end of CO. In the right-hand panel, ejection fraction was reduced at the end of CO. The diastolic LV pressure-volume relation at the end of CO was superimposable on the terminal portion of the diastolic LV pressure-volume relation at rest and the diastolic LV pressure-volume relation following pacing was shifted upward.

A similar interaction between systolic performance and diastolic distensibility changes was observed when analyzing regional LV function. Figure 17–4 shows diastolic LV pressure-radial length plots of the ischemic segment observed in three patients, again representing extremes of responses to PI and to CO. In the left panel, the diastolic LV pressure-radial length plot shows a marked upward shift immediately following pacing. At the end of CO, it falls

on the REST curve. Following pacing, the upward shift of the diastolic LV pressure-radial length plot of the ischemic segment is accompanied by preserved systolic shortening, whereas at the end of CO, systolic shortening is greatly reduced. In the upper right panel, the LV pressure-radial length plots following pacing and at the end of CO both coincide with the LV pressure-radial length plot at REST. In this patient, systolic shortening of the ischemic segment was profoundly impaired both following pacing tachycardia and at the end of CO. In the bottom panel, upward shifting of the left ventricular pressure-radial length plot is seen, both following pacing and at the end of CO. In this patient, systolic shortening of the ischemic segment was well preserved in both conditions. The shifts of the diastolic left ventricular pressure-radial length plots of the ischemic segments were quantified by a P_m value or a mean pressure value, over which overlapping portions of the diastolic LV pressure-radial

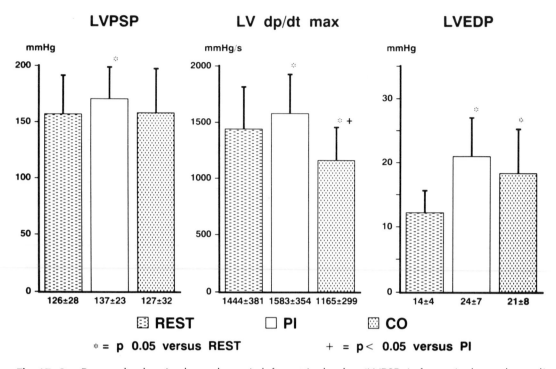

Fig. 17–2. Bar graphs showing hemodynamic left ventricular data (LVPSP: Left ventricular peak systolic pressure; LV dp/dt max: Maximal rate of left ventricular pressure rise; LVEDP: Left ventricular end-diastolic pressure) obtained at rest (REST), during pacing-induced ischemia (PI) and at the end of balloon coronary occlusion (CO). PI induced a significant rise of LVPSP, LV dp/dt max, and LVEDP with respect to REST data. CO caused a significant fall of LV dp/dt max with respect to both REST and PI data and a significant rise of LVEDP with respect to REST data.

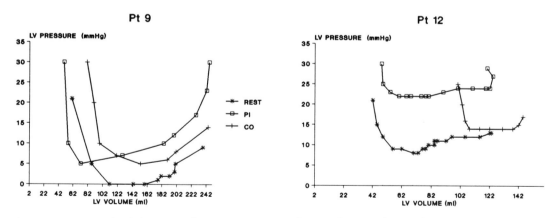

Fig. 17–3. Diastolic left ventricular (LV) pressure-volume relations observed in two patients at rest (REST), during pacing-induced ischemia (PI) and at the end of balloon coronary occlusion (CO). In the left-hand panel, LV stroke volume was well preserved during both PI and CO, and an upward shift of the diastolic LV pressure-volume relation was observed with respect to the REST curve during both PI and CO. In the right-hand panel, LV stroke volume was well preserved during PI but not during CO, and an upward shift of the diastolic LV pressure-volume relation was observed during PI but not during CO. Reproduced with permission from Bronzwaer JGF, et al.: Comparative effects of pacing-induced and balloon coronary occlusion ischemia on left ventricular diastolic function in man. Circulation 84: 211, 1991.

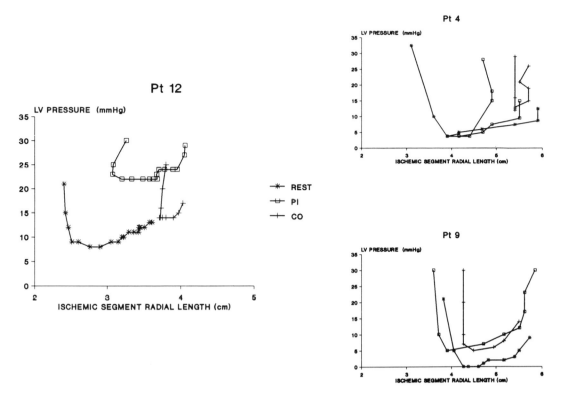

Fig. 17–4. Diastolic left ventricular (LV) pressure-radial length plots of the ischemic segment observed in 3 patients at rest (REST), during pacing-induced ischemia (PI) and at the end of balloon coronary occlusion (CO). In the left panel, PI resulted in a small drop of systolic shortening of the ischemic segment and an upward shift of the diastolic LV pressure-radial length relation, whereas CO caused a profound depression of systolic shortening and no shift of the diastolic LV pressure-radial length relation. In the right panel, both PI and CO induced severe reductions of systolic shortening of the ischemic segment and no shifts of the diastolic LV pressure-radial length relations. In the bottom panel, systolic shortening of the ischemic segment was well preserved during both PI and CO and both interventions resulted in an upward shift of the diastolic LV pressure-radial length relation.

length plots had moved upward. The higher the P_m, the lower the regional diastolic distensibility. Following pacing, P_m equaled 7 ± 5 mm Hg and at the end of CO, P_m equaled 3 ± 2 mm Hg ($p < 0.05$). At the end of CO, a correlation was observed between the upward shift of the diastolic LV pressure-radial length plot of the ischemic segment, quantified by P_m, and systolic shortening of the ischemic segment, expressed as a fraction of the value at rest (fSS) ($P_m = 7.6 \times$ fSS $+ 1.8$; r $= 0.64$; $p < 0.03$). For the pooled patient data, % systolic shortening of the ischemic segment fell from $40.1 \pm 10.6\%$ at rest to $25.8 \pm 8.6\%$ immediately following pacing ($p < 0.01$) and to $6.4 \pm 8.6\%$ at the end of CO ($p < 0.01$).

Metabolic Alterations during Pacing-Induced and Balloon Coronary Occlusion Ischemia in Humans (n = 11)

Concentrations of H^+, K^+, and lactate were determined on blood samples drawn from a coronary sinus catheter and from the side-arm of an arterial sheath. Sampling was performed before initiation of the pacing stress test, during the last 15 seconds of each pacing step, 10, 30 and 120 seconds after cessation of pacing, before balloon CO, after 30 seconds of balloon CO, and 10, 30, and 120 seconds after deflation of the balloon. During pacing, lactate extraction changed to lactate production during the second pacing step; significant lactate production was observed

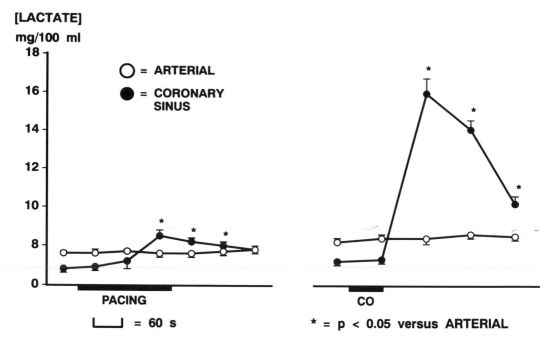

Fig. 17–5. Concentrations of lactate in coronary sinus and arterial blood at 1-minute intervals before, during, and after pacing stress test (left-hand panel) and before, during and after angioplasty balloon coronary occlusion (CO) (right-hand panel). During the pacing stress test, lactate extraction changed to lactate production. This implied washout of tissue metabolites at the time of hemodynamic data procurement upon cessation of pacing. At the end of CO, there was persistent lactate extraction. This implied absence of washout of tissue metabolites at the time of hemodynamic data procurement at the end of CO.

during the two last pacing steps and continued for 90 seconds after cessation of pacing (Fig. 17–5). Lactate concentration in the coronary sinus was lower than in arterial blood during balloon coronary occlusion. Immediately upon deflation of the angioplasty balloon, a sharp rise in coronary sinus lactate concentration was observed, and persisted for 120 seconds after balloon deflation (Fig. 17–5). Similar patterns were observed for H^+ and K^+ concentrations in the coronary sinus and arterial blood samples.

Comparative Effects of Hypoxia and Ischemia on Left Ventricular Diastolic Function in Humans (n = 11)

The LV effects of no-flow ischemia and of hypoxia were investigated in humans by comparing LV function at the end of a balloon CO to LV function at the end of an equally long (51 ± 12 seconds) balloon CO,

during which saline was perfused at a flow rate of 1 ml/s through the distal lumen of the balloon catheter. The bar graphs of Figure 17–6 show hemodynamic data at REST, at the end of a balloon CO, and at the end of a balloon CO with maintained hypoxic perfusion (CO + PER). LVEDP rose from 18 ± 9 mm Hg at REST to 29 ± 6 mm Hg ($p < 0.01$) at the end of balloon CO and to 36 ± 8 mm Hg ($p < 0.01$ versus REST; $p < 0.01$ versus CO) at the end of CO + PER. LVEDVI showed a similar rise at the end of balloon CO and at the end of balloon CO + PER (REST: 71 ± 13 mL/m^2; CO: 75 ± 15 mL/m^2; CO + PER: 75 ± 14 mL/m^2). A higher LVEDP at the end of balloon CO + PER than at the end of balloon CO despite equal LVEDVI is consistent with induction of a straight upward shift of the end-diastolic left ventricular pressure-volume relation by maintenance of hypoxic coronary perfusion during balloon CO. Left ventricular peak systolic

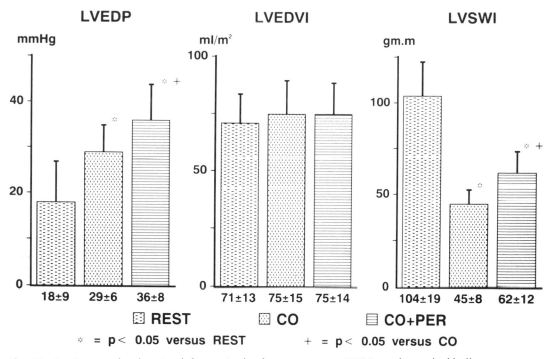

Fig. 17–6. Bar graphs showing left ventricular function at rest (REST), at the end of balloon coronary occlusion (CO), and at the end of balloon coronary occlusion with saline perfusion through the distal lumen of the balloon catheter (CO + PER). At the end of CO + PER, the rise in left ventricular end-diastolic pressure (LVEDP) was significantly larger than at the end of CO despite similar changes in left ventricular end-diastolic volume index (LVEDVI). Left ventricular stroke work index (LVSWI) was less depressed at the end of CO + PER than at the end of CO.

pressure (LVPSP) and left ventricular stroke work index (LVSWI) were higher during CO + PER than during CO (LVPSP-CO + PER: 163 ± 28 mm Hg; LVPSP-CO: 149 ± 28 mm Hg; p < 0.01) (LVSWI-CO + PER: 62 ± 12 g.m; LVSWI-CO: 45 ± 8 g.m; p < 0.01). Hence, maintenance of hypoxic coronary perfusion during balloon CO results in better preservation of LV systolic performance and a larger decrease in LV diastolic distensibility.

DISCUSSION

Comparative Analysis of Global and Regional Left Ventricular Diastolic Distensibility in Different Types of Ischemia in Humans

Clinical Observations

These studies (14–16) are the first to compare in humans diastolic distensibility of the same left ventricular anterior wall segment during pacing-induced ischemia and at the end of balloon coronary occlusion. LVEDP rose to similar levels during pacing-induced ischemia and at the end of balloon coronary occlusion, but only at the end of balloon coronary occlusion was LVEDVI significantly larger than the control value. These findings were consistent with an upward shift of the end-diastolic left ventricular pressure-volume relation during pacing-induced ischemia and an upward and rightward shift of the same relation at the end of balloon coronary occlusion. Regional left ventricular diastolic distensibility of the ischemic anterior wall segment changed in a manner similar to that of global left ventricular diastolic distensibility. Overlapping portions of the diastolic left ventricular pressure-radial length plot shifted upward to a greater extent during pacing-induced ischemia than at the end of balloon coronary occlusion.

Previous studies investigating the initial

effects of ischemia on global and regional left ventricular diastolic distensibility in man looked at a single type of ischemic insult: pacing-induced ischemia (20–22), exercise-induced ischemia (23, 24), spontaneous coronary spasm (25), and angioplasty balloon coronary occlusion (9, 10, 18, 26). In patients with triple-vessel coronary disease, pacing-induced angina caused an upward shift of the global diastolic left ventricular pressure-volume relation (20–22), of the diastolic left ventricular pressure-radial length relation (17), and of the diastolic left ventricular pressure-wall thickness relation (27) of the ischemic myocardium. Exercise-induced angina caused similar changes, although less pronounced at end-diastole with a trend of the exercise related diastolic left ventricular pressure-length relation to converge toward the resting curve (24). Spontaneous angina at rest induced an upward shift of the global diastolic left ventricular pressure-volume relation (25). At the end of balloon coronary occlusion, most studies (10, 18) except one (26) observed an upward shift of both the global diastolic left ventricular pressure-volume relation and the diastolic left ventricular pressure-radial length relation of the ischemic segment. Hence, in humans the initial effects of myocardial ischemia appeared to be similar, irrespective of the type of ischemic insult imposed.

This contradiction between previous studies on balloon coronary occlusion ischemia and the present comparative study could be explained by the inverse correlation observed in the present study and in previous animal experiments (6) between a decrease in global and regional diastolic left ventricular distensibility and preservation of global and segmental systolic left ventricular performance. In the present study, a significant correlation was indeed observed at the end of balloon coronary occlusion between the upward shift of the diastolic left ventricular pressure-radial length plot and segmental shortening expressed as a fraction of the resting value. On interstudy comparison, a similar correlation becomes evident. Wijns et al. (10) and Kass et al. (28) observed respectively a 20% decrease in systolic segmental shortening and a fall in ejection fraction from

69 ± 8% to 54 ± 12%. They reported an upward shift of the diastolic left ventricular pressure-radial length plot and of the diastolic left ventricular pressure-volume relation. Bertrand et al. (26) and the present studies observed a larger decrease in ejection fraction (from 72 ± 6% to 46 ± 10% and from 77 ± 7% to 47 ± 11%) and respectively observed no significant change in radial stiffness modulus and an up- and rightward shift of the diastolic left ventricular pressure-volume relation. These differences in depression of left ventricular systolic performance during balloon coronary occlusion ischemia are related to presence or absence of clinical or objective (e.g., ECG) evidence of myocardial ischemia during the balloon inflation, unequal balloon inflation time, recruitment of collaterals during balloon inflation, and variable procurement of data during either first or subsequent balloon inflations. In the study by Wijns et al. (10), average balloon occlusion time was short (± 30 seconds) and the balloon inflation, during which the left ventricular angiogram was obtained varied from a third to a tenth balloon inflation. In the present study, all patients had angina and ischemic ST segment changes at the end of the balloon inflation period, balloon inflation time equaled 60 seconds, coronary wedge pressure during balloon inflation was low (29 ± 11 mm Hg), and the balloon inflation studied was either a fourth (Protocol 1) or a second (Protocols 2 and 3) balloon inflation.

Previous reports examined the effects of pacing angina on diastolic left ventricular distensibility in patients with triple-vessel coronary disease (20–22). In these studies, pacing-induced ischemia resulted in an upward shift of the entire left ventricular pressure-volume relation or of the entire left ventricular pressure-wall thickness relation (27). In the present study, patients with single-vessel coronary disease were studied. The smaller amount of myocardium at risk in these patients could explain shifts of the diastolic left ventricular pressure-volume relation or of the diastolic left ventricular pressure-radial length relation, which were sometimes limited to early and mid-diastole. A similar upward shift limited to early and mid-diastole was recently reported in conscious dogs with a single-vessel coronary stenosis of the left circumflex artery (29). Despite the presence of single vessel disease, pacing-induced ischemia sometimes resulted in profound depression of left ventricular performance (Figs. 17–3 and 17–4). In these patients, in whom systolic performance was severely depressed following pacing, the diastolic pressure-volume relation and the diastolic pressure-radial length relation failed to change. A similar subset of patients, who have depressed systolic performance and unaltered diastolic distensibility during pacing induced ischemia, has been reported by other investigators (17). Hence, during both pacing-induced ischemia and balloon coronary occlusion ischemia, severely reduced systolic shortening seems to preclude decreases in both global and regional distensibility of ischemic myocardium.

In the present studies, left ventricular diastolic distensibility was also investigated at the end of a balloon coronary occlusion and at the end of an equally long balloon coronary occlusion, during which saline was perfused through the distal lumen of the balloon catheter at a rate of 1 mL/sec. This set-up allowed an assessment in man of the comparative effects of ischemia and of hypoxia on left ventricular function. Continuous saline perfusion during balloon coronary occlusion caused (at the end of the occlusion episode) no change in LVEDVI but a marked rise in LVEDP, when compared to an equally long balloon coronary occlusion without saline perfusion. These findings are consistent with induction of decreased left ventricular diastolic distensibility, when saline perfusion is superimposed on balloon coronary occlusion ischemia. The decrease in left ventricular diastolic distensibility at the end of the balloon occlusion with continuous saline perfusion was accompanied by better preservation of systolic performance, as evident from comparing left ventricular stroke work index at the end of both balloon occlusion episodes. Hence, comparative analysis of the myocardial effects of ischemia and of hypoxia in man revealed an interaction between diastolic distensibility and systolic performance, which was similar to the observations performed during

regular balloon coronary occlusions and during pacing-induced ischemia.

Methodologic Limitations

In the present and similar studies on regional left ventricular wall motion during ischemia, left ventricular volumes and radial lengths of ischemic and nonischemic segments were derived from single-plane right anterior oblique left ventricular angiograms and a moving reference point angiographic method. These limitations influence wall motion measurement because of motion of the center of mass toward the area of akinesia during the ischemic stress episode. This artifact leads to overestimation of systolic shortening of the ischemic segment, underestimation of systolic shortening of the nonischemic segment, and reduction of an eventual rightward shift of the diastolic left ventricular pressure-radial length relation as previously observed in numerous coronary ligation animal experiments (30–32).

The present comparison of the effects of different types of ischemia on left ventricular function implies sequential ischemic episodes and assumes reproducibility of sequential balloon inflations. This was indeed observed in a study for all consecutive balloon inflations of equal duration except for the first one, which caused more ischemia than the following balloon inflations probably because of subocclusion of the coronary stenosis by the deflated balloon before the actual inflation period (33). Opposing evidence was, however, recently provided by Deutsch et al. (13), who observed adaptation to ischemia during sequential coronary balloon inflations suggestive of myocardial preconditioning to ischemic stress by previous balloon inflations. This raises the issue of whether a similar preconditioning effect can be induced by a foregoing low flow-high demand ischemia episode as in the present study.

In the present study, similar episodes of coronary occlusion ischemia resulted in a variable depression of segmental shortening of ischemic myocardium, probably because of variable recruitment of collateral flow. Such a recruitment occurred despite the absence of visible collaterals on contralateral coronary injection at the time of the diagnostic study and justifies measurement of coronary wedge pressure during balloon inflation as a more accurate measure of collateralization (34, 35).

Experimental Evidence on Diastolic Left Ventricular Distensibility in Different Types of Ischemia

Anesthetized Dogs and Pigs

Serizawa et al. (36) were the first to reproduce in an anesthetized dog with two-vessel coronary stenoses and open pericardium the upward shift of the diastolic left ventricular pressure-volume relation, which had previously been observed in humans during pacing angina (20–22). These experiments countered assertions that the upward shift of the diastolic left ventricular pressure-volume relation during pacing angina was unrelated to altered diastolic tone of the ischemic muscle but attributable to pericardial constraints (37) or to ventricular interaction through the shared interventricular septum (32). The upward shift of the diastolic left ventricular pressure-volume relation observed in these experiments was opposite to the downward and rightward shift observed previously by numerous investigators during brief coronary occlusions (30–32, 38). The way in which myocardial blood flow was reduced appeared to be of critical importance to reproduce in an anesthetized dog the diastolic left ventricular dysfunction of human pacing-induced angina. The reduction of myocardial blood flow to the left ventricle was achieved by creating metal-clip coronary stenoses on both left anterior descending and left circumflex coronary arteries, which reduced antegrade coronary blood flow in each vessel by ±50%. This resulted in: (1) a large amount of left ventricular myocardium at risk; (2) no impairment of resting function of the jeopardized myocardium; (3) absence of reactive hyperemia during pacing; and (4) subendocardial ischemia during pacing producing ST segment depression on the surface electrocardiogram. Nonadherence to these four criteria explains most of the experimental studies that failed to observe a decrease in diastolic left ventricular distensibility during pacing-induced ischemia. In a right-heart bypass preparation (39), global myocardial ischemia resulted in a depressed left ventricular function at rest. In this model, a further increase in myocardial oxygen demand by pacing had no effect on diastolic left ventricular distensibility (40). In conscious dogs with single-vessel coronary stenosis of the left circumflex coronary artery, increased myocardial oxygen demand by exercise resulted in an upward shift limited to the early portion of the left ventricular diastolic pressure-volume (29) relation, probably because of a smaller amount of myocardium at risk than in the two-vessel coronary stenosis model. In an anesthetized two-vessel coronary stenosis model (41), reduction of coronary blood flow in each vessel to a level that just avoided regional left ventricular dysfunction at rest resulted in transmural myocardial ischemia after 3 minutes of pacing and not in subendocardial myocardial ischemia as observed during demand angina in humans. In this model, there was profound impairment of systolic performance and no decrease in regional diastolic left ventricular distensibility after pacing.

This angina physiology model of pacing-stress superimposed on two vessel coronary stenoses was subsequently compared to the more classical coronary occlusion model (6, 7). From this comparison, it became evident that the "low flow-high demand" ischemia of pacing-induced angina and the "no-flow ischemia" of coronary occlusion exerted opposite effects on systolic and diastolic function of ischemic myocardium. During pacing-induced ischemia, segmental systolic shortening was slightly reduced (from 16.7 ± 2.6% to 12.7 ± 1.5%) and diastolic distensibility of the ischemic segment was decreased, as is evident from an upward shift of the diastolic left ventricular pressure-segment length and the diastolic left ventricular pressure-wall thickness relations. When regional diastolic distensibility was correlated with regional systolic shortening of different experiments and of different segments during pacing-induced ischemia, it also became evident that the upward shift of the diastolic left ventricular pressure-segment length relation was absent or small when systolic performance was severely depressed during pacing-induced ischemia (6). Procurement of transmural biopsies on cessation of pacing and after 3 minutes of pacing tachycardia revealed similar depression of adenosine triphosphate in both types of ischemia (7). Implantation of a hydrogen ion-selective membrane in the subendocardium showed a small decline in myocardial pH (-0.14) after pacing tachycardia and a striking fall (-0.33) after coronary occlusion (7). Regional myocardial blood flow measured by microsphere technique confirmed the presence of subendocardial ischemia after pacing tachycardia and of transmural ischemia during brief coronary occlusion (7). To overcome the critique of assessing regional left ventricular diastolic distensibility on the diastole of a single beat, caval occlusions were performed at rest and after pacing tachycardia in the presence of coronary stenoses. This allowed construction of wide range diastolic pressure-segment length relations composed of multiple end-diastolic left ventricular pressure-segment length points obtained during a single caval occlusion run (42). These wide-range end-diastolic pressure-segment length relations were shifted upward during pacing-induced ischemia in a way similar to the curves derived from single beat analysis. The angina physiology model of pacing tachycardia superimposed on coronary stenosis has also been reproduced in pigs (43). Because of absent collateral flow, only a single coronary stenosis was required, and antegrade coronary blood flow needed to be reduced by 25% and not by 50% as in the dog model to elicit the hemodynamic changes characteristic of pacing-induced angina in man. In the pig model, low flow-high demand ischemia of pacing-induced angina and no-flow ischemia of coronary occlusion induced opposite effects on segmental diastolic distensibility of ischemic myocardium, similar to the observations previously reported in the dog model. Moreover, the authors ruled out left ventricular segmental dyssynchrony as the cause of the observed decrease in diastolic left ventricular distensibility during pacing-induced ischemia because coronary occlusion ischemia failed to induce a decrease in diastolic distensibility despite larger dyssynchrony between ischemic and normal segments during coronary occlusion ischemia than during pacing-induced ischemia.

From all these experiments, it became obvious that the upward shift of the diastolic left ventricular pressure-volume relation originally described in humans during pacing-induced angina was (1) unrelated to pericardial constraints because it could be reproduced in open-chest, open-pericardium animal models, (2) unrelated to early diastolic viscous effects because it could be reproduced from multiple end-diastolic left ventricular pressure-volume points obtained during a caval occlusion run, (3) unrelated to dyssynchrony between ischemic and nonischemic segments, and therefore (4) related to altered diastolic tone of ischemic myocardium. This relation to diastolic tone led to experimental attempts to pharmacologically modulate the response of myocardium to low flow-high demand ischemia by agents administered during or before the ischemia episode. The decrease in diastolic left ventricular distensibility observed during pacing-induced ischemia was augmented by administration of caffeine (44), an agent known to interfere with calcium homeostasis mainly by reducing calcium reuptake of the sarcoplasmic reticulum and by increasing calcium sensitivity of the myofilaments. Both the decreased diastolic left ventricular distensibility observed during demand angina and its potentiation by administration of caffeine could not be prevented by pretreatment with verapamil (45). These pharmacologic effects support the notion that demand ischemia leads to a decrease in diastolic distensibility of the ischemic segment through impairment of sarcoplasmic reticular calcium uptake, through altered myofilamentary calcium sensitivity and not through augmented slow channel calcium influx.

Isovolumic Rodent Hearts

From the experiments performed in anesthetized dogs, it appeared that increased myocardial oxygen demand superimposed on a reduction of myocardial blood flow resulted in decreased regional diastolic distensibility only when myocardial perfusion remained above a critical limit. Once myocardial blood flow dropped below this critical limit, the effects of decreased vascular turgor and of accumulation of metabolites could abolish the effect of tissue hypoxia on regional diastolic distensibility. These complex and opposite interactions on left ventricular diastolic distensibility of tissue hypoxia, accumulation of metabolites (H^+, inorganic phosphate . . .) and vascular turgor have been elucidated in isolated, isovolumically beating and retrogradely perfused guinea-pig, rat and rabbit hearts (4). In the isovolumic guinea-pig and rabbit heart (5, 46), a switch from aerobic to hypoxic perfusion at equal coronary flow induced within 5 minutes a progressive decline in developed tension and a rise in resting tension. Under isovolumic conditions, a rise in resting tension implied a decrease in diastolic distensibility. Increasing heart rate during hypoxic perfusion prompted the rise in resting tension. In the isovolumic, blood-perfused rabbit heart, a 6-minute reduction in coronary perfusion pressure from 100 mm Hg to 20 mm Hg caused no change in diastolic left ventricular distensibility when heart rate was maintained at baseline level but a decrease in diastolic left ventricular distensibility when pacing tachycardia was superimposed on the reduction in coronary perfusion pressure (low flow-high demand ischemia) (47). In the isovolumic rat heart, a complete interruption of coronary flow (= no flow ischemia) produced within 3 minutes a total loss of developed tension and a fall in resting tension, consistent with increased diastolic left ventricular distensibility (48). The isovolumic rodent heart therefore resembles the anaesthetized dog model: during the initial stages of ischemia, a loss of systolic performance precludes a decrease in diastolic distensibility.

Pathophysiologic Mechanisms

Comparative studies on the myocardial effects of low flow-high demand and of no-flow ischemia in humans and in several experimental models revealed that low flow-high demand ischemia causes a smaller reduction of systolic left ventricular performance and a larger decrease in global and regional diastolic left ventricular distensibility than no-flow ischemia. Pathophysiologic mechanisms, which could contribute to this divergent mechanical

performance of myocardium subjected to different types of ischemia, include: (1) absence or presence of tissue metabolites during the initial stages of ischemia, (2) vascular turgor during the ischemic episode and hyperemic response during initial relief of the ischemic stress, (3) loss of synchronicity between ischemic and nonischemic zones, and (4) unequal intensity of the ischemic stress episode.

Absence or Presence of Tissue Metabolites

Hypoxia, low flow-high demand ischemia, and no-flow ischemia all cause an imbalance between myocardial demand and supply for oxygen and substrates but exert profoundly different effects on washout or buildup of tissue metabolites as shown in Figure 17–7. During hypoxia and to a lesser extent during low flow-high demand ischemia, such as occurs in pacing-induced angina, there is continuous washout of metabolites (e.g., H^+ and inorganic phosphate). During no-flow ischemia such as occurs during coronary ligation and balloon coronary occlusion in the absence of coronary collaterals, tissue concentrations of metabolites rise. Divergent metabolic effects of pacing-induced ischemia and of coronary occlusion ischemia have indeed been demonstrated by implantation of a hydrogen-selective membrane in the subendocardium of anesthetized dogs (7) and in the present studies by determination of concentrations of H^+, K^+, and lactate in the coronary sinus in patients with single-vessel tight proximal left anterior descending stenosis. (See Chap. 1.)

The buildup of tissue metabolites in no-flow ischemia leads to a cascade of alterations of myocardial metabolism and of calcium handling, which ultimately result in absence of contractile activity before significant ATP depletion. These alterations include: (1) Acidosis-induced drive of the creatine kinase reaction (49) with replenishment of ATP stores, depletion of creatine phosphate (7) and production of inorganic phosphate, which induces contractile failure by reducing calcium sensitivity of myofilaments (50); (2) Increased amplitude of the calcium transient (51–54) as

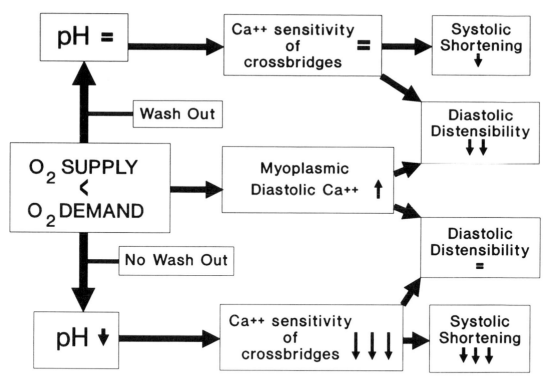

Fig. 17–7. Modulation of the myocardial effects of an ischemic episode by presence or absence of tissue metabolites. When an imbalance between myocardial oxygen supply and demand is accompanied by washout of tissue metabolites, tissue pH and tissue concentration of inorganic phosphate remain unaltered and calcium sensitivity of crossbridges therefore remains unchanged. This leads to better preservation of systolic performance during the ischemic episode and, because of increased diastolic myoplasmic calcium, to diastolic crossbridge cycling and decreased diastolic distensibility. When an imbalance between myocardial oxygen supply and demand is not accompanied by washout of tissue metabolites, tissue concentrations of H+ and of inorganic phosphate rise and calcium sensitivity of crossbridges therefore decrease. This leads to loss of systolic shortening and, despite high diastolic myoplasmic calcium, to absence of diastolic crossbridge cycling and unaltered diastolic distensibility.

a result of an enhanced parallel operation of Na^+-Ca^{2+} and Na^+-H^+ exchangers, which overcome a direct inhibitory action of acidosis on sarcoplasmic reticulum function. This calcium overload does not affect contractile performance in situ because of simultaneous desensitization of myofilaments (55, 56) but becomes evident through enhanced mechanical performance when ischemic muscle is subsequently transferred to an organ bath and compared to nonischemic control (57).

Complete washout of tissue metabolites such as occurs during hypoxia or partial washout of tissue metabolites such as occurs during pacing-induced angina could reverse this interaction between calcium overload and desensitization of myofila-

ments during the initial stages of oxygen deprivation. Washout of metabolites could lead to partially maintained calcium sensitivity of myofilaments and therefore better preservation of systolic performance. It could also lead to diastolic crossbridge cycling because of a diastolic cytosolic calcium overload, which is of smaller amplitude than during no-flow ischemia (58) but which succeeds in expressing itself mechanically because of the concomitant partial preservation of myofilamentary calcium sensitivity. Hence, presence or absence of an inhibitory effect on myofilaments by tissue metabolites explains both the unequal effects on systolic performance and on diastolic distensibility of different types of myocardial ischemia (4, 59).

vations in left ventricular end-diastolic pressure as a result of both ischemic stress episodes. Despite these similar elevations in left ventricular filling pressures, left ventricular ejection fractions and left ventricular end-diastolic volume indexes were significantly different. This finding is incompatible with unequal severity of ischemia modulating the same type of left ventricular failure during both ischemic stress episodes and is more likely to be explained by different types of left ventricular failure during pacing-induced and balloon occlusion ischemia. Moreover, the use of left ventricular end-diastolic pressure as a measure for the severity of ischemic stress rests on the assumption that the left ventricle is always operating on the same left ventricular compliance curve irrespective of the type of ischemic intervention; however, this assumption is precisely the subject of investigation of these comparative studies on the left ventricular effects of different types of ischemia. The severity of ischemia in different types of ischemic interventions is probably more accurately measured by adenosine triphosphate and by creatine phosphate contents of ischemic myocardium, as performed in dogs in different types of ischemia by Momomura et al. using a transmural biopsy drill (7) and as measured noninvasively during handgrip-induced angina in humans using nuclear-magnetic-resonance spectroscopy (78).

CONCLUSIONS

In the present studies, diastolic left ventricular pressure-volume and diastolic left ventricular pressure-radial length relations were compared in patients with single-vessel proximal tight left anterior descending coronary stenosis immediately after pacing (low flow-high demand ischemia), during balloon coronary occlusion (no-flow ischemia) and during balloon coronary occlusion with maintained hypoxic perfusion distal to the occlusion (hypoxia). Immediately after pacing and during balloon coronary occlusion with distal hypoxic perfusion, global left ventricular distensibility and regional diastolic distensibility of the ischemic segment showed a larger decrease than during a regular balloon coronary occlusion. This larger decrease in diastolic

distensibility was accompanied by better preservation of systolic performance and continuous washout of tissue metabolites. These divergent mechanical effects of the different types of ischemia in humans could be related to presence or absence of tissue metabolites in ischemic myocardium and to unequal stretching of sarcomeres by coronary vascular turgor, both of which modulate contractile performance of myofilaments. Differences of contractile performance of myofilaments in these different types of ischemia explain not only the unequal systolic performance but also the unequal change of diastolic distensibility because of different degrees of diastolic cross-bridge cycling in the presence of high diastolic myoplasmic calcium.

REFERENCES

1. Ross J Jr: Assessment of ischemic regional myocardial dysfunction and its reversibility. Circulation 74:1186, 1986.
2. Ross J Jr: Myocardial perfusion-contraction matching. Implications for coronary heart disease and hibernation. Circulation 83:1076, 1991.
3. Marban E: Myocardial stunning and hibernation: The physiology behind the colloquialisms. Circulation 83:681, 1991.
4. Apstein CS, Grossman W: Opposite initial effects of supply and demand ischemia on left ventricular diastolic compliance: The ischemia-diastolic paradox. J Mol Cell Cardiol 19:119, 1987.
5. Serizawa T, Vogel WM, Apstein CS, Grossman W: Comparison of acute alterations in left ventricular relaxation and diastolic chamber stiffness induced by hypoxia and ischemia. J Clin Invest 64:91, 1981.
6. Paulus WJ, et al.: Different effects of two types of ischemia on myocardial systolic and diastolic function. Am J Physiol 248:H719, 1985.
7. Momomura S, et al.: The relationships of high energy phosphates, tissue pH, and regional blood flow to diastolic distensibility in the ischemic dog myocardium. Circ Res 57:822, 1985.
8. Murry CE, Jennings RB, Reimer KA: Preconditioning with ischemia: A delay of lethal cell injury in ischemic myocardium. Circulation 74:1124, 1986.
9. Serruys PW, et al.: Left ventricular performance, regional blood flow, wall motion, and lactate metabolism during transluminal angioplasty. Circulation 70:25, 1984.
10. Wijns W, et al.: Effect of coronary occlusion

during percutaneous transluminal angioplasty in humans on left ventricular chamber stiffness and regional diastolic pressure-radius relations. J Am Coll Cardiol 7: 455, 1986.

11. Labovitz AJ, et al.: Evaluation of left ventricular systolic and diastolic dysfunction during transient myocardial ischemia produced by angioplasty. J Am Coll Cardiol 10: 748, 1987.

12. Kern MJ, Deligonul U, Labovitz A: Influence of drug therapy on the ischemic response to acute coronary occlusion in man: Supply-side economics. Am Heart J 118: 361, 1989.

13. Deutsch E, et al.: Adaptation to ischemia during percutaneous transluminal coronary angioplasty. Circulation 82:2044, 1990.

14. Bronzwaer JGF, de Bruyne B, Ascoop CAPL, Paulus WJ: Comparative effects of pacing-induced and balloon coronary occlusion ischemia on left ventricular diastolic function in man. Circulation 84:211, 1991.

15. de Bruyne B, et al.: Pacing angina and balloon coronary occlusion: Divergent effects on LV wall motion and wash-out of tissue metabolites in man. Circulation 82(Suppl III):III-122, 1990.

16. de Bruyne B, Heyndrickx GR, De Vriese J, Paulus WJ: Saline perfusion distal to balloon coronary occlusion reduces diastolic distensibility of the ischaemic left ventricle. Eur Heart J 12(Abstr Suppl):59, 1991.

17. Sasayama S, et al.: Changes in diastolic properties of the regional myocardium during pacing-induced ischemia in human subjects. J Am Coll Cardiol 5:599, 1985.

18. Carlson EB, Hinohara T, Morris KG: Recovery of systolic and diastolic left ventricular function after a 60-second coronary arterial occlusion during percutaneous transluminal coronary angioplasty for angina pectoris. Am J Cardiol 60:460, 1987.

19. Weiss JL, Frederiksen JW, Weisfeldt ML: Hemodynamic determinants of the time course of fall in canine left ventricular pressure. J Clin Invest 58:751, 1970.

20. Dwyer EM Jr: Left ventricular pressure-volume alterations and regional disorders of contraction during myocardial ischemia induced by atrial pacing. Circulation 42: 1111, 1970.

21. Barry WH, Brooker JZ, Alderman EL, Harrison DC: Changes in diastolic stiffness and tone of the left ventricle during angina pectoris. Circulation 49:255, 1974.

22. Mann T, Goldberg S, Mudge GH, Grossman W: Factors contributing to altered left ventricular diastolic properties during angina pectoris. Circulation 59:14, 1979.

23. Carroll JD, Hess OM, Hirzel HO, Krayenbuehl HP: Exercise-induced ischemia: The influence of altered relaxation on early diastolic pressures. Circulation 67:521, 1983.

24. Nonogi H, et al.: Left ventricular pressure-length relation during exercise-induced ischemia. J Am Coll Cardiol 13:1062, 1989.

25. Sharma B, et al.: Left ventricular diastolic properties and filling characteristics during spontaneous angina pectoris at rest. Am J Cardiol 52:704, 1983.

26. Bertrand ME, et al.: Left ventricular systolic and diastolic function during acute coronary artery balloon occlusion in humans. J Am Coll Cardiol 12:341, 1988.

27. Bourdillon PD, et al.: Increased regional myocardial stiffness of the left ventricle during pacing induced angina in man. Circulation 67:316, 1983.

28. Kass DA, Midei M, Brinker J, Maughan WL: Influence of coronary occlusion during PTCA on end-systolic and end-diastolic pressure-volume relations in humans. Circulation 81:447, 1990.

29. Miyazaki S, et al.: Changes of left ventricular diastolic function in exercising dogs without and with ischemia. Circulation 81: 1058, 1990.

30. Tyberg JV, et al.: An analysis of segmental ischemic dysfunction utilizing the pressure-length loop. Circulation 49:748, 1974.

31. Theroux P, Franklin D, Ross J Jr, Kemper WS: Regional myocardial function during acute coronary artery occlusion and its modification by pharmacological agents in the dog. Circ Res 35:896, 1974.

32. Hess OM, et al.: Diastolic myocardial wall stiffness and ventricular relaxation during partial and complete coronary occlusions in the conscious dog. Circ Res 52:387, 1983.

33. Perry RA, et al.: Balloon occlusion during coronary angioplasty as a model of myocardial ischemia: Reproducibility of sequential inflations. Eur Heart J 10:791, 1989.

34. Meier B, et al.: Coronary wedge pressure in relation to spontaneously visible and recruitable collaterals. Circulation 75:906, 1987.

35. De Bruyne B, et al.: Potential protective effect of high coronary wedge pressure on left ventricular function after coronary occlusion. Circulation 78:566, 1988.

36. Serizawa T, Carabello BA, Grossman W: Effect of pacing induced ischemia on left ventricular diastolic pressure-volume relations in dogs with coronary stenoses. Circ Res 46:430, 1980.

37. Glantz SA, Parmley WW: Factors which affect the diastolic pressure-volume curve. Circ Res 42:171, 1978.

38. Wong BYS, Toyama M, Reis RL, Goodyer AVN: Sequential changes in left ventricular compliance during acute coronary occlusion in the isovolumic working canine heart. Circ Res 43:274, 1978.

39. Palacios I, Newell JB, Powell WJ Jr: Left ventricular end-diastolic pressure-volume relationships with experimental acute global ischemia. Circulation 39:735, 1976.

40. Lorell BH, et al.: Right ventricular distension and left ventricular compliance. Am J Physiol 240:H87, 1981.

41. Applegate RJ, Walsh RA, O'Rourke RA: Comparative effects of pacing-induced and flow-limited ischemia on left ventricular function. Circulation 81:1380, 1990.

42. Momomura SI, Bradley AB, Grossman W: Left ventricular diastolic pressure-segment length relations and end-diastolic distensiblity in dogs with coronary stenoses: An angina physiology model. Circ Res 55:203, 1984.

43. Takahashi T, Levine MJ, Grossman W: Regional diastolic mechanics of ischemic and nonischemic myocardium in the pig heart. J Am Coll Cardiol 17:1203, 1991.

44. Paulus WJ, Serizawa T, Grossman W: Altered left ventricular diastolic properties during pacing-induced ischemia in dogs with coronary stenoses: Potentiation by caffeine. Circ Res 50;218, 1982.

45. Bourdillon PD, Paulus WJ, Serizawa T, Grossman W: Effects of verapamil on regional myocardial diastolic function in pacing-induced ischemia in dogs. Am J Physiol 251:H834, 1986.

46. Nayler WG, Yepez CE, Poole-Wilson PA: The effect of β-adrenoreceptor and Ca^{2+} antagonist drugs on the hypoxia-induced increase in resting tension. Cardiovasc Res 12:666, 1978.

47. Isoyama S, et al.: Acute decrease in left ventricular diastolic chamber distensibility during simulated angina in isolated hearts. Circ Res 61:925, 1987.

48. Wexler LF, Weinberg EO, Ingwall JS, Apstein CS: Acute alterations in diastolic left ventricular chamber distensibility: mechanistic differences between hypoxemia and ischemia in isolated perfused rabbit and rat hearts. Circ Res 59:515, 1986.

49. Schwartz GS, et al.: Myocardial high-energy phosphates in reactive hyperemia. Am J Physiol 259:H1190, 1990.

50. Kusuoka H, et al.: Mechanism of early contractile failure during hypoxia in intact ferret heart. Evidence for modulation of maximal Ca^{2+} activated force by inorganic phosphate. Circ Res 59:270, 1986.

51. Allen DG, Orchard CH: The effects of changes of pH on intracellular calcium transients in mammalian cardiac muscle. J Physiol (Lond) 335:555, 1983.

52. Allen DG, Orchard CH: Myocardial contractile function during ischemia and hypoxia. Circ Res 60:153, 1987.

53. Lee H, et al.: Effect of ischemia on calcium-dependent fluorescence transients in rabbit hearts containing indo-1. Circulation 78:1047, 1988.

54. Koretsune Y, Marban E: Relative roles of Ca^{2+}-dependent and Ca^{2+}-independent mechanisms in hypoxic contractile dysfunction. Circulation 82:528, 1990.

55. Katz AM, Hecht HH: The early "pump" failure of the ischemic heart. Am J Med 47:497, 1969.

56. Barry WH: Mechanical dysfunction of the heart during and after ischemia. Circulation 82:652, 1990.

57. Schouten VJA, et al.: Paradox of enhanced contractility in postischemic rat hearts with depressed function. Am J Physiol 260:H89, 1991.

58. Kihara Y, Grossman W, Morgan JP: Direct measurement of changes in intracellular calcium transients during hypoxia, ischemia and reperfusion of the intact mammalian heart. Circ Res 65:1029, 1989.

59. Paulus WJ: Upward shift and outward bulge: The divergent myocardial effects of pacing angina and of brief coronary occlusion. Circulation 81:1436, 1990.

60. Salisbury PF, Cross CE, Rieben PA: Influence of coronary pressure on myocardial elasticity. Circ Res 8:794, 1960.

61. Gaasch WH, et al.: The influence of acute alterations in coronary blood flow on left ventricular diastolic compliance and wall thickness. Eur J Cardiol 7(Suppl):147, 1978.

62. Vogel WM, et al.: Acute alterations in left ventricular diastolic chamber stiffness. Role of the "erectile" effect of coronary arterial pressure and flow in normal and damaged hearts. Circ Res 51:465, 1982.

63. Olson CO, et al.: The coronary pressure-flow determinants of left ventricular compliance in dogs. Circ Res 49:856, 1981.

64. Poche R, Arnold G, Gahlen D: Uber den Einfluss des Perfusionsdruckes im Coronarsystem des stillgestellten, aerob perfundierten, isolierten Meerschweinchenherzens auf Stoffwechsel und Feinstruktur des Herzmuskels. Virchows Arch (Cell Pathol) 8:252, 1971.

65. Koretsune Y, Corretti MC, Kusuoka H, Marban E: Mechanism of early ischemic contractile failure. Inexcitability, metabo-

lite accumulation or vascular collapse? Circ Res 68:255, 1991.

66. Babu A, Sonnenblick E, Gulati J: Molecular basis for the influence of muscle length on myocardial performance. Science 240:74, 1988.

67. Brutsaert DL, Meulemans AL, Sipido KR, Sys SU: Effects of damaging the endocardial surface on the mechanical performance of isolated cardiac muscle. Circ Res 62:358, 1988.

68. Gallagher KP, et al.: Myocardial blood flow and function with critical coronary stenosis in exercising dogs. Am J Physiol 243:H698, 1982.

69. Gallagher KP, et al.: Isoproterenol-induced myocardial dysfunction in dogs with coronary stenoses. Am J Physiol 242:H260, 1982.

70. Ross J Jr: Is there a true increase in myocardial stiffness with acute ischemia? Am J Cardiol 63:87E, 1989.

71. Aroesty JM, et al.: Simultaneous assessment of left ventricular systolic and diastolic dysfunction during pacing-induced ischemia. Circulation 71:889, 1985.

72. Brutsaert DL, Rademakers FE, Sys SU: Triple control of relaxation: Implications in cardiac disease. Circulation 69:190, 1984.

73. Jaski BE, Serruys PW, ten Katen H, Meij S: Epicardial wall motion and left ventricular function during coronary graft angioplasty in humans. J Am Coll Cardiol 6:695, 1985.

74. Dawson JR, Gibson DG: Left ventricular filling and early diastolic function at rest and during angina in patients with coronary artery disease. Br Heart J 61:248, 1989.

75. Nakamura Y, et al.: Effects of pacing-induced ischemia on early left ventricular filling and regional myocardial dynamics and their modification by nifedipine. Circulation 76:1232, 1987.

76. McKay RG, et al.: The pacing stress reexamined: Correlation of pacing-induced hemodynamic changes with the amount of myocardium at risk. J Am Coll Cardiol 3:1469, 1984.

77. Fifer MA, Bourdillon PD, Lorell BH: Altered left ventricular diastolic properties during pacing-induced angina in patients with aortic stenosis. Circulation 74:675, 1986.

78. Weiss RG, Bottomley PA, Hardy CJ, Gerstenblith G: Regional myocardial metabolism of high-energy phosphates during isometric exercise in patients with coronary artery disease. N Engl J Med 323:1593, 1990.

Chapter 18

LEFT VENTRICULAR REMODELING AND DIASTOLIC DYSFUNCTION IN CHRONIC ISCHEMIC HEART DISEASE

Howard A. Rockman and Wilbur Y. W. Lew

Acute myocardial infarction produces complex alterations in regional ventricular function in both infarcted and noninfarcted regions, resulting in changes in global left ventricular (LV) shape and geometry. The time course for these changes varies by region and infarct size. Acutely, the most dramatic changes occur in the infarct region, whereas chronically (weeks to months), the alterations occur predominantly in noninfarcted regions as the heart adapts to the global impairments in cardiac function. Regional changes in ventricular structure and function, along with global changes in LV cavity volume, shape and myocardial muscle mass, have been collectively termed "ventricular remodeling" (1).

Although ventricular remodeling is an adaptive process, some changes may be maladaptive. After acute ischemia, the ischemic region develops paradoxical systolic expansion and performs little effective work (2). The progressive increase in LV end-diastolic pressure and volume helps to restore systolic function by the Frank-Starling mechanism. During the first week, the infarct zone may undergo progressive regional thinning and dilation unrelated to further myocardial necrosis, a process termed "infarct expansion" (3). Because the increase in LV volume is caused primarily by changes in the infarct zone, there is little hemodynamic benefit from this LV dilation. In fact, these changes may be deleterious because infarct expansion is associated with several complications and increased mortality (3–5). Overall survival following acute myocardial infarction is inversely related to the extent of LV dilation (6).

This chapter reviews the pathophysiology of infarct expansion and ventricular remodeling. The structural changes in both infarct and noninfarcted regions underlying LV dilation will be examined. The influence of ventricular remodeling on LV diastolic performance early and late after myocardial infarction will be reviewed. Finally, factors that modify ventricular remodeling and may affect the outcome from acute myocardial infarction will be examined.

PATHOPHYSIOLOGY OF CARDIAC ENLARGEMENT

Infarct Expansion

Infarct expansion occurs in up to 70% of transmural myocardial infarctions (7), but is rare with nontransmural infarcts (8, 9). Infarct expansion may begin within the first day, but the incidence and extent progress over the first 2 weeks after myocardial infarction (4, 8). Dilation of the LV chamber begins within days following a transmural myocardial infarction (10, 11) and is primarily a result of infarct expansion with lengthening of segments in the infarct region (12). An example of infarct expansion is shown in Figure 18–1.

A major determinant of infarct expansion is the presence of transmural necrosis with an infarct above a critical size (8, 9). Infarct expansion and LV dilation occur more often with anterior wall infarcts (4, 10, 11, 13, 14). The LV apex is particularly vulnerable to infarct expansion (15), which may be related to the thinner wall and higher wall stress in this region (16). The importance of wall stress in infarct expansion is also suggested by the finding that chronic increases in afterload increase the degree of expansion (17, 18). Infarct ex-

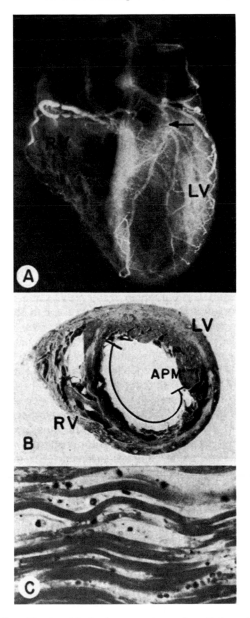

Fig. 18–1. Marked expansion of a 7-day-old transmural myocardial infarct. *A,* postmortem arteriogram with an occlusion of the left anterior descending coronary artery (arrow). *B,* cross section of right (RV) and left (LV) ventricles showing a large anterior septal infarct *(line)* with marked thinning relative to posterior and lateral surviving myocardium. Expansion of the infarct has displaced the anterior papillary muscle (APM) complex to a lateral position. *C,* the infarcted myocardium with thin wavy fibers and apparent disruption of necrotic cells. (Hematoxylin-eosin × 400). Reproduced with permission from Hutchins GM, Bulkley BH: Infarct expansion versus extension: Two different complications of acute myocardial infarction. Am J Cardiol 41:1127, 1978.

pansion may serve as a substrate for LV aneurysm formation (5, 19) and LV rupture (20). The development of infarct expansion is correlated with hemodynamic deterioration (21) and an increase in mortality (4, 5, 17).

Geometry Changes in Noninfarcted Regions

Changes in the topography of the normal, noninfarcted regions have an important role in the development of progressive LV enlargement. Although infarct expansion produces early LV dilation, generalized LV dilation develops over several months after myocardial infarction (10, 11) because of progressive lengthening of myocardial segments in noninfarcted regions (22–24). Dilation of noninfarcted regions may begin within an hour of acute transmural infarction and is associated with an increase in LV end-diastolic pressure (25). Over the next several months, noninfarcted segments may lengthen by as much as 20% (23, 24), contributing to the progressive increase in LV chamber volume. Lengthening and wall thinning of adjacent and remote noninfarcted myocardial regions occur primarily in hearts that develop infarct expansion, but does not appear to depend on infarct size (23, 26). Although these remodeling changes are associated with improved hemodynamics (e.g., increased stroke volume from a lower LV filling pressure), this occurs at the expense of an increase in LV chamber volume (24). It has been hypothesized that remodeling of noninfarcted regions is due to an increase in diastolic wall stress, analogous to the eccentric hypertrophy that develops in response to chronic volume overload (24, 27).

MECHANISMS OF CARDIAC ENLARGEMENT

Myocardial Fiber Rearrangement

The heart is composed of myocardial fibers with a transmural distribution of fiber orientations (the predominant direction is circumferential, particularly in the midwall) (28). Myocardial fibers are arranged in bundles to form cleavage planes that are oriented perpendicular to the endocardial surface (29). When LV volume increases, the wall thins because of an internal rearrangement of fibers without a change in the transmural distribution of fiber orientations (29). With larger ventricular volumes, the number of fibers across the wall decreases because of a shift in the cleavage plane from perpendicular to more acute angles. This indicates that the wall thins from an internal rearrangement of fibers, rather than by simple myocardial fiber stretching. This is postulated to occur by sliding planes between groups of muscle fibers (29).

Infarct expansion is a disproportionate wall thinning and regional dilatation of the infarct region. Early wall thinning is not a result of loss of myocytes because infarct expansion occurs before resorption of necrotic myocardium. There is no evidence of intramyocardial rupture which would explain infarct expansion (30). The wall thinning in infarct expansion is associated with a decreased number of myocytes across the wall, and an increase in cell density of approximately 20%. There is also a small increase in sarcomere lengths in the ischemic region with infarction (30). However, only part of the increased cell density is caused by cell stretch (as assessed by a decrease in myocyte cross-sectional area and an increase in sarcomere length) (30). A significant portion of wall thinning in the infarct region is related to a translation of myocardial fiber bundles (side to side myocyte slippage), so that cleavage planes that are normally perpendicular to the endocardial surface form a more acute angle (30).

Cell slippage accounts for nearly all of the wall thinning in noninfarcted regions which leads to significant increases in LV chamber diameter (30) and alterations in the global geometry in such a way that the shape of the ventricle is more cylindrical (31). These global changes, along with the transmural decrease in myocyte and capillary density, produce marked (e.g., 7-8 fold) increases in calculated diastolic wall stress, with smaller increases in systolic wall stress (31, 32). This results in significant myocyte cellular hypertrophy in noninfarcted regions (32). Similar remodeling changes may be observed with acute nonocclusive coronary artery constriction that produce ventricular dilation with wall thinning primarily due to cell slippage, resulting in elevated diastolic (and more modest systolic) wall stress (33).

The mechanisms for myocardial fiber rearrangement which may contribute to infarct expansion are illustrated in Figures 18–2 and 18–3.

Extracellular Matrix Remodeling

The extracellular matrix is composed of collagen struts that connect myocytes to adjacent myocytes and capillaries (34). (See Chap. 8.) The collagen struts mechanically couple myocytes, preventing slippage as well as maintaining relatively uniform sarcomere lengths. Groups of myocytes are enclosed in a collagen web network with long collagen bundles or cables connecting different web networks (34). The radial cleavage planes that separate groups of fibers in the form of septae (34), facilitate rearrangement of muscle bundles with increases in load. This rearrangement decreases the cleavage angle between the muscle bundles relative to the endocardial surface, accounting for the transmural decrease in cell number with wall thinning in both infarct and noninfarcted regions (30).

Alterations in the collagen matrix occur with myocardial ischemia. After 40 minutes of ischemia, there is breakdown and loss of collagen fibrils, microfilaments, and elastic fibers (35). Changes initially occur in the endocardium, but become transmural and more extensive with prolonged ischemia (35, 36). Increased activity of collagenase, neutral proteinases (36) and infiltration of inflammatory cells into the necrotic tissue (37) all contribute to the collagen degradation during acute myocardial ischemia. The extracellular collagen matrix may be damaged even without irreversible cell injury. Myocardial stunning produced by repeated episodes of coronary artery occlusion and reperfusion cause breakdown and loss of collagen struts and cables and disrupt the collagen weave (38) as demonstrated in Figure 18–4.

Damage to the extracellular collagen causes loss of mechanical coupling, which may contribute to the ventricular dilation with myocardial ischemia (38). There is a correlation between the degree of infarct

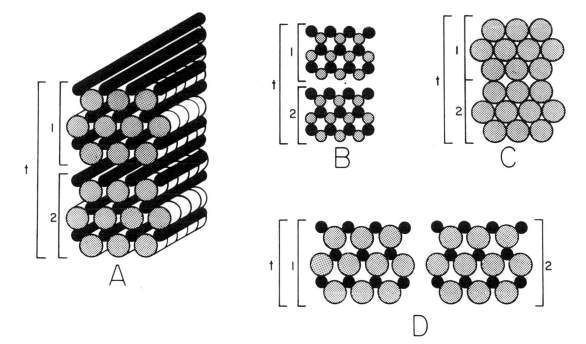

Fig. 18–2. Schematic drawing of possible mechanisms of infarct expansion. *A,* Myocytes (stippled cylinders) and capillaries (solid cylinders) are shown as being arranged in discrete bundles (1 and 2). *A* is a three-dimensional perspective diagram of a hypothetical preinfarct ventricular wall. In subsequent panels, only the two-dimensional cross-sectional view is shown. For illustrative purposes, cross-sections of only two bundles are shown composing the total wall thickness (t). *B,* With cell stretch, the total number of cells across the wall and capillary dimension remain unchanged, but the number of cells per unit length (cell density) increases as the wall thins. *C,* Collapse of the microvascular space results in tighter packing of the myocytes, also producing an increase in cell density and hence wall thinning. *D,* With rearrangement of myocyte bundles, fewer cells make up the thickness of the wall, but the number of cells per unit length is unchanged. Reproduced with permission from Weisman HF, et al.: Cellular mechanisms of myocardial infarct expansion. Circulation 78:186, 1988.

expansion and the extent of collagen damage and loss of collagen struts (39). The collagen content is important for preventing myocardial rupture during acute ischemia (39). During the chronic healing phase, collagen synthesis increases as part of the repair and healing processes, and this structural remodeling of the collagen matrix may contribute to increased diastolic wall stiffness in the infarcted area (40, 41).

Compensatory Myocyte Hypertrophy

Geometric alterations in noninfarcted regions, such as segment lengthening with LV dilation, help to maintain stroke volume by the Frank-Starling mechanism but at the expense of an increase in diastolic wall stress (24). Early after large myocar-

dial infarction, LV end-diastolic pressures remain elevated and the volume of viable myocardium increases approximately 30% because of increases in both myocyte cell length and diameter (42). Later events after myocardial infarction are characterized by chamber enlargement associated with lengthening of the noninfarcted contractile segment (43), which occurs in part from the increase in myocyte length by the addition of sarcomeres in series (44). These cellular responses are consistent with combined pressure and volume overload hypertrophy (42).

Chronically after myocardial infarction, the degree of hypertrophy in noninfarcted regions is directly related to the infarct size (45–47). Although hypertrophy of noninfarcted regions can fully restore the mass

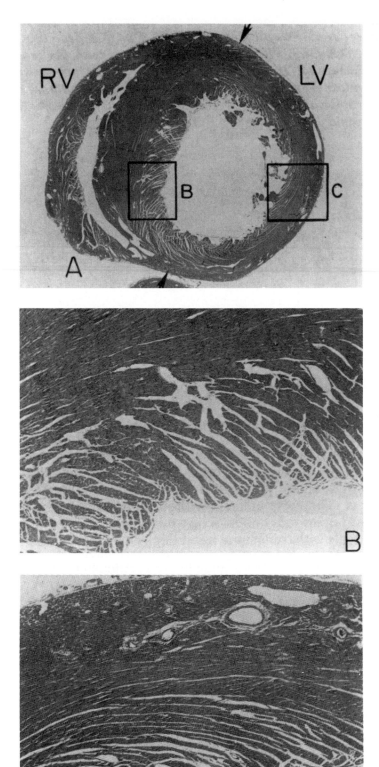

Fig. 18–3. *A,* Transverse section from middle third of long axis of rat heart with large 1-day infarction showing 2+ expansion. Borders of infarct are marked by arrows. Infarct region is thinned and dilated, and overall cavity size is increased. In the septum, inner fiber bundles and cleavage planes have some perpendicular alignment with endocardial surface as was seen in control hearts (original magnification, ×9). *B,* Portion of septum enclosed at higher magnification (original magnification ×50). Within infarct zone, angle of inner muscle bundles and cleavage planes relative to endocardial surface is more acute, as can be seen in greater detail in higher magnification view of the boxed region of the infarct (*C*) (original magnification, ×50). This translation of muscle bundles smooths the endocardial contour, RV = right ventricle LV = left ventricle. Reproduced with permission from Weisman HF, et al.: Cellular mechanisms of myocardial infarct expansion. Circulation 78:186, 1988.

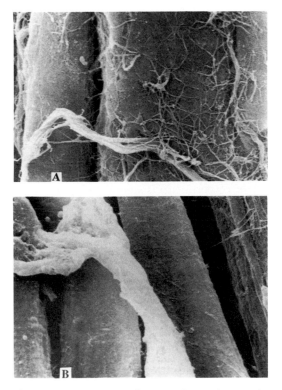

Fig. 18–4. Scanning electron photomicrographs of normal myocardium *(A)* (× 4000) and myocardium subjected to repeated episodes of ischemia *(B)* (× 2000). Reproduced with permission from Covell JW: Factors influencing diastolic function: Possible role of the extracellular matrix. Circulation 81:III-155, 1990.

of functioning myocardium with small infarcts, this mechanism is unable to fully compensate for losses sustained during large infarcts that affect approximately >30 to 40% of the LV (45–47). The growth in the capillary bed is not proportional to the degree of myocyte hypertrophy, particularly with large infarcts (47). As a result, there are deficits in capillary lumen and surface density, as well as an increase in the distance from the capillary wall to the surrounding tissue (increasing the diffusion distance for oxygen) (47). Inadequate adaptation of capillary growth may increase the vulnerability to further ischemic damage (47).

Elevated diastolic wall stress may provide the stimulus of compensatory hypertrophy, which may partially explain the greater hypertrophy response with large

compared with small infarcts (46, 47). The myocyte hypertrophy response is greater in noninfarcted regions that border rather than are remote from the infarcted area (46). This is consistent with theoretical predictions of a two- to fourfold amplification of wall stress in nonischemic border zones (48, 49). The high wall stress, along with local tethering effects, produces a narrow border zone where function is impaired despite normal coronary blood flow (50).

Despite cellular growth in nonischemic areas, these processes are inadequate for normalizing the high diastolic wall stresses with large infarcts (46). High wall stresses and ventricular remodeling may provide the stimuli for biochemical alterations. Three weeks after experimental myocardial infarction, the actomyosin ATPase activity in the surviving myocardium decreases and remains depressed for up to 11 weeks (51). There is a shift from the predominance of V1 myosin isoenzyme to significant expression of the V3 myosin isoform in direct relation to infarct size after experimental infarction in rats (51). This shift is partially reversed by treatment with an angiotensin converting enzyme (ACE) inhibitor (52).

INFLUENCE OF VENTRICULAR REMODELING ON DIASTOLIC PERFORMANCE

Myocardial infarction alters LV diastolic function in a complex manner because the time course and direction of regional diastolic alterations are different in the infarct and noninfarcted regions, producing a complicated sequence of changes in LV geometry and shape. In addition, it is difficult to quantitate diastolic changes and separate the direct and indirect effects of myocardial ischemia and ventricular remodeling because of the complex interaction between numerous factors that influence diastolic function (53, 54).

The pathologic sequence of events in the ischemic zone includes an early inflammatory response followed by progressive resorption of necrotic tissue and scar formation (55). Chamber enlargement may occur with infarct expansion caused by cell slippage and rearrangement (and to a lesser extent by cell stretch) (3). Cell slippage in nonischemic areas leads to wall thinning (30) and elevated diastolic wall stress, which may serve as a stimulus for compensatory hypertrophy (32). Thus dynamic changes in regional contractility (which directly and indirectly influence inactivation processes) and regional changes in wall thickness as well as the material properties of the wall (which affect wall stiffness) develop with time courses that differ for the infarct and noninfarct regions. These regional alterations produce global changes in chamber size and geometry that alter several diastolic processes including relaxation, viscoelasticity, passive elastic properties, and ventricular interaction.

Early Changes in Diastolic Function

Acute myocardial ischemia alters regional and global LV diastolic properties resulting in a slower rate of LV pressure fall, slower rate of diastolic filling, and alterations in passive elastic properties of the LV (56). Within minutes of acute myocardial ischemia, there is a slower rate of LV pressure fall, increased viscous resistance during early diastolic filling, and an upward shift in the diastolic pressure-volume relationship (57). These global changes are caused by delayed relaxation, increased wall stiffness, and an increase in resting muscle length in the ischemic zone (57).

Increased muscle lengths in the ischemic region are largely caused by a phenomenon termed creep (58). Creep refers to a time-dependent change in muscle length under constant load. It is assessed experimentally by measuring the resting muscle length (L_0) or volume (V_0) under conditions of zero stress, which is approximated by zero transmural pressure (e.g., during a transient decrease in venous return). Acute ischemia induces diastolic creep with a 16% increase in L_0 (58), which correlates with systolic dysfunction and can be reversed by reperfusion (59). It is important to assess creep changes to properly evaluate changes in muscle or LV chamber compliance (or its inverse, stiffness). Strain provides a more accurate measure of deformation than either length or volume because strain measurements are normalized to the appropriate reference configuration of L_0 or V_0. Therefore strain measures the

change in length or volume relative to the length or volume under zero stress. The rightward shift in passive pressure-length and pressure-volume relationships with acute ischemia (i.e., increased muscle length and LV volume at a matched LV diastolic pressure) does not necessarily indicate an increase in compliance (decreased stiffness) because the passive pressure-strain relationship, which takes into account the large increase in L_0, is not shifted rightward. In fact, the pressure-strain relationship is steeper after acute ischemia, indicating decreased compliance or increased stiffness (57). The increase in stiffness early during myocardial infarction can be reversed with early reperfusion (60).

The rate of LV pressure fall is slower with acute myocardial ischemia (57), normalizes within one hour, and remains normal for several days after myocardial infarction (61). This does not necessarily reflect normalization of myocardial relaxation because indices of LV pressure fall (e.g., the time constant of LV pressure decay, tau) underestimate the severity of local impairments in myocardial relaxation (62). Furthermore, a slower rate of LV pressure fall does not necessarily reflect the direct effects of ischemia on myocardial relaxation because ischemia induces several indirect effects (e.g., decreased contractility, altered loading conditions, and increased nonuniformity) which slow the rate of LV pressure fall by independent mechanisms (63).

Decreased myocardial relaxation, increased nonuniformity, and increased myocardial stiffness may all contribute to lower diastolic filling rates (53, 64). Diastolic filling rates may be normalized by elevating left atrial pressure, which commonly occurs with myocardial ischemia. Thus a normal early filling pattern does not necessarily indicate normal diastolic function (64). Acute myocardial ischemia attenuates the normal intraventricular pressure gradient that occurs early during rapid filling (65). This may be caused by regional wall motion abnormalities with loss of elastic recoil (65). The combination of decreased early diastolic filling, LV chamber enlargement, and dyskinetic wall motion of the LV apex alters blood inflow patterns that predispose to hemostasis and thrombus formation in the LV apex (66).

Left ventricular filling pressures are frequently elevated in acute myocardial infarction (67). This is caused by a combination of larger LV end-diastolic and end-systolic volumes (a result of LV dilation and less effective emptying), impaired myocardial relaxation, and increased myocardial and LV chamber stiffness. Regional and global ventricular function improve with elevations in LV end-diastolic pressure caused by increased utilization of the Frank-Starling mechanism in nonischemic regions and increased ischemic zone stiffness, which reduces paradoxic systolic expansion (bulge) and the mechanical disadvantage imposed by the ischemic zone (68). However, the cost of elevating LV filling pressures is increased diastolic wall stress, which may lead to pulmonary venous congestion, increased infarct size, ventricular dilation, and detrimental LV remodeling changes. The changes in the diastolic pressure-volume relation early and late after myocardial infarction are shown in Figure 18–5.

Late Changes in Diastolic Function

During the healing phase, progressive remodeling in both infarct and noninfarcted regions results from scar formation in infarcted areas and compensatory hypertrophy in noninfarcted regions. (See Chap. 14.) LV filling pressures are normal with small infarcts, but remain persistently elevated with larger infarcts (69). Myocardial stiffness, which had increased during the acute phase, decreases during the chronic phase of myocardial infarction so that LV compliance is greater than normal (61, 70, 71). This is partially related to LV dilation with ventricular remodeling, which causes a disproportionate increase in LV cavity volume relative to wall volume (61, 71). The LV may dilate progressively over several months after myocardial infarction (11). LV dilation produces a progressive rightward shift in the passive LV pressure-volume relationship from days to weeks to months after myocardial infarction (70, 71) (Fig. 18–5). The magnitude of this rightward shift is greater with large infarct sizes (70, 71). Although LV cham-

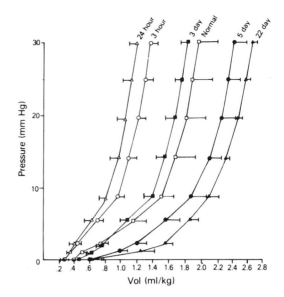

Fig. 18–5. Mean left ventricular pressure-volume relation in control rats (□) and in 3 hours (○), 24 hours (△), 3 days (■), 5 days (●), and more than 22 days (▲) after infarction. With acute infarction, there is a shift of the pressure-volume relation to the left. In the healing stages, there is progressive rightward displacement of the pressure-volume relation. Reproduced with permission from Raya TE, et al.: Serial changes in left ventricular relaxation and chamber stiffness after large myocardial infarction in rats. Circulation 77:1424, 1984.

ber stiffness decreases, stiffness may increase in papillary muscles from noninfarcted regions during the chronic phase (72) (Fig. 18–6). This may be related to the myocyte hypertrophy and/or increased collagen content in nonischemic areas following large infarcts (72).

The rate of LV pressure fall, which initially slowed and then normalized during the acute phase, becomes slower again during the chronic phase (61). This is not entirely caused by regional nonuniformity (63) because both patients with and without asynergy have slower rates of LV pressure fall after myocardial infarction (73). These abnormalities may be related to higher wall stress during isovolumetric relaxation in both infarcted and ischemic regions (the latter defined as regions supplied by a stenotic coronary artery but without electrocardiographic evidence of an infarct) (62). Regional relaxation in infarcted regions occurs at a rate similar to the rate of LV pres-

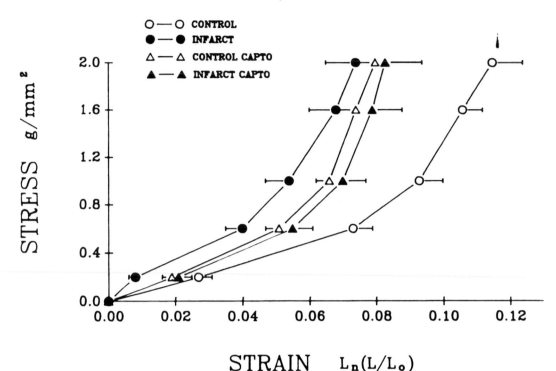

Fig. 18–6. Passive stress-strain relations of papillary muscles in control, large infarct, captopril-treated control, and captopril-treated infarct rats. Error bars are SEM. Curves for the large infarct, captopril-treated control, and captopril-treated infarct muscles are shifted to the left and have steeper slopes than the control muscles. Curve for the moderate-sized infarct group is very close to that of the control group and is not shown for purposes of clarity. Reproduced with permission from Litwin SE, et al.: Contractility and stiffness of noninfarcted myocardium after coronary ligation in rats. Circulation 83:1028, 1991.

sure fall, whereas relaxation in ischemic regions is slower (62).

LEFT VENTRICULAR ANEURYSM

Ventricular aneurysm formation is a common complication of acute myocardial infarction, particularly after transmural anterior wall infarcts (5, 74). Approximately 20% of patients develop an LV aneurysm after their first myocardial infarction (74). This is associated with an increase in mortality that is independent of the ejection fraction and is particularly high in patients who develop aneurysms within the first few days after myocardial infarction (5, 74). Early shape changes that develop in the LV wall within 48 to 72 hours following acute myocardial infarction reflect expansion of necrotic myocardium, and predisposes to the development of true LV aneurysms over the next 3 months (5, 19). Aneurysms are less likely to develop when

the coronary artery supplying the infarct region is patent (by spontaneous or successful therapeutic thrombolysis) and/or when there is adequate collateral circulation (75, 76).

Ventricular aneurysms adversely affect ventricular function. Theoretical models predict that the ejection fraction decreases in direct proportion to the size of the LV aneurysm (77). Compliant aneurysms impose a greater mechanical disadvantage than stiff fibrous aneurysms (77). This is related to paradoxic systolic expansion of the aneurysm which reduces LV mechanical efficiency. Paradoxic thinning of the aneurysm occurs during isovolumetric systole (78), analogous to the paradoxic expansion of acutely ischemic myocardium (68). Because noninfarcted regions expend or "waste" a significant amount of work in paradoxically stretching the ischemic zone or aneurysm during isovolumetric systole, the amount of work available for ventricular ejection is reduced. An ischemic region with paradoxic systolic expansion imposes a mechanical disadvantage on normal LV areas in direct proportion to the size (79) and compliance (68) of the ischemic area.

Chronic LV aneurysms are predicted to adversely influence function in the adjacent, normal myocardium (80). This is caused by a restraining effect that reduces the end-diastolic length in the adjacent normal myocardium, reducing peak tension development because of decreased utilization of the Frank-Starling mechanism (80). Wall stress amplification occurs in normal border regions, an effect which increases with increased compliance of the ischemic zone (48, 49).

Loading conditions influence the development of LV aneurysms. An increase in afterload causes an irreversible increase in muscle length in ischemic and infarcted myocardium (81). Although acutely ischemic myocardium is most susceptible, myocardial tissue early (24 hours) and late (3 and 15 weeks) after myocardial infarction are also susceptible to irreversible increases in length with increased afterload (81) (Fig. 18–7). This suggests that pharmacologic interventions that reduce afterload after myocardial infarction may re-

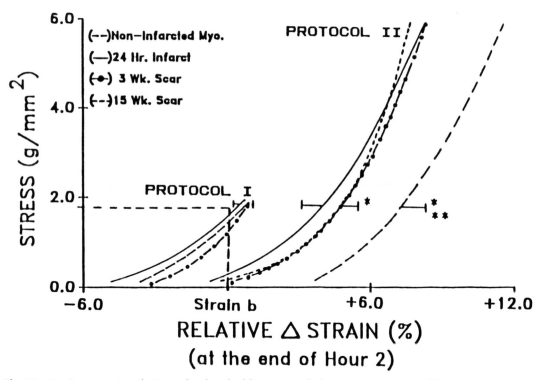

Fig. 18–7. Stress-strain relations of isolated rabbit myocardial tissue strips early and late after myocardial infarction. Tissue strips were cut along the long axis of the ventricle and repetitively stretched at physiologic stresses for 1 hour (strain b, protocol I). During a second hour, peak stress was tripled (afterload stress) and the increase in strip length (strain) was measured (protocol II). Tissue strips from acutely ischemic and healed infarction showed a significant increase in tissue elongation with application of an afterload stress that was irreversible following return to physiologic peak stress (data not shown). Relative Δ strain is expressed as a % [ln(L/Lo) × 100, where L is instantaneous length and Lo is initial length of unloaded strips] and measures the changes in strain relative to strain b. Noninfarcted myo. = acutely ischemic tissue, 24 Hr. infarct = acutely infarcted tissue, 3 and 15 Wk. Scar = healed infarction. Reproduced with permission from Connelly CM, et al.: Reversible and irreversible elongation of ischemic, infarcted, and healed myocardium in responses to increases in preload and afterload. Circulation 84: 387, 1991.

duce infarct expansion and thus reduce the likelihood of developing an LV aneurysm.

MODIFICATION OF LEFT VENTRICULAR REMODELING

The increased mortality associated with infarct expansion (4, 5) and LV dilation (6) has led to investigation of factors that may modify the extent of left ventricular remodeling following acute myocardial infarction. Although efforts aimed at reducing infarct sized are important during the acute phase, significant LV remodeling also develops late after myocardial infarction. The extent of LV remodeling can be modified by the degree of coronary perfusion, loading conditions, and pharmacologic agents that influence healing processes.

Vessel Patency

Successful thrombolysis early during the course of an acute myocardial infarction improves survival by limiting the extent of myocardial necrosis and improving regional and global LV function (82–85). The LV size is smaller after thrombolysis (82, 85) and remains smaller 6 months after myocardial infarction (84). This is not entirely the result of myocardial salvage because the LV size tends to be smaller in treated than in untreated patients who have a similar extent of regional wall motion abnormality (84). Reperfusion 2 hours after experimental coronary artery occlusion inhibits infarct expansion even though the reperfusion is too late for myocardial salvage and reducing infarct size (86). Late thrombolysis (4 to 8 hours after the onset of symptoms) limited infarct expansion in one study (87) but did not limit LV dilation in another study (10). With or without thrombolytic therapy, LV dilation is more likely to occur with total occlusion of the infarct vessel and less likely to occur with a patent coronary artery and/or with coronary collateral blood flow (88, 89). The benefits of a patent infarct vessel on limiting progressive chamber dilation occurs both early (89) and late (90) after myocardial infarction and are independent of infarct size (88, 91). The severity of the baseline residual stenosis of the infarct related artery is an important predictor of subse-

quent ventricular dilatation (90). Similarly, a patent infarct vessel and/or collateral blood flow reduces the risk of LV aneurysm formation (75). Thus, adequate perfusion during the healing phase of myocardial infarction may not reduce infarct size, but may decrease the extent of infarct expansion and LV dilation.

Exercise Training

The role of exercise training after myocardial infarction is controversial. Exercise training following experimental transmural myocardial infarction increases the ventricular fibrillation threshold (92), reverses the chronotropic incompetence, and partially reverses the downregulation of myosin isozyme back towards the fast ATPase V1 isoform (93). Exercise during the first week following an experimental myocardial infarction did not influence infarct expansion in one study (94), but another group found that exercise during the healing phase resulted in significant scar thinning and infarct expansion (95, 96). In patients with marked LV asynergy, low-level exercise training started well into the healing phase (15 weeks after infarction) exacerbates the extent of infarct expansion, wall thinning and local shape distortion (97). Thus, despite the conflicting literature as to the role of exercise training, exercise may adversely affect LV remodeling following large transmural myocardial infarctions.

Glucocorticosteroids and Nonsteroidal Antiinflammatory Drugs

High doses of glucocorticosteroids given early during experimental myocardial infarction cause scar thinning without altering the collagen content (as assessed by hydroxyproline content), resulting in reduced regional function (98). Glucocorticosteroids primarily enhance early infarct expansion within the first 3 days of myocardial infarction (before new collagen deposition) primarily by promoting myocyte cell slippage in the infarct region (99).

Nonsteroidal antiinflammatory drugs also modify LV remodeling. Ibuprofen (100, 101) and indomethacin (102) produce a scar thinning without altering the collagen content (assessed by hydroxyproline content). Aspirin does not affect infarct healing (100). Regional function decreases in direct proportion to the extent of infarct expansion, whether expansion occurs spontaneously or is induced by indomethacin (103). Ibuprofen promotes infarct thinning and expansion despite its effect on reducing infarct size (101).

The mechanisms by which glucocorticosteroids and nonsteroidal antiinflammatory drugs modify LV remodeling are not entirely known. Because collagen content in the thinned scars does not change and significant infarct expansion occurs early after myocardial infarction, a delay in collagen deposition or scar stretching do not appear to be major factors. It has been postulated that these agents reduce early tissue edema and inflammatory cell infiltration, thereby promoting infarct expansion (99, 103). It has been demonstrated that glucocorticosteroids promotes cell slippage which predisposes to infarct expansion (99).

Hemodynamic Factors

Transient increases in afterload early during experimental myocardial infarction result in infarct expansion and scar thinning, with histologic evidence of delayed healing (104). Sustained increases in afterload with LV hypertrophy (produced by aortic banding) predisposes to infarct expansion independently of its effects on infarct size (18). Both acutely ischemic and chronically infarcted myocardium are lengthened irreversibly by increases in afterload (but not by increases in preload), which may be a precursor of infarct expansion and LV aneurysms formation (81). Clinical hypertension is more common in patients with than without infarct expansion (17).

Low-dose nitroglycerin given early after an experimental myocardial infarction (decreasing mean arterial pressure by 10%) decreases infarct expansion (101). This may be caused by a decrease in infarct size, decreased preload and afterload, decreased wall stress and myocardial oxygen demands, increased collateral blood flow, and increased collagen content in the infarct region (101). Low-dose nitroglycerin given to patients early during an acute

myocardial infarction also decreases infarct size and decreases infarct expansion (105).

Angiotensin Converting Enzyme Inhibitors

Angiotensin converting enzyme (ACE) inhibitors can modify the extent of ventricular remodeling. Chronic captopril treatment for 6 weeks to 3 months after an experimental myocardial infarction decreases LV end-diastolic pressure and volume, while increasing ejection fraction and maximum stroke volume index, when compared to animals without treatment but with comparable size infarcts (106, 107). These effects are not solely a result of the acute hemodynamic benefits of captopril. (See Chap. 20.) Captopril attenuates the rightward shift in the passive LV pressure-volume relationship following myocardial infarction (106). This is associated with improved 1-year survival (108). Thus captopril attenuates ventricular remodeling and improves survival in experimental myocardial infarction.

Clinical studies have yielded similar results. Three randomized, double-blind, placebo-controlled trials have evaluated the effects of captopril, started within 1 to 3 weeks and continued for 6 months to 1 year after acute myocardial infarction (109–111). Patients from these trials had reduced ejection fractions (<45%) without clinical heart failure. Captopril decreased LV end-diastolic pressure (109) and attenuated the LV dilation that developed in untreated patients (109, 111). In two of the studies, captopril produced a marked decrease in LV end-systolic and end-diastolic volume in addition to increases in both stroke volume index and ejection fraction; benefits not observed with furosemide treatment (110) or in placebo control patients (110, 111). Deterioration in diastolic function as measured by peak mitral inflow velocities was prevented with captopril therapy (111). In an unblinded, randomized, placebo-controlled trial, treatment with captopril resulted in less left ventricular dilation than did digitalis 1 year after anterior myocardial infarction (112). The beneficial effects of captopril on LV remodeling are accompanied by less infarct expansion (113) and improved exercise duration (109).

Three recent large multicenter trials have evaluated whether ACE inhibitors also reduce mortality from heart failure. The Survival and Ventricular Enlargement (SAVE) Trial randomized 2231 patients who survived the first 3 days of myocardial infarction to either placebo to captopril (114). Patients were randomized within 3 to 16 (mean 11) days after myocardial infarction and followed for an average of 42 months. All patients had ejection fractions ≤40% but no symptoms of congestive heart failure. Therapy with captopril reduced total and cardiovascular mortality, recurrent myocardial infarction and hospitalization for heart failure by ~20% (114).

The Cooperative New Scandinavian Enalapril Survey Study (CONSENSUS II) trial randomized 6090 patients to placebo or enalapril within 24 hours after myocardial infarction (115). All patients were eligible for randomization regardless of ejection fraction. There was no significant reduction in mortality after six months. The study was terminated prematurely because of a trend suggesting an adverse effect of enalapril on mortality, especially in patients who developed hypotension with the drug. These results suggest that the early use of ACE inhibitors may promote unfavorable ventricular remodeling (115). It is possible that a longer follow-up than 6 months would be required to demonstrate benefits of ACE inhibition, such as the 42-month follow-up period in the SAVE trial. Furthermore, all patients in the SAVE trial had reduced ejection fractions which may preselect those at greatest risk for the deleterious effects of LV dilation and remodeling.

Treatment with ACE inhibitors reduces mortality in patients with congestive heart failure (116–118). In the recent Studies of Left Ventricular Dysfunction (SOLVD) Prevention Trial, over 4200 patients with reduced ejection fractions but without symptoms of congestive heart failure were randomized to receive placebo or enalapril and followed for an average of 37 months (119). In contrast to the benefits in symptomatic heart failure (116–118), treatment with enalapril does not reduce mortality in patients with asymptomatic left ventricular dysfunction (119). This provides indirect evidence that the reductions in mortality in

the SAVE trial (114) were related to the beneficial effects of ACE inhibitors on ventricular remodeling following myocardial infarction, rather than any benefit of reducing mortality in asymptomatic left ventricular dysfunction.

In the near future, results will become available from other large randomized, double-blind, placebo controlled, multicenter trials. Several other trials identified by the acronyms CATS (Captopril and Thrombolysis Study Trial), CAPTIN (Captopril plus tPA following Acute Myocardial Infarction), SMILE (Survival of Myocardial Infarction Long-term Evaluation), ISIS-4 (Fourth International Study of Infarct Survival), and GISSI-III (Gruppo Italiano per lo Studie Selks Streptochinasi nell'Infarto Miocardico) will examine the benefits of early ACE inhibitor therapy on survival in the first few months following myocardial infarction (120).

The mechanisms by which ACE inhibitors minimize LV remodeling after myocardial infarction are not entirely understood. Although captopril is an arterial vasodilator, the use of hydralazine in doses that produce a similar decrease in mean arterial pressure does not attenuate LV remodeling following myocardial infarction (121). The venodilation effects of captopril may play an important role in decreasing LV end-diastolic pressure and volume following myocardial infarction by decreasing blood volume and increasing venous compliance, effects that are not observed with hydralazine (121). However, a decrease in preload cannot entirely explain the beneficial effects of ACE inhibitors. Decreasing blood volume with furosemide does not attenuate LV remodeling in patients with myocardial infarction (110). Low-dose nitroglycerin decreases infarct expansion, but nitroglycerin also decreases afterload, decreases infarct size, and increases collateral blood flow (101). Finally, other vasodilators, such as milrinone (a phosphodiesterase inhibitor with positive inotropic effects) do not have significant preload effects, yet attenuate LV remodeling after myocardial infarction (122). Interestingly, milrinone does not affect the renin-angiotensin system.

Although most of the attention has focused on the hemodynamic effects, ACE inhibitors may attenuate LV remodeling by other mechanisms. The ACE inhibitor perindopril attenuates several of the hormonal and protein abnormalities that develop with myocardial infarction, including the increase in atrial natriuretic factor, increase in atria and right ventricular mass, and shift in isomyosin from V1 to V3 (52). Captopril has cardioprotective effects, which may be related to the free-radical scavenging properties of ACE inhibitors with a sulphydryl group (123). Early administration of captopril can limit infarct size, reduce reperfusion injury (myocardial stunning), and limit early infarct expansion and dilation (123). Although these mechanisms may be important early during ischemia, experimental and clinical studies clearly demonstrate that ACE inhibitors attenuate LV remodeling even when administered late (e.g., during the healing phase) after myocardial infarction.

Recently, it has been shown that several tissues, including the heart, possess a local renin-angiotensin system (124). (See Chaps. 1 and 20.) Although the physiologic function remains to be defined, ACE inhibitors may influence LV remodeling by modulating the cardiac renin-angiotensin system. In any case, the local effects of angiotensin II (produced intrinsically and/or delivered from extracardiac sources) may play an important role in LV remodeling. Angiotensin II has important direct inotropic and growth-promoting effects (125). The role of inotropic state on LV remodeling is unknown. As noted, milrinone, which has both vasodilator and positive inotropic properties, attenuates LV remodeling (122). Propranolol causes greater LV dilation following myocardial infarction and blunts the compensatory hypertrophy that normally develops in noninfarcted regions (126). Although captopril inhibits the direct inotropic effects of angiotensin II, LV remodeling is attenuated, not increased. Thus it seems unlikely that an inotropic mechanism explains the attenuation of LV remodeling with captopril.

Recent attention has focused on the role of angiotensin II as a growth factor in ventricular hypertrophy (124, 125). Captopril and other ACE inhibitors attenuate LV remodeling in part by blocking the compensatory hypertrophy that develops in nonin-

farcted regions. Angiotensin II may also play an important role in collagen synthesis and deposition. ACE inhibitors may interfere or alter the function of angiotensin II in the healing process of acute myocardial infarction, and thus modulate the extent of LV remodeling. Although several of these mechanisms remain speculative at this time, it seems unlikely that alterations in loading conditions can solely explain the beneficial effects of ACE inhibitors in attenuating LV remodeling following myocardial infarction.

CONCLUSION

Acute transmural myocardial infarction may result in LV dilation that results from two processes that involve both the ischemic and nonischemic myocardium. Infarct expansion is characterized by thinning and dilation in the chronic infarct area, which most often occurs in large transmural myocardial infarction and develops over hours to days. Early LV dilation results from myocyte slippage in both necrotic and remote areas, caused partly by damage of collagen structures. With infarct healing, fibrosis develops and, within a period of 2 to 3 weeks, the process of infarct expansion is stabilized. With reduced contractile function, LV end-diastolic volume and end-diastolic fiber length in the normal myocardium is increased both in the acute and chronic setting depending on the infarct size. This tends to augment fiber shortening and normalize stroke volume by the Frank-Starling mechanism, however, at the expense of LV enlargement. Increased LV end-diastolic pressure and cavity volume result in increased diastolic wall tension, which promotes myocyte slippage, reduced LV compliance, and further increases in LV end-diastolic pressure. According to the law of Laplace, LV wall stress is augmented because of the increase in both LV end-diastolic pressure and radius. Reactive hypertrophy of viable myocardium ensues to normalize wall tension. Ultimately, myocardial hypertrophy tends to reduce fiber shortening, which promotes further LV enlargement and reduced ejection fraction. Heightened activity of both the sympathetic and renin angiotensin systems is found following myocardial infarction. Although these mechanisms are invoked to preserve myocardial contractility and perfusion pressure, wall stress and LV remodeling are adversely effected. Collateral blood flow, vessel patency, and ACE inhibitors have all been shown to favorably affect infarct expansion and LV remodeling.

REFERENCES

1. Pfeffer MA, Braunwald E: Ventricular remodeling after myocardial infarction. Circulation 81:1161, 1990.
2. Tennant R, Wiggers CJ: The effect of coronary occlusion on myocardial contraction. Am J Physiol 112:351, 1935.
3. Wiesman HF, Healy B: Myocardial infarction expansion, infarct extension, and reinfarction: Pathophysiologic concepts. Prog Cardiovasc Dis 30:73, 1987.
4. Eaton LW, et al.: Regional cardiac dilatation after acute myocardial infarction. N Engl J Med 300:57, 1979.
5. Meizlish JL, et al.: Functional left ventricular aneurysm formation after acute anterior transmural myocardial infarction. N Engl J Med 311:1001, 1984.
6. White HD, et al.: Left ventricular end-systolic volume as the major determinant of survival after recovery from myocardial infarction. Circulation 76:44, 1987.
7. Hutchins GM, Bulkley BH: Infarct expansion versus extension: Two different complications of acute myocardial infarction. Am J Cardiol 41:1127, 1978.
8. Hochman JS, Bulkley BH: Expansion of acute myocardial infarction: An experimental study. Circulation 65:1446, 1982.
9. Eaton LW, Bulkley BH: Expansion of acute myocardial infarction: Its relationship to infarct morphology in a canine model. Circ Res 49:80, 1981.
10. Warren SE, et al.: Time course left ventricular dilation after myocardial infarction: influence of infarct-related artery and success of coronary thrombolysis. J Am Coll Cardiol 11:12, 1988.
11. Jeremy RW, et al.: Patterns of left ventricular dilation during the six months after myocardial infarction. J Am Coll Cardiol 13:304, 1989.
12. Erlebacher JA, et al.: Early dilation of the infarcted segment in acute transmural myocardial infarctin: Role of infarct expansion in acute left ventricular enlargement. J Am Coll Cardiol 4:201, 1984.
13. Pirolo JS, Hutchins GM, Moore GW: Infarct expansion: Pathologic analysis of 204 patients with a single myocardial infarct. J Am Coll Cardiol 7:349, 1986.
14. Gadsboll N, et al.: Late ventricular dilatation in survivors of acute myocardial infarction. Am J Cardiol 64:961, 1989.
15. Picard MH, Wilkins GT, Ray PA, Weyman AE: Natural history of left ventricular size and function after acute myocardial infarction. Circulation 82:484, 1990.
16. Role L, Bogen D, McMahon TA, Abelmann WH: Regional variations in calculated diastolic wall stress in rat left ventricle. Am J Physiol 235:H247, 1978.
17. Pierard LA, et al.: Hemodynamic profile of patients with acute myocardial infarction at risk of infarct expansion. Am J Cardiol 60:5, 1987.
18. Nolan SE, et al.: Increased afterload aggravates infarct expansion after acute myocardial infarction. J Am Coll Cardiol 12:1318, 1988.
19. Hochman JS, Bulkley BH: Pathogenesis of left ventricular aneurysms: An experimental study in the rat model. Am J Cardiol 50:83, 1982.
20. Schuster EH, Bulkley BH: Expansion of transmural myocardial infarction: A pathophysiologic factor in cardiac rupture. Circulation 60:1532, 1979.
21. DeFelice A, Frering R, Horan P: Time course of hemodynamic changes in rats with healed severe myocardial infarction. Am J Physiol 257:H289, 1989.
22. Sasayma S, et al.: Regional left ventricular wall thickness early and late after coronary occlusion in the conscious dog. Am J Physiol 240:H293, 1981.
23. Erlebacher JA, et al.: Late effects of acute infarct dilation on heart size: A two dimensional echocardiographic study. Am J Cardiol 49:1120, 1982.
24. McKay RG, et al.: Left ventricular remodeling after myocardial infarction: A corollary to infarct expansion. Circulation 74:693, 1986.
25. Kass DA, et al.: Disproportionate epicardial dilation after transmural infarction of the canine left ventricle: Acute and chronic differences. J Am Coll Cardiol 11:177, 1988.
26. Weisman HF, Bush DE, Mannisi JA, Bulkley BH: Global cardiac remodeling after acute myocardial infarction: A study in the rat model. J Am Coll Cardiol 5:1355, 1985.
27. Grossman W: Cardiac hypertrophy: Useful adaptation or pathologic process? Am J Med 69:576, 1980.
28. Streeter DD, et al.: Fiber orientation in the canine left ventricle during diastole and systole. Circ Res 24:339, 1969.

29. Spotnitz HM, et al.: Cellular basis for volume related wall thickness changes in the rat left ventricle. J Mol Cell Cardiol 6:317, 1974.

30. Weisman HF, et al.: Cellular mechanisms of myocardial infarct expansion. Circulation 78:186, 1988.

31. Capasso JM, Li P, Zhang X, Anversa P: Heterogeneity of ventricular remodeling after acute myocardial infarction in rats. Am J Physiol 262:H486, 1992.

32. Olivetti G, Capasso JM, Sonnenblick EH, Anversa P: Side-to-side slippage of myocytes participates in ventricular wall remodeling acutely after myocardial infarction in rats. Circ Res 67:23, 1990.

33. Capasso JM, et al.: Ventricular remodeling induced by acute nonocclusive constriction of coronary artery in rats. Am J Physiol 257:H1983, 1989.

34. Caulfield JB, Borg TK: The collagen network of the heart. Lab Invest 40:364, 1979.

35. Sato S, Ashraf M, Millard RW, Fujiwara H, Schwartz A: Connective tissue changes in early ischemia of porcine myocardium: An ultrastructural study. J Mol Cell Cardiol 15:261, 1983.

36. Takahashi S, Barry AC, Factor SM: Collagen degradation in ischaemic rat hearts. Biochem J 265:233, 1990.

37. Cannon III RO, et al.: Early degradation of collagen after acute myocardial infarction in the rat. Am J Cardiol 52:390, 1983.

38. Zhao M, et al.: Profound structural alterations of the extracellular collagen matrix in postischemic dysfunctional ("stunned") but viable myocardium. J Am Coll Cardiol 10:1322, 1987.

39. Whittaker P, Boughner DR, Kloner RA: Role of collagen in acute myocardial infarct expansion. Circulation 84:2123, 1991.

40. Lerman RH, et al.: Myocardial healing and repair after experimental infarction in the rabbit. Circ Res 53:378, 1983.

41. Carroll EP, Janicki JS, Pick R, Weber KT: Myocardial stiffness and reparative fibrosis following coronary embolisation in the rat. Cardiovasc Res 23:655, 1989.

42. Anversa P, Loud AV, Levicky V, Guideri G: Left ventricular failure induced by myocardial infarction. I. Myocyte hypertrophy. Am J Physiol 248:H876, 1985.

43. Mitchell GF, Lamas GA, Vaughan DE, Pfeffer MA: Left ventricular remodeling in the year after anterior myocardial infarction: A quantitative analysis of contractile segment lengths and ventricular shape. J Am Coll Cardiol 19:1136, 1992.

44. Gerdes AM, et al.: Structural remodeling of cardiac myocytes in patients with ischemic cardiomyopathy. Circulation 86:426, 1992.

45. Rubin SA, Fishbein MC, Swain HJC, Rabines A: Compensatory hypertrophy in the heart after myocardial infarction in the rat. J Am Coll Cardiol 1:1435, 1983.

46. Olivetti G, et al.: Cellular basis of chronic ventricular remodeling after myocardial infarction in rats. Circ Res 68:856, 1991.

47. Anversa P, Beghi C, Kikkawa Y, Olivetti G: Myocardial infarction in rats. Circ Res 58:26, 1986.

48. Bogen DK, et al.: An analysis of the mechanical disadvantage of myocardial infarction in the canine left ventricle. Circ Res 47:728, 1980.

49. Bogen DK, Needleman A, McMahon TA: An analysis of myocardial infarction: The effect of regional changes in contractility. Circ Res 55:805, 1984.

50. Gallagher KP, et al.: The distribution of functional impairment across the lateral border of acutely ischemic myocardium. Circ Res 58:570, 1986.

51. Geenen DL, Malhotra A, Scheuer J: Regional variation in rat cardiac myosin isoenzymes and ATPase activity after infarction. Am J Physiol 256:H745, 1989.

52. Michel JB, et al.: Hormonal and cardiac effects of converting enzyme inhibition in rat myocardial infarction. Circ Res 62:641, 1988.

53. Lew WYW: Evaluation of left ventricular diastolic function. Circulation 79:1393, 1989.

54. Gilbert JC, Glantz SA: Determinants of left ventricular filling and of diastolic pressure-volume relation. Circ Res 64:827, 1989.

55. Fishbein MC, Maclean D, Maroko PR: Experimental myocardial infarction in the rat. Am J Pathol 90:57, 1978.

56. Lew WYW, LeWinter MM: Acute myocardial infarction: Pathophysiology. Chapter 8, Volume 2. *In* Cardiology. Edited by Parmley WW, Chatterjee K. Philadelphia, JB Lippincott Co., 1990.

57. Hess OM, et al.: Diastolic myocardial wall stiffness and ventricular relaxation during partial and completed coronary occlusions in the conscious dog. Circ Res 52:387, 1983.

58. Edwards CH, et al.: Effects of ischemia on left ventricular regional function in the conscious dog. Am J Physiol 240:H413, 1981.

59. Glower DD, et al.: Relation between reversal of diastolic creep and recovery of sys-

tolic function after ischemic myocardial injury in conscious dogs. Circ Res 60:850, 1987.

60. Kurnik PB, Courtois MR, Ludbrook PA: Diastolic stiffening induced by acute myocardial infarction is reduced by early reperfusion. J Am Coll Cardiol 12:1029, 1988.

61. Raya TE, et al.: Serial changes in left ventricular relaxation and chamber stiffness after large myocardial infarction in rats. Circulation 77:1424, 1988.

62. Pouleur H, Rousseau MF, VanEyll C, Charlier AA: Assessment of regional left ventricular relaxation in patients with coronary artery disease: importance of geometric factors and changes in wall thickness. Circulation 69:696, 1984.

63. Lew WYW, Rasmussen CM: Influence of nonuniformity on rate of left ventricular pressure fall in the dog. Am J Physiol 256: H222, 1989.

64. Yellin EL, Nikolic S, Frater RWM: Left ventricular filling dynamics and diastolic function. Prog Cardiovasc Dis 32:247, 1990.

65. Courtois M, Kovács SJ, Ludbrook PA: Physiological early diastolic intraventricular pressure gradient is lost during acute myocardial ischemia. Circulation 81:1688, 1990.

66. Beppu S, et al.: Abnormal blood pathways in left ventricular cavity in acute myocardial infarction. Circulation 78:157, 1988.

67. Forrester JS, Diamond G, Chatterjee K, Swan HJC: Medical therapy of acute myocardial infarction by application of hemodynamic subsets (first of two parts). N Engl J Med 295:1356, 1976.

68. Lew WYW, Ban-Hayashi E: Mechanisms of improving regional and global ventricular function by preload alterations during acute ischemia in the canine left ventricle. Circulation 72:1125, 1985.

69. Pfeffer MA, et al.: Myocardial infarct size and ventricular function in rats. Circ Res 44:503, 1979.

70. Fletcher PJ, Pfeffer JM, Pfeffer MA, Braunwald E: Left ventricular diastolic pressure-volume relations in rats with healed myocardial infarction. Circ Res 49: 618, 1981.

71. Pfeffer JM, Pfeffer MA, Fletcher PJ, Braunwald E: Progressive ventricular remodeling in rat with myocardial infarction. Am J Physiol 260:H1406, 1991.

72. Litwin SE, et al.: Contractility and stiffness of noninfarcted myocardium after coronary ligation in rats. Circulation 83:1028, 1991.

73. Hirota Y: A clinical study of left ventricular relaxation. Circulation 62:756, 1980.

74. Visser CA, et al.: Incidence, timing and prognostic value of left ventricular aneurysm formation after myocardial infarction: A prospective, serial echocardiographic study of 158 patients. Am J Cardiol 57:729, 1986.

75. Forman MB, et al.: Determinants of left ventricular aneurysm formation after anterior myocardial infarction: A clinical and angiographic study. J Am Coll Cardiol 8:1256, 1986.

76. Hirai T, et al.: Importance of collateral circulation for prevention of left ventricular aneurysm formation in acute myocardial infarction. Circulation 79:791, 1989.

77. Parmley WW, et al.: In vitro length-tension relations of human ventricular aneurysms. Am J Cardiol 32:889, 1973.

78. Nicolosi AC, Spotnitz HM: Quantitative analysis of regional systolic function with left ventricular aneurysm. Circulation 78: 856, 1988.

79. Lew WYW: Influence of ischemic zone size on nonischemic area function in the canine left ventricle. Am J Physiol 252: H990, 1987.

80. Janz RF, Waldron RJ: Predicted effect of chronic apical aneurysms on the passive stiffness of the human left ventricle. Circ Res 42:255, 1978.

81. Connelly CM, McLaughlin RJ, Vogel WM, Apstein CS: Reversible and irreversible elongation of ischemic, infarcted, and healed myocardium in response to increases in preload and afterload. Circulation 84:387, 1991.

82. Serruys PW, et al.: Preservation of global and regional left ventricular function after early thrombolysis in acute myocardial infarction. J Am Coll Cardiol 7:729, 1986.

83. Sheehan FH, et al.: Early recovery of left ventricular function after thrombolytic therapy for acute myocardial infarction: An important determinant of survival. J Am Coll Cardiol 12:289, 1988.

84. Marino P, et al.: Effect of streptokinase on left ventricular modeling and function after myocardial infarction: The GISSI (Gruppo Italiano per lo Studio della Streptochinasi nell'Infarto Miocardico) Trial. J Am Coll Cardiol 14:1149, 1989.

85. White HD, et al.: Effect of intravenous streptokinase on left ventricular function and early survival after acute myocardial infarction. N Engl J Med 317:850, 1987.

86. Hochman JS, Choo H: Limitation of myocardial infarct expansion by reperfusion independent of myocardial salvage. Circulation 75:299, 1987.

87. Bonaduce D, et al.: Effects of late administration of tissue-type plasminogen activator on left ventricular remodeling and function after myocardial infarction. J Am Coll Cardiol 16:1561, 1990.

88. Jeremy RW, et al.: Infarct artery perfusion and changes in left ventricular volume in the month after acute myocardial infarction. J Am Coll Cardiol 9:989, 1987.

89. Siu SC, et al.: The effect of late patency of the infarct-related coronary artery on left ventricular morphology and regional function after thrombolysis. Am Heart J 124:265, 1992.

90. Leung WH, Lau CP: Effects of severity of the residual stenosis of the infarct-related coronary artery on left ventricular dilation after acute myocardial infarction. J Am Coll Cardiol 20:307, 1992.

91. Touchstone DA, et al.: Effects of successful intravenous reperfusion therapy on regional myocardial function and geometry in humans: A tomographic assessment using two-dimensional echocardiography. J Am Coll Cardiol 13:1506, 1989.

92. Posel D, et al.: Exercise training after experimental myocardial infarction increases the ventricular fibrillation threshold before and after the onset of reinfarction in the isolated rat heart. Circulation 80:138, 1989.

93. Musch TI, et al.: Cardiac adaptations to endurance training in rats with a chronic myocardial infarction. J Appl Physiol 66:712, 1989.

94. Hochman JS, Healy B: Effect of exercise on acute myocardial infarction in rats. J Am Coll Cardiol 7:126, 1986.

95. Kloner RA, Kloner JA: The effect of early exercise on myocardial infarct scar formation. Am Heart J 106:1009, 1983.

96. Hammerman H, Schoen FJ, Kloner RA: Short-term exercise has a prolonged effect on scar formation after experimental acute myocardial infarction. J Am Coll Cardiol 2:979, 1983.

97. Jugdutt BI, Michorowski BL, Kappagoda CT: Exercise training after anterior Q wave myocardial infarction: Importance of regional left ventricular function and topography. J Am Coll Cardiol 12:362, 1988.

98. Hammerman H, et al.: Dose-dependent effects of short-term methylprednisolone on myocardial infarct extent, scar formation, and ventricular function. Circulation 68:446, 1983.

99. Mannisi JA, et al.: Steroid administration after myocardial infarction promotes early infarct expansion. J Clin Invest 79:1431, 1987.

100. Brown EJ, et al.: Scar thinning due to ibuprofen administration after experimental myocardial infarction. Am J Cardiol 51:877, 1983.

101. Jugdutt BI: Delayed effects of early infarct-limiting therapies on healing after myocardial infarction. Circulation 72:907, 1985.

102. Hammerman H, et al.: Indomethacin induced scar thinning after experimental myocardial infarction. Circulation 67:1290, 1983.

103. Hammerman H, Schoen FJ, Braunwald E, Kloner RA: Drug induced expansion of infarct: morphologic and functional correlations. Circulation 69:611, 1984.

104. Hammerman H, et al.: Effects of transient increased afterload during experimentally induced acute myocardial infarction in dogs. Am J Cardiol 55:566, 1985.

105. Jugdutt BI, Warnica JW: Intravenous nitroglycerin therapy to limit myocardial infarct size, expansion and complications. Circulation 78:906, 1988.

106. Pfeffer JM, Pfeffer MA, Braunwald E: Influence of chronic captopril therapy on the infarcted left ventricle of the rat. Circ Res 57:84, 1985.

107. Jugdutt BI, Schwarz-Michorowski BL, Khan MI: Effect of long term captopril therapy on left ventricular remodeling and function during healing of canine myocardial infarction. J Am Coll Cardiol 19:713, 1992.

108. Pfeffer MA, Pfeffer JM, Steinberg C, Finn P: Survival after an experimental myocardial infarction: Beneficial effects of long-term therapy with captopril. Circulation 72:406, 1985.

109. Pfeffer MA, et al.: Effect of captopril on progressive ventricular dilatation after anterior myocardial infarction. N Engl J Med 319:80, 1988.

110. Sharpe N, Smith H, Murphy J, Hannan S: Treatment of patients with symptomless left ventricular dysfunction after myocardial infarction. Lancet 1:255, 1988.

111. Gotzsche CO, Sogaard P, Ravkilde J, Thygesen K: Effects of captopril on left ventricular systolic and diastolic function after acute myocardial infarction. Am J Cardiol 70:156, 1992.

112. Bonaduce D, et al.: Effect of captopril treatment on left ventricular remodeling and function after anterior myocardial infarction: comparison with digitalis. J Am Coll Cardiol 19:858, 1992.

113. Oldroyd KG, et al.: Effects of early captopril administration on infarct expansion,

left ventricular remodeling and exercise capacity after acute myocardial infarction. Am J Cardiol 68:713, 1991.

114. Pfeffer MA, et al.: Effect of captopril on mortality and morbidity in patients with left ventricular dysfunction after myocardial infarction. Results of the survival and ventricular enlargement trial. N Engl J Med 327:669, 1992.

115. Swedberg K, et al.: Effects of the early administration of enalapril on mortality in patients with acute myocardial infarction. Results of the Cooperative New Scandinavian Enalapril Survival Study II (CONSENSUS II). N Engl J Med 327:678, 1992.

116. Cohn JN, Archibald DG, Ziesche S, et al.: Effect of vasodilator therapy on mortality in chronic congestive heart failure: Results of a Veterans Administration Cooperative Study. N Engl J Med 314:1547, 1986.

117. The CONSENSUS Trial Study Group. Effects of enalapril on mortality in severe congestive heart failure: Results of the Cooperative North Scandinavian Enalapril Survival Study (CONSENSUS). N Engl J Med 316:1429, 1987.

118. The SOLVD Investigators. Effect of enalapril on survival in patients with reduced left ventricular ejection fractions and congestive heart failure. N Engl J Med 325:293, 1991.

119. The SOLVD Investigators: Effect of enalapril on mortality and the development of heart failure in asymptomatic patients with reduced left ventricular ejection fractions. N Engl J Med 327:685, 1992.

120. Pfeffer MA, Braunwald E: Ventricular enlargement following infarction is a modifiable process. Am J Cardiol 68:127D, 1991.

121. Raya TE, Gay RG, Aguirre M, Goldman S: Importance of venodilation in prevention of left ventricular dilatation after chronic large myocardial infarction in rats: A comparison of captopril and hydralazine. Circ Res 64:330, 1989.

122. Jain P, et al.: Effects of milrinone on left ventricular remodeling after acute myocardial infarction. Circulation 84:796, 1991.

123. Mehta PM, Przyklenk K, Kloner RA: Cardioprotective effects of captopril in myocardial ischaemia, ischaemia/reperfusion and infarction. Eur Heart J 11(B):94, 1990.

124. Lindpaintner K, Ganten D: The cardiac renin-angiotensin system: An appraisal of present experimental and clinical evidence. Circ Res 68:905, 1991.

125. Morgan HE, Baker KM: Cardiac hypertrophy: Mechanical, neural and endocrine dependence. Circulation 83:13, 1991.

126. Fishbein MC, Lei LQ, Rubin SA: Long-term propranolol administration alters myocyte and ventricular geometry in rat hearts with and without infarction. Circulation 78:369, 1988.

Chapter 19

ANGIOGRAPHIC AND ECHOCARDIOGRAPHIC EVALUATION OF SEGMENTAL LEFT VENTRICULAR DISEASE

Derek G. Gibson

Disturbed left ventricular diastolic function is becoming increasingly recognized as a mechanism of disease. It is usually assessed from its overall effects on the ventricle: the rate of pressure decline, peak filling velocity, cavity compliance or end-diastolic pressure (1). Because diseases may be local as well as generalized in their distribution, the same is likely to apply to their effects. Even generalized disease may manifest itself locally; a high end-diastolic pressure in patients with dilated cardiomyopathy leads to preferential ischemia affecting the subendocardium. To demonstrate impaired systolic function, it is necessary only to show that the local amplitude of wall motion is reduced between end-diastole and end-systole. Disturbances of diastole are more difficult to document. They may manifest themselves as abnormalities in the timing or velocity of wall motion, or of local changes in wall stiffness. These local disturbances can only be defined against the background of normal function, which itself is characteristically nonuniform. Disease may unmask mechanisms that are unobtrusive in normal persons, leading to complicated patterns of wall motion that cannot be easily explained in terms of simple loss of local function. Local disturbances affect overall ventricular function; indeed, this is a major reason for studying them. However, they cannot be unambiguously distinguished from generalized disturbances by simple measurements of pressure, volume, or compliance. Regional involvement can be detected only by an imaging process. This chapter discusses the strengths and weaknesses of contrast left ventriculography and echocardiography for this purpose.

TECHNICAL PROBLEMS

Twenty years' experience has not solved the technical problems associated with measuring regional left ventricular wall motion. Regional ventricular function is usually assessed from changes in endocardial position or wall thickness. Apart from the left side of the septum, the inner surface of the left ventricle is trabeculated. At end-diastole, these trabeculae are widely separated, so that it is the endocardium between them that is detected by contrast angiography and M-mode echo as the "endocardium." However, at end-systole, when cavity size is small, the trabeculae approximate to one another, so that their inner surfaces now form the apparent boundary of the cavity. The anatomic basis of the cavity outline has thus changed between end-systole and end-diastole. Whether this change occurs continuously throughout filling, or whether, as seems more likely, it occurs mainly during isovolumic relaxation and early filling has not been determined.

Local wall thickness may also be difficult to measure. There are several anatomic structures surrounding ventricular myocardium. These include epicardium or the visceral layer of the serous pericardium, the pericardial space, the parietal layer of serous pericardium, and finally the fibrous pericardium. There may be additional layers of fat beneath the epicardium and outside the fibrous pericardium. The modern M-mode echocardiograph has adequate depth resolution and dynamic range to separate these layers, but this does not apply to contrast angiography or apical cross-sectional echocardiography working in range resolution. Once epi- and endocardium have been localized, their motion must be determined. The motion of a target on the endocardium can only be described relative to some reference point. It remains uncertain whether a point internal or external to the heart should be used. It is also uncertain whether the same reference point applies for all parts of the ventricle, and throughout the cardiac cycle. Even if these questions could be resolved in the normal person, there is no reason to believe that the results could be applied to patients with heart disease. Numerous arbitrary solutions have therefore been applied. The end-diastolic cavity centroid is often used (2). A long axis (3) can readily be defined if cavity shape is normal, but if the outline becomes globular, its exact position may vary significantly from frame to frame, depending on the algorithm used to locate it. An alternative convention is to use a fixed external reference point (4). Local motion may be assessed towards the centroid (2), perpendicular to the long axis (3), or towards a point defined from the motion of endomyocardial markers (5). Localized area rather than linear change may be measured (6). Alternatively, account may be taken of local curvature, and wall motion be assessed along trajectories defined as the shortest distances between end-diastolic and end-systolic outlines (7), perpendicular to a "center line" between these two outlines (8, 9), or along paths defined from actual trajectories of identifiable points on the endocardium in normal subjects (10). None of these conventions solve the problem of distinguishing a change in endocardial position from overall movement of the heart in space (translation). Perhaps the most satisfactory solution is to measure distances between two intracardiac landmarks, such as wall thickness or cavity dimension.

Lateral or rotational motion of the heart in space may cause the anatomic structure causing the apparent boundary of the cavity to change. This effect cannot easily be allowed when the analysis depends on defining the cavity outline. An extenuating factor is that clinically significant regional wall motion disturbances are usually large in comparison with the extent of this motion. Analysis-based errors and inconsistencies are commoner when small altera-

tions in regional amplitude or velocity are being assessed, and less so for major disturbances in the direction or timing of motion. Fortunately, it is the latter that are common in clinically significant disease.

When the velocity and timing of wall motion are being studied, the repetition rate of the imaging process becomes important. The normal isovolumic relaxation time is 60 to 80 msec, and may be considerably less when end-diastolic pressure is high (11). It is a period of great significance for diastolic function because it is frequently a time of strikingly incoordinate wall motion that has major effects on subsequent filling. It is obviously desirable to acquire at least three images during this period, suggesting a repetition rate of 50 to 60/sec as a minimum. That of M-mode echocardiography, 1000/sec, is much more satisfactory, whereas this period cannot be studied at all with a repetition rate of 20/sec or less.

Displaying Asynchronous Wall Motion

If local diastolic wall motion is to be studied objectively, its timing and amplitude must be displayed in a way that can be readily appreciated. The simplest approach has been to present two cavity outlines at specified times within the cardiac cycle—for example, at aortic valve closure and at mitral opening (12, 13). Although multiple cavity outlines can be easily superimposed, they cross one another when wall motion is at all abnormal, and the underlying pattern is lost (Fig. 19–1). When only a small number of outlines are being considered, each can be coded with a different color (14). Methods based on time-motion plots have proved much more versatile. A series of such plots from around the cavity outline give a comprehensive picture of regional motion. They can be stacked vertically (15), related to a schematized cavity outline to show their origin (10), or integrated to generate more complex patterns (7, 16, 17) (Fig. 19–2B). A contour display is another variant (7, 16, 17) that again produces easily recognizable patterns (Fig. 19–2C). A final approach is to assume that regional wall motion can be described as a single sinusoidal curve, and display regional differences in the phase of this fundamental frequency (18). It has been occasionally ap-

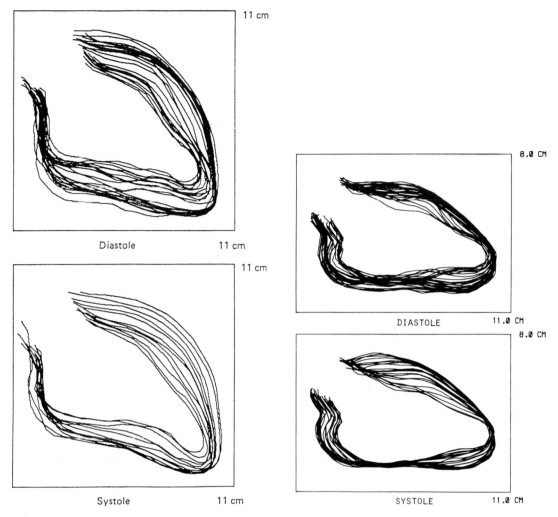

Fig. 19–1. Superimposed cavity outlines from successive frames of a contrast left ventriculogram of a normal subject *(A)*, and a patient with right coronary artery disease *(B)*. End-systolic frame corresponds to that with the smallest area. Note that the normal symmetrical pattern of inward and outward wall motion is adequately shown by this simple method. However, the results are ambiguous in the patient with coronary artery disease, particularly along the inferior wall, where the systolic frames appear to show akinesis, whereas the diastolic ones show a normal amplitude of motion. Reproduced with permission from Gibson DG, Prewitt TA, Brown DJ: Analysis of left ventricular wall movement during isovolumic relaxation and its relation to coronary artery disease. Br Heart J 38:1010, 1976.

plied to contrast angiograms, but is discussed in more detail in the section on nuclear cardiology (See Chap. 11.)

ISOVOLUMIC RELAXATION

Normal Events

Isovolumic relaxation is the period from aortic valve closure to mitral cusp separation and the onset of ventricular filling (19). These latter two landmarks are not identical; the onset of flow normally follows mitral cusp separation by approximately 25 msec and by 50 msec or more in disease (20).

Although the volume of the ventricle is constant during this period, cavity shape may change. Indeed, this was the reason why the term isometric relaxation, originally proposed by Wiggers, was abandoned

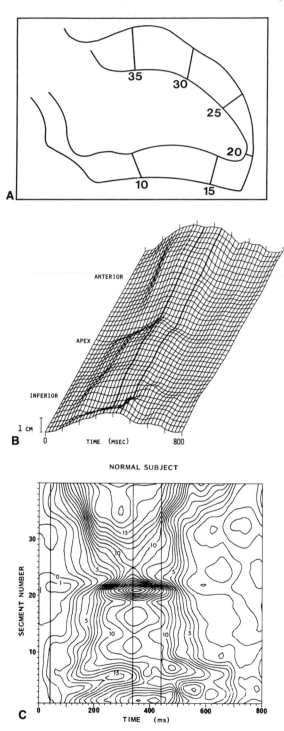

Fig. 19–2. Analysis of regional left ventricular wall motion. *A,* End-diastolic and end-systolic cavity outlines are superimposed with respect to an external reference point. Forty equally spaced points are identified around the end-diastolic perimeter, and from each, a chord is constructed to the nearest point on the end-systolic outline. Six representative chords are shown in this diagram. *B,* Plots of regional endocardial position against time are plotted for each of the 40 chords. They have been stacked in an isometric display, with inward motion shown as upward displacement. The diagonal lines connect points on each curve occurring synchronously (i.e., they are isochrones). The accentuated isochrones represent the times of aortic closure and mitral opening. *C,* Contour display based on Figure 19–2B. Each contour represents inward or outward motion of endocardium by 1 mm from its end-diastolic position. Vertical lines represent the timing of aortic closure (340 msec), and mitral opening (420 msec). Note the synchronous inward motion during ejection and outward motion during filling, with lack of motion anywhere around the cavity outline during isovolumic relaxation. Reproduced with permission from Gibson DG, Prewitt TA, Brown DJ: Analysis of left ventricular wall movement during isovolumic relaxation and its relation to coronary artery disease. Br Heart J 38:1010, 1976.

(19). On contrast angiography, isovolumic relaxation time is taken as starting at the time of aortic valve cusp closure and ending with the first appearance of unopacified blood from the left atrium within the left ventricular cavity. In "normal" subjects, there is a consistent increase in apparent cavity volume of up to 10 mL during this time (21). Its basis is uncertain. It may be the result of the mitral cusps doming into the cavity before they separate. At least part of it is the effect of blood entering the spaces between the trabeculae as the ventricle begins to relax. Up to 5 mm outward motion may occur along the free wall and up to 2 mm along the inferior wall, in the RAO projection (22). Outward wall motion starts on the midportion of the anterior wall, and the most delayed, approximately 50 msec later, is the posterior-inferior segment. These changes in endocardial position are not simply the result of translation of the heart in space (23) because they are accompanied by significant changes in cavity shape (7) and are reflected in local wall thickness (24). In a minority of patients, particularly those with mitral prolapse, they may be so marked as to lead to characteristic appearance of the ventricular cavity at end-systole (ballerina's foot) (25). Early outward movement along the anterior wall

has been given the name segmental early relaxation phenomenon (SERP) (26).

Changes in major and minor axis of the left ventricle have also been studied by M-mode echocardiography (Fig. 19–3), isovolumic relaxation being taken, in these studies, as ending with mitral cusp separation. Time intervals and peak velocities can be measured much more easily if records are digitized. Long axis is characteristically unchanged during isovolumic relaxation, whereas minor axis shortens by 1 ± 2 mm at chordal level (27). Again, differences in timing can be demonstrated within the ventricle. At midcavity level, peak inward motion of endocardium follows that of epicardium by 30 ± 15 msec, although this difference is not apparent at the base or below the insertion of the chordae (28). At the level of the standard M-mode echocardiogram, therefore, minimum cavity di-

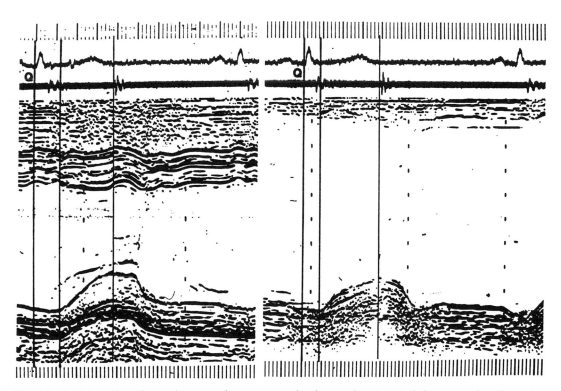

Fig. 19–3. M-mode echocardiograms from a normal subject, showing *A*, left ventricular dimension changes in transverse (left panel) and long (right panel) axes. Vertical lines represent the onset of the QRS complex, mitral closure and aortic closure *(A2)*. Note the synchronous motion in the two directions. Reproduced with permission from Jones CJH, Raposo L, Gibson DG: Functional importance of the long axis dynamics of the human left ventricle. Br Heart J 63:215, 1990.

mension coincides to 10 ± 10 msec with mitral valve cusp separation.

Coronary Artery Disease

Incoordinate regional wall motion with concomitant changes in left ventricular cavity shape during isovolumic relaxation are common in patients with coronary artery disease. This abnormal motion is somewhat similar to changes that may occur in normal subjects, so that their pathologic nature can be established only when normal limits have been defined. Wall motion during an isovolumic period is necessarily restrained because, by definition, cavity volume and myocardial mass are both constant, and blood is incompressible. Abnormal movement in one part of the ventricle must therefore be accompanied by equal and opposite motion elsewhere. Of these two components of the shape change, only one need be the direct result of local disease; the other, which may be equally striking in terms of the extent or velocity of displacement of endocardium, can be purely secondary (Fig. 19–4).

The changes in cavity shape occurring in patients with coronary artery disease prove, in fact, to be remarkably uniform. An example is shown in Figures 19–2B and 19–5C. Isovolumic relaxation can be recognized as the period between aortic valve closure and mitral opening. The two components of the shape change are clearly identified: both are outside the 95% confidence limits of normal. There is early outward motion in the anterior part of the ventricle of 7 mm, so that by the time the mitral opens, the endocardium is effectively in its end-diastolic position. Along the inferior wall, there is 4 mm inward motion, followed by normal outward movement during filling. The amplitude of systolic wall motion is normal in the anterior region, whereas on the inferior wall, inward movement starts late, and its overall amplitude is reduced, in line with the right coronary artery disease present in this patient. Prolonged inward motion is characteristically associated with reduced systolic function, whereas early outward motion is not. In addition, in patients with single-vessel disease, regions showing inward motion during isovolumic relaxation were consis-

ISOVOLUMIC RELAXATION

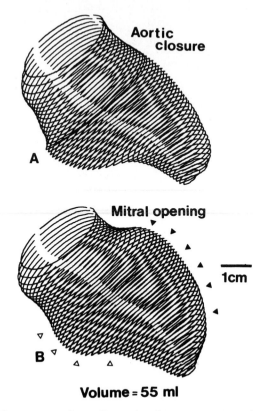

Fig. 19–4. Three-dimensional reconstruction of the change in left ventricular cavity shape during isovolumic relaxation based on biplane angiograms from a patient with coronary artery disease. Note the inward motion of the inferior wall and outward motion of the anterior wall between aortic closure *(A)* and mitral opening *(B)*.

tently in the region of the affected coronary artery (7). They frequently arise during isovolumic contraction, and persist throughout ejection (29) (Fig. 19–6). This close relation between wall motion and arterial stenosis has subsequently been confirmed using a variety of angiographic approaches (12, 13, 30, 31). Using a video intensity technique, Bhagarva et al. (31) demonstrated that the combination of a regional delay in peak inward motion along with a reduced outward velocity could be used as a marker of the effects of coronary stenosis with specificities and sensitivities of 80 to 90%. There was usually an associated disturbance of systolic wall motion; an isolated systolic abnormality was unusual, and a totally normal pattern was seen in only 2 out of 80 patients. The same relationship between abnormal wall motion and coronary artery disease is seen early after acute coronary occlusion: regions subtended by the thrombosed artery showed abnormal inward motion during isovolumic relaxation, whereas early outward motion was characteristically a distant phenomenon (32) (Fig. 19-7). In contrast to simple akinesis or hypokinesis, delayed inward movement in the region of the affected coronary artery was a potent marker of subsequent reversibility, following thrombolysis, provided that perfusion was re-established (33).

The frequency with which wall motion in each of the 40 segments fell outside the 95% confidence limits of normal in 90 patients with triple vessel disease is plotted as a frequency histogram in Figure 19-8, to show the distribution of prolonged inward motion (34). It is not random, as might be expected from the distribution of the coronary artery disease, but was much more common along the inferior wall. The distri-

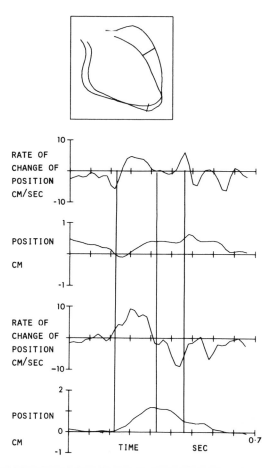

Fig. 19-6. Displays from the contrast angiogram of a patient with a disturbance of isovolumic contraction involving the inferior wall. Vertical lines represent the times of aortic closure (220 msec), aortic closure (420 msec), and mitral opening (560 msec). The upper pair of traces represent the inferior segment, whose position is indicated in the top panel. It moves outward during isovolumic contraction and early ejection. Its overall duration of inward motion is normal, so it continues to move inward during isovolumic relaxation. By contrast, the other segment, from the anterior wall, shows early outward motion before mitral valve opening. Reproduced with permission from Gibson DG, et al.: Abnormal left ventricular wall movement during early systole in patients with angina pectoris. Br Heart J 40:758, 1984.

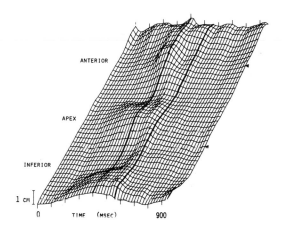

Fig. 19-5. Isometric display of the contrast angiogram represented in Figure 19-1B, from a patient with right coronary artery disease. Note that, in the anterior region of the cavity, motion is normal until aortic valve closure. Following this, there is striking outward motion during isovolumic relaxation, so that by the time of mitral valve opening, the endocardium has already reached its end-diastolic position. In the inferior region, the amplitude of systolic motion is reduced, but during isovolumic relaxation, there is inward motion of 4 mm.

bution of segments showing abnormal outward motion is even more remarkable, being confined to the free wall, particularly to its midportion. These findings suggest that the distribution of coronary artery lesions is not the only factor determining this

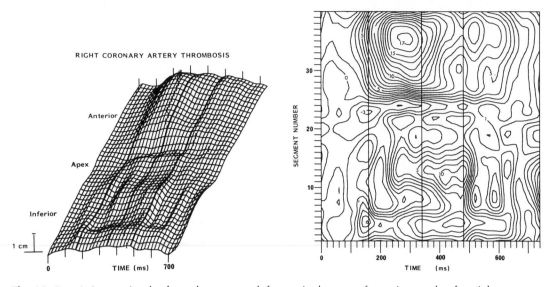

RIGHT CORONARY ARTERY THROMBOSIS

Fig. 19–7. *A,* Isometric plot from the contrast left ventriculogram of a patient early after right coronary artery occlusion, immediately before intracoronary thrombolysis. Note delayed inward motion during isovolumic relaxation, preceded by outward movement during isovolumic contraction and early ejection. Anteriorly, there is abnormal outward motion during isovolumic relaxation. *B,* Contour display from the same data. Accentuated isochrones correspond to aortic opening (160 msec), aortic closure (340 msec), and mitral opening (480 msec). Reproduced with permission from Gibson DG, et al.: Asynchronous left ventricular wall motion early after coronary thrombosis. Br Heart J 55:4, 1986.

abnormal wall motion during isovolumic relaxation: others, apparently related to position within the left ventricle itself, are also involved.

Incoordinate wall motion can also be studied by M-mode echocardiography (35, 36). Figure 19–9 shows left ventricular dimension increasing between A2 and mitral valve opening, caused by early thinning of the posterior wall. This behavior is exactly the same as that of the free wall as demonstrated by angiography, and is thus likely to be secondary to a primary disturbance elsewhere. Only when the ischemic disturbance directly affects the posterior left ventricular wall can the primary disturbance of prolonged inward motion be detected

by the standard M-mode echocardiogram. Much more commonly, however, the ventricular long axis shows the expected primary change, continuing to shorten or maintain tension throughout the period of isovolumic relaxation (Fig. 19–9) (27). The high repetition rate of M-mode echocardiography and its ability to demonstrate epi- and pericardial layers make it possible to use this method to investigate wall motion in these regions showing an early dimension increase. The dimension increase is always caused by wall thinning, not by any motion of the epicardium. The wall thinning itself is premature. Like many other systolic time intervals, the interval from Q wave to peak wall thickness depends on

Fig. 19–8. *A,* Distribution of delayed inward motion during isovolumic relaxation in patients with triple vessel coronary artery disease. Note that, in spite of uniform coronary artery involvement, this abnormality is much commoner in segments 5 through 15, corresponding to the inferior wall of the ventricle. *B,* Distribution of early outward motion during isovolumic relaxation in the same group of patients. Note that the abnormality is effectively confined to segments 20 through 40, corresponding to the free wall of the ventricle. Reproduced with permission from Greenbaum RA, Gibson DG: Regional non-uniformity of left ventricular wall movement in man. Br Heart J 45:29, 1981.

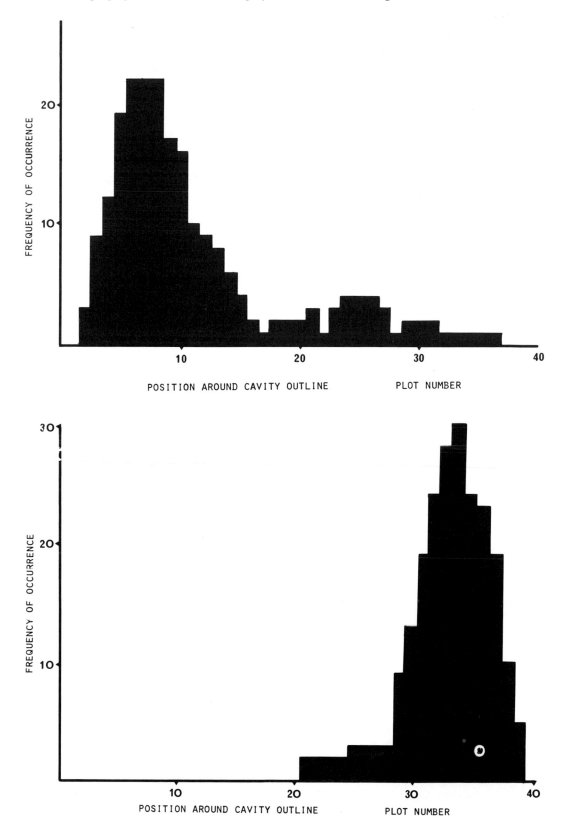

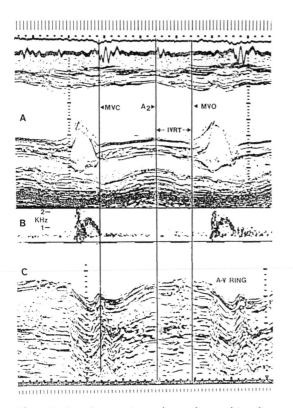

Fig. 19–9. Composite echocardiographic display from a patient with coronary artery disease, showing M-mode echocardiogram of minor axis of left ventricular cavity *(A),* transmitral Doppler *(B),* and long axis changes *(C).* Ventrical lines represent mitral valve closure (MVC), A2, and mitral valve opening (MVO). Note that mitral valve opening is greatly delayed, with an isovolumic relaxation time (IVRT) of 200 msec. On the minor axis of the ventricle, there is an increase in transverse ventricular dimension during this period. The onset of long axis shortening is delayed at the start of systole, and long axis changes are very abnormal during diastole, when the onset of lengthening is delayed until atrial systole. Note also that the onset of transmitral flow is delayed for a further 100 msec after mitral cusp separation.

heart rate (37). When allowance is made for this effect, the onset of thinning in these abnormal segments is consistently 80 to 100 msec early. The normal high velocity of thinning is, however, maintained even though the mitral valve has not yet opened.

On the basis of these observations, a coherent picture of these events can be developed. As might be expected from experimental studies, the onset of contraction is delayed in ischemic segments, peak systolic

force is reduced, and overall contraction is prolonged. Tension thus persists in affected segments when the rest of the ventricle is relaxing, and pressure, a function of overall ventricular function, is falling. The maximum shortening of these abnormal segments thus occurs as their afterload is falling, i.e., during isovolumic relaxation. This abnormal behavior is most commonly shown by longitudinally directed fibers, which dissection shows to be in the subendocardium, and to a lesser extent in the subepicardium (38). The former, in particular, is known to be uniquely subject to ischemia. Prolonged long axis shortening manifests itself on a standard RAO angiogram as inward movement at the apex and proximal inferior wall. Compensatory outward motion is confined to the midportion of the free wall on angiograms, suggesting specialization of function within the ventricle, possibly based on its complex fiber architecture. In patients with coronary artery disease, rapid wall thinning may be complete before mitral valve opening, demonstrating that it is not uniquely the result of rapid filling. Although it is normally coupled to filling, therefore, rapid thinning appears to be an autonomous process whose behavior has much in common that that of elastic restoring forces (39). (See Chap. 5.) The tendency of this same region of the ventricular wall to move outward during isovolumic relaxation even in normal subjects is thus not unexpected. It appears to be the basis of the normal segmental early relaxation phenomenon (SERP) (40). However, it is attractive to postulate that, when inward motion is abnormally prolonged elsewhere in the ventricle, its extent is much greater. Early outward wall motion occurring during isovolumic relaxation in patients with coronary artery disease is thus rather unusual. It is not the direct effect of local ischaemia, nor is it even a simple compensatory phenomenon. Rather, it can be seen as occurring because specialized processes normally coupled to rapid filling are unbalanced. A striking feature throughout the literature on SERP has been the uncertainty as to whether it is a normal or an abnormal finding (40, 41). This can be satisfactorily explained once the idea of disruption of a normal complex mechanism is adopted. It is only when 95%

confidence limits of normal are established, and the whole pattern analyzed in detail using suitable methods of display, that these rather complex interrelations become apparent.

Like many other aspects of left ventricular function, incoordinate wall motion during isovolumic relaxation is load-dependent (42). Its overall extent varies directly with the duration of the isovolumic relaxation period itself. Thus an increase in left atrial pressure, which shortens isovolumic relaxation time, also reduces the extent of wall motion before mitral valve opening, whereas a reduction in preload, caused, for example, by nitroglycerin administration, has the reverse effect.

Although these effects were originally described in chronic coronary artery disease, they are common in the acute phase of myocardial infarction, and may also be seen in approximately half of patients with left ventricular hypertrophy, whether primary or secondary (43).

The ultimate test of these ideas would be to measure wall tension directly in affected areas, and confirm its asynchronous decline. This has not been undertaken in humans. Instead, regional wall stress has been calculated from local curvature, wall thickness, and ventricular pressure (44). With this approach, regional reductions in the rate of stress decline can be demonstrated and quantified as an increased time constant in patients with coronary artery disease (45) or hypertrophic cardiomyopathy (46). Such time constants are characteristically longer than those of the ventricular pressure itself, from which wall tension is derived. Although the method has not been validated directly, it gives values in the normal dog that approximate to within 25% of those obtained from a simple finite element analysis. These results, although suggestive, are not conclusive. It follows from this rather simple derivation of wall stress that the local time constant of stress reduction can only become dissociated from that of overall pressure decline and drop more slowly in regions where local curvature increases and wall thickness falls during the course of isovolumic relaxation. Paradoxically, in a region that thickens as pressure falls, i.e., one that is likely to be the seat of the primary disturbance, calculated

local wall stress will actually fall faster than pressure. This paradox arises because any computation of systolic wall stress based on Laplace's law assumes that the stress is the consequence of intracavity pressure rather than the reverse. In this complex field, therefore, it seems preferable to confine oneself to direct observation, rather than deal in derived quantities.

LEFT VENTRICULAR FILLING

The time course of left ventricular filling is usually divided into three phases: rapid early diastolic filling, when approximately 70% of the stroke volume enters, a period of diastasis, when volume alters little, and finally atrial systole, which accounts for the remaining 20 to 30% of the stroke volume. Mechanisms underlying these three phases are quite different, as is the nature of their involvement in disease. They are therefore considered separately, although interactions between them can, of course, occur, and, in particular, disturbances of one phase frequently have a "knock-on" effect on those occurring later.

Rapid Filling

Left ventricular filling can be taken as starting at the time of mitral valve cusp separation, followed 25 msec or so later in normal subjects by the onset of forward flow detectable by pulsed Doppler (2). A possible basis for this discrepancy is apparent on color flow M-mode. With the echo beam directed along the left ventricular inflow, it can be used to study the column of blood moving into the ventricle. This column does not start to move synchronously at all levels within the ventricle, but rather, the onset of flow is propagated into the ventricle from base to apex with a finite velocity of 50 cm/sec, as shown by the line OF (Fig. 19–10). The normal value is approximately 50 ± 10 cm/sec. Higher values are seen in patients with restrictive filling, and strikingly low ones in those with severe dilated cardiomyopathy. The onset of ventricular filling is thus regional in nature even in normal subjects, in whom it is delayed by approximately 20 msec per cm from the mitral ring towards the apex. Doppler estimates of isovolumic relaxation time that depend on timing the onset of

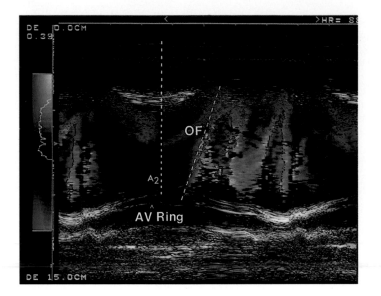

Fig. 19–10. Color flow M-mode directed along the inflow tract of the left ventricle of a normal subject, showing the finite propagation velocity of early diastolic flow into the left ventricle (OF). It is apparent that the time interval from A2 to the onset of flow depends on the depth within the ventricle that the measurement is made. (LV = left ventricle, LA = left atrium).

flow thus depend critically on the level within the ventricle at which the sample volume is set .

Peak early diastolic filling rate is often reduced in patients with coronary artery disease. This is seen whether filling rate is expressed in absolute values (cc/sec) derived from a contrast angiogram (47), or in cm/sec from pulsed Doppler. (See Chap. 12.) The question arises as to whether outward left ventricular wall motion is uniformly slowed or is asynchronous. Contrast left ventriculography has demonstrated a series of regional disturbances to filling in these patients. A full-thickness scar causes loss of inward motion during systole and outward motion during diastole. Local outward motion during filling may also be absent because it has already occurred during isovolumic relaxation (see Fig. 19–5). Asynchronous wall motion is common in patients with coronary artery disease, even when peak resting filling velocity itself is normal (48). The nature of this asynchrony

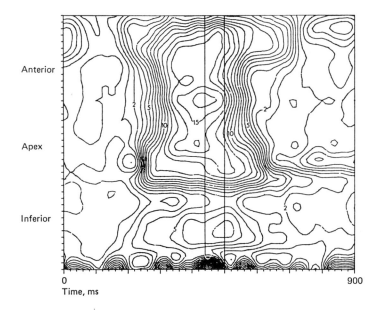

Fig. 19–11. Contour display derived from the contrast left ventriculogram of a patient with an inferior scar. Note that the overall amplitude of inferior wall motion is greatly reduced, but that both systolic and diastolic wall motion elsewhere within the ventricle is quite normal.

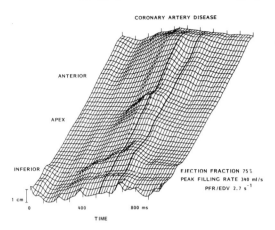

Fig. 19–12. Isometric plot from the contrast left ventriculogram of a patient with coronary artery disease, showing asynchronous outward wall motion during diastole. The characteristic sequence of anterior motion preceding that toward the apex, which itself precedes that along the inferior wall, is demonstrated. Accentuated isochrones represent the timing of aortic closure (520 msec) and mitral opening (640 msec).

is clear from regional plots of outward wall motion, on which the onset, peak rate and end of rapid early diastolic motion can be detected (Figs. 19–11 and 19–12). Normally, each of these occurs within 50 msec of one another in different regions of the ventricle. In patients with coronary artery disease, however, the time interval between the earliest and latest region to move, the dispersion, can be greatly increased to 120 msec or more. The nature of dispersion is characteristic. Delayed segments are not necessarily ischemic ones. In patients with triple vessel coronary artery disease, when asynchrony occurred, it was because outward motion always started on the free wall and was followed by that at the apex, and finally inferiorly. The extent of this dispersion was greater when overall filling velocity was reduced, and when changes in cavity shape during isovolumic relaxation were extensive. In a minority of patients, particularly those in whom outward wall motion on the free wall had been extensive, the ventricular wall actually moved inwards during filling effectively leading to an oscillation with a frequency of 3–4 Hz (Fig. 19–13). The basis of these consistent patterns is likely to be the same as that causing

abnormal wall motion during isovolumic relaxation.

On the basis of these findings, it is tempting to suggest that this incoordinate wall motion is the direct cause of the slow filling in patients with coronary artery disease. However, this is not certain. Even in normal subjects, there is dispersion in outward movement between the different regions of the ventricle. If outward wall motion were uniformly slowed, therefore, one would expect this dispersion to be correspondingly increased. To establish the fact that incoordination might contribute directly to slow filling, therefore, peak regional velocities of outward motion should be normal or only slightly reduced, but the timing of peak values should be asynchronous. Even this, however, may not be enough. Ventricular filling rate is reduced in patients with mitral stenosis (49), a reduction generally assumed to be caused by a stenosed mitral valve. In spite of this, wall motion shows a pattern of asynchrony almost identical to that seen in patients with coronary artery disease. Conversely, wall motion may be asynchronous after acute myocardial infarction, yet filling rate may

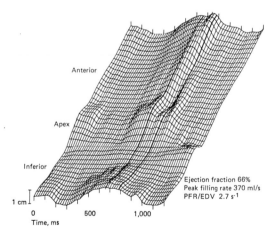

Fig. 19–13. Isometric plot from the contrast left ventriculogram of a patient with coronary artery disease, showing a diastolic oscillation. There is early outward motion during isovolumic relaxation, particularly obvious toward the apex. After the mitral valve opens, there is localized inward movement in this region. Accentuated isochrones represent aortic closure (660 msec) and mitral opening (780 msec). Reproduced with permission from Jones CJH, Song GJ, Gibson DG: An echocardiographic assessment of atrial mechanical behaviour. Br Heart J 65:31, 1991.

be within normal limits (32), probably because left atrial pressure is high. (See Chap. 13.) In hypertrophic cardiomyopathy, wall motion is almost invariably asynchronous, although filling rate varies greatly among patients. (See Chap. 22.)

Early diastolic filling rates are determined by the atrioventricular pressure gradient modified by frictional effects at the mitral valve (50). (See Chap. 5.) These are difficult to determine comprehensively in humans, and are only inadequately reflected in measures of left atrial or left ventricular diastolic pressures. However, much evidence shows the powerful effect of events during isovolumic relaxation on ventricular filling pattern, based on angiographic and Doppler measurements. Two effects appear to be involved: the duration of isovolumic relaxation time, and, as a separate variable, the extent of incoordinate wall motion during this time. Isovolumic relaxation time itself is powerfully affected by left atrial pressure, but only to a minor extent by aortic pressure, so presumably it is the former that is responsible for the first of these interrelations. A possible mechanism of the interrelation between incoordinate relaxation and the subsequent course of filling is apparent from isometric plots of regional wall motion. In Figure 19–5, for example, the normal pattern of wall motion after mitral valve opening has been disrupted around the greater part of the cavity outline as the result of premature outward movement before mitral valve opening. Not surprisingly, incoordinate wall motion during isovolumic relaxation reduces the rate of left ventricular pressure fall (12, 51) and prolongs both isovolumic relaxation time and the time constant of pressure fall (12, 51), illustrating that none of these overall measurements can be used to distinguish slow from incoordinate relaxation.

Diastasis and Regional Wall Stiffness

Measuring the passive properties of the whole ventricle depends on the relation between pressure and volume during the mid-diastolic period of diastasis. This period is limited. Early in diastole, pressure falls throughout the greater part of rapid filling, behavior that is not passive. During atrial systole, the mechanism of increase in ventricular volume is fundamentally dif-

ferent from that earlier in diastole, involving external work on the ventricle by the atrium (section 12), so that again, conditions are not those of passive filling. Ventricular stiffness may be assessed in terms of either the compliance of the cavity, represented by the slope of the pressure volume curve at any point during filling, or, if wall thickness is also known, mean values of myocardial elastic modulus can be calculated. Difficulties in assessing these quantities in the intact heart are compounded when regional stiffness is being assessed. Several approaches have been used. Sasayama et al. (52) have defined regional stiffness from the local pressure-displacement curve. Endocardial position with respect to the end-diastolic centroid of the cardiac cycle is plotted against cavity pressure, and the slope of this relation is a measure of local resistance of the endocardium to deformation. A single cavity pressure is used, so that any regional differences are caused by the extent and timing of regional wall motion. Clearly, there are problems in defining the zero position from which measurements of endocardial position are made. It is not clear whether the end-diastolic centroid of the cavity is physiologically valid for all parts of the myocardium, or whether of the whole heart in space occurs during systole, which would summate with local endocardial motion. Because the amplitude of the latter is frequently 5 mm or less, even 1 to 2 mm of translation would lead to major error. In patients with coronary artery disease (53) or hypertrophic cardiomyopathy (54), regional "distensibility" has been assessed from regional variation in peak filling rate. Although overall filling rate cannot be used as an index of overall distensibility, overall forces acting on the blood in different regions of the cavity are similar, so that regional differences in filling velocity would seem to reflect local difference in some myocardial property. Estimates of local filling velocity are subject to the same limitations of those of local ejection fraction, in that endocardium itself bounds only a small part of the volume that is being measured; the greater part is defined by lines or planes constructed with respect to the long axis or the centroid of the ventricle, and thus is subject to the limitations discussed previously. Conditions of passive stiffness do not apply during rapid filling, so the "regional distensibility" calculated is not local elastic stiffness but probably more closely related to regional relaxation rate or restoring forces (53). (See Chap. 4.)

Estimating regional myocardial stiffness or elastic modulus has proved even more difficult. Posterior wall stress can be estimated from simultaneous left ventricular cavity M-mode echocardiograms and high fidelity pressure recordings. The relation between wall stress and cavity circumference is complex (55, 56). During early filling, wall stress falls sharply as cavity size increases. This is followed by a mid-diastolic period when the relation is often flat, i.e., cavity circumference increases without measurable change in wall stress. This unexpected behavior occurs during rapid wall thinning. It is followed by a third phase during which stress and strain increase together, when stiffness and elastic modulus can be assessed. This last phase, however, usually accounts for less than 10% of the total change in circumference occurring with filling. It has been pointed out that these results are much more compatible with the activity of restoring forces than a simple elastic model (56). The late diastolic slope is characteristically increased in patients with left ventricular hypertrophy (55). In those with hypertrophic cardiomyopathy, nifedipine administration may cause a downward shift of the late diastolic pressure-dimension relation (57). (See Chap. 28.)

A series of studies have used data from angiograms in finite element models of the left ventricle to assess local elastic modulus. To review this complex field would be beyond the scope of the present chapter. These approaches require complex computing equipment, and their effectiveness is greatly reduced by the limited available data concerning wall thickness, pericardial forces, myocardial structure, trabecular anatomy, and internal cavity shape. At present, their contribution to a clinical understanding of diastolic events has been limited.

Regional Left Ventricular Diastolic Function in Angina Pectoris

It is well recognized that overall left ventricular diastolic function becomes abnormal during an attack of angina pectoris (58). One of the earliest manifestations of local ischaemia is an increase in end-diastolic pressure. Several mechanisms appear to cause this (59–61). End-diastolic volume may increase without any change in the slope of the pressure-volume relation. The pressure-volume relation itself may become steeper, i.e., cavity compliance may fall. Finally, the pressure-volume curve may be displaced upward, so that cavity pressure is higher at each volume, although the slope itself is unchanged. This last effect is often referred to as "reduced distensibility." These changes are presumably the direct result of regional ischemia, although intervening mechanisms are not clear. Regional function has therefore been studied in an attempt to elucidate them.

In pacing-induced angina occurring in patients with coronary artery disease, the overall amplitude of motion of the affected region is often reduced. (See Chap. 16.) Frequently such regions show impaired systolic function under control conditions. Simultaneous M-mode cardiograms and high-fidelity pressure measurements show the relation between local wall thickness and cavity pressure as displaced upwards (62). Peak thinning rate of the posterior wall falls, and the time constant of isovolumic left ventricular fall increases. Following mitral valve opening, left ventricular pressure is higher than that derived from extrapolation of the isovolumic pressure decline. This has been explained as being due to a residual wall stress increasing cavity pressure. A fall in overall systolic work in affected areas was noted by Sasayama et al. (52) with end-diastolic length remaining unchanged. Diastolic pressure was higher at any given segment length, and the diastolic pressure-length curve was shifted upward, suggesting regional alterations in the properties of ischaemic myocardium. In normal segments, by contrast, end-diastolic segment length increased and moved up a single passive displacement-pressure curve. Although local external work is reduced in these hypokinetic segments, local mechanical efficiency is well maintained. In a minority of cases, striking asynchrony occurs with angina (63). Inward motion is greatly prolonged, and persists throughout rapid ventricular filling. Systolic function is normal under control conditions in these segments. Regional wall motion may thus be abnormal in angina. The extent to which these local disturbances contribute to the well-known changes in overall ventricular behavior, however, has yet to be determined.

Left Atrial Systole

Approximately one third of the stroke volume normally enters the left ventricle during left atrial systole. This increase in volume is not symmetrically distributed around the cavity outline (Fig. 19–14). Changes in minor axis are small, whereas outward wall motion is most prominent

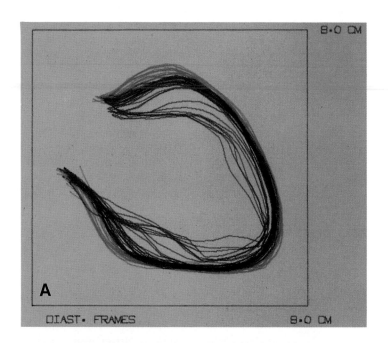

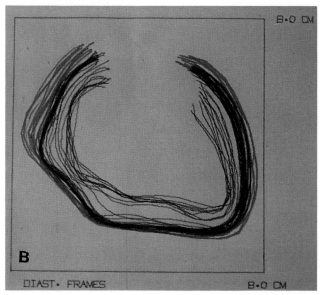

Fig. 19–14. Superimposed endocardial outlines from the contrast left ventriculogram of a normal subject in PA *(A)* and lateral *(B)* projections. Outlines during rapid filling and diastasis are shown in black and those during atrial systole in red. Note that the volume increase during atrial systole is not symmetrical, but is accommodated by a selective increase in the long axis, particularly by backward motion of the plane of the mitral valve.

along the long axis of the ventricle, and particularly in the region of the mitral ring. The anatomic basis for this asymmetrical distribution was uncovered as long ago as 1910 by Keith (64), who demonstrated how it depended on left atrial anatomy. The left atrium is supported by mediastinal structures superiorly, laterally, and posteriorly. When left atrial muscle contracts, therefore, left atrial cavity size falls as the aortic root is pulled backward and the mitral ring upward. Effectively, therefore, a significant volume of blood is within the left atrium at the end of diastasis, but with motion of the valve ring finds itself effectively within the left ventricle with atrial systole (Fig. 19–15). This blood shows no motion with respect to the chest wall, and is thus not detected by Doppler. Clinically, this

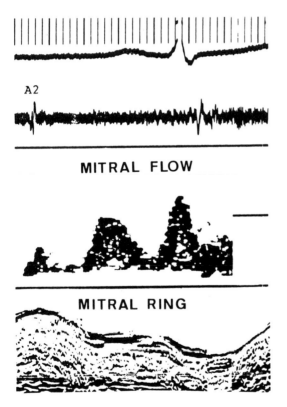

Fig. 19–15. Relation between changes in mitral ring position and Doppler transmitral flow velocities. Note that, early in diastole, ring motion precedes the Doppler, whereas during atrial systole, they are synchronous. Reproduced with permission from Jones CJH, Song GJ, Gibson DG: An echocardiographic assessment of atrial mechanical behaviour. Br Heart J 65:31, 1991.

mechanism can be documented by M-mode echo as well as by angiography. The effects of the normal atrial systole are not prominent on a normal transverse record of the left ventricular cavity, but are obvious when the long axis is studied (65). The extent of ring motion with atrial systole is characteristically increased with left ventricular hypertrophy, both in absolute terms, and also as a proportion of the total long axis lengthening occurring with diastole. Similar changes are common in patients with coronary artery disease, particularly those subject to angina of effort. The pattern of long axis lengthening characteristically returns towards normal after successful PTCA. Finally, in some patients with dilated cardiomyopathy, long axis changes during atrial systole may be reduced or absent altogether. This is not usually a result of atrial "failure" because a pressure A wave can usually be demonstrated. The combination of loss of a wave on the Doppler and the mitral ring with a pressure A wave indicating mechanical atrial activity is strong evidence that left ventricular end-diastolic volume is fixed. This combination is seen in about one third of cases of end-stage dilated cardiomyopathy.

CONCLUSION

Overall ventricular function is no more than the sum of its parts. Studying regional behavior in normal subjects and in patients with heart disease might therefore have been expected to explain many of the disturbances seen in disease. This has not proved to be the case, and as many new problems have been raised as have been solved. In spite of this, however, the importance of synchronous wall motion to normal function, and the profound effects of its loss in disease, are becoming clear. The subject is a difficult one, beset with technical as well as conceptual uncertainties. Nevertheless, it seems certain that diastolic left ventricular function will never be completely understood until its regional manifestations have been fully elucidated.

REFERENCES

1. Little WC, Downes TR: Clinical evaluation of left ventricular diastolic performance. Progr Cardiovasc Dis 32:273, 1990.

2. Mancini GBJ, Norris SL, Peterson KL, et al.: Quantitative assessment of segmental wall motion abnormalities at rest and after atrial pacing using digital intravenous ventriculography. J Am Coll Cardiol 2:70, 1983.

3. Altieri PI, Wilt SM, Leighton RF: Left ventricular wall motion during the isovolumic relaxation period. Circulation 48:499, 1973.

4. Chaitman BR, Bristow JD, Rahimtoola SH: Left ventricular wall motion assessed by using fixed external reference systems. Circulation 48:1043, 1973.

5. Ingels Jr NB, Daughters II GT, Stinson EB, Alderman EL: Evaluation of methods for quantitating left ventricular segmental wall motion in man using segmental markers as a standard. Circulation 61:966, 1980.

6. Gelberg HJ, Brundage BH, Glantz S, Parmley WW: Quantitative left ventricular wall motion analysis: A comparison of area, chord and radial methods. Circulation 59:991, 1979.

7. Gibson DG, Prewitt TA, Brown DJ: Analysis of left ventricular wall movement during isovolumic relaxation and its relation to coronary artery disease. Br Heart J 38:1010, 1976.

8. Bolson EL, Kliman S, Sheehan F, Dodge HT: Left ventricular segmental wall motion—a new method using local direction information. *In* Computers in Cardiology. Los Angeles, IEEE Computer Society, 1980, pp. 245–248.

9. Sheehan FH, Bolson EL, Dodge HT, et al.: Advantages and applications of the centerline method for characterizing regional ventricular function. Circulation 74:293, 1986.

10. Slager CJ, Hooghoudt TEH, Reiber JCH, et al.: Left ventricular contour segmentation from anatomical landmark trajectories and its application to wall motion analysis. *In* Computers in Cardiology. Los Angeles, IEEE Computer Society, 1980, pp. 253–256.

11. Mattheos M, Shapiro E, Oldershaw PJ, et al.: Non-invasive assessment of changes in left ventricular relaxation by combined phono-, echo-, and mechanography. Br Heart J 47:253, 1982.

12. Vanoverschelde J-L, Wijns W, Michel X, Cosyns J, Detry J-M: Asynchronous (segmental early) relaxation impairs left ventricular filling in patients with coronary artery disease and normal systolic function. J Am Coll Cardiol 18:1251, 1991.

13. Holman BL, Wynne J, Idoine J, Neill J: Disruption in the temporal sequence of regional ventricular contraction. I. Characteristics and incidence in coronary artery disease. Circulation 61:1075, 1980.

14. Ludbrook PA, Byrne JD, Tiefenbrunn AJ. Association of asynchronous protodiastolic segmental wall motion with impaired left ventricular relaxation. Circulation 64:1201, 1981.

15. Rickards AF, Seabra-Gomes R, Thurston P. The assessment of regional abnormalities of the left ventricle by angiography. Eur J Cardiol 5:167, 1977.

16. Fujita M, Sasayama S, Kawai C, et al.: Automatic processing of cineventriculograms for analysis of regional myocardial function. Circulation 63:1065, 1981.

17. Gotsman MS, Welber S, Sapoznikov D, et al.: Spatial and temporal variations in regional left ventricular function in isolated disease of the left anterior descending coronary artery. Cardiology 73:22, 1986.

18. Sunnerhagen KS, Smith SDC, Jaski BE, Bhargava V: Ischemic heart disease and regional left ventricular wall motion: A study comparing radial, centerline and a video intensity based slope technique. Int J Card Imag 6:85, 1991.

19. Wiggers CJ: Studies on the duration of the consecutive phases of the cardiac cycle. I. The duration of the consecutive phases of the cardiac cycle and criteria for their precise determination. Am J Physiol 56:415, 1921.

20. Lee CH, Vancheri F, Josen MS, Gibson DG: Discrepancies in the measurement of isovolumic relaxation time: a study comparing M-mode and Doppler echocardiography. Br Heart J 64:214, 1990.

21. Ruttley MS, Adams DF, Cohn PF, Abrams HL: Shape and volume changes during "isovolumetric relaxation" in normal and asynergic ventricles. Circulation 50:306, 1974.

22. Hammermeister K, Gibson DG, Hughes D: Regional variation in the timing and extent of left ventricular wall motion in normal subjects. Br Heart J 56:226, 1986.

23. Klausner SC, Blair TJ, Bulawa WF, et al.: Quantitative analysis of segmental wall motion throughout systole and diastole in the normal human left ventricle. Circulation 65:580, 1982.

24. Gibson DG, Traill TA, Brown DJ: Changes in left ventricular free wall thickness in patients with ischaemic heart disease. Br Heart J 39:1312, 1977.

25. Gooch AS, Vicencio F, Maranhao V, Goldberg H: Arrhythmias and left ventricular asynergy in the prolapsing mitral leaflet syndrome. Am J Cardiol 29:611, 1972.

26. Altieri PI, Wilt SM, Leighton RF: Left ventricular wall motion during the isovolumic relaxation period. Circulation 48:499, 1973.

27. Jones CJH, Raposo L, Gibson DG: Functional importance of the long axis dynamics of the human left ventricle. Br Heart J 63: 215, 1990.

28. Shapiro E, Marier DL, St John Sutton MG, Gibson DG: Regional non-uniformity of wall dynamics in the normal left ventricle. Br Heart J 45:1264, 1980.

29. Gibson DG, Doran JH, Traill TA, Brown DJ: Abnormal left ventricular wall movement during early systole in patients with angina pectoris. Br Heart J 40:758, 1978.

30. Sasayama S, Nonogi H, Fujita M, et al.: Analysis of asynchronous wall motion by regional pressure-length loops in patients with coronary artery disease. J Am Coll Cardiol 4:259, 1984.

31. Bhagarva V, Sunnerhagen KS, Rasshwan M, et al.: Detection and quantification of left ventricular ischemic dysfunction using a new video intensity technique for regional wall motion evaluation. Am Heart J 120: 1058, 1990.

32. Gibson D, Mehmel H, Schwarz F, et al.: Asynchronous left ventricular wall motion early after coronary thrombosis. Br Heart J 55:4, 1986.

33. Gibson D, Mehmel H, Schwarz F, et al.: Changes in left ventricular regional asynchrony after intracoronary thrombolysis in patients with impending myocardial infarction. Br Heart J 56:121, 1986.

34. Greenbaum RA, Gibson DG: Regional non-uniformity of left ventricular wall movement in man. Br Heart J 45:29, 1981.

35. Upton MT, Gibson DG: The study of left ventricular function from digitized echocardiograms. Prog Cardiovasc Dis 20:359, 1978.

36. Lawson WE, Brown Jr EJ, Swinford RD, et al.: A new use for M-mode echocardiography in detecting left ventricular diastolic dysfunction in coronary artery disease. Am J Cardiol 52:210, 1986.

37. Von Bibra H, Gibson DG, Nityanandan K: Effects of propranolol on left ventricular wall movement in patients with ischaemic heart disease. Br Heart J 43:293, 1980.

38. Greenbaum RA, Ho SY, Gibson DG, et al.: Left ventricular fibre architecture in man. Br Heart J 45:248, 1981.

39. Nikolic S, Yellin EL, Tamura K, et al.: Passive properties of canine left ventricle: diastolic stiffness and restoring forces. Circ Res 62:1210, 1988.

40. Wilson CS, Krueger S, Forker AD, Weaver WF: Correlation between segmental early relaxation of the left ventricular wall and coronary occlusive disease. Am Heart J 89: 474, 1975.

41. Gaasch WH, Blaustein AS, Bing OHL: Asynchronous (segmental early) relaxation of the left ventricle. J Am Coll Cardiol 5: 891, 1985.

42. Hall RJC, Doran J, Pusey C, et al.: The effect of nitroglycerin, beta blockade with acebutalol and isometric stress on incoordinate left ventricular function. Eur Heart J 3:23, 1982.

43. Gibson DG, Sanderson JE, Traill TA, et al.: Regional left ventricular wall movement in hypertrophic cardiomyopathy. Br Heart J 40:1327, 1978.

44. Janz RF: Estimation of local myocardial stress. Am J Physiol (H) 242:875, 1982.

45. Pouleur H, Rousseau MF, van Eyll C, Charlier AA. Assessment of regional left ventricular relaxation in patients with coronary artery disease: Importance of geometrical factors and changes in wall thickness. Circulation 69:696, 1984.

46. Hayashida W, Kumada T, Kohno F, et al.: Left ventricular regional relaxation and its nonuniformity in hypertrophic nonobstructive cardiomyopathy. Circulation 84: 1461, 1991.

47. Hammermeister KE, Warbasse JR: The rate of change of left ventricular volume in man. II. Diastolic events in health and disease. Circulation 49:739, 1974.

48. Hui WKK, Gibson DG: Mechanisms of reduced left ventricular filling rate in coronary artery disease. Br Heart J 50:362, 1983.

49. Hui WKK, Lee PK, Chow JSF, Gibson DG: Analysis of regional left ventricular wall motion during diastole in mitral stenosis. Br Heart J 50:231, 1983.

50. Ishida Y, Meisner JS, Tsujioka K, et al.: Left ventricular filling dynamics: Influence of left ventricular relaxation and left atrial pressure. Circulation 74:187, 1986.

51. Fioretti P, Brower RW, Meester GT, Serruys PW: Interaction of left ventricular relaxation and filling during early diastole in human subjects. Am J Cardiol 46:197, 1980.

52. Sasayama S, Nonogi H, Miyazaki S, et al.: Changes in diastolic properties of the regional myocardium during pacing-induced ischemia in human subjects. J Am Coll Cardiol 5:599, 1985.

53. Pouleur H, Rousseau MF, van Eyll C, et al.: Impaired regional diastolic distensibility in coronary artery disease: Relation with dynamic compliance. Am Heart J 112:721, 1986.

54. Hayashida W, Kumada T, Kohno F, et al.: Left ventricular regional relaxation and its

nonuniformity in hypertrophic nonobstructive cardiomyopathy. Circulation 84: 1461, 1991.

55. Gibson DG, Brown DJ: Relation between diastolic left ventricular wall stress and strain in man. Br Heart J 36:1066, 1974.

56. Sabbah HN, Stein PD: Pressure-diameter relations during early diastole in dogs. Incompatibility with the concept of passive left ventricular filling. Circ Res 48:357, 1981.

57. Lorell BH, Paulus W, Grossman W, et al.: Modification of abnormal left ventricular diastolic properties by nifedipine in patients with hypertrophic cardiomyopathy. Circulation 65:499, 1982.

58. Grossman W: Why is left ventricular diastolic pressure increased during angina pectoris? J Am Coll Cardiol 5:607, 1985.

59. Mann T, Goldberg S, Mudge GH, Grossman W: Factors contributing to altered left ventricular diastolic properties during angina pectoris. Circulation 59:14, 1979.

60. Gilbert JC, Glantz SA: Determinants of left ventricular filling and of the diastolic pressure-volume relation. Circ Res 64:827, 1989.

61. Wijns W, Serruys PW, Slager CJ, et al.: Effect of coronary occlusion during percutaneous transluminal angioplasty in humans on left ventricular chamber stiffness and regional diastolic pressure radius relations. J Am Coll Cardiol 7:455, 1986.

62. Bourdillon PD, Lorell BH, Mirsky I, et al.: Increased regional myocardial stiffness of the left ventricle during pacing-induced ischemia. Circulation 67:316, 1983.

63. Dawson JR, Gibson DG: Regional left ventricular wall motion in pacing induced angina. Br Heart J 59:309, 1988.

64. Keith A: An account of the structures concerned in production of the jugular pulse. J Anat Physiol 42:1, 1907.

65. Jones CJH, Song GJ, Gibson DG: An echocardiographic assessment of atrial mechanical behavior. Br Heart J 65:31, 1991.

Chapter 20

LEFT VENTRICULAR HYPERTROPHY: THE CONSEQUENCES FOR DIASTOLE

Beverly H. Lorell

Diastolic dysfunction is a major cause of congestive heart failure in patients with left ventricular hypertrophy. In patients with chronic left ventricular hypertrophy, predominant diastolic dysfunction frequently occurs in the presence of adequate preservation of systolic shortening. In such patients, diastolic heart failure is defined as an increased resistance to filling of the ventricle during diastole in such a way that the left ventricle cannot fill with a normal diastolic volume at a normal diastolic filling pressure. When the resistance to diastolic filling is moderate, the predominant hemodynamic finding may be the elevation of left ventricular diastolic pressure and pulmonary venous pressure. In this situation, the clinical manifestations range from exertional dyspnea to frank pulmonary edema. As the resistance to left ventricular diastolic filling becomes more severe, the extent of diastolic filling may be insufficient to produce adequate myofiber stretch, resulting in the depression of stroke volume and ultimately cardiac output (1–3). This chapter will discuss the alterations in gene expression and cardiac remodelling that occur in response to chronic pressure overload and the mechanisms that appear to contribute to impaired diastolic function in patients with cardiac hypertrophy.

PRESSURE OVERLOAD HYPERTROPHY: BENEFICIAL AND DELETERIOUS ASPECTS OF REMODELLING

Cardiac hypertrophy is an adaptation that occurs in response to overload of the myocardium. The exact mechanisms responsible for the signal transduction of an increase in wall stretch to the end-point of coordinated changes in gene expression and protein synthesis are the subject of intense active research. Current studies suggest that mechanogenic transduction may involve myocyte deformation and subsequent activation of intracellular signals such as phosphoinositide second messengers (4–6). The alterations in protein synthesis that accompany the adaptive response to the sustained increase in work of the heart include a *quantitative* increase in the synthesis of the contractile proteins themselves and subsequent enlargement of existing myocytes. After fetal development, the potential adaptation of cell division of myocytes cannot be invoked. The left ventricle remodels in a pattern that is distinctive for the underlying stress. In response to chronic pressure overload, the left ventricle gradually remodels in a pattern of concentric hypertrophy characterized by the parallel addition of myofibrils and thickening of the left ventricular walls with little change in cavity size, whereas chronic volume overload is characterized by eccentric hypertrophy in which the increase in left ventricular mass is associated with the serial addition of myofibrils and the subsequent enlargement of the left ventricular cavity with relatively less increase in wall thickness (7). In patients with chronic pressure overload caused by aortic stenosis or chronic hypertension, the geometric remodelling of concentric hypertrophy has the adaptive benefit of normalizing systolic wall stress and preserving normal systolic shortening (8–10). However, the adaptation of cardiac hypertrophy has deleterious consequences on diastolic function in most patients.

Diastolic Dysfunction in Patients with Left Ventricular Hypertrophy

Pressure overload hypertrophy consistently results in progressive impairment of left ventricular diastolic distensibility, defined as an increase in left ventricular diastolic filling pressure relative to diastolic volume (1, 11–13). In patients with pressure overload hypertrophy, it is controversial whether this change in distensibility of the left ventricular chamber is caused partly by an alteration of myofibril distensibility (intrinsic myocardial stiffness) as well as changes in left ventricular geometry and regional dysynchrony of contraction. In patient studies using simultaneous pressure and ultrasound measurements, changes in left ventricular chamber distensibility appear to be predominantly related to changes in left ventricular geometry and the extent of wall thickness (12, 14). (See Chap. 9.) However, analyses of the left ventricular stress-strain relationship in patients with hypertrophy caused by aortic stenosis support the notion that there is also an increase in intrinsic myocardial stiffness in some patients (15, 16). Advanced hypertrophy in patients is also associated with slowing of left ventricular isovolumic relaxation (15, 17–20). These abnormalities of slowed relaxation and decreased diastolic distensibility can occur in both children and adults with pressure overload hypertrophy and clearly do not depend on the presence of coexisting systolic failure (17, 19–21). Similar abnormalities of diastolic function are important in the etiology of congestive heart failure in elderly patients with severe hypertrophy caused by chronic hypertension (hypertensive hypertrophic cardiomyopathy) (22) as well as in patients with idiopathic hypertrophic cardiomyopathy, with or without left ventricular outflow gradients (23, 24). In rare patients with very severe hypertrophy, the time course of left ventricular relaxation is sufficiently aberrant that the left ventricular wave form shows a continuous sluggish decay of pressure into mid- or late diastole (23).

It is important to recognize that a slowed rate and reduced extent of diastolic relaxation may itself reduce the gradient between the left atrium and left ventricle in early diastole after mitral valve opening and contribute to an abnormal rate of early diastolic filling and limit the extent of filling (25, 26). The adverse effects of impaired diastolic filling on systolic pump function are especially apparent during exercise and tachycardia, when the duration of diastole and the time available for atrial emptying and ventricular filling is shortened. Previously, the importance of diastolic dysfunction as the proximate cause of both pulmonary congestion as well as "systolic symptoms" of fatigue and exercise intolerance in patients with cardiac hypertrophy was often unrecognized. Many patients were often ineffectually treated with aggressive diuresis that worsened left ventricular filling or with drugs such as digitalis aimed at stimulating contractile function.

Thus, alterations in left ventricular geometry per se related to the increase in protein synthesis and subsequent increase in wall thickness may contribute to changes in left ventricular distensibility and filling (14, 21, 27–29). However, an increase in left ventricular mass or wall thickness per se is not likely to be the only factor responsible for abnormal diastolic function in patients with hypertrophy because cardiac hypertrophy in healthy athletes does not appear to be associated with impaired ventricular relaxation and filling (30, 31).

Altered Gene Isoform Expression

In addition to quantitative changes in protein synthesis that account for the increase in left ventricular mass, pressure overload hypertrophy is accompanied by changes in gene isoform expression, which simulate the fetal pattern of cardiac isoform programming (32). The adaptive response to sustained pressure work includes the altered expression of isoforms of multigene families which regulate synthesis of components of the contractile proteins, such as α-skeletal actin and tryponin. The intriguing switch from the fast to slow myosin ATPase isoform that occurs in rats with pressure overload does not appear relevant to humans because the slow isoform is predominant in the normal human heart (32). It is not yet clear what effects these *switches in isoform expression* of components of the contractile proteins have on systolic and diastolic function in the intact human heart. In addition, cardiac hypertrophy is accompanied by *altered quantitative expression of single genes,* which encode enzymes important for the regulation of intracellular ion homeostasis.

Abnormal Calcium Homeostasis

Altered quantitative synthesis of enzymes critical for the regulation of intracellular calcium contributes to slowed diastolic relaxation in the hypertrophied heart. (See Chap. 1.) The time course of the calcium transient is prolonged in hypertrophied cardiac tissue from both humans and experimental animals with chronic cardiac hypertrophy (33, 34). This alteration of the time course of the calcium transient results in the prolonged availability of high levels of activating calcium. The prolongation of the availability of activating calcium may be beneficial in systole in the well-oxygenated heart which is beating at a slow-normal heart rate because it promotes a high level of sustained force development to meet the increased systolic pressure work imposed by hypertension or aortic stenosis. However, the prolongation of the calcium transient also has the consequence of the prolongation of myofilament crossbridge cycling and slowed force inactivation in diastole. It is likely that this change in diastolic calcium regulation is a contributing factor to the slowed left ventricular relaxation that is characteristic of patients and animal models with advanced pressure overload hypertrophy.

These changes in intracellular calcium regulation appear to be related to a reduced expression of sarcoplasmic reticulum calcium ATPase pumps, which results in impaired calcium reuptake by the sarcoplasmic reticulum during diastole, and to the altered expression and altered activity of sarcolemmal cation pumps (35–37). Studies suggest that advanced cardiac hypertrophy with myocardial failure is accompanied by a deficiency of cyclic AMP (38). This intracellular messenger modifies the relaxation process by stimulating the phosphorylation of the regulatory protein phospholamban, an enzyme that stimulates sarcoplasmic reticulum calcium uptake. In advanced cardiac hypertrophy with myo-

cardial failure, alterations in this critical cyclic AMP signalling pathway appear to involve changes in the expression of β-adrenergic receptors, alterations in the relative expression of stimulatory versus inhibitory G-proteins, and possibly depressed expression of the gene which encodes the regulatory protein phospholamban itself (39–41). In patients with severe hypertrophy caused by hypertrophic cardiomyopathy, β-adrenergic stimulation with isoproterenol, despite provoking ischemia, improves left ventricular relaxation and distensibility (42).

Altered Collagen Synthesis

In addition to alterations in expression of gene families that encode components of contractile proteins and individual genes that encode critical enzymes involved in ion homeostasis, cardiac hypertrophy is also accompanied by altered collagen synthesis. (See Chap. 8.) In certain animal models of cardiac hypertrophy and in advanced severe cardiac hypertrophy in patients, pressure overload is accompanied by an increase in total collagen that is synthesized by fibroblasts within the left ventricular myocardium. It is clear that changes in myocardial distensibility may occur independent of major increases in collagen content (43). Nonetheless, an increase in collagen content within the hypertrophied left ventricular wall can be an additive factor that contributes to impaired left ventricular distensibility and relaxation. Correlative studies of left ventricular biopsy histologic analyses and hemodynamic data derived during cardiac catheterization in patients with cardiac hypertrophy suggest that myocardial fibrosis contributes to the elevation of left ventricular diastolic pressure and modifies myocardial distensibility once the amount of fibrous tissue exceeds about 20% (16). In models of experimental hypertrophy, the development of hypertrophy appears to be associated not only with an increase in total collagen content, but also with changes in collagen subtype and the pattern of crosslinkage (44).

Activation of the Cardiac Renin-Angiotensin System

Interestingly, in experimental hypertension in rats, myocyte hypertrophy appears

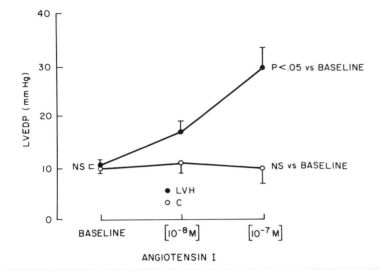

Fig. 20–1. Effects of angiotensin I infusion on LVEDP in isolated perfused hypertrophied (LVH) and control (C) rat hearts. The cardiac conversion of angiotensin I to II was enhanced in the LVH hearts. In this setting, although angiotensin I infusion had minimal effect on diastolic function in the normal (C) hearts, there was a dose-related deterioration of diastolic function in the LVH hearts. Reproduced with permission from Schunkert H, Dzau VJ, Tang SS, et al.: J Clin Invest 86:1913, 1990.

to be predominantly related to the magnitude of ventricular loading, whereas activation of the circulating renin-angiotension system appears to regulate the accumulation of collagen (45). (See Chap. 8.) In this regard, recent studies in experimental pressure overload models suggest that compensatory pressure-overload hypertrophy is accompanied by an increased activation of the local cardiac renin-angiotensin system (46, 47). Activation of the cardiac renin-angiotensin system in pressure overload hypertrophy may play a partial role in the modulation and promotion of the hypertrophic process itself (4, 48). However, consistent with many biologic adaptations, the increased activation of the cardiac renin-angiotensin system carries adverse consequences as well. Experiments in isolated hypertrophied rat hearts suggest that the enhanced activation of cardiac angiotensin II promotes coronary vasoconstriction as well as severe and reversible depression of left ventricular diastolic relaxation (46, 49) (Fig. 20–1). It is not yet known whether an enhanced activation of the cardiac renin-angiotensin system occurs in humans with chronic pressure overload hypertrophy, and whether such activation may contribute to impaired diastolic function.

THE INTERPLAY OF ISCHEMIA AND HYPERTROPHY

The changes in gene expression and protein synthesis that accompany the development of left ventricular hypertrophy appear to make the hypertrophied left ventricle extremely susceptible to further deterioration of diastolic function in response to ischemia or hypoxia. Patients with pressure overload hypertrophy are at risk for developing myocardial ischemia from two mechanisms: coexisting atherosclerotic coronary artery disease and impaired coronary vasodilator reserve. Impaired coronary vasodilator reserve with relative subendocardial hypoperfusion has been demonstrated in both animal models of experimental left ventricular hypertrophy and in humans with pressure overload hypertrophy (50–53). It is well recognized that patients with hypertrophy caused by aortic stenosis or hypertension commonly develop both angina and dyspnea in response to stress of exercise. The changes in diastolic function that occur during angina have been studied during cardiac catheterization in patients with severe left ventricular hypertrophy caused by aortic stenosis (20). During angina induced by brief pacing tachycardia, these patients developed a marked increase in left ventricular end-diastolic pressure (Fig. 20–2), associated with slowing of left ventricular relaxation, as well as an upward shift of the left ventricular pressure-dimension relation indicative of an abrupt impairment of left ventricular diastolic distensibility. (See Chap. 17.)

Multiple experimental studies in animals with experimental pressure overload hy-

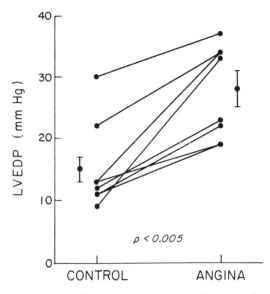

Fig. 20–2. Effects of ischemia on left ventricular end-diastolic pressure (LVEDP) in patients with chronic left ventricular hypertrophy and impaired coronary reserve due to aortic stenosis. Angina induced by brief pacing tachycardia was associated with a significant elevation in left ventricular end-diastolic pressure measured during angina immediately postpacing. Reproduced with permission from Fifer MA, Bourdillon PD, Lorell BH: Circulation 74:675, 1986.

pertrophy support the hypothesis that the hypertrophied left ventricle is more susceptible than the nonhypertrophied heart to developing severe impairment of diastolic function in response to brief hypoxia or ischemia (54, 55) (Fig. 20–3). Studies using nuclear magnetic resonance spectroscopy to study high energy phosphate levels during hypoxia indicate that the hypertrophied left ventricle develops more severe diastolic dysfunction for any level of myocardial ATP depletion relative to control hearts (56).

The mechanisms responsible for the enhanced sensitivity to hypoxia and ischemia-induced diastolic dysfunction in the hypertrophied heart are not yet fully defined. It is likely that there is an adverse interplay between the intrinsic alteration in myocyte calcium regulation that is characteristic of the hypertrophied heart and the superimposition of calcium overload that occurs in response to ischemia and hypoxia. An increase in cytosolic levels of calcium has been shown to occur very early during myocardial ischemia and myocardial hypoxia. Multiple studies using the fluorescent calcium indicator Indo-1 AM (57, 58), the luminescent indicator aequorin (59), and nuclear magnetic resonance spectroscopy (60, 61) all support the notion that an

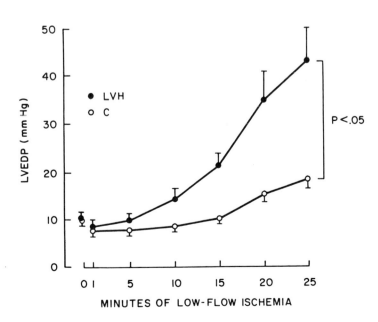

Fig. 20–3. Effects of low-flow global ischemia on left ventricular end-diastolic pressure (LVEDP) in isolated isovolumic blood-perfused hearts from aortic-banded rats (LVH) and control (C) rats. The ischemic increase in isovolumic LVEDP was earlier and more severe in the hypertrophied hearts compared with controls despite similar levels of coronary flow per gram and myocardial ATP depletion. Reproduced with permission from Lorell BH, Grice WN, Apstein CS: Circulation 80:II-97, 1989.

increase in cytosolic calcium occurs during early ischemia, hypoxia or metabolic inhibition. In the presence of intrinsic prolongation of the calcium transient in the setting of pressure overload hypertrophy, the imposition of an additional increase in cytosolic free calcium during ischemia would be expected to cause a more severe level of calcium overload and impaired force inactivation at any level of ATP depletion in hypertrophied versus normal myocardium.

Glycolytic ATP Production

Additional factors may also contribute to the susceptibility of the hypertrophied heart to ischemic diastolic dysfunction. The capacity of the hypertrophied myocyte to recruit anaerobic glycolysis may be a factor. (See Chap. 1.) There is substantial inferential evidence that cytosolic ATP produced by glycolysis may be preferentially utilized by ATP-dependent membrane pumps and is of critical importance in preserving myocardial relaxation during hypoxia and ischemia (62, 63). In a hypertensive rat model of pressure overload hypertrophy, myocardial lactate production during hypoxia, which is a stoichiometric marker of cytosolic ATP production by anaerobic glycolysis, was impaired (64). Myocardial lactate production and, presumably, glycolytic ATP production during ischemia, has also been demonstrated to be impaired in canine hypertrophied hearts with cardiac failure during ischemia (65). However, impaired generation of glycolytic ATP does not appear to be characteristic of all models of experimental hypertrophy in response to hypoxic or ischemic stress (66, 67). Further studies are needed to determine if the capacity to utilize anaerobic glycolysis during transient ischemia is impaired in humans with advanced pressure overload hypertrophy.

An additional factor that may modify the development of ischemic diastolic dysfunction of the hypertrophied heart is the enhanced activation of the intrinsic cardiac renin-angiotensin system. In this regard, a beneficial effect of the inhibition of angiotensin-converting enzyme (ACE) has been demonstrated in nonhypertrophied rat hearts during ischemia-reperfusion injury

(68). Studies in isolated, perfused hypertrophied rat hearts suggest that the specific cardiac ACE inhibition protects against exaggerated diastolic dysfunction during ischemia in comparison with control hearts (67). Further studies are needed to test the hypothesis that activation of a "primed" cardiac renin-angiotensin system in hypertrophied hearts during ischemia has a direct adverse effect on diastolic function, which can be modified by inhibition of cardiac angiotensin converting enzyme (ACE) or by angiotensin II receptor antagonists.

Ventricular Hypertrophy after Infarction

In patients who have experienced myocardial infarction, the development of a thin regional scar is accompanied by compensatory hypertrophy of the non-infarcted segments of the ventricle. (See Chap. 18.) Following acute myocardial infarction, the changes in regional wall stress imposed on the noninfarcted segments result in extensive remodelling of the left ventricle which is characterized by dilation of the left ventricular chamber and by an increase in wall thickness and expansion of the perimeter of the non-infarcted region. The compensatory left ventricular hypertrophy that rapidly occurs after myocardial infarction has been observed both in animal models and in patients after myocardial infarction (69, 70). Both the presence of fibrotic noncontracting scar in the infarcted region as well as regional hypertrophy appear to contribute to the decrease in left ventricular chamber distensibility and slowed myocardial relaxation that occurs in this setting (70, 71). In addition, tissue-specific activation of cardiac ACE and enhanced local synthesis of angiotensin II has been demonstrated in rat hearts with compensatory hypertrophy and remodelling following myocardial infarction (72). In the setting of cardiac hypertrophy in postinfarction remodelling, an increased production of cardiac angiotensin II may participate in the hypertrophic process via its growth-promoting effects and contribute to alterations in diastolic properties.

In summary, cardiac hypertrophy that occurs as an adaptation to a sustained increase in work of the heart is accompanied by changes in left ventricular geometry and in the expression of genes that encode enzymes that regulate intracellular ion homeostasis. Although these adaptations may have a net beneficial effect on the preservation of systolic force development during well oxygenated conditions, these alterations in gene expression appear to play a critical role in promoting diastolic dysfunction in hypertrophied heart. Further work is needed to unravel the contribution of altered gene expression and synthesis of critical proteins to diastolic physiology in the isolated myocyte and in the intact heart. These insights are needed to better understand and ultimately treat diastolic dysfunction in patients with cardiac hypertrophy.

REFERENCES

1. Lorell BH: Significance of diastolic dysfunction of the heart. Ann Rev Med 42:411, 1991.
2. Grossman W: Diastolic function in congestive heart failure. Circulation 81(Suppl. III):III1, 1990.
3. Stauffer JC, Gaasch WH: Recognition and treatment of left ventricular diastolic dysfunction. Prog Cardiovasc Dis 32:319, 1990.
4. Morgan HE, Baker KM: Cardiac hypertrophy: Mechanical, neural, and endocrine dependence. Circulation 83:13, 1991.
5. Kent RL, Hoober JK, Cooper G IV: Load responsiveness of protein synthesis in adult mammalian myocardium: Role of cardiac deformation linked to sodium influx. Circ Res 64:74, 1989.
6. Harsdorf RV, Lang RE, Fullerton M, Woodcock EA: Myocardial stretch stimulates phosphatidyl inositol turnover. Circ Res 65:494, 1989.
7. Grossman W, Jones D, McLaurin LP: Wall stress and patterns of hypertrophy in the human left ventricle. J Clin Invest 56:56, 1975.
8. Fifer MA, et al.: Myocardial contractile function in aortic stenosis as determined from the rate of stress development during isovolumic systole. Am J Cardiol 44:1318, 1979.
9. Gunther S, Grossman W: Determinants of ventricular function in pressure overload hypertrophy in man. Circulation 59:679, 1979.
10. Anversa P, Ricci R, Olivetti G: Quantitative structural analysis of the myocardium during physiologic growth and induced cardiac hypertrophy: A review. J Am Coll Cardiol 7:1140, 1986.
11. Gaasch WH, et al.: Left ventricular stress and compliance in man: with special reference to normalized ventricular function curves. Circulation 46:746, 1972.
12. Grossman W, McLaurin LP, Moos SP, Stefadouros MA: Left ventricular stiffness associated with chronic pressure and volume overloads in man. Circ Res 35:793, 1974.
13. Mirsky I: Assessment of diastolic function: Suggested methods and future considerations. Circ Res 69:836, 1984.
14. Grossman W, et al.: Wall thickness and diastolic properties of the left ventricle. Circulation 49:129, 1974.
15. Peterson KL, et al.: Diastolic left ventricular pressure-volume and stress-strain relations in patients with valvular aortic stenosis and left ventricular hypertrophy. Circulation 58:77, 1978.
16. Krayenbuehl HP, et al.: Influence of pressure and volume overload on diastolic compliance. *In* Diastolic Relaxation of the Heart. Edited by W Grossman and BH Lorell. Boston, Martinez-Nijhoff, 1987, p. 143–150.
17. Eichhorn P, et al.: Left ventricular relaxation in patients with left ventricular hypertrophy secondary to aortic valve disease. Circulation 65:1395, 1982.
18. Smith VE, et al.: Rapid ventricular filling in left ventricular hypertrophy. Pathologic hypertrophy. J Am Coll Cardiol 5:869, 1985.
19. Diver DJ, et al.: Diastolic function in patients with aortic stenosis: Influence of left ventricular load reduction. J Am Coll Cardiol 12:642, 1988.
20. Fifer AM, Bourdillon PD, Lorell BH: Altered left ventricular diastolic properties during pacing-induced angina in patients with aortic stenosis. Circulation 74:675, 1986.
21. Fifer M, Borow K, Colan S, Lorell BH: Early diastolic left ventricular function in children and adults with aortic stenosis. J Am Coll Cardiol 5:1147, 1985.
22. Topol EJ, Trail TA, Fortuin NJ: Hypertensive hypertrophic cardiomyopathy of the elderly. N Engl J Med 312:277, 1985.
23. Lorell BH, et al.: Modification of abnormal left ventricular diastolic properties by nifedipine in patients with hypertrophic cardiomyopathy. Circulation 65:499, 1982.
24. Bonow RO, et al.: Effects of verapamil on left ventricular systolic function and diastolic filling in patients with hypertrophic cardiomyopathy. Circulation 64:787, 1981.
25. Zile MR, Gaasch WH: Mechanical leads and

the isovolumic and filling indices of left ventricular relaxation. Prog Cardiovasc Dis 32:333, 1990.

26. Cheng C-P, et al.: Effect of loading conditions, contractile state, and heart rate on early left ventricular filling in conscious dogs. Circ Res 66:814, 1990.

27. Thidemann KU, Holubarsch CH, Medugorac I, Jacob R: Connective tissue content and myocardial stiffness in pressure overload hypertrophy. Basic Res Cardiol 78: 140, 1983.

28. Shapiro LM, McKinnon WJ: Left ventricular hypertrophy. Relation of structure to diastolic function in hypertension. Br Heart J 51:637, 1984.

29. Schwartz F, Flameng W, Schaper J, Hehrlein F: Correlation between myocardial structure and diastolic function of the heart in chronic aortic valve disease: Effects of corrective surgery. Am J Cardiol 42:895, 1978.

30. Colan SD, Sanders SP, McPherson D, Borow KM: Left ventricular diastolic function in elite athletes with physiologic cardiac hypertrophy. J Am Coll Cardiol 6:545, 1985.

31. Granger CB, et al.: Rapid ventricular filling in left ventricular hypertrophy: Physiologic hypertrophy. J Am Coll Cardiol 5:862, 1985.

32. Izumo S, et al.: Myosin heavy chain messenger RNA and protein isoform transitions during cardiac hypertrophy. J Clin Invest 79:970, 1987.

33. Morgan JP, Morgan KG: Calcium and cardiovascular function: intracellular calcium levels during contraction and relaxation of mammalian cardiac and vascular smooth muscle as detected with aequorin. Am J Med 77(Suppl. 5A):33, 1984.

34. Gwathmey JK, Morgan JP: Altered calcium handling in experimental pressure-overload in the ferret. Circ Res 57:836, 1985.

35. de la Bastie D, et al.: Function of the sarcoplasmic reticulum and expression of its Ca^{2+}-ATPase gene in pressure overload-induced cardiac hypertrophy in the rat. Circ Res 66:554, 1990.

36. Dixon IM, et al.: Sarcolemmal calcium transport in congestive heart failure due to myocardial infarction in rats. Am J Physiol 262:H1387, 1992.

37. Hanf R, Drubaix I, Lelievre L: Rat cardiac hypertrophy: Altered sodium-calcium exchange in sarcolemmal vesicles. FEBS Letts. 236:145, 1988.

38. Feldman MD, et al.: Deficient production of cyclic AMP: Pharmacologic evidence of an important cause of contractile dysfunction in patients with end-stage heart failure. Circulation 75:331, 1987.

39. Bristow MR, et al.: β_1 and β_2 adrenergic receptor subpopulations in nonfailing and failing human myocardium: Coupling of both receptor subtypes to muscle contraction and selective β_1 receptor down-regulation in heart failure. Circ Res 59:297, 1986.

40. Feldman AM, et al.: Increase of the 40,000-mol wt. pertussis toxin substrate (G-protein) in the failing human heart. J Clin Invest 82:189, 1988.

41. Feldman AM: Preliminary Communication. Alterations in G-proteins in human and animal models of heart failure: methodological considerations and interpretation of results. American Heart Association Scientific Conference on Heart Failure: Adaptive and Maladaptive Processes. Portsmouth, New Hampshire, August 4–7, 1991.

42. Udelson JE, et al.: β-adrenergic stimulation with isoproterenol enhances left ventricular diastolic performance in hypertrophic cardiomyopathy despite potentiation of myocardial ischemia. Circulation 79:371, 1989.

43. Thidemann KB, Hollubars CH, Medugorac I, Jacob R: Connective tissue content and myocardial stiffness in pressure overload hypertrophy. Basic Res Cardiol 78: 140, 1983.

44. Mukherjee D, Sen S: Collagen phenotypes during development and regression of myocardial hypertrophy in spontaneously hypertensive rats. Circ Res 67:1474, 1990.

45. Brilla CG, et al.: Remodelling of the rat right and left ventricles in experimental hypertension. Circ Res 67:1355, 1990.

46. Schunkert H, et al.: Increased rat cardiac angiotensin converting enzyme activity and mRNA expression in pressure overload left ventricular hypertrophy: effects on coronary resistance, contractility, and relaxation. J Clin Invest 86:1913, 1990.

47. Baker KM, Cherin MI, Wixson SK, and Aceto JF: Renin-angiotensin system involvement in pressure overload hypertrophy in rats. Am J Physiol 259:H324, 1990.

48. Komuro I, et al.: Angiotensin II induces hypertrophy and oncogene expression in cultured rat heart myocytes (Abstr.) Circulation 80(Suppl. II):2, 1989.

49. Schunkert H, et al.: Distribution and functional significance of cardiac angiotensin converting enzyme in hypertrophied rat hearts. Circulation, In press, 1993.

50. Bache RJ, Arentzen CE, Simon AB, Vrobel TR: Abnormalities in myocardial perfusion during tachycardia in dogs with left ventricular hypertrophy: metabolic evidence of ischemia. Circulation 69:409, 1984.

51. Tomanek RJ, et al.: Morphology of canine coronary arteries, arterioles and capillaries during hypertension in left ventricular hypertrophy. Circ Res 58:38, 1986.

52. Marcus ML, et al.: Decreased coronary reserve. A mechanism for angina pectoris in patients with aortic stenosis and normal coronary arteries. N Engl J Med 307:1362, 1982.

53. Pichard AD, et al.: Coronary flow studies in patients with left ventricular hypertrophy of the hypertensive type. Am J Cardiol 47:547, 1981.

54. Lorell BH, et al.: The influence of pressure overload left ventricular hypertrophy on diastolic properties during hypoxia in isovolumically contracting rat hearts. Circ Res 58:653, 1986.

55. Lorell BH, Grice WN, and Apstein CS: Influence of hypertension with minimal hypertrophy during demand ischemia. Hypertension 13:361, 1989.

56. Wexler LF, et al.: Enhanced sensitivity to hypoxia-induced diastolic dysfunction in pressure overload hypertrophy in the rat: Role of high energy phosphate depletion. Circ Res 62:766, 1988.

57. Lee HC, et al.: Effect of ischemia on calcium-dependent fluorescence transience in rabbit hearts containing Indo-1. Correlation with monophasic action potentials and contraction. Circulation 78:1047, 1988.

58. Barry WH, Peeters CAF, Rasmussen JR, and Cunningham MJ: Role of changes in $[Ca^{2+}]_i$ in energy deprivation contracture. Circ Res 61:726, 1987.

59. Kihara Y, Grossman W, and Morgan JP: Direct measurement of changes in $[Ca^{2+}]_i$ during hypoxia, ischemia, and reperfusion of intact mammalian heart. Circ Res 65: 1029, 1989.

60. Steenbergen C, Murphy E, Levy L, London RE: Elevation in cytosolic free calcium concentration early in myocardial ischemia in perfused rat hearts. Circ Res 60:700, 1987.

61. Steenbergen C, Murphy E, Watts JA, London RE: Correlation between cytosolic free calcium, contracture, ATP, and irreversible ischemic injury in perfused rat heart. Circ Res 66:135, 1990.

62. Owen P, Dennis S, Opie LH: Glucose flux regulates onset of ischemic contracture in globally underperfused rat hearts. Circ Res 66:344, 1990.

63. Eberli FR, et al.: Protective effect of increased glycolytic substrate resistance from prolonged global underperfusion and reperfusion in isolated rabbit hearts perfused with erythrocyte suspensions. Circ Res 68: 466, 1991.

64. Cunningham MJ, et al.: Influence of glucose and insulin on exaggerated diastolic and systolic dysfunction of hypertrophied rat hearts during hypoxia. Circ Res 66:406, 1990.

65. Gaasch WH, et al.: Tolerance of the hypertrophic heart to ischemia. Studies in compensated and failing dog hearts with pressure overload hypertrophy. Circulation 81: 1644, 1990.

66. Anderson PG, et al.: Increased ischemic injury but decreased hypoxic injury in hypertrophied rat hearts. Circ Res 67:984, 1990.

67. Eberli FR, Apstein CS, Ngoy S, Lorell BH: Exacerbation of left ventricular ischemic diastolic dysfunction by pressure overload hypertrophy: Modulation by specific inhibition of cardiac angiotensin converting enzyme. Circ Res 70:931, 1992.

68. Van Gilst WH, de Graeff PA, Wesseling H, DeLangen CDJ: Reduction of reperfusion arrhythmias in ischemic isolated rat heart by angiotensin converting enzyme inhibitors: A comparison of captopril, enalapril, and HOE 498. J Cardiovasc Pharmacol 8: 722, 1986.

69. Pfeffer JM, Pfeffer MA, Braunwald E: Influence of chronic captopril therapy on the infarcted left ventricle of the rat. Circ Res 57:84, 1985.

70. McKay RG, et al.: Left ventricular remodelling following myocardial infarction: A corollary to infarct expansion. Circulation 74: 693, 1986.

71. Pouleur H, Rousseau MF, Van Eyll C, Charlier AA: Assessment of regional left ventricular relaxation in patients with coronary disease: Importance of geometric factors and change in wall thickness. Circulation 69:696, 1984.

72. Hirsch AT, et al.: Tissue-specific activation of cardiac angiotensin converting enzyme in experimental heart failure. Circ Res 69: 475, 1991.

Chapter 21

DIASTOLIC FUNCTION IN HYPERTENSIVE HEART DISEASE

Brian D. Hoit and Richard A. Walsh

Systemic arterial hypertension is a major cause of cardiovascular morbidity and mortality. Although it is well established that congestive heart failure caused by systolic ventricular dysfunction may complicate hypertension, only recently has the importance of diastolic abnormalities of ventricular function been recognized. Interest in diastolic function in patients with hypertensive heart disease is related to several related developments in clinical cardiology. First, noninvasive (ultrasound and nuclear) techniques that quantitatively assess diastolic function have been developed and validated, permitting study of patients early in the course of their disease. Second, using these methods, it has become apparent that ventricular diastolic function is frequently impaired in patients with hypertension and that, in many instances, diastolic abnormalities occur in the absence of detectable left ventricular hypertrophy and systolic dysfunction (1–4). Third, the development of effective antihypertensive drugs has led to the realization that regression of left ventricular hypertrophy may be associated with normalization of abnormal diastolic function and clinical improvement (5–9). Finally, the presence of diastolic abnormalities may help risk stratify patients with hypertension (10, 11) and provide clues to the pathophysiology of hypertensive heart disease (12, 13).

Despite this renewed enthusiasm, several conceptual, methodologic, and analytic difficulties have complicated the study of diastolic function in clinical hypertensive heart disease. Abnormalities of left ventricular diastolic function are classified as either those related to left ventricular relaxation and early ventricular filling or those associated with altered left ventricular pressure-volume and stress-strain rela-

tionships. However, many factors are known to influence both early left ventricular filling and compliance; in patients with hypertension, the effects of altered hemodynamics, ventricular hypertrophy, and myocardial ischemia may each contribute to an impairment of diastolic function. Dissecting these effects is often difficult and frequently impossible in human studies.

This chapter reviews briefly the principal determinants of diastolic function and the methodologic limitations of the various diagnostic diastolic filling indices, discusses human and animal studies of diastolic function in hypertensive heart disease in the framework of altered hemodynamics, left ventricular hypertrophy and myocardial ischemia, and outlines implications for therapy.

DIASTOLIC FUNCTION IN PATIENTS WITH HYPERTENSIVE HEART DISEASE

The fundamental determinants of myocardial relaxation in the isolated papillary muscle are load, inactivation, and the temporal and spatial nonuniform distribution of inactivation and load (14). Although it is conceptually attractive to extrapolate findings from isolated muscle to the intact left ventricle, data in this regard remain controversial. For example, several groups have reported that, in intact animal preparations, the rate and duration of isovolumic relaxation depend on preload and after load (15–18); however, the rate of isovolumic relaxation was relatively insensitive to altered loading conditions in conscious humans (19). Nonetheless, these concepts have proven useful in understanding the complexities of left ventricular relaxation. For example, both an inability to normalize wall stress (afterload mismatch) by virtue of increased systolic loading (elevated arterial pressure and systolic wall stress) and decreased diastolic loading (decreased wall stress at the time of mitral valve opening and decreased coronary turgor) may slow left ventricular relaxation (14). In general, however, hemodynamic loading is not considered to be the major determinant of diastolic function in patients with hypertension and left ventricular hypertrophy. Myocardial inactivation (dissipation of force-generating sites—i.e., actin-myosin crossbridges) may be impaired by intrinsic defects in sarcoplasmic reticulum calcium transport by ischemia or hypoxia-induced sarcoplasmic reticulum dysfunction, or by a subtle interplay of intrinsic and induced abnormalities (20, 21). Changes in the composition of the left ventricular wall (e.g., connective tissue, contractile elements, intracellular connections) and altered geometry of the hypertrophied heart presumably increases nonuniformity of load and inactivation which further contributes to slowed left ventricular relaxation (14). (See Chaps. 4 and 20.)

The determinants of the passive diastolic pressure-volume relation are complex and include left ventricular volume, mass, and geometry, myocardial stiffness and external constraint (e.g., pericardial effects and right ventricular interaction) (Table 21–1). The relative importance of these factors in the patient with hypertension depends on the level of arterial pressure and its rate of

development, the magnitude of the ventricular hypertrophic response, coronary vascular reserve, concomitant disease (e.g., coronary artery disease) and pharmacologic therapy. Although reduced diastolic distensibility may accompany pressure overload hypertrophy, controversy exists as to whether shifts of the diastolic pressure-volume relation are caused by changes in intrinsic myocardial stiffness and fibrosis or to increased wall thickness and chamber geometry (22–24). (See Chap. 9.)

There are several hemodynamic and clinical consequences of diastolic dysfunction. Impaired left ventricular relaxation decreases early ventricular filling and shifts the burden of maintaining an adequate end-diastolic volume (preload) to atrial contraction. If end-diastolic volume is reduced, stroke volume and cardiac output fall by virtue of the Frank-Starling relation. Reduced left ventricular compliance causes increased ventricular diastolic pressures for any level of ventricular filling, which may result in pulmonary venous congestion and symptoms of exertional dyspnea and paroxysmal nocturnal dyspnea. These mechanisms are not independent of one another; for example, slowed left ventricular relaxation adversely influences the passive pressure-volume relation of the left ventricle. Loss of effective atrial contraction because of atrial systolic failure (afterload mismatch, decreased inotropic state) or atrial arrhythmia, further compromises left ventricular filling and cardiac output and increases left atrial pressure.

Table 21–1. Factors Influencing Left Ventricular Chamber Stiffness*

Physical Properties of the Left Ventricle
• Left ventricular chamber volume and mass
• Composition of the left ventricular wall
• Viscosity, stress relaxation, and creep

Intrinsic Factors
• Myocardial relaxation
• Coronary turgor

Extrinsic Factors
• Pericardial restraint
• RV interaction
• Atrial contraction
• Pleural and mediastinal pressure

* Reproduced with permission from Gaasch WH: Basic and clinical aspects. *In* The Ventricle. Edited by HJ Levine, WH Gaasch. Boston, Martinus Nijhoff Publishing, 1985.

METHODOLOGIC CONSIDERATIONS

The noninvasive techniques used to characterize diastolic function have been of limited value for diagnostic decisions. Although these approaches have improved the ability to rapidly, simply, and repetitively identify and quantify abnormalities of diagnostic filling in groups of patients (otherwise impractical or impossible with invasive methods), modalities such as imaging and Doppler echo and radionuclide ventriculography have generated a considerable number of descriptive diastolic indices with wide ranges of normal values and considerable overlap between normal

Table 21–2. Indices of LV Diastolic Function in Hypertension

	Change	Reference
*Imaging Echocardiography**		
IVRT	↑	8, 35, 36, 38
Rate of LV enlargement	↓	36, 38
Rate of posterior wall thinning	↓	36, 50
Doppler Echocardiography†		
E/A (velocity and vti)	↓	39, 42, 73
E (velocity and vti)	↓	40, 41
A (velocity and vti)	↑	3, 39, 40
Atrial filling fraction	↑	3, 73
Radionuclide Ventriculogram‡		
Peak filling rate	↓	1, 2, 8
Filling fractions (½, ⅓)	↓	1, 2, 93
IVRT	↑	6
Time to peak filling rate	↑	2, 9, 93
Cardiac Catheterization		
Relaxation time constant	↑	50, 51, 54
LV compliance	↓	24, 51
	↔	51, 54

* Other indices include relaxation time, duration of early diastolic filling period
† Other indices include early deceleration slope, filling fractions and peak filling rate
‡ Other indices include mean diastolic filling rate and peak filling rate/peak ejection rate
IVRT = isovolumic relaxation time, E = early transmitral velocity, A = late transmitral velocity, vti = velocity time integral

individuals and patients with cardiovascular disease (Table 21–2). Moreover, they have little relationship to invasive measures of diastolic function (25–28), and there are only modest correlations between similar indices (e.g., peak filling rate, atrial contribution to left ventricular filling) derived from Doppler echo and radionuclide techniques (29, 30). Importantly, the majority of the noninvasive indices are age, load and heart rate dependent. Finally, there are no established criteria for what constitutes "abnormal diastolic function."

Symptoms of effort intolerance and dyspnea are substantially related to pulmonary venous pressure, which is only one determinant of left ventricular filling. The factors that influence the peak left ventricular filling rate are complex and include the rate of left ventricular relaxation, the extent of systolic ventricular deformation, atrial and ventricular compliance, visco-

elastic effects, coronary turgor, pericardial restraint, ventricular interaction, and the atrioventricular pressure gradient (31–34). The timing and vigor of atrial systole must also be considered when using indices that measure relative early left ventricular filling, such as Doppler E/A ratios. Moreover, abnormalities of relaxation and chamber stiffness have opposing effects on the pattern of left ventricular filling (28). In patients with normal left ventricular relaxation, left ventricular chamber stiffness correlated directly with Doppler peak early filling velocity and inversely with the atrial filling fraction; in contrast, in patients with impaired left ventricular relaxation, Doppler variables were not correlated with chamber stiffness, but early filling velocity correlated inversely and atrial filling fraction correlated directly with the time constant of relaxation, tau. Thus, patients with coronary disease and concomitant left ventricular hypertrophy had Doppler left ventricular filling patterns that closely resembled patterns in control patients (28). Coexisting abnormalities of load, hypertrophy, and myocardial ischemia are common in hypertensive heart disease and may, by their discordant effects on the determinants of left ventricular filling, decrease the sensitivity of ventricular diastolic filling indices. The methods used to measure diastolic function have been described in detail previously; their value and limitations in patients with hypertensive heart disease are discussed subsequently.

Imaging and Echo Doppler

Digitized M-mode images of the left ventricle and Doppler velocity profiles of transmitral flow are generally used to evaluate diastolic function. (See Chap. 12.) Two-dimensional echocardiography lacks the temporal resolution necessary for interval based indices, but is useful insofar as left ventricular volume can be estimated and combined with invasively determined pressure data to compute compliance (34). The isovolumic relaxation time (IVRT) measured from digitized M-mode echo tends to increase directly with the level of blood pressure (35) and left ventricular filling and posterior wall thinning rates are decreased in pressure overload left ventricular hypertrophy (36, 37). The IVRT may prolong early in the course of hypertension and correlates with decreased peak rapid filling, increased left ventricular mass, and LA size (8). Improvement in M-mode indices of diastolic function has been reported in patients with regression of left ventricular hypertrophy (38).

M-mode echo analysis of diastolic function has the advantages of high temporal resolution (sampling rate 1000/sec) and the ability to measure rates of wall thinning. This approach is limited by the inability to measure global left ventricular function or abnormalities in regions of myocardium not sampled by the ultrasound beam and the need for digitization, which may be time-consuming and relatively expensive. For these reasons, measurement of diastolic transmitral blood flow velocity (which mirrors the diastolic atrioventricular pressure gradient) using pulsed wave Doppler echo has superseded the use of digitized M-mode in clinical practice (Fig. 21–1). Although various velocity and time interval indices have been developed, the ratio of early to late peak velocity (E/A) is easiest to obtain and is most often used. Patients with hypertension characteristically show increased late (A) velocity, decreased E/A ratios, and variable reductions in the early (E) velocity (39–41). These abnormalities may occur early, before slowed peak rates of chamber enlargement are detected by M-mode echo and do not necessarily correlate with the presence or magnitude of left ventricular hypertrophy (3, 42, 43). Doppler indices have the advantages of assessing global ventricular diastolic function and ready accessibility, but are seriously compromised by their marked sensitivity to a variety of physiologic (e.g., heart rate, age, respiration, left atrial pressure), pathophysiologic (e.g., mitral regurgitation and atrial fibrillation) and technical factors (e.g., sample volume location) (44–46). Furthermore, Doppler measures transmitral velocity, not flow; measurement of instantaneous transmitral flow and peak filling rate requires an accurate estimate of the corresponding mitral valvular cross-sectional area (47).

Radionuclide Ventriculography

Global and regional time-activity curves can be derived from gated equilibrium radionuclide angiography. Peak filling rates, filling fractions, and isovolumic relaxation times can be derived from these curves (Fig. 21–2A). (See Chap. 11.) Evidence of left ventricular diastolic dysfunction manifest by decreased peak filling rate, increased time to peak filling rate, decreased third and one-half filling fractions are reported in patients with hypertension (Fig. 21–2B) (1, 2, 8, 26). Although first-pass studies may be used to generate ventricular volume curves, low signal-to-noise limits their utility in assessing diastolic function. Radionuclide-determined peak filling rate was correlated with the Doppler E velocity and the Doppler E/A ratio correlated well with percent left ventricular filling during both early rapid filling and filling caused by atrial contraction (29). Instantaneous transmitral flow derived from combined mitral valve M-mode and transmitral Doppler velocities more closely resembled the time course and shape of radionuclide left ventricular filling curves than mitral velocities alone (47).

In addition to the factors that may alter Doppler transmitral velocity waveforms, radionuclide-derived indices are influenced by the region of interest selected, the choice of background activity, image frame rate, count statistics, the method of selecting R-R intervals, curve fitting and smoothing algorithms, and the method of normalization (26, 48). We have shown that the radionuclide one-half filling fraction (but not the absolute and normalized peak filling rate) is independent of loading conditions in the anesthetized dog (unpublished data).

Cardiac Catheterization

The most rigorous assessment of diastolic function requires measurement of left ventricular pressure and volume, which presently can be determined only by invasive techniques. Although pressure measured with fluid-filled catheters is usually sufficient for clinical decisions, precise measurement of left ventricular pressure during diastole requires the use of a high-fidelity micromanometer. Accurate assess-

A

NORMAL

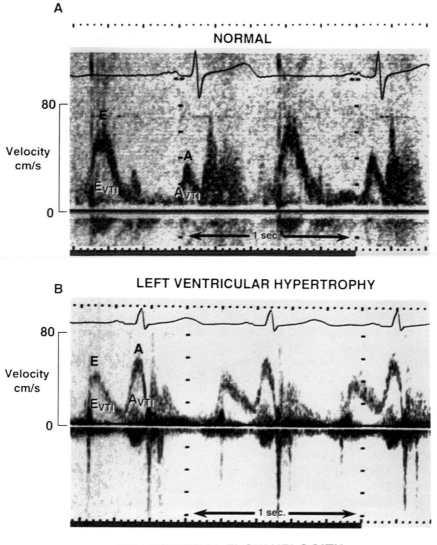

B

LEFT VENTRICULAR HYPERTROPHY

**TRANSMITRAL FLOW VELOCITY
AND INSTANTANEOUS LA—LV GRADIENT**

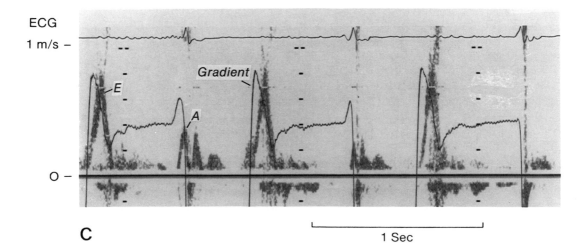

C

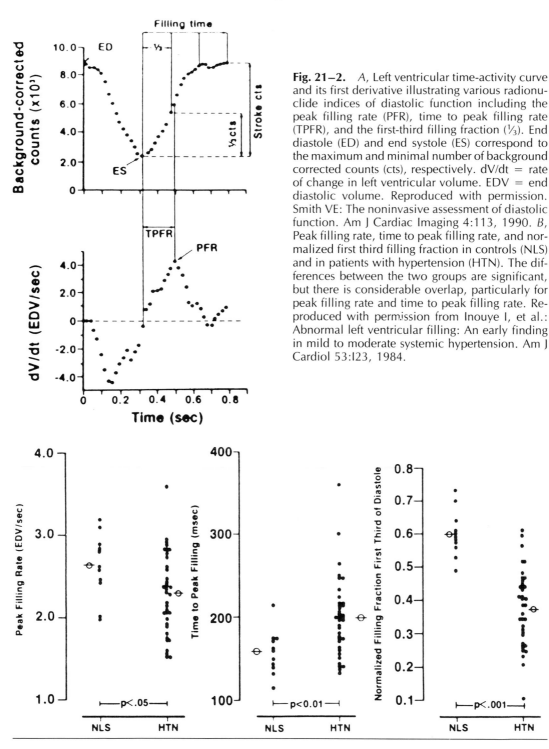

Fig. 21–2. *A,* Left ventricular time-activity curve and its first derivative illustrating various radionuclide indices of diastolic function including the peak filling rate (PFR), time to peak filling rate (TPFR), and the first-third filling fraction ($\frac{1}{3}$). End diastole (ED) and end systole (ES) correspond to the maximum and minimal number of background corrected counts (cts), respectively. dV/dt = rate of change in left ventricular volume. EDV = end diastolic volume. Reproduced with permission. Smith VE: The noninvasive assessment of diastolic function. Am J Cardiac Imaging 4:113, 1990. *B,* Peak filling rate, time to peak filling rate, and normalized first third filling fraction in controls (NLS) and in patients with hypertension (HTN). The differences between the two groups are significant, but there is considerable overlap, particularly for peak filling rate and time to peak filling rate. Reproduced with permission from Inouye I, et al.: Abnormal left ventricular filling: An early finding in mild to moderate systemic hypertension. Am J Cardiol 53:123, 1984.

Fig. 21–1. Doppler mitral flow velocities from a normal subject *(A)* and a patient with hypertensive heart disease *(B).* Note that the normal ratio of peak early (E) to late (A) transmitral velocity is reversed in the patient with hypertensive heart disease. In *(C),* the instantaneous left atrial-left ventricular gradient is superimposed on the Doppler waveform. Note the striking similarity between Doppler and gradient waveforms. E_{VTI} = early velocity time integral; A_{VTI} = late velocity time integral. Panel C reproduced with permission from Hoit BD, et al.: Pericardial influences on right and left ventricular filling dynamics. Circ Res 68:199, 1991.

ment of passive left ventricular diastolic properties requires simultaneous measurement of left ventricular volume with sufficient precision and temporal resolution. Pressure-volume data of the left ventricle are usually approximated by a monoexponential model, and therefore, left ventricular chamber stiffness (dP/dV) depends on operating pressure and volume. (See Chap. 9.) Accordingly, comparisons of chamber stiffness should be performed at comparable (or normalized) volumes over a similar range of pressures (49). Unlike chamber stiffness, myocardial stiffness (the slope of the stress-strain relation) is not dependent on chamber size and geometry. Although it is often assumed that left ventricular compliance is reduced in hypertensive hypertrophy, data in this regard are conflicting (23, 24, 50, 51).

The time constant of left ventricular relaxation (Tau) can be derived from a monoexponential curve fit of isovolumic left ventricular pressure from peak negative dp/dt to left ventricular pressure 5 to 10 mm above left ventricular end diastolic pressure of the preceding beat, assuming either a zero or variable asymptotic pressure (52, 53). Despite different theoretical assumptions, tau determined by these different methods changes in a directionally similar manner (53). In conscious patients, the time constant of isovolumic relaxation is minimally affected by altered loading conditions, suggesting that changes in this parameter partly represent intrinsic changes in isovolumic myocardial relaxation (Fig. 21–3). It is not surprising, therefore, that pressure overload hypertrophy has been associated with prolongation of the time constant of relaxation (50, 54).

Clinical Study Design

In addition to the conceptual, methodologic, and analytic difficulties described

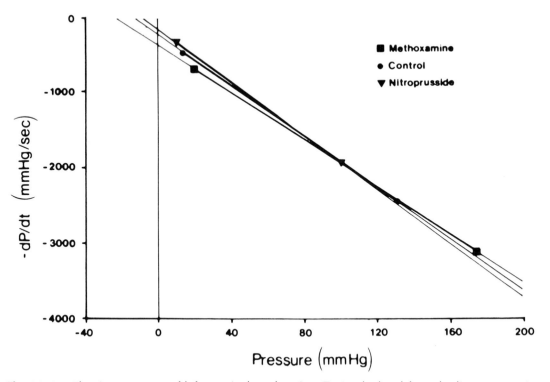

Fig. 21–3. The time constant of left ventricular relaxation (Tau) calculated from the linear regression of instantaneous (−) dP/dt vs. pressure in 14 conscious humans. The time constant of left ventricular relaxation was unaffected by changes in load with methoxamine and nitroprusside infusions. Reprinted with permission of the American Heart Association. Walsh RA: Noninvasive assessment of diastolic function. Am J Cardiac Imaging 4:142, 1990.

previously, clinical investigations of diastolic function in hypertension are hampered by inherent limitations of study design. By necessity, most investigators employ a cross-sectional analysis in which patients are studied during a single time frame of their disease. Thus, patients differ with respect to the magnitude, duration, and treatment of hypertension, loading conditions, and hypertrophic responses. The influence of concomitant intrinsic and environmental factors is often unknown.

Relation of Left Ventricular Hypertrophy and Pressure

Left ventricular hypertrophy can be viewed as an adaptive response that normalizes left ventricular wall stress and preserves systolic function at the expense of prolonged left ventricular relaxation, reduced diastolic distensibility, and impaired coronary vascular reserve. The recognition of the independent prognostic influence of left ventricular hypertrophy and the ability to quantitate left ventricular hypertrophy noninvasively have intensified interest in the functional consequences of hypertrophy in patients with hypertension (10, 11).

The influence of left ventricular hypertrophy on left ventricular filling parameters is complex. Investigators have reported correlations between impaired left ventricular filling and hypertensive (1, 8, 36) but not physiological hypertrophy (55, 56), and indices of diastolic function are abnormal in some patients with hypertension and no left ventricular hypertrophy (2, 3). Moreover, the relation between arterial pressure and left ventricular hypertrophy is poor, even when long-term monitoring of blood pressure is employed (57). Although more precise measures of afterload, such as end-systolic wall stress or aortic impedance, may be better related to left ventricular hypertrophy than systolic pressure, many factors modulate the relationship between blood pressure and hypertrophy (Table 21–3).

In summary, evaluation of diastolic function in patients with hypertensive heart disease requires a thorough knowledge of pathophysiology and the difficult methods of measurement and their limitations. In-

Table 21–3. Potential Factors Modulating the Relationship Between Systemic Arterial Pressure and Left Ventricular Hypertrophy

1. Age
2. Sex
3. Genetic factors
4. Dietary factors—e.g., sodium intake
5. Hemodynamic factors, e.g., end-systolic wall stress
6. Sympathetic nervous system activation
7. Humoral factors
   - Norepinephrine
   - Angiotensin II
8. Associated diseases, e.g., coronary artery disease, valvular heart disease

terpretation of clinical studies demands an appreciation of the various factors determining the relation between left ventricular hypertrophy and blood pressure and the limitations inherent in cross-sectional studies of a heterogeneous disease. For these reasons, studies of hypertension of known severity and duration are needed in well-defined, rigorously controlled animal models.

STUDIES OF DIASTOLIC FUNCTION IN HYPERTENSIVE HEART DISEASE

The discussion of clinical and animal studies that follows is organized according to the major determinant of diastolic dysfunction in hypertensive heart disease, i.e., elevated blood pressure, left ventricular hypertrophy, and coronary vascular reserve. It should be recognized that such a classification is artificial in that diastolic abnormalities complicating hypertensive heart disease probably result from a complex interplay of these variables. (See Chap. 13.)

Elevated Blood Pressure

Numerous hemodynamic factors influence early left ventricular filling, including left atrial pressure, afterload, inotropic state, heart rate, and sympathetic tone (58). Although several of these hemodynamic variables may be altered in patients with hypertensive heart disease, elevation of arterial pressure, or afterload, is the most consistent abnormality. In hypertrophied papillary muscles, imposing a load during isotonic contraction causes both a decrease in the extent of shortening and the rate of lengthening (59). In the intact heart, the effect of increased afterload on left ventricular relaxation depends on experimental conditions and whether acute or steady-state increases are produced (15, 19, 60). Difficulties in defining the role of arterial pressure in clinical studies include the disparate direct and reflex effects of drugs on the heart (61), fluctuations in blood pressure, and interactions between various hemodynamic variables. For example, the effect of beta blockers on left ventricular filling depends on whether arterial pressure is altered: peak filling rate decreases if the blood pressure is unchanged but increases if arterial pressure is lowered (62).

Afterload mismatch (caused by the failure to normalize systolic wall stress) may account for impaired relaxation in pressure overload states (Fig. 21–4), but is probably not the major cause (1, 31, 63). Patients with aortic stenosis and normal or low wall stress and excellent systolic function have impaired early filling and wall thinning rates compared to age-matched controls (64). In one study little correlation was found between the level of arterial blood pressure and the isovolumic relaxation time measured by apex cardiography and M-mode echo; however, the relaxation time tended to increase with increased wall thickness and reduced left ventricular distensibility (Fig. 21–5) (35). In another study, patients with hypertension but no left ventricular hypertrophy had borderline significant reductions in peak filling rate compared to normotensives (1). Diastolic filling abnormalities have been identified in hypertensive adults (2) and children (3) without detectable hypertrophy. Other clinical studies report a correlation between systolic blood pressure and isovolumic relaxation time measured with M-mode-phonoechocardiography (8).

In chronically instrumented conscious dogs with perinephritic hypertension, animals with developing hypertension (2 to 4 weeks of hypertension) had increased peak filling rate, a normal time constant of left ventricular relaxation and increased myocardial stiffness (54). Similar increases in myocardial and chamber stiffness appeared in control dogs with phenylephrine-induced hypertension, but vanished when diastolic indices were examined at

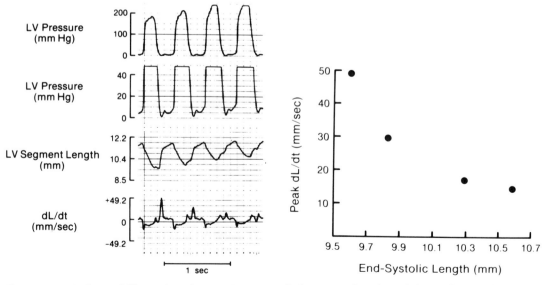

Fig. 21–4. *A,* Record illustrating changes in myocardial segment length and the peak rate of segment lengthening (dL/dt) during an abrupt descending aortic occlusion. Note that, as left ventricular pressure increases, left ventricular end systolic dimension increases and the peak lengthening rate decreases. *B,* Curvilinear relationship between end-systolic segment length and peak lengthening rate derived from data in *A.*

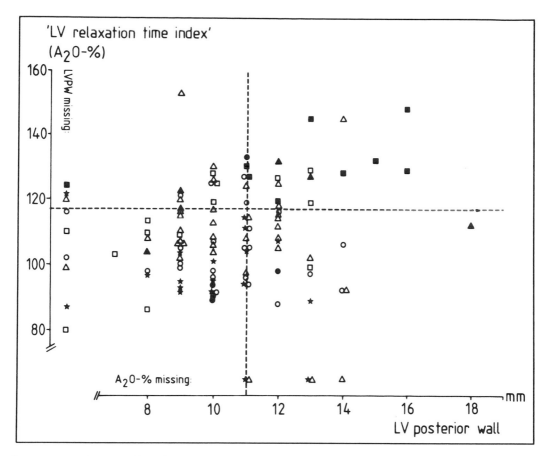

Fig. 21–5. Left ventricular relaxation time index plotted against left ventricular posterior wall thickness in patients with hypertension and in normal controls. The dashed lines indicate cut-off values for normal wall thickness (> 11 mm) and left ventricular relaxation time index (≥ 117%). An a/H ratio (ratio of "a" wave to total deflection on an apex cardiogram) >15% indicates reduced left ventricular distensibility. Note that the relaxation time index tends to increase with increased wall thickness and decreased left ventricular distensibility. However, several patients with a normal left ventricular posterior wall thickness and left ventricular distensibility have a prolonged left ventricular relaxation time. Reproduced with permission from Borer JS, et al.: Systolic function of the hypertrophied left ventricle: Hypertension and aortic stenosis. *In* Heart and Hypertension. Edited by F. Messerli. 1987, p. 133.

comparable levels of preload and afterload. In animals with stable hypertension (14 weeks of hypertension), the time constant of isovolumic relaxation was prolonged and peak filling rate and myocardial stiffness returned to normal (Fig. 21–6). Thus, in this model of developing hypertension, altered loading conditions were primarily responsible for altered diastolic function (54). One should extrapolate these results cautiously to patients with longstanding hypertension and hypertrophy. Generally, correlations between indices of diastolic function and systolic

blood pressure in patients with hypertension are weak at best; this may partly reflect the inability of cross-sectional studies to detect an increase in left ventricular hypertrophy (above baseline) in an individual whose calculated left ventricular mass falls in the normal range.

Left Ventricular Hypertrophy

Many investigators have found an inverse relation between left ventricular mass and peak filling rate in patients with hypertension (1, 3, 8, 37, 65, 66). However, it

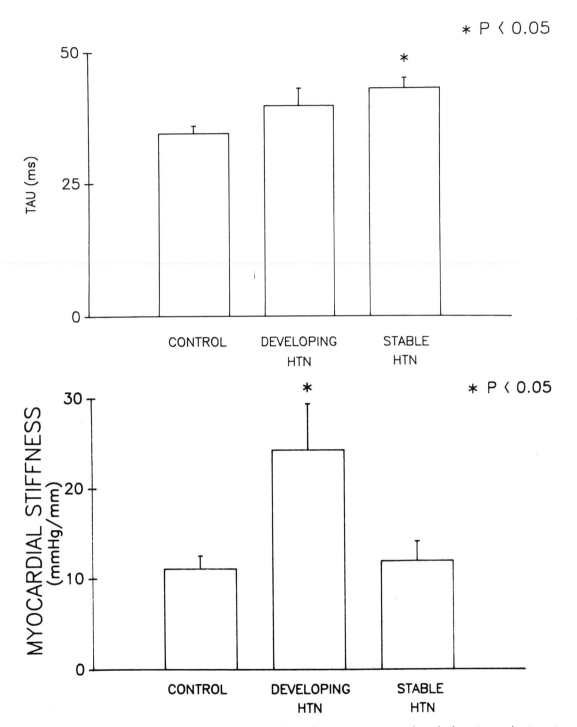

Fig. 21–6. *A,* The time constant of left ventricular relaxation (TAU) in dogs before (control), 2 to 4 weeks after induction of perinephritic hypertension (developing HTN), and in a separate group of dogs after 14 weeks of hypertension (stable HTN). Tau was significantly longer in dogs with stable hypertension. HTN = hypertension. Reproduced with permission from Gelpi RJ, et al.: Diastolic function in developing and stable hypertension. Circ Res 68:562, 1991. *B,* Myocardial stiffness (left ventricular end-diastolic stress/diameter ratio) in the three groups of dogs described in *A*. Myocardial stiffness increased in developing hypertension, but returned to control levels in stable hypertension. Reproduced with permission from Gelpi RJ, et al.: Diastolic function in developing and stable hypertension. Circ Res 68:560, 1991.

is well recognized that top-class endurance swimmers with increased left ventricular mass (physiologic hypertrophy) have normal indices of left ventricular diastolic function (55). Thus, other factors, such as chamber geometry (i.e., the wall thickness/ dimension ratio), ischemia (67, 68) and fibrosis (22, 54) rather than hypertrophy per se, may be responsible for impaired ventricular diastolic filling. In addition, not only the type of hypertrophy, but the type and stage of hypertension may be important. For example, peak filling rates are increased in patients with hypertension and a hyperkinetic circulation (69). In another study, peak filling rate normalized for ejection rate was *increased* early (3 to 6 weeks) after bilateral renal arterial constriction and returned towards normal with the appearance of left ventricular hypertrophy (13).

Left ventricular hypertrophy is associated with intrinsic changes in cytosolic calcium transport. Abnormal sarcoplasmic reticulum function has been reported in both spontaneous hypertensive rats and rats with renovascular hypertension (70). In a ferret model of chronic pressure overload hypertrophy, the time course of the intracellular calcium transient measured with the aequorin injection technique was increased and was associated with prolongation of the development and decay of myocardial tension (71). In addition, isolated sarcoplasmic reticulum from hearts with mild left ventricular hypertrophy exhibits increased calcium transport, whereas sarcoplasmic reticulum from hearts with advanced left ventricular hypertrophy exhibits depressed calcium transport (20, 72). Taken together, these data have been interpreted to support an association between left ventricular hypertrophy and a decreased rate of reuptake and release of calcium by the sarcoplasmic reticulum.

Data suggest that hypertrophy per se may have a detrimental effect on left ventricular diastolic function. M-mode and Doppler echo indices of diastolic function were impaired with progressive hypertrophy in a conscious canine model of perinephritic hypertension (50, 73). In that model, there was a 26% increase in left ventricular mass (at 12 weeks), which was associated with a reduced transmitral flow E/A

ratio, increased atrial filling fraction, decreased peak rate of wall thinning and cavity enlargement, and a prolongation of the time constant of left ventricular relaxation compared to control dogs (50). Postmortem studies revealed a transmural increase in myocyte fiber diameter but no differences in percent fibrosis or morphometrically measured fibrotic volume. Moreover, there was a significant inverse relation between both peak filling rate and the time constant of isovolumic relaxation and myocyte fiber size (50).

Coronary Vascular Reserve

There is a limitation of coronary vascular capacity in left ventricular hypertrophy that results from inadequate growth of new vessels and vascular hypertrophy in the coronary arteries (67, 68). Hypertrophy alone (i.e., in the absence of increased aortic and coronary arterial pressure) was associated with increased minimum coronary vascular resistance and impaired subendocardial perfusion during pacing stress in dogs with surgically created aortic stenosis (74). Factors influencing the interaction between the magnitude of left ventricular hypertrophy and structural changes in the coronary arterial bed include the intensity, type (i.e., pressure versus volume overload hypertrophy), and timing of the hypertrophic stimulus. In general, pressure overload hypertrophy in animal models is associated with normal coronary blood flow per gram of myocardium at rest and mildly impaired coronary vascular reserve (67). Interestingly, coronary vascular reserve is normal in greyhounds with physiologic hypertrophy (75). Compared to the increase in human patients, the increase in left ventricular mass in experimental models of left ventricular hypertrophy is relatively small and the duration of hypertension is not as great. In contrast, coronary vascular reserve markedly decreases in humans with left ventricular pressure overload hypertrophy (67). It should be emphasized that, in clinical hypertensive heart disease, myocardial ischemia may be caused by the impaired coronary reserve that accompanies left ventricular hypertrophy per se, and/or concomitant atherosclerotic coronary artery disease.

In patients and animals without left ventricular hypertrophy, transient ischemia or hypoxia impairs the rate and extent of left ventricular relaxation and decreases diastolic distensibility of the left ventricle (76, 77). The hypertrophied ventricle is susceptible to the development of impaired relaxation in response to interventions such as ischemia and hypoxia, which further reduce sarcoplasmic reticulum function and cause high-energy phosphate depletion (78, 79). (See Chaps. 1 and 20.) In isolated rabbit hearts with hypertensive hypertrophy, a severe impairment of diastolic function developed in response to demand ischemia (pacing tachycardia) when compared to control (79). Similarly, abnormalities of relaxation were more pronounced in the hypertrophied rat heart for any level of high energy phosphate depletion and acidosis compared to control hearts (78). In another study, baseline diastolic function and myocardial stiffness were normal in conscious dogs with pressure overload hypertrophy; with pacing stress, dogs developed diastolic dysfunction manifest by elevated left ventricular end-diastolic pressure and stress and increased myocardial stiffness that was associated with reduced subendocardial coronary reserve (80, 81).

IMPLICATIONS FOR TREATMENT

The concept that elevated arterial pressure, left ventricular hypertrophy, and myocardial ischemia each contribute to diastolic dysfunction has important implications for treating patients with hypertensive heart disease. Whether normalization of impaired diastolic function should itself be a therapeutic goal is an issue of considerable public health and economic importance. Such efforts are directed towards optimizing arterial blood pressure and systolic wall stress, reducing left ventricular mass and correction of myocardial ischemia. (See Chaps. 14 and 26.)

Studies of patients with hypertensive hypertrophy have shown that impaired left ventricular diastolic filling returns to normal as left ventricular hypertrophy regresses (6, 8, 38). In a recent study, verapamil, but not atenolol, taken for 6 months decreased left ventricular mass in a group of elderly patients with hypertension (9). The peak radionuclide filling rate and peak filling rate normalized to the ejection rate were significantly higher in patients whose left ventricular mass decreased; diastolic filling was unchanged in those patients whose left ventricular hypertrophy did not regress (9) (Fig. 21–7). Similarly, normalization of M-mode diastolic indices occurred in patients whose left ventricular hypertrophy regressed with aldomet, but diastolic indices were unchanged in patients without reductions of left ventricular mass (38). Improvements in left ventricular diastolic function lasted at least one month after left ventricular hypertrophy regressed by treatment with the nonselective beta blocker, tertanolol (82). It should be emphasized that studies in patients are difficult to interpret because the effects of hypertrophy regression are not readily separated from the favorably altered loading conditions and other effects of antihypertensive therapy.

Regression of left ventricular hypertrophy in spontaneously hypertensive rats treated with aldomet was associated with a correction of decreased sarcoplasmic reticulum calcium uptake (70); this improvement was related to regression of left ventricular hypertrophy because a reduction of arterial pressure alone with the vasodilator hydralazine failed to correct the abnormality. The reasons for improvement in left ventricular diastolic function with regression of left ventricular hypertrophy are not entirely clear, but it may be the result of a direct effect on calcium kinetics, myocardial and interstitial remodelling (83, 84), or perhaps a restoration of the ratio between capillary cross-sectional area to myofibrillar mass and mitochondrial to myofibril volume ratio (85). In spontaneously hypertensive rats, 12 weeks of treatment with the angiotensin-converting enzyme inhibitor lisinopril resulted in regression of left ventricular hypertrophy and interstitial fibrosis, which was associated with normalization of myocardial stiffness, and remodeling of the intramyocardial coronary arteries associated with normalization of the coronary vasodilator response to adenosine (83). It is important to recognize that regression of left ventricular hypertrophy (like its development) is

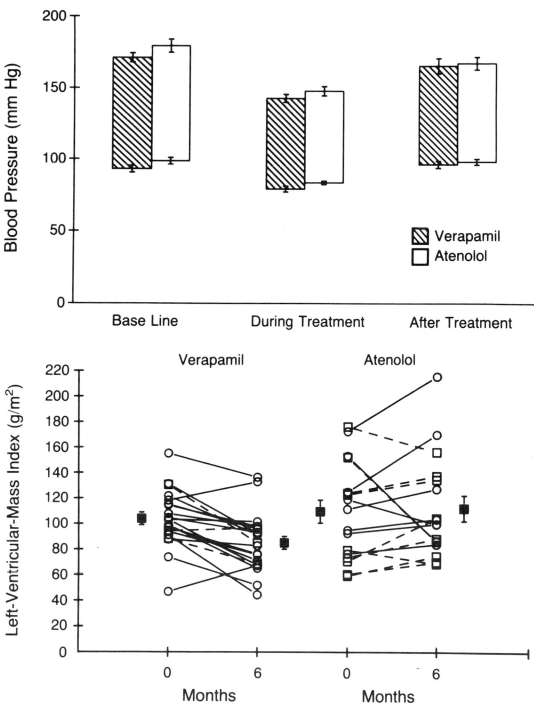

Fig. 21–7. *A,* Systolic and diastolic blood pressures in patients at base line, after 1 month, and 1 to 2 weeks after the withdrawal of therapy with either verapamil (n = 21) or atenolol (n = 18). I bars indicate standard errors. Reproduced with permission from Schulman SP, et al.: The effects of antihypertensive therapy on left ventricular mass in elderly patients. N Engl J Med 322:1351, 1990. *B,* Changes in left ventricular mass index from baseline to 6-month follow-up. Open squares with dashed lines indicate that a diuretic was added to the regimen. Solid squares and bars represent mean ± standard error. After 6 months of treatment, left ventricular mass index decreased significantly after verapamil, but not after atenolol. Reproduced with permission from Schulman SP, et al.: The effects of antihypertensive therapy on left ventricular mass in elderly patients. N Engl J Med 322:1352, 1990.

not only related to a change in load, but is modulated by age, sex, end systolic wall stress (57), adrenergic drive (86), dietary sodium intake (87), and humoral factors such as the renin-angiotensin system (88).

A favorable effect on left ventricular diastolic function is more difficult to demonstrate by correction of elevated arterial blood pressure alone. The time to peak filling rate was significantly reduced by a single dose of an angiotensin-converting enzyme inhibitor in patients with hypertensive hypertrophy (89, 90). Acute administration of calcium blockers, on the other hand, had either no effect on time to peak filling rate (91) or effects that could be explained by changes in heart rate (89). In one study, calcium blockers resulted in small but significant improvements in mean diastolic filling rate and the isovolumic relaxation time (91). In contrast, radionuclide-determined peak filling rate increased in response to acute administration of intravenous verapamil (6), and 3 months of verapamil improved diastolic function as assessed by Doppler echo (92). Despite similar reductions in blood pressure, nifedipine but not propanolol increased rest and exercise first-pass radionuclide peak filling rate, half-filling fraction, and decreased time to peak filling and atrial filling volume (93). Normalization of left ventricular diastolic filling was also seen in elderly patients with hypertensive hypertrophy treated with either beta blockers or calcium antagonists (5).

Regression of left ventricular hypertrophy may have favorable effects on diastolic function owing to improved coronary vascular reserve and myocardial perfusion. Regression of left ventricular hypertrophy in rats with renovascular hypertension increased coronary reserve, but did not alter resting flow (94). Reducing blood pressure without a corresponding reduction in left ventricular mass decreased maximal myocardial perfusion, suggesting that pharmacologic reductions in systemic arterial pressure without regression of left ventricular hypertrophy may compromise coronary reserve and result in myocardial ischemia (94). However, the relation between hypertrophy regression and coronary reserve is complex because the calcium blocker nitrendipine regressed left ventricular hypertrophy in animals with renovascular hypertension and increased resting coronary blood flow, but failed to improve coronary vascular reserve (95).

Diastolic abnormalities failed to reverse in several patients receiving adequate antihypertensive therapy with beta blockers, calcium blockers, diuretics (3, 96), and chronic clonidine therapy (97), suggesting that irreversible changes in left ventricular diastolic function may occur in patients with systemic hypertension. Moreover, in conscious dogs, direct intracoronary administration of calcium blockers was associated with an *impairment* of left ventricular relaxation (61). However, most available information indicates that diastolic abnormalities in patients with hypertensive heart disease are reversible and are favorably influenced by a reduction in left ventricular mass and, to a lesser extent, by correction of elevated arterial pressure. Unfortunately, little is known regarding the long-term effects of regression on diastolic (or systolic) function or coronary vascular reserve.

REFERENCES

1. Fouad FM, Slominski M, Tarazi RC: Left ventricular diastolic function in hypertension: Relation to left ventricular mass and systolic function. J Am Coll Cardiol 3:1500, 1984.
2. Inouye I, et al.: Abnormal left ventricular filling: an early finding in mild to moderate systemic hypertension. Am J Cardiol 53:120, 1984.
3. Snider AR, et al.: Doppler evaluation of left ventricular diastolic filling in children with systemic hypertension. Am J Cardiol 56:921, 1985.
4. Soufer R, et al.: Intact systolic left ventricular function in clinical congestive heart failure. Am J Cardiol 55:1032, 1985.
5. Topol EJ, Traill EA, Fortuin NJ: Hypertensive hypertrophic cardiomyopathy of the elderly. N Engl J Med 312:277, 1985.
6. Betocchi S, et al.: Effects of intravenous verapamil administration on left ventricular diastolic function in systemic hypertension. Am J Cardiol 59:624, 1987.
7. Fouad-Tarazi FM, Liebson PR: Echocardiographic studies of regression of left ventricular hypertrophy in hypertension. Hypertension 9:II-65, 1987.
8. Smith VE, White WB, Meeran MK, Karimeddini MK: Improved left ventricular

filling accompanies reduced left ventricular mass during therapy of essential hypertension. J Am Coll Cardiol 8:1449, 1986.

9. Schulman SP, et al.: The effects of antihypertensive therapy on left ventricular mass in elderly patients. N Engl J Med 322:1350, 1990.

10. Koren MJ, et al.: Relation of left ventricular mass and geometry to morbidity and mortality in uncomplicated essential hypertension. Ann Intern Med 114:345, 1991.

11. Levy D, et al.: Prognostic implications of echocardiographically determined left ventricular mass in the Framingham Heart Study. N Engl J Med 322:1561, 1990.

12. Fouad-Tarazi FM: Left ventricular diastolic dysfunction and cardiovascular regulation in hypertension. Am J Med 87:6B, 1989.

13. Fouad-Tarazi FM: Ventricular diastolic function of the heart in systemic hypertension. Am J Cardiol 65:85G, 1990.

14. Brutsaert DL, Rademakers FE, Stanislas US: Triple control of relaxation: implications in cardiac disease. Circulation 69:190, 1984.

15. Su JB, Hittinger L, Laplace M, Crozatier B: Loading determinants of isovolumic pressure fall in closed-chest dogs. Am J Physiol 260:H690, 1991.

16. Gaasch WH, et al.: Myocardial relaxation. II. Hemodynamic determinants of rate of left ventricular isovolumic pressure decline. Am J Physiol 239:H1, 1980.

17. Karliner JS, et al.: Pharmacologic and hemodynamic influences on the rate of isovolumic left ventricular relaxation in the normal conscious dog. J Clin Invest 60:511, 1977.

18. Raff GL, Glantz SA: Volume loading slows left ventricular isovolumic relaxation rate. Circ Res 48:813, 1981.

19. Starling MR, et al.: Load independence of the rate of isovolumic relaxation in man. Circulation 76:1274, 1987.

20. Sordahl LA, McCollum WB, Wood WG, Schwartz A: Mitochondria and sarcoplasmic reticulum function in cardiac hypertrophy and failure. Am J Physiol 224:497, 1978.

21. Walsh RA: Sympathetic control of diastolic function in congestive heart failure. Circulation 82(Suppl I):I-52, 1990.

22. Weber KT, et al.: Collagen remodeling of the pressure-overloaded, hypertrophied nonhuman primate myocardium. Circ Res 62:757, 1988.

23. Hess OM, et al.: Diastolic function and myocardial structure in patients with myocardial hypertrophy. Circulation 63:360, 1981.

24. Grossman W, McLaurin LP, Stefadourous MA: Left ventricular stiffness associated with chronic pressure and volume overloads in man. Circ Res 35:793, 1974.

25. Lin SL, et al.: Comparison of Doppler echocardiographic and hemodynamic indexes of left ventricular diastolic properties in coronary artery disease. Am J Cardiol 62:882, 1988.

26. Iskandrian AS, et al.: Left ventricular diastolic function: Evaluation by radionuclide angiography. Am Heart J 115:924, 1988.

27. Appleton CA, Hatle LK, Popp RL: Relation of transmitral flow velocity patterns to left ventricular diastolic function: New insights from a combined hemodynamic and Doppler echocardiographic study. J Am Coll Cardiol 12:426, 1988.

28. Stoddard MF, et al.: Left ventricular diastolic function: Comparison of pulsed Doppler echocardiographic and hemodynamic indexes in subjects with and without coronary artery disease. JACC 13:327, 1989.

29. Spirito P, Maron BJ, Bonow RO: Noninvasive assessment of left ventricular diastolic function: Comparative analysis of Doppler echocardiographic and radionuclide angiographic techniques. J Am Coll Cardiol 7:518, 1986.

30. Pearson AC, et al.: Comparison of pulsed Doppler echocardiography and radionuclide angiography in the assessment of left ventricular filling. Am J Cardiol 61:446, 1988.

31. Bahler RC, Martin P: Effects of loading conditions and inotropic state on rapid filling phase of left ventricle. Am J Physiol 248:H523, 1985.

32. Ishida Y, et al.: Left ventricular filling dynamics: influence of left ventricular relaxation and left atrial pressure. Circulation 74:187, 1986.

33. Hoit BD, LeWinter M, Lew WYW: Independent influence of left atrial pressure on regional peak lengthening rates. Am J Physiol 259:H480, 1990.

34. Hoit BD, Dalton N, Bhargava V, Shabetai R: Pericardial influences on right and left ventricular filling dynamics. Circ Res 68:197, 1991.

35. Hartford M, et al.: Diastolic function of the heart in untreated primary hypertension. Hypertension 6:329, 1984.

36. Shapiro LM, McKenna WJ: Left ventricular hypertrophy. Relation of structure to diastolic function in hypertension. Br Heart J 51:637, 1984.

37. Crawford MH, et al.: Echocardiographic left ventricular mass and function in the hypertensive baboon. Hypertension 10:339, 1987.

38. Agati L, et al.: Left ventricular filling pattern in hypertensive patients after reversal of myocardial hypertrophy. Int J Cardiol 17:177, 1987.

39. Phillips RA, et al.: Doppler echocardiographic analysis of left ventricular filling in treated hypertensive patients. J Am Coll Cardiol 9:317, 1987.

40. Kitabatake A, et al.: Transmitral blood flow reflection diastolic behavior of the left ventricle in health and disease. A study by pulsed Doppler technique. Jpn Circ J 46:92, 1982.

41. Genovesi-Ebert A, et al.: Left ventricular filling: Relationship with arterial blood pressure, left ventricular mass, age, heart rate and body build. Hypertension 9:345, 1991.

42. Pearson AC, et al.: Assessment of diastolic function in normal and hypertrophied hearts: Comparison of Doppler echocardiography and M-mode echocardiography. Am Heart J 113:1417, 1987.

43. Szlachcic J, Tubau JF, O'Kelly B, Massie BM: Correlates of diastolic filling abnormalities in hypertension: A Doppler echocardiographic study. Am Heart J 120:386, 1990.

44. Thomas JD, Newell JB, Choong CYP, Weyman AE: Physical and physiological determinants of transmitral velocity: numerical analysis. Am J Physiol 260:H1718, 1991.

45. Plotnick GD: Changes in diastolic function—difficult to measure, harder to interpret. Am Heart J 118:637, 1989.

46. Gardin JM, Dabestani A, Takenaka K: Effect of imaging view and sample volume location on evaluation of mitral flow velocity by pulsed Doppler technique. Am J Cardiol 57:1335, 1986.

47. Hoit BD, et al.: Instantaneous transmitral flow using Doppler and M-mode echocardiography: Comparison with radionuclide ventriculography. Am Heart J 118:308, 1989.

48. Bacharach SL, et al.: Left ventricular peak ejection rate, filling rate, and ejection fraction—Frame rate requirements at rest and exercise. J Nucl Med 20:189, 1979.

49. Mirsky I: Assessment of passive elastic stiffness of cardiac muscle: mathematical concepts, physiologic and clinical considerations, direction of future research. Prog Cardiovasc Dis 18:277, 1976.

50. Douglas PS, Tallant B: Hypertrophy, fibrosis and diastolic dysfunction in early canine experimental hypertension. J Am Coll Cardiol 17:530, 1991.

51. Yamakado T, Nakano T: Left ventricular systolic and diastolic function in the hypertrophied ventricle. Jpn Circ J 54:554, 1990.

52. Weiss JL, Frederiksen JW, Weisfeldt ML: Hemodynamic determinants of the time-course of fall in canine left ventricular pressure. J Clin Invest 58:751, 1976.

53. Starling MR, et al.: The relationship of various measures of end-systole to left ventricular maximum time varying elastance in man. Circulation 76:32, 1987.

54. Gelpi RJ, et al.: Changes in diastolic cardiac function in developing and stable perinepritic hypertension in conscious dogs. Circ Res 68:555, 1991.

55. Colan SD, Sander SP, McPherson D, Borow KM: Left ventricular diastolic function in elite athletes with physiologic cardiac hypertrophy. J Am Coll Cardiol 6:545, 1985.

56. Granger CB, et al.: Rapid ventricular filling in left ventricular hypertrophy: I. Physiologic hypertrophy. J Am Coll Cardiol 5:862, 1985.

57. Sugishita Y, Iida K, Yukisada K, Ito I: Cardiac determinants of regression of left ventricular hypertrophy in essentially hypertension with antihypertensive treatment. J Am Coll Cardiol 15:665, 1990.

58. Fouad FM: Left ventricular diastolic function in hypertensive patients. Circulation 75(Suppl I):I-48, 1987.

59. Lecarpentier Y, Martin JL, Gastineau P, Hatt PY: Load independence of mammalian heart relaxation during cardiac hypertrophy and heart failure. Am J Physiol 242:H855, 1981.

60. Gaasch WH, et al.: Asynchronous (segmental early) relaxation of the left ventricle. J Am Coll Cardiol 5:891, 1985.

61. Walsh RA, O'Rourke RA: Direct and indirect effects of calcium entry blocking agents on isovolumic left ventricular relaxation in conscious dogs. J Clin Invest 75:1426, 1985.

62. Fouad FM, Slominski MJ, Tarazi RC, Gallagher J: Alterations in left ventricular filling with beta adrenergic blockade. Am J Cardiol 51:161, 1983.

63. Lorrell BH, Grossman W: Cardiac hypertrophy: The consequences for diastole. J Am Coll Cardiol 9:1189, 1987.

64. Piter M, Borow K, Colan S, Lorell B: Early diastolic left ventricular function in children and adults with aortic stenosis. J Am Coll Cardiol 5:1147, 1985.

65. Hanrath P, Mathey DG, Siegert R, Bleifeld W: Left ventricular relaxation and filling pattern in direct forms of left ventricular hypertrophy: An echocardiographic study. Am J Cardiol 45:15, 1980.

66. Smith VE, White WB, Karimeddini MF: Echocardiographic assessment of left ventricular diastolic performance in hyperten-

sive subjects. Correlation with changes in left ventricular mass. Hypertension 9:II-81, 1987.

67. Marcus ML, et al.: Abnormalities in coronary circulation secondary to cardiac hypertrophy. Perspect Cardiovasc Res 8:273, 1983.

68. Marcus ML, et al.: Decreased coronary reserve. A mechanism for angina pectoris in patients with aortic stenosis and normal coronary arteries. N Engl J Med 307:1362, 1982.

69. Fouad FM, et al.: Abnormal left ventricular relaxation in hypertensive patients. Clin Sci 59:S411, 1980.

70. Limas CJ, Spier SS: Effect of antihypertensive therapy on calcium transport by cardiac sarcoplasmic reticulum of SHR's. Cardiovasc Res 14:692, 1980.

71. Gwathmey JK, Morgan JP: Altered calcium handling in experimental pressure-overload hypertrophy in the ferret. Circ Res 57:836, 1985.

72. Malholtra A, Penpargkul S, Schaible T, Scheuer J: Contractile proteins and sarcoplasmic reticulum in physiologic cardiac hypertrophy. Am J Physiol 241:H263, 1981.

73. Douglas PS, Berko B, Lesh M, Reichek N: Alterations in diastolic function in response to progressive left ventricular hypertrophy. J Am Coll Cardiol 13:461, 1989.

74. Alyono D, et al.: Alterations of myocardial blood flow associated with experimental canine left ventricular hypertrophy secondary to valvular aortic stenosis. Cir Res 58:47, 1986.

75. Cohen MV, et al.: Coronary vascular reserve in the greyhound with left ventricular hypertrophy. Cardiol Res 20:182, 1986.

76. McLaurin LP, Rolett EL, Grossman W: Impaired left ventricular relaxation during pacing-induced ischemia. Am J Cardiol 32:751, 1973.

77. Serizawa T, Vogel WM, Apstein CS, Grossman W: Comparison of acute alterations in left ventricular diastolic chamber stiffness induced by hypoxia and ischemia. J Clin Invest 68:91, 1981.

78. Lorell BH, et al.: The influence of pressure overload left ventricular hypertrophy on diastolic properties during hypoxia in isovolumically contracting rat hearts. Circ Res 58:653, 1986.

79. Lorell BH, Grice WN, Apstein CS: Influence of hypertension with minimal hypertrophy on diastolic function during demand ischemia. Hypertension 13:361, 1989.

80. Fujii AM, Gelpi RJ, Mirsky I, Vatner SF: Systolic and diastolic dysfunction during atrial pacing in conscious dogs with left ventricular hypertrophy. Circ Res 62:462, 1988.

81. Vatner SF, Shannon R, Hittinger L: Reduced subendocardiol coronary reserve. A potential mechanism for impaired diastolic function in the hypertrophied and failing heart. Circulation 81:III8, 1990.

82. Trimarco B, et al.: Improvement of diastolic function after reversal of left ventricular hypertrophy induced by long-term antihypertensive treatment with tertatolol. Am J Cardiol 64:745, 1989.

83. Brilla CG, Janicki JS, Webert KT: Cardioreparative effects of lisinopril in rats with genetic hypertension and left ventricular hypertrophy. Circulation 83:1771, 1991.

84. Monrad ES, et al.: Time course of regression of left ventricular hypertrophy after aortic valve replacement. Circulation 77:1345, 1988.

85. Anversa P, Ricci R, Olivetti G: Quantitative structural analysis of the myocardium during physiologic growth and induced cardiac hypertrophy: A review. J Am Coll Cardiol 7:1140, 1986.

86. Ayobe MH, Tarazi RC: Reversal of changes in myocardial β-receptors and inotropic responsiveness with regression of cardiac hypertrophy in renal hypertensive rats (RHR). Circ Res 54:125, 1984.

87. Lindpaintner K: Role of sodium in hypertensive cardiac hypertrophy. Circ Res 57:610, 1985.

88. Tarazi RC: Regression of left ventricular hypertrophy: Partial answers for persistent questions. J Am Coll Cardiol 3:1349, 1984.

89. Traub YM, et al.: Comparison of the acute effects of captopril and of nifedipine on left ventricular diastolic function in elderly hypertensive patients. Jpn Heart J 31:799, 1990.

90. Marmor A, et al.: A single dose of cilazapril improves diastolic function in hypertensive patients. Am J Med 87:6B-61S, 1989.

91. Opie JH, Commerford PJ, Adnams C: Effects of calcium antagonists on hypertension and diastolic function. S Afr Med J 76:89, 1989.

92. Grainer P, et al.: Improvement in left ventricular hypertrophy and left ventricular diastolic function following verapamil therapy in mild to moderate hypertension. Eur J Clin Pharmacol 39 (Suppl 1):S45, 1990.

93. Zusman RM, et al.: Nifedipine, but not propranolol, improves left ventricular systolic and diastolic function in patients with hypertension. Am J Cardiol 64:51F, 1989.

94. Wicker P, Tarazi RC, Kobayashi K: Coronary blood flow with reversal of cardiac hypertrophy. Am J Cardiol 51:1744, 1983.
95. Kobayashi K, Tarazi RC: Effect of nitrendipine on coronary flow and ventricular hypertrophy in hypertension. Hypertension 5 (supp II):II-45, 1983.
96. Inouye IK, et al.: Failure of antihypertensive therapy with diuretic, beta-blocking, and calcium channel-blocking drugs to consistently reverse left ventricular diastolic filling abnormalities. Am J Cardiol 53: 1583, 1984.
97. Huting J, et al.: Left ventricular muscle mass and diastolic function in patients with essential hypertension under long-term clonidine monotherapy. Clin Cardiol 14: 134, 1991.

Chapter 22

DIASTOLIC DYSFUNCTION IN HYPERTROPHIC CARDIOMYOPATHY

E. Douglas Wigle

Although two nineteenth-century French pathologists (1, 2) and an early twentieth-century German pathologist (3) described the gross pathologic anatomy of hypertrophic cardiomyopathy (HCM), it remained for the virtual simultaneous reports of Brock (4) and Teare (5) to draw modern attention to this entity. In the 1960s and 1970s, the dynamic obstruction to left ventricular outflow was the focus of attention and intense investigative interest (6, 7), and continues to be the most important pathophysiologic abnormality in systole in HCM (8, 9). From the beginning, however, it was appreciated that diastolic dysfunction was also a very important component of the pathophysiology of HCM. Initially, the elevated left (6, 7) and right (7) ventricular end-diastolic pressures in these patients were attributed to decreased compliance of those chambers. It was appreciated that "HCM could disable a patient more from poor ventricular filling in diastole than from obstruction to outflow in systole." (7) Subsequently, our understanding of the pathophysiology of diastolic dysfunction has been greatly enhanced by several factors. First, myocardial relaxation has been recognized as one of the principal determinants of diastolic filling, largely as the result of the basic work of Brutsaert (10–12) and others. This understanding led to the necessity to distinguish between the passive compliance or stiffness of the ventricle versus active relaxation (see Chapter 14). Second, numerous new investigative techniques in cardiology have permitted assessment of the dynamics of diastolic function. Thus, techniques such as Doppler echocardiography, echophonocardiography, nuclear angiography, mi-cromanometry, and cineventriculography, alone and in combination, may be used to assess the dynamics of diastolic function. Finally, pericardial constraint and ventricular interaction are beginning to be appreciated as important factors in determining diastolic filling characteristics in many clinical circumstances.

HCM may be defined as ventricular hypertrophy without identifiable cause, that is usually, but not always, associated with microscopic evidence of myocardial fiber disarray (Figures 22–1 to 22–3, Table 22–1). Although the left ventricle is the predominant site of involvement, right ventricular involvement may occur in apparent isolation or in association with left-sided involvement. The known varieties of HCM are listed in Table 22–1 and illustrated in Figures 22–1 and 22–2. Approximately 95% of all cases of HCM encountered at the author's institution have shown evidence of asymmetric hypertrophy, asymmetric ventricular septal hypertrophy being by far the commonest variety (Fig. 22–1, Table 22–1). In this discussion, we equate HCM with ventricular septal hypertrophy, unless we specify otherwise. Patients with this form of HCM may suffer from one or more of the following: obstruction to left ventricular outflow, diastolic dysfunction, end-stage deterioration of left ventricular function both in systole and diastole, and atrial and ventricular arrhythmias.

In discussing diastolic dysfunction in HCM, it is important to appreciate a number of features in this condition:

1. The hypertrophy is usually asymmetric (nonuniform) (Figures 22–1 and 22–2, Table 22–1).

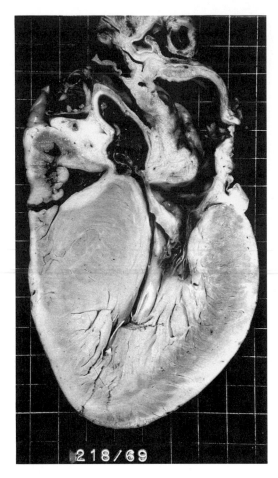

Fig. 22–1. Longitudinal section of the heart from a patient with obstructive HCM. Note the asymmetrical hypertrophy of the septum and to a lesser extent, the free wall of the left ventricle. The extent of myocardial fiber disarray was greatest at the base of the septum, but extended for the full length of the septum and into the free wall of the left ventricle. Reproduced with permission from Horlick, L.: Cardiovascular Pathology. New York, Churchill Livingston, 1983, p. 499.

Table 22–1. Types of Hypertrophic Cardiomyopathy

Type	Approximate Incidence (%)*	
Left ventricular involvement		
Asymmetrical hypertrophy:	95	
Ventricular septal hypertrophy		90
Midventricular hypertrophy		1
Apical hypertrophy		3
Posterior and/or lateral wall hypertrophy		1
Symmetrical (concentric) hypertrophy	5	
Right ventricular involvement		

* At the Toronto General Hospital, Toronto, Ontario, Canada. The incidence of the different types of hypertrophic cardiomyopathy varies considerably among centers.

2. The extent of hypertrophy is extremely variable. Some patients may have very localized hypertrophy and normal diastolic function, whereas others have very extensive hypertrophy and significant diastolic dysfunction (8). The extent of hypertrophy in the patient with HCM can be determined noninvasively by means of two-dimensional echocardiography or magnetic resonance imaging.

3. In HCM, areas of myocardial fiber disarray are interspersed with loose, intercellular connective tissue, myocardial fibrosis, or both (Fig. 22–3). In other areas, the myocardium may be normal. In the late stages of the disease, interstitial fibrosis may be extensive (Fig. 22–3B). The myocardial cells in areas of myocardial fiber disarray are short and plump and run in various directions (Fig. 22–3A). Thus the gross and microscopic pathologic findings in HCM reveal marked nonuniformity, which is now recognized to be an important determinant of active relaxation of the ventricle.

4. The obstruction to left ventricular outflow during systole may affect diastolic left ventricular filling in HCM (8). Surgical relief of the obstruction (and of the concomitant mitral regurgitation) may normalize left ventricular end-diastolic pressure, provided that the hypertrophy is not too extensive (13).

DETERMINANTS OF DIASTOLIC FILLING

The principal determinants of diastolic filling of the left ventricle are chamber stiffness (or its inverse, compliance), active relaxation of the ventricle, pericardial con-

ASYMMETRICAL HYPERTROPHY OF LEFT VENTRICLE

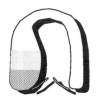 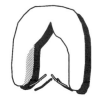

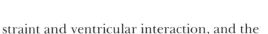

Septal Hypertrophy   **Apical Hypertrophy**   **Midventricular Hypertrophy**

Fig. 22–2. Diagrammatic representation of three common varieties of asymmetric hypertrophy in HCM, as they would be seen in the apical four-chamber view of a two-dimensional echocardiogram. Reproduced with permission from Wigle et al.: Hypertrophic Cardiomyopathy. The importance of the site and the extent of hypertrophy. A review. Prog Cardiovasc Dis 28:1, 1985.

straint and ventricular interaction, and the extent of hypertrophy.

The following is an attempt to examine the way in which diastolic filling of the left ventricle may be affected by these factors in HCM (8, 14). The effect of various pharmacologic agents will be discussed when this is important to the understanding of mechanisms.

Chamber Stiffness

The passive elastic properties of the left ventricular chamber are perhaps best envisaged by discussing chamber stiffness (dp/dv) rather than its inverse, chamber compliance (dv/dp). Chamber stiffness is directly related to the stiffness of the myocardium itself and to myocardial mass, and inversely proportional to left ventricular chamber volume (15) (see Chapter 9). Myocardial stiffness would be increased in HCM by the amount of intercellular connective tissue or fibrosis (see Chapter 8), and possibly by the presence of areas of myocardial fiber disarray. Myocardial mass would obviously be increased in HCM in direct relation to the extent of hypertrophy (Fig. 22–1). Left ventricular volume in HCM would be decreased by the extent of increase in myocardial mass. Thus, in HCM the increase in myocardial stiffness and mass and the decrease in ventricular volume all act to increase chamber stiffness (i.e., to decrease compliance) (Fig. 22–4). The relative importance of these three factors in determining chamber stiffness in any given case of HCM can vary consider-

ably, depending on the extent of hypertrophy, the degree of myocardial fibrosis and the volume of the left ventricle.

These passive elastic characteristics of the diastolic left ventricle in HCM are obviously of importance in determining the diastolic pressure-volume relationship. Although the significance in healthy persons of the viscous and inertial properties of the left ventricular wall is not known (16), it seems that these factors may come into play in diastole in HCM, considering the abnormal amounts of intercellular connective tissue and fibrosis, as well as the myocardial fiber disarray that occurs in these hearts (8, 14) (Fig. 22–3).

An increase in chamber stiffness results in the diastolic pressure volume curve being shifted upward and to the left, so that, for any increase in diastolic volume, the diastolic pressure rises to a greater extent than it would in the normal ventricle. When active relaxation of the ventricle is also impaired, as it is in HCM, the left ventricular diastolic pressure-volume relationship is shifted further to the left. Thus, the left ventricular diastolic pressure-volume relationship in HCM reflects not only the passive chamber stiffness, but also impairment of active relaxation of the ventricle (see Chapter 14).

Active Relaxation

Brutsaert and colleagues have recently defined three basic factors that affect diastolic relaxation: load, inactivation, and nonuniformity of load and inactivation in

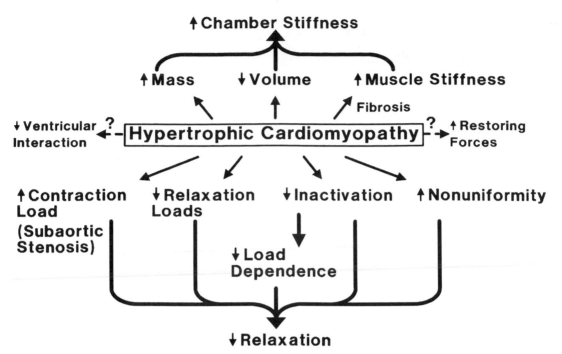

Fig. 22–4. In HCM, the increase in muscle mass and the concomitant decrease in ventricular volume, as well as the increase in muscle stiffness caused by myocardial fibrosis, all act to increase left ventricular chamber stiffness. The effect of the hypertrophic process on left ventricular relaxation is shown in the bottom half of the figure. The subaortic stenosis would act as a contraction load, to impair relaxation. The degree of hypertrophy as well as other factors would diminish the principle relaxation loads (coronary filling and ventricular filling loads) which would also impair relaxation. Diminished inactivation by primary or ischemic calcium overload would impair relaxation and would also diminish the load dependence of relaxation, thus having a doubly adverse effect. The nonuniformity of load and inactivation would also impair relaxation. Thus, the factors that are the principal determinants of relaxation (load, inactivation, nonuniformity) act to impair relaxation in HCM. It is also possible that, with extensive hypertrophy, increased restoring forces would be generated and pericardial constraint could become a factor (see text). Reproduced with permission from Wigle et al.: Hypertrophic Cardiomyopathy. The importance of the site and the extent of hypertrophy. A review. Prog Cardiovasc Dis 28:1, 1985.

the obstruction, occurs after 55% of systole, no obstruction or pressure gradient develops. Thus, there is no evidence at present that late systolic loading plays any significant role in the active relaxation of the left ventricle in HCM (8).

End-Systolic Deformation Load (Restoring Forces). External restoring forces are generated during contraction and stored as potential energy (interfascicular tension) in the connections between muscular and connective tissue (17). The magnitude of these restoring forces that could be released during the isovolumic relaxation period is related to the degree of systolic deformation. In HCM, these forces could be greater than normal by virtue of the small

end-systolic volume (greater systolic deformation) and the amount of connective tissue, myocardial fiber disarray, and hypertrophy in the ventricular wall. All of these factors could result in the generation of greater external restoring forces for release during early diastole (Fig. 22–5).

Internal restoring forces result from shortening of muscle fibers below slack length, and tend to elongate the muscle fibers back to slack length. These forces are not thought to be of any significance in the normal heart, but could conceivably be important in HCM, particularly in areas of myocardial fiber disarray (see Fig. 22–3). Thus, restoring forces, both internal and external, could be increased in HCM and

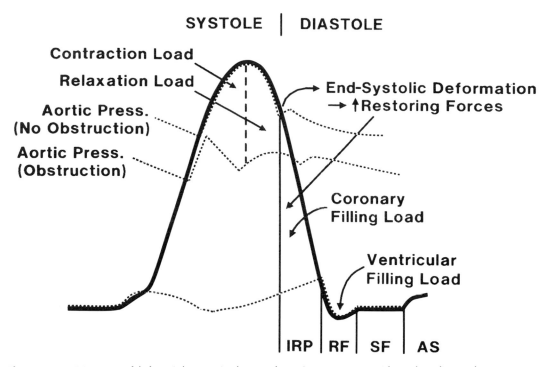

Fig. 22–5. Diagram of left atrial, ventricular, and aortic pressures (with and without obstruction to outflow), together with the various loads that may effect diastolic relaxation in HCM. A contraction load (the obstruction) applied in the first half of systole would delay the onset and slow the rate of relaxation. There is no evidence to suggest that a relaxation load in the last half of systole is of any significance in HCM. Exaggerated end-systolic deformation, caused by extensive hypertrophy, could generate increased restoring forces that would be released principally during isovolumic relaxation (IRP). The coronary filling load (during IRP) and the ventricular filling load (during rapid filling (RF)) are reduced in HCM as the result of the extent of hypertrophy and other factors (see text). SF = slow filling period. AS = atrial systolic filling. Reprinted with permission from Wigle et al.: Hypertrophic Cardiomyopathy. The importance of the site and the extent of hypertrophy. A review. Prog Cardiovasc Dis 28:1, 1985.

would act to improve relaxation. It is possible that these forces are responsible for the exaggerated changes in diameter and shape that are noted during isovolumic relaxation in HCM (18, 19). However, because relaxation is characteristically impaired in HCM, they are unlikely to be of great importance. In some cases of HCM, however, massive hypertrophy and marked end-systolic deformation occurs, yet left ventricular end-diastolic pressure is normal. Increased restoring forces could possibly be important in explaining this apparent paradox (8, 14).

Coronary Filling Load. The degree of filling of the coronary arterial tree during isovolumic relaxation represents a third load that may augment diastolic relaxation by applying an intramural load to the already relaxing muscle (10–12) (Fig. 22–5, Table 22–2). This "coronary kick" could be considerably blunted in HCM. Thus, coronary perfusion pressure would be variably reduced because of low aortic diastolic pressure and high left ventricular end-diastolic pressure. Intramyocardial blood flow could be reduced by small vessel disease, by the decreased capillary-fiber ratio of hypertrophy, by septal perforator artery compression, and by a decreased coronary vasodilator capacity (8, 20). The hypertrophy itself would lessen the impact of the coronary filling load. Decreased myocardial relaxation from any cause would also reduce coronary filling during the isovolumic relaxation period, particularly in areas of the myocardium in which systolic compression of the coronary arteries occur

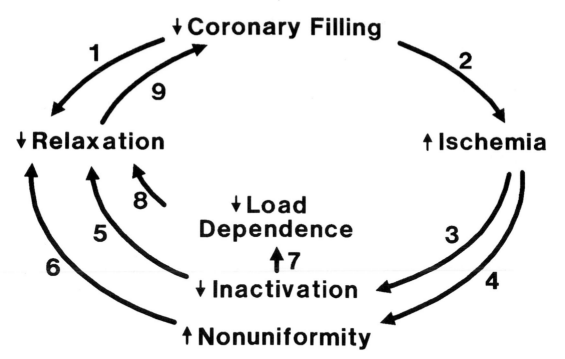

Fig. 22–6. Vicious cycle of the effect of decreased coronary filling and myocardial ischemia on left ventricular relaxation in HCM. Decreased coronary filling during the isovolumic relaxation period would impair relaxation by the decreased load (1), as well as by producing myocardial ischemia (2), which in turn would decrease inactivation (3) and increase nonuniformity (4), both of which would act to slow the rate of relaxation (5 and 6). Decreased inactivation would also decrease load dependency (7), which would further impair relaxation (8). Finally, impaired relaxation itself would reduce coronary filling (9) during the isovolumic relaxation period, and this would complete the vicious cycle by further reducing the coronary filling load (1), and producing more myocardial ischemia (2) (see text). Reproduced with permission from Wigle et al.: Hypertrophic Cardiomyopathy. The importance of the site and the extent of hypertrophy. A review. Prog Cardiovasc Dis 28:1, 1985.

(Fig. 22–6). Consideration of all these factors leads to the conclusion that the coronary filling load that is applied to the myocardium during isovolumic relaxation is reduced in HCM (8, 14).

Ventricular Filling Load. The fourth relaxation load on the left ventricle in diastole is caused by ventricular filling after mitral valve opening. The degree of ventricular filling is determined by the tension in the left ventricular wall, as indicated by the La Place relationship, $(T = Pxr/2h)$ (10–12) (Fig. 22–5, Table 22–2). Some authors prefer to think of this load as the left atrial-left ventricular pressure gradient in early diastole. In healthy subjects, although filling pressure (P) is low, the rapid decrease in wall thickness (h) and increase in left ventricular radius (r) result in an increased tension (T) or load on the left ventricular wall and ensure rapid diastolic filling. In HCM, however, wall thickness is increased, the rate of thinning of the wall is reduced (18, 19, 21), and the radius is reduced; all these factors would decrease the wall tension or load that normally aids relaxation. These effects would, to some extent, be counteracted by the elevated left atrial (filling) pressure, which would increase the load on the LV wall and promote relaxation. Appropriately, this elevation of filling pressure is greatest in patients with HCM, who have the greatest abnormalities of diastolic filling. This is particularly true in patients with obstructive HCM, because of the concomitant mitral regurgitation, that would elevate left atrial pressure, and particularly the "v" wave, thus further augmenting the filling pressure and the relaxation load on the left ventricle once the

Table 22–2. Measurable Indexes of Relaxation and Relaxation Loads According to Diastolic Period

Diastolic Period	Load	Indexes of Relaxation
Isovolumic relaxation	Restoring forces	Isovolumic relaxation time
	Coronary filling	Relaxation time index
		Time constant of isovolumic pressure decline
		Peak—dP/dt
		LV pressure waveform
Rapid filling	Ventricular filling	PFR
		Time to PFR
		Posterior wall thinning
		Minor diameter lengthening
		Rapid-filling volume
		Rapid-filling duration
		LV pressure waveform
Slow filling		Slow-filling duration
Atrial systole		Atrial systolic volume

LV = left ventricular; PFR = peak filling rate

mitral valve opens (8, 14). These elevated filling pressures would partially compensate for, but not overcome, the effects of increased wall thickness and diminished radius, which act to diminish the hemodynamic ventricular filling load, during rapid ventricular filling in HCM.

In summary, the contraction load in obstructive HCM and a reduction in the principle relaxation loads, (coronary and ventricular filling loads) are believed to be important considerations in explaining impaired relaxation in HCM. Increased restoring forces that would improve relaxation may be important in certain circumstances in HCM and would act to limit the impairment of relaxation caused by other factors. There is no evidence that the late systolic relaxation load plays an important role in HCM.

Inactivation

Inactivation is the second major factor affecting relaxation of the left ventricle; the term refers specifically to the deactivation of the force-generating sites, the actin-myosin crossbridges, in the myocardium (10–12) (see Chapters 1 and 2). This deactivation process is generally attributed to the reuptake of myoplasmic calcium by the sarcoplasmic reticulum, which is an energy-dependent process, and to the extrusion of calcium to the extracellular space through the sarcolemma. With unchanging loads on the left ventricle, the rate of inactivation of the contractile process is a principal determinant of the rate of myocardial relaxation (10–12). Factors known to retard inactivation, and hence relaxation, are ischemia, calcium overload, caffeine, and the absence of an active sarcoplasmic reticulum. All of these factors impair relaxation by elevating myoplasmic calcium concentration and slowing the rate of deactivation of the force-generating sites.

There is mounting evidence that there may be a primary calcium overload in HCM. This has been supported by the studies using the calcium-sensitive bioluminescent protein aequorin, in studying HCM tissue removed at the time of myectomy surgery or following transplantation (22, 23). In these studies, action potentials, calcium transients and isometric contraction and relaxation were markedly prolonged when compared to controls (23). These abnormalities were lessened by Verapamil, which would lower myoplasmic calcium, and were worsened by increasing the calcium concentration in the bath, or digitalis glycosides (which would also increase myoplasmic calcium). If there is a primary calcium overload in HCM, it might be related to increased trans-sarcolemmal calcium flux, as the result of altered calcium channel regulation (24, 25) although this has been challenged (26). It is to be noted that these abnormalities of myoplasmic calcium seen in HCM, may be a reflection of the hypertrophy process per se, rather than being specific for HCM (23).

Of interest is the fact that isoproterenol and forskolin also increased intracellular calcium, but improve rather than impair relaxation, possibly by stimulating cyclic AMP, which in turn would enhance calcium reuptake by the sarcoplasmic reticulum (23). Isoproterenol has also been demonstrated to improve relaxation in patients with HCM, in spite of increasing the contraction load (the subaortic obstruction) and producing myocardial ischemia, both of which should impair relaxation (27).

Myocardial ischemia may also impede reuptake of calcium by the sarcoplasmic reticulum, thereby retarding inactivation and relaxation. Metabolic studies have demonstrated evidence of myocardial ischemia in HCM, both at rest and during pacing, (20) suggesting that ischemia-induced delay in inactivation may be a contributing factor in the slow relaxation observed in these patients. The same factors that contribute to a diminished coronary filling load during isovolumic relaxation in HCM would contribute to ischemia, namely, decreased coronary perfusion pressure, small vessel disease, reduced capillary-myocardial fiber ratio, septal perforator artery compression, and diminished vasodilator reserve. Delayed relaxation during the isovolumic relaxation period would of itself impede coronary filling and promote myocardial ischemia, particularly in areas of septal perforator-artery compression. Thus, a vicious cycle is set up, in which diminished coronary filling and myocardial perfusion cause ischemia and impaired inactivation and relaxation, which in turn further impede coronary filling, leading to further ischemia and so on (8, 14) (Fig. 22–6).

Deactivation of the force-generating sites not only affects relaxation directly, but also determines how sensitive myocardial relaxation is to the prevailing relaxation load (10–12). A reduction in the inactivation process, leads to diminution of load dependency. Thus, diminished inactivation is doubly adverse with respect to relaxation, affecting it both directly and indirectly, through diminished load dependency. This twofold effect would have particularly severe consequences in patients with HCM, in whom the principle relaxation loads are already diminished (8–14) (Fig. 22–4). As indicated previously, pharmacologic agents that increase cyclic AMP such as isoproterenol or forskolin, as well as the phosphodiesterase inhibitors, amrinone and mirinone, improve relaxation by causing the phosphorylation of phospholamban, the regulatory protein for the sarcoplasmic reticulum calcium pump, thereby accelerating uptake of calcium during diastole (23). It has also been demonstrated in hypertrophied left ventricular myocardium from rats, subjected to experimental aortic stenosis, that there is a significant increase in the concentration of messenger RNA for angiotensin-converting enzyme and the corresponding increase in the conversion of circulating angiotensin I to angiotensin II (28). The latter substance appears to produce marked diastolic dysfunction in the hypertrophied left ventricle of rats, which can be blocked by pretreatment with an angiotensin converting enzyme inhibitor (28). The cellular mechanism of this type of diastolic dysfunction is currently unknown, but also may involve altered homeostasis of intracellular calcium.

At the present time, it is not known whether there are any abnormalities of cyclic AMP levels or angiotensin metabolism in the abnormal muscle seen in HCM. It is evident, however, that various metabolic abnormalities seen in hypertrophied myocardium may alter diastolic function and impair relaxation through their effects on intracellular calcium.

Non-Uniformity of Load and Inactivation

The third major factor affecting diastolic relaxation is the nonuniform temporal and regional distribution of load and inactivation (10–12). Physiologic nonuniformity is believed to be present in the normal human heart. Ample evidence suggests that pathologic nonuniformity is an important feature in cardiac hypertrophy, particularly in HCM. The essence of both the gross and microscopic pathology of HCM is asymmetry and nonuniformity (Figs. 22–1 through 22–3, Table 22–1). Evidence suggests that contraction and relaxation loading in HCM are nonuniform in distribution, and the same is undoubtedly true of the inactivation process. Thus, the inflow and apical regions of the left ventricle would be subjected to the contraction load caused by the obstruction to outflow, whereas the outflow tract myocardium would not. In cases with extensive septal hypertrophy and septal perforator artery compression, the coronary filling load would be particularly diminished in the septal region in comparison with other areas of the left ventricle. During rapid ventricular filling, wall tension would be nonuniform because of the variable site and extent of the hypertrophic process in the different types of HCM (Fig. 22–2). There is no absolute evidence with regard to the possibility of nonuniform inactivation, but it is known that myoplasmic calcium concentration is higher than normal in areas of myocardial fiber disarray. Similarly, ischemia-impaired inactivation would be expected to be nonuniform. Thus, there may be significant nonuniformity in the distribution of the various loads, and in the inactivation process in HCM (8, 14).

In addition, incoordinate or asynchronous systolic and diastolic wall motion abnormalities have been reported in HCM and have been associated with impaired global left ventricular relaxation (29). It has been reported that drug-induced (30) or disease-induced (31) regional wall motion asynchrony in humans and animals results in global left ventricular relaxation abnormalities that are virtually identical to those seen in HCM. Finally, studies by Bonow and colleagues have indicated that improvement in global left ventricular relaxation in HCM after administration of Verapamil is associated with a decrease in the asynchrony of contraction and relaxation (29). All of these observations suggest that regional nonuniformity of load and inactivation in space and time may play a major role in determining global left ventricular relaxation abnormalities in HCM.

In summary, there is evidence that abnormalities of left ventricular relaxation in HCM are due to a combination of altered load, impaired inactivation, and increased nonuniformity of load and inactivation in space and time. Thus, all three factors involved in the triple control of relaxation (10–12) are significantly altered in HCM.

Pericardial Constraint and Ventricular Interaction

Recently evolved concepts suggest that pericardial constraint may, in certain circumstances, have a significant effect on diastolic pressure-volume relationships of the left and right ventricles (see Chapter 6). If one assumes uniform pericardial pressure over both ventricles, the pericardial surface pressure has been found to equal right ventricular diastolic pressure or right atrial pressure (32, 33). Under such circumstances, the effective left ventricular filling pressure becomes the left ventricular transmural pressure, which is equal to left ventricular diastolic pressure, minus the pericardial pressure, the latter being equal to right ventricular diastolic pressure (32, 33).

In some circumstances, pericardial constraint may be of importance in HCM. First, right ventricular diastolic pressures may be considerably elevated in some cases, and the effective left ventricular filling pressure would then be considerably less than the measured left ventricular diastolic pressure. Second, the onset of atrial fibrillation in HCM is often accompanied by drastic elevations in ventricular diastolic and atrial pressures. Although there are ample reasons for this, the increased atrial size associated with atrial fibrillation may result in an increased degree of pericardial constraint and in an even greater rise in atrial and ventricular diastolic pressures. Third, the decrease in left ventricular end-diastolic pressure after successful ventriculomyectomy may be the result of abolition of the contraction load, with improvement in left ventricular relaxation; but a postoperative decrease in atrial size, as well as the fact that the pericardium is left partially open, could contribute to a decrease in left ventricular diastolic pressure through lessened pericardial constraint (8–14).

Changes in ventricular pressure can affect the pressure volume relationship in the opposite ventricle, through the phenomenon of ventricular interaction. We have suggested that, in HCM, with ventricular septal hypertrophy, the septum may be relatively immobile, and thus these hearts may be less susceptible to ventricular interaction (14).

Extent of Hypertrophy

Figure 22–4 illustrates how the extent of hypertrophy in HCM could affect chamber stiffness and myocardial relaxation, as well as possibly affecting the degree of pericardial constraint and the magnitude of restoring forces (8–14).

CLINICAL MEASURES OF IMPAIRED RELAXATION

Indices of left ventricular diastolic relaxation in HCM have been measured by means of many different techniques over the past decade or more. Table 22–2 lists these relaxation indices according to the diastolic period in which they are measured, and indicates the relaxation loads that apply during these different time intervals (see Chapter 13).

Numerous abnormalities have been described during the isovolumic relaxation period in HCM. This period, measured by echophonocardiography as the interval between aortic valve closure and mitral valve opening is prolonged (33, 34), as is the relaxation-time index, measured by angiography or echocardiography, as the time from minimal ventricular size to mitral valve opening (18, 19). It is important to note, however, that the isovolumic relaxation period may be abnormally short in HCM patients, with severe obstruction to left ventricular outflow (35). This phenomenon is believed to be caused by the prolonged ejection time, delaying aortic valve closure, and by the elevated left atrial pressure, causing early opening of the mitral valve (8, 14). The use of micromanometers to measure left ventricular pressure in HCM has indicated that peak negative dp/dt during isovolumic relaxation is decreased and the time constant of the isovolumic pressure decline is increased, both reflecting impaired relaxation (30, 36, 37). An interesting but unexplained phenomenon is the exaggerated increase in left ventricular diameter that occurs during the isovolumic relaxation period in HCM (34). We have speculated whether this might be caused by the release of augmented restoring forces at this time (8).

Another interesting phenomenon that is observed in the isovolumic relaxation period in patients with HCM are the different directions of intracavitary isovolumic flow. In normal subjects and in patients with ventricular septal hypertrophy, flow is from base to apex during the isovolumic relaxation period. However, in patients with apical HCM, isovolumic flow may occur in the apex to base direction, and this may be because of impaired relaxation of the hypertrophied apex (38).

Numerous other measurements have indicated impaired left ventricular relaxation during the rapid filling phase. Reduced rates of posterior wall thinning and minor diameter lengthening, measured by echocardiography and reflecting the rate of rapid filling, have been repeatedly observed (19, 21, 35) (see Chapter 19). A reduced peak filling rate and prolonged time to peak filling, measured by nuclear angiographic techniques, have also been observed (39) (see Chapter 11) (Fig. 22–7). Echocardiographic, nuclear angiographic, and Doppler measurements have indicated a reduced filling velocity and volume during the rapid filling phase, together with a compensatory increase in atrial systolic filling (39, 40) (Fig. 22–7). In interpreting these noninvasive studies measuring the velocity and volume of ventricular filling during the rapid and atrial filling periods, it is important to recognize their load dependence, and the fact that alterations in the ventricular filling load may dramatically affect these indices (41).

Nuclear angiographic techniques have also demonstrated a marked asynchrony of relaxation and filling, particularly during the rapid filling period, and this has been correlated with impaired global relaxation (29). Micromanometric measurements of left ventricular diastolic pressure wave form also reflects the dynamics of impaired relaxation in HCM (36, 37). Several studies have demonstrated a continual fall of left ventricular diastolic pressure during the period of rapid filling, an observation that could be explained only by slow and continued relaxation, well into the diastolic interval.

Many of the observations that reflect ab-

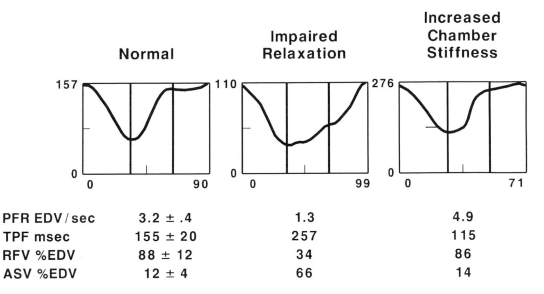

	Normal	Impaired Relaxation	Increased Chamber Stiffness
PFR EDV / sec	3.2 ± .4	1.3	4.9
TPF msec	155 ± 20	257	115
RFV %EDV	88 ± 12	34	86
ASV %EDV	12 ± 4	66	14

Fig. 22–7. Nuclear diastolic function (time/activity) curves in a healthy subject (left) and in two patients with HCM, one with impaired relaxation and the other with increased chamber stiffness. Impaired relaxation results in a reduced peak filling rate (PFR) and a prolonged time to peak filling (TPF), as well as reduced rapid filling volume (RFV) and, in compensation, an increased atrial systolic volume (ASV). Increased chamber stiffness results in an increased PFR, a shortened TPF, a normal or increased RFV, and a normal or decreased ASV. These diametrically opposite forms of ventricular filling account for the different clinical manifestation and response to atrial fibrillation in these two types of diastolic dysfunction (see text).

normal diastolic filling in HCM indicate that impaired left ventricular relaxation may affect not only the isovolumic relaxation and rapid filling phase, but may also profoundly affect diastasis and atrial systolic filling, periods of diastole that are usually thought to reflect the passive-elastic properties (stiffness) of the left ventricle. When relaxation is impaired, the rate and volume of rapid filling are reduced, the rapid filling phase itself is prolonged, diastasis is shortened or even abolished, and atrial systolic filling is increased in compensation for the reduced volume of rapid filling. Thus, relaxation may affect all phases of diastole. This fact may require a rethinking of what the passive-elastic properties of the left ventricle truly are (8, 14).

EFFECT OF CALCIUM ANTAGONISTS ON LEFT VENTRICULAR RELAXATION

The calcium antagonists verapamil, nifedipine, and diltiazem are capable of reversing many of the abnormal relaxation indices in HCM. Thus, during the isovo-lumic relaxation period, these agents decrease the time of isovolumic relaxation (34, 36) and the time constant of isovolumic pressure decline, while increasing peak negative dp/dt (36, 37). In addition, they reduce the abnormal width and shape changes that occur during this period (35). During the rapid filling phase, the rate and volume of filling are increased by calcium antagonists and the time to peak filling is decreased (34, 39), and this has been correlated with a decreased degree of asynchrony during the rapid filling phase (29). As a result of the increased rate and volume of ventricular filling during the rapid filling phase, this phase of diastole is shortened, diastasis is lengthened and there is an offsetting decrease in atrial systolic filling (39). The left ventricular diastolic pressure wave form is returned to a more normal configuration (36, 37).

Calcium antagonists could improve left ventricular relaxation in HCM by altering load, inactivation, or the uniformity of contraction and relaxation. By means of peripheral vasodilation and change in impedance, they could alter the balance between contraction and relaxation loading in systole. By the negative inotropic effect, they could reduce the contraction load in obstructive cases as well as the degree of end-systolic deformation, hence affecting the restoring forces. The coronary filling load during isovolumic relaxation could be increased by coronary vasodilation, which might also reduce ischemia and thereby improve inactivation and restore load dependency. These drugs could also reduce myoplasmic calcium concentration and improve inactivation by direct action on the myocardial cell. They have been shown to lessen the degree of asynchronous contraction and relaxation, an effect that is associated with improved indices of global relaxations (29). Altered loading conditions have not been thought to be the principal mode of action of calcium antagonists on left ventricular relaxation in HCM, in that at least one pure vasodilating agent did not affect relaxation (42). A direct myocardial effect in relieving ischemic or primary calcium overload, decreased asynchrony of contraction and relaxation, or both are the favored modes by which calcium antagonists have been thought to improve left ventricular relaxation in HCM (see Chapter 28).

A note of caution in the use of calcium antagonists in obstructive HCM is warranted. We believe that nifedipine is contraindicated in obstructive HCM because of the potential for its powerful vasodilating action to worsen the outflow tract obstruction. In obstructive HCM, verapamil is given for its negative inotropic action to lessen the outflow obstruction. However, at times the vasodilating action of this drug predominates and leads to unpredictable intensification of the outflow obstruction, and several patients have died as a result of this. It is our policy not to use calcium antagonists in obstructive HCM for the above reasons.

ATRIAL FIBRILLATION

The occurrence of atrial fibrillation in HCM appears to be related principally to left atrial size. We have noted left atrial enlargement to be six times more frequent in patients with obstructive HCM than in those with nonobstructive HCM (8). We believe this to be caused by the mitral regurgitation, which invariably accompanies the obstruction to left ventricular outflow (8). When left atrial enlargement occurs in nonobstructive HCM, it is caused by impaired relaxation, increased chamber stiffness, or a combination thereof.

In the presence of impaired relaxation, the onset of atrial fibrillation in HCM is often accompanied by drastic rises in ventricular diastolic and atrial pressures with resultant pulmonary edema. This sequence is seen in the presence of impaired relaxation because rapid atrial fibrillation does not allow sufficient time for relaxation to occur. In addition, atrial systolic filling, the most important compensatory mechanism for impaired relaxation, is absent. For these reasons, it is mandatory to attempt restoration of sinus rhythm in patients with HCM and impaired relaxation, by whatever medical or surgical means are necessary. We believe that the occurrence of atrial fibrillation in obstructive HCM is an indication for consideration of surgery because a successful ventriculomyectomy not only relieves the outflow tract obstruction, but also the concomitant mitral regurgitation (8, 9). This results in a reduction in left atrial size and restoration of sinus rhythm in patients under age 45. Older patients are better able to tolerate atrial fibrillation in the absence of obstruction to left ventricular outflow and the concomitant mitral regurgitation. In these patients, however, atrial size is infrequently reduced by surgery.

IMPAIRED RELAXATION VERSUS INCREASED CHAMBER STIFFNESS

Impairment of relaxation is characterized by a reduced rate of early diastolic rapid filling and by exaggerated atrial systolic filling (Fig. 22–7). The latter is often accompanied by a loud and palpable fourth heart sound, in keeping with this being a ventricular distention sound (9, 14) (see Chapter 26). It should be noted that the literature suggests that a fourth heart sound is caused by a stiff or noncompliant ventricle, but we suggest that a loud and palpable fourth heart sound is far more frequently an indication of impaired ventricular relaxation.

In contradistinction to the ventricular filling pattern seen with impaired relaxation is that encountered in the presence of a restrictive filling defect when there is increased chamber stiffness (Fig. 22–7). In the latter, the rate and volume of rapid filling are increased rather than decreased. The rapid filling phase is shortened rather than lengthened. Diastasis tends to be prolonged rather than shortened, and atrial systole makes a normal, or at times reduced, contribution to end-diastolic volume (14). Under these circumstances, a loud third heart sound is characteristic, and is in keeping with such a sound being a ventricular distention sound (9, 14). Thus, the type of diastolic filling defect caused by impaired relaxation is opposite to the filling defect caused by restriction or increased passive chamber stiffness (Fig. 22–7). Under these circumstances, the type of ventricular filling sound may therefore be diagnostically important. In our experience, a loud and palpable fourth heart sound is characteristically heard in the presence of impaired relaxation, as a result of exaggerated atrial systolic filling, whereas the third heart sound is characteristic of a restrictive filling defect, in which the rapid filling phase is exaggerated. These observations warrant a rethinking of the significance of third and fourth heart sounds in the presence of diastolic dysfunction. On the other hand, a loud third heart sound has often been seen in patients with stiff or noncompliant ventricles.

As previously indicated, the onset of atrial fibrillation in patients with impaired relaxation often results in dramatic rises in left atrial pressure and pulmonary edema, because the rapid rate of fibrillation does not permit time for ventricular relaxation and there is a loss of atrial systole, the most important compensatory mechanism for the impaired early diastolic filling. Quite the opposite is the case, however, when diastolic filling is restricted as a result of increased chamber stiffness. In these circumstances, the onset of atrial fibrillation often goes unrecognized by the patient, and we believe that this is the case because rapid filling is fast and short, and atrial systole

does not contribute significantly to the ventricular end-diastolic volume (14).

SUMMARY

HCM is characterized by obstruction to left ventricular outflow in systole, by abnormalities of diastolic filling, and by atrial and ventricular arrhythmias. Evidence now suggests that impairment of relaxation may be the most important cause of diastolic dysfunction in HCM although chamber stiffness is also increased. The calcium antagonist drugs offer the greatest hope for improvement of left ventricular relaxation in these patients.

Patients with impaired relaxation have a reduced volume of rapid filling with a compensatory increase in atrial systolic filling that is often accompanied by a loud and palpable atrial gallop sound. These patients tolerate atrial fibrillation poorly. In contradistinction, patients with increased chamber stiffness have exaggerated rapid filling, accompanied by a loud third heart sound and normal or subnormal atrial systolic filling and a better tolerance of atrial fibrillation. Both types of diastolic dysfunction may be present in HCM.

REFERENCES

1. Liouville H: Retrécissement cardiaque sous aortique. Gaz Med Paris 24:161, 1869.
2. Hallopeau L: Retrécissement ventriculo-aortique. Gaz Med Paris 24:683, 1869.
3. Schmincke A: Ueber linksseitige muskulose conusstenosen. Dtsch Med Wochenschr 33:2082, 1907.
4. Brock RC: Functional obstruction of the left ventricle. Guys Hosp Rep 106:221–238, 1957.
5. Teare RD: Asymmetrical hypertrophy of the heart in young adults. Br Heart J 20:1, 1958.
6. Braunwald E, Morrow AG, Cornell WP, et al.: Idiopathic hypertrophic subaortic stenosis. Am J Med 29:924, 1960.
7. Wigle ED, Heimbecker RO, Gunton RW: Idiopathic ventricular septal hypertrophy causing muscular subaortic stenosis. Circulation 26:325, 1962.
8. Wigle ED, Sasson Z, Henderson MA, et al.: Hypertrophic cardiomyopathy. The importance of the site and the extent of hypertrophy. A review. Prog Cardiovasc Dis 28:1, 1985.
9. Wigle ED: Hypertrophic cardiomyopathy:

A 1987 viewpoint (editorial). Circulation 75:311, 1987.

10. Brutsaert DL, Housmans PR, Goethais MA: Dual control of relaxation. Its role in the ventricular function in the mammalian heart. Circ Res 47:637, 1980.

11. Brutsaert DL, Rademakers FE, Sys SU: Triple control of relaxation: Implications in cardiac disease. Circulation 69:190, 1984.

12. Brutsaert DL, Sys SU: Relaxation and diastole of the heart. Physiol Rev 69:1228, 1989.

13. Wigle ED, Chrysohou A, Bigelow W: Results of ventriculomyotomy in muscular subaortic stenosis. Am J Cardiol 11:572, 1963.

14. Wigle ED, Wilansky S: Diastolic dysfunction in hypertrophic cardiomyopathy. Heart Failure 3:82, 1987.

15. Gaasch WH, Levine HJ, Quinones MA, et al.: Left ventricular compliance: Mechanisms and clinical implications. Am J Cardiol 38:645, 1976.

16. Grossman W, McLaurin LP: Diastolic properties of the left ventricle. Ann Intern Med 84:316, 1976.

17. Rushmer RF, Crystal DK, Wagner C: The functional anatomy of ventricular contraction. Circ Res 1:162, 1953.

18. Hanrath P, Mathey DG, Siegert R, et al.: Left ventricular relaxation and filling pattern in different forms of left ventricular hypertrophy. An echocardiographic study. Am J Cardiol 45:15, 1980.

19. Sanderson JE, Traill TA, St. John Sutton MG, et al.: Left ventricular relaxation and filling in hypertrophic cardiomyopathy. An echocardiographic study. Br Heart J 40:596, 1978.

20. Cannon RO, Rosing DR, Maron BJ et al.: Myocardial ischemia in hypertrophic cardiomyopathy: Contribution of inadequate vasodilator reserve and elevated left ventricular pressures. Circulation 71:234, 1985.

21. St. John Sutton MG, Tajik AJ, Gibson DG, et al.: Echocardiographic assessment of left ventricular filling and septal and posterior wall dynamics in idiopathic hypertrophic subaortic stenosis. Circulation 57:512–520, 1978.

22. Morgan MP, Morgan KG: Intracellular calcium levels during contraction and relaxation of mammalian cardiac vascular smooth muscle as detected with aequorin. Am J Med 77:33, 1984.

23. Gwathmey JK, Warren SE, Briggs GM, et al.: Diastolic dysfunction in hypertrophic cardiomyopathy. Effect on active force generation during systole. J Clin Invest 87:1023, 1991.

24. Wagner JA, Reynolds IJ, Weisman HF, Dudeck P, Weisfeldt ML, Snyder SH: Calcium antagonist receptors in cardiomyopathic hamsters. Selective increases in heart, muscle, brain. Science (Wash DC) 232:515, 1986.

25. Wagner JA, Sax FL, Weisman HF, et al.: Calcium-antagonist receptors in the atrial tissue of patients with hypertrophic cardiomyopathy. N Engl J Med 320:755, 1989.

26. O'Neil Sen. LM, Marsh JD, Smith TW: Inotropic and calcium kinetic effect of calcium channel agonist and antagonist in isolated cardiac myocytes from cardiomyopathic hamsters. Circ Res 67:599, 1990.

27. Udelson JE, Cannon III RO, Bacharach SL, et al.: B-adrenergic stimulation with isoproterenol enhances left ventricular diastolic performance in hypertrophic cardiomyopathy despite potentiation of myocardial ischemia. Comparison to rapid atrial pacing. Circulation 79:371, 1989.

28. Schunkert H, Dzau VJ, Tang SS, et al.: Increased rat cardiac angiotensin converting enzyme activity and mRNA expression in pressure overload left ventricular hypertrophy: effects on coronary resistance, contractility, and relaxation. J Clin Invest 86:1913, 1990.

29. Bonow RO, Vitale DF, Maron BJ, et al.: Regional left ventricular asynchrony and impaired global ventricular filling in hypertrophic cardiomyopathy: Effect of verapamil. J Am Coll Cardiol 9:1108, 1987.

30. Pagani M, Pizzinelli P, Gussoni M, et al.: Diastolic abnormalities of hypertrophic cardiomyopathy reproduced by asynchrony of the left ventricle in conscious dogs (abstract). J Am Coll Cardiol 1:641, 1983.

31. Ludbrook PA, Byrne JD: Influence of asynchronous early diastolic left ventricular relaxation on diastolic function (abstract). Am J Cardiol 45:392, 1980.

32. Smiseth DA, Refsum H, Tyberg JV: Pericardial pressure assessed by right atrial pressure: A basis for calculation of left ventricular transmural pressure. Am Heart J 108:603, 1984.

33. Tyberg JV: Ventricular interaction and the pericardium: In The Ventricle. Edited by Levine HJ, Gaasch WH. Boston, Martinus-Nijhoff, 1985, pp. 171–184.

34. Hanrath P, Mathey DG, Kremer P, et al.: Effect of verapamil on left ventricular isovolumic relaxation time and regional left ventricular filling in hypertrophic cardiomyopathy. Am J Cardiol 45:1258, 1980.

35. Alvares RF, Shaver JA, Gamble WH, et al.: Isovolumic relaxation period in hypertrophic cardiomyopathy. J Am Coll Cardiol 3:71, 1984.

36. Lorell BH, Paulus WJ, Grossman W: Modification of abnormal left ventricular diastolic properties by nifedipine in patients with hypertrophic cardiomyopathy. Circulation 65:499, 1982.

37. Bonow RD, Ostrow HG, Rosing DR, et al.: Effects of verapamil on left ventricular systolic and diastolic function in patients with hypertrophic cardiomyopathy: Pressure-volume analysis with nonimaging scintillation probe. Circulation 68:1062, 1983.

38. Sasson Z, Hatle L, Rakowski H, et al.: Patterns of LV isovolumic relaxation an diastolic filling in apical hypertrophy. Circulation 76:IV-249, 1987 (Abstract).

39. Bonow RO, Frederick RM, Bacharach SL, et al.: Atrial systole and left ventricular filling in hypertrophic cardiomyopathy. Effect of verapamil. Am J Cardiol 51:1386, 1983.

40. Maron BH, Spirito P, Green KJ, et al.: Noninvasive assessment of left ventricular diastolic function by pulsed Doppler echocardiography in patients with hypertrophic cardiomyopathy. J Am Coll Cardiol 10:733, 1987.

41. Appleton C, Hatle LK, Popp RL: Relation of transmitral flow velocity patterns to left ventricular diastolic function: New insights from a combined hemodynamic and Doppler echocardiographic study. JACC 12:426, 1988.

42. Paulus WJ, Lorell BH, Craig WE, et al.: Comparison of the effects of nitroprusside and nifedipine on diastolic properties in patients with hypertrophic cardiomyopathy: Altered left ventricular loading or impaired muscle inactivation? J Am Coll Cardiol 2:879, 1983.

Chapter 23

DIASTOLIC DYSFUNCTION IN RESTRICTIVE AND CONSTRICTIVE HEART DISEASE

Liv Hatle

Limitation to filling of the heart is the main feature of both restrictive and constrictive heart disease, resulting in similar symptoms and often similar clinical and hemodynamic findings. Restriction may result from myocardial and/or endocardial lesions, including infiltrative disorders (1). Constriction is most often caused by chronic constrictive pericarditis, but can also occur in acute or subacute pericarditis. The limitation to filling results in elevated venous pressures and, when pronounced, signs of pulmonary congestion as well as hepatomegalia, edema and ascites. The severity of symptoms and elevation of pressure is mainly a result of the severity of constriction or decrease in myocardial compliance, but depends also on the actual ventricular chamber sizes.

RESTRICTIVE HEART DISEASE

Etiology

Restrictive heart disease is a common term for nondilated ventricles with reduced distensibility resulting in abnormal pressure increase with filling. The diagnosis of *restrictive cardiomyopathy* is used when no specific cause is found, myocardial biopsies usually showing increase in fibrosis as well as hypertrophy (1–4). Familial cases have been described (3, 5), as well as an intermediate form with predominant restrictive features but also some dilation (6). *Restrictive physiology* can be seen in end-stage hypertrophic cardiomyopathy with extensive fibrosis, sometimes without an increase in myocardial mass (7). Restrictive physiology can also be seen following radiation and in cardiac transplants, with myocardial biopsies showing increase in fibrosis (8, 9), and it may result from other myocar-

dial lesions, including infiltrative and storage diseases as amyloid, sarcoid, Fabry's disease, and glycogen storage diseases (10, 11). Restrictive physiology caused by endocardial changes include endomyocardial fibrosis and hypereosinophilic syndrome (12–16) as well as carcinoid.

Pathophysiology

When ventricular distensibility is reduced, ventricular filling results in abnormal increases in diastolic pressures. This is followed by an increase in atrial pressures and often marked dilation of the atria that are initially less affected by the disease process. Elevated atrial pressures lead to dilation also of the central veins, and to pulmonary congestion, hepatic enlargement, edema and ascites. With marked atrial enlargement, annulus dysfunction may occur and cause significant tricuspid and/or mitral regurgitation. Although the main problem is a decrease in ventricular compliance (1, 17, 18), a reduced rate of relaxation or ventricular pressure fall can also be present (19). This is likely to occur in the presence of amyloid, ventricular hypertrophy or systolic dysfunction (20–22), but a reduced rate of relaxation has also been shown in the absence of such disease (19). The resulting filling pattern depends on the balance between the abnormal relaxation and the decrease in compliance, and on the level of atrial pressure (23, 24) (see Chapters 12 and 13).

Systolic function may be normal or near normal, but may also become markedly reduced in some of the conditions showing restrictive physiology. In the presence of systolic dysfunction, a more marked abnormal relaxation may modify the filling pattern, especially at an early stage with less elevated diastolic pressures.

Clinical Features

A reduced exercise tolerance with dyspnea is followed by elevated central venous pressures and signs of both left and right heart failure. With significant biatrial enlargement, atrial fibrillation is common, and emboli from atrial or ventricular thrombi may occur. In restrictive cardiomyopathy the condition may be stable or show only a slow progression (3, 4), whereas some of the other lesions showing restrictive physiology as amyloid may deteriorate more rapidly (25).

The ECG may show left ventricular hypertrophy or nonspecific ST-T changes. Bundle branch block may be present (Fabry's disease); atrial fibrillation is a frequent finding; in amyloid heart disease, low voltage is usually present. On x-ray, heart size may vary from normal to markedly enlarged, usually because of marked biatrial enlargement.

Hemodynamics

The decrease in compliance results in an abnormal pressure/volume curve with a steep rise in ventricular pressures during filling. With marked restriction, a rapid rise in pressure results in a dip and plateau pattern similar to that in constrictive pericarditis, and although diastolic pressure in the left ventricle is often higher than in the right, equal diastolic pressures in both ventricles can be seen. At an early stage, the abnormal pressure increase may occur only in late diastole, and a fluid challenge may then result in abnormal pressure rise earlier in diastole. A reduced rate of left ventricular pressure fall can be present (18).

Ventricular Filling

A marked pressure rise in early diastole results in mainly early diastolic filling. In lesions with a reduced rate of LV pressure fall, and in which LV diastolic pressures are not yet markedly increased, normal or even more late diastolic filling may be seen as in the early stage of amyloid disease (21). Various techniques have been used to assess left ventricular filling, especially

attempting to differentiate between restrictive cardiomyopathy and constrictive pericarditis, including angiography, radionuclear techniques, digitized echocardiograms, or Doppler echocardiography (8, 24, 26–29).

In atrial pressure curves as well as in the jugular veins a more prominent Y- than X-descent is usually seen, even in sinus rhythm, and indicates mostly early diastolic filling. The inspiratory increase in filling of the right heart may result in abnormal increases in atrial as well as ventricular diastolic pressures, indicating restriction to filling (8).

Echocardiography/Doppler

Echocardiography usually shows normal-sized ventricles with normal wall thickness and normal systolic shortening. In diastole, a flat posterior wall motion is characteristic of early cessation of filling. Biatrial enlargement is regularly present and ventricular or atrial thrombi may be seen. The latter are most likely to be visualized by transesophageal echocardiography. In endomyocardial fibrosis, increased endocardial echoes may be present, as well as obliteration of the apical areas of one or both ventricles (14, 15). Dilation of pulmonary, caval, and hepatic veins also indicates elevated atrial pressures, and a decreased inspiratory reduction in the diameter of the inferior vena cava has been shown to correlate with increased right atrial pressures (30).

Atrioventricular Flow Velocities

With pulsed Doppler recording of the flow velocities across the atrioventricular (A-V) valves, the relation between early and late diastolic filling can be clearly shown (Fig. 23–1). In normal young subjects, most of the filling occurs in early diastole. In the elderly, the rate of relaxation may be slower (20, 29); this results in a longer isovolumic relaxation time, a longer duration of early diastolic filling with a longer deceleration time and more filling with atrial contraction as seen in Figure 23–1B. When reduction in ventricular compliance results in a marked rise in early diastolic pressure, this leads to abbreviation of early diastolic filling and a shortening of

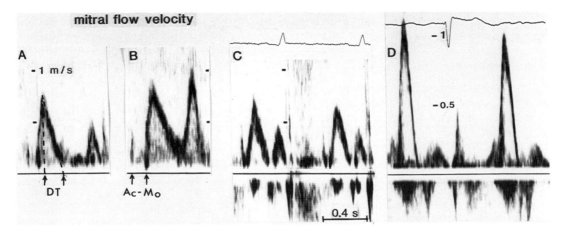

Fig. 23–1.   The mitral flow velocity in *A* and *B* is recorded from normal subjects and shows mainly early diastolic filling in A (age 18 years). In *B* (age 65 years), the isovolumic relaxation time (Ac-Mo) and the deceleration time (DT) are both longer than in *A* (120 vs 65 ms and DT 240 vs 155 ms), and there is more filling with atrial contraction. *C* and *D* are recorded from patients with restriction and both isovolumic relaxation time and deceleration times are shortened (DT 120 msec in C and 80 msec in D). In addition, there is mid-diastolic flow reversal, and in C, filling at atrial contraction is abbreviated.

the deceleration time (Figure 23–1C and D). The degree of shortening correlates with the size of the rapid filling wave in the ventricles (24), but clinically this has to be related to the patient's age and to other factors that may have the opposite effect on early diastolic filling, for example ventricular hypertrophy. Peak velocity may be normal or even increased, and the isovolumic relaxation time normal or shortened because of elevated left atrial pressure. When ventricular diastolic pressure prior to atrial contraction is high, forward flow at atrial contraction may be reduced, even if atrial function is still good (31, 32). Both the velocity and the duration of forward flow at atrial contraction is reduced and diastolic flow reversals may be present during or even before atrial contraction (Fig. 23–1C and Fig. 23–2) as ventricular diastolic pressure may exceed atrial pressure (32) (see Chapters 5, 10, and 12).

Table 23–1 shows mitral flow velocities in normal children and adults and in patients with restrictive cardiomyopathy and constrictive pericarditis. The deceleration time (DT) and the duration of filling in early diastole and at atrial contraction were shortened in both restriction and constriction.

With only a moderate decrease in compliance and an abnormal pressure increase

during atrial contraction, the forward flow velocities across the A-V valves can appear normal, except for abbreviation of forward flow at atrial contraction. The abnormal pressure increase may, however, result in increased flow reversal in pulmonary and systemic veins (32).

In the right heart, the inspiratory increase in filling serves as a volume test. In the presence of restriction, an inspiratory increase in filling results in shortening of the deceleration time and increase in flow reversals (Fig. 23–2), corresponding to an inspiratory increase in the A- and/or V-waves in the right atrial pressure curve. Pulmonary regurgitation is often present, and a marked dip in the velocity of the regurgitation can indicate an abnormal increase in right ventricular pressure in early diastole or at atrial contraction.

Venous Flow Velocities.

Recording of central venous flow velocities may show mainly diastolic filling and with shortened duration, corresponding to prominent Y-descents in atrial pressures. This is often followed by increased flow reversals, even before atrial contraction as indicated in Figure 23–2C (8, 33, 34). Systolic filling may be well seen in early stages, but is most often reduced, even in the presence

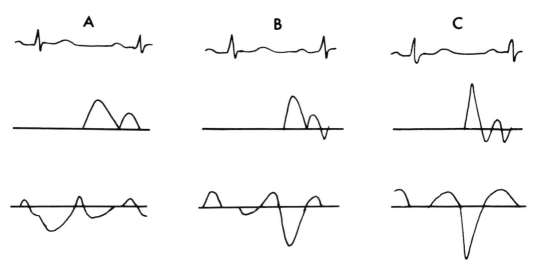

Fig. 23–2. The schematic shows ECG, tricuspid and hepatic venous flow velocities in a normal subject (A) and the patterns observed in moderate (B) and severe (C) restriction to filling. In the presence of restriction, the deceleration time of early tricuspid flow shortens and the velocity and duration of filling at atrial contraction are reduced. In the hepatic veins, forward flow is recorded away from the transducer and seen below the zero line. In the presence of restriction, systolic filling is reduced. The deceleration time of diastolic filling shortens and is followed by more pronounced flow reversals, which can be seen also before or in the absence of atrial contractions. The change from B and C can be seen with progression, but also following volume loading or the inspiratory increase in right heart filling.

of sinus rhythm, corresponding to a reduced or absent X-descent in the pressure curves. This may be caused by several factors, including reduced atrial and ventricular systolic function as well as significant A-V valve regurgitation and a reduced atrial compliance. Marked end-systolic flow reversals can indicate abnormal V-waves.

With inspiration, an increase in forward flow velocity in the hepatic and superior caval veins can be clearly seen; in the presence of restriction this is usually followed by an increase in flow reversals *during* inspiration. This increase in flow reversal occurs on a beat-to-beat basis and may therefore be well seen even without a simultaneous recording of respiration as indicated in Figure 23–3. With a slower heart rate and/or a more rapid respiration, however, a respiratory trace may be necessary to distinguish between an inspiratory increase in flow reversals caused by restriction, and the normal expiratory increase in flow reversal.

A-V Valve Regurgitation

The presence of severe mitral or tricuspid regurgitation may cause higher for-

Table 23–1.   Left Ventricular Filling

	Normal Subjects		Constriction	Restriction
Number	26	36	12	20
Age (years)	13 ± 6	45 ± 18	41 ± 18	44 ± 17
E Velocity (cm/s)	91 ± 10	86 ± 11	63 ± 18	85 ± 29
A Velocity (cm/s)	49 ± 11	62 ± 15	41 ± 10	44 ± 17
Dec Time (ms)	144 ± 20	178 ± 21	93 ± 21	120 ± 38
E Filling (ms)	202 ± 33	249 ± 23	137 ± 44	156 ± 44
A duration (ms)	109 ± 11	143 ± 14	101 ± 23	89 ± 15

E = early diastolic, A = atrial contraction, Dec = deceleration, ms = milliseconds

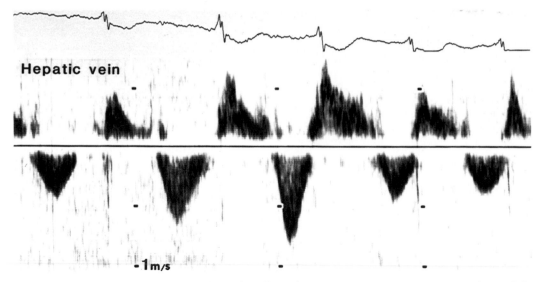

Fig. 23–3. In this hepatic vein recording, the effect of inspiration is seen as increase in forward flow velocity (below the zero line) in the second and third diastole. The increase in flow reversal in the second beat indicates inspiratory increase in right atrial pressure and restriction to filling, the increased reversal in the third beat could also be caused by onset of expiration.

ward flow velocity across that A-V valve, but in the presence of restriction, the deceleration times will still be shortened; in addition there will be diastolic flow reversals both across the A-V valve and in the central veins. This is in contrast to the normal deceleration time in severe regurgitation with dilated ventricles, in which a "functional" restriction may be indicated from the pressure curves.

In restriction, the presence of significant tricuspid and/or mitral regurgitation may result in more pronounced holosystolic flow reversal in the central veins because of reduced atrial compliance, but inspiratory increase in reversals may still be seen.

When the regurgitations are recorded with continuous wave Doppler, the negative dp/dt can be estimated (35), indicating whether abnormal ventricular pressure fall is present. With marked elevation of atrial pressures, however, this is likely to be less apparent.

Treatment

Except for the surgical treatment of endomyocardial fibrosis, and transplantation in end-stage disease, treatment is symptomatic, including diuretics and anticoagulation for the prevention of thromboembo-

lism. Calcium channel blockers may be deleterious in some patients, especially in advanced stages. Rapid heart rates are not well tolerated because of the short filling period. Extremely slow rates are not tolerated because of the limited stroke volume and its impact on cardiac output.

CONSTRICTIVE PERICARDITIS

Etiology

Chronic constrictive pericarditis may result from viral or bacterial infections, including tuberculosis. It is also seen in connective tissue diseases or after radiation or cardiac surgery; however, in a significant number no specific etiology is detected (36, 37). Subacute effusive/constrictive pericarditis has been described as an intermediate form between acute and chronic constrictive pericarditis, with both some effusion as well as a thickened pericardium, limiting filling and progressing to chronic constriction in some (38). Constriction that develops during acute pericarditis can be reversible (39, 40).

Pathophysiology

The normal pericardium has been shown to influence filling, with a steeper pressure/volume curve than when the pericardium is removed (41). It is also shown to enhance the interaction between the two ventricles (see Chapter 6). With a thickened and less elastic or a rigid pericardium a steeper pressure/volume curve is seen and with increased ventricular interaction (42, 43). Constriction most often limits filling of the whole heart, occasionally some areas are less affected, resulting in differences between the chambers.

The limitation to filling results in elevated diastolic pressures, increased venous pressures, dilated central veins, and signs and symptoms of congestive heart failure with hepatic enlargement, ascites, and edema. The more prominent signs of right-sided congestion compared to the rare occurrence of pulmonary edema may be related to a relatively low atrial naturetic factor (ANF) in the pulmonary circulation that might be a result of less stretch of the right than the left atrium (44).

Systolic function is often normal, and with the combination of normal ventricular relaxation and elevated left atrial pressure, there is rapid filling in early diastole; early cessation of filling occurs because the limit for the rigid pericardium is reached (43, 45–46). With significant constriction, the diastolic pressures often show a dip and plateau pattern, and because of increased ventricular interaction, diastolic pressures are nearly equal in both atria and ventricles as well as in the pulmonary artery.

The intracardiac diastolic and right atrial pressures show less respiratory variation than normal, possibly because of limited transmission of intrathoracic pressures (43, 47). The intrathoracic pressure changes therefore result in a lower pressure gradient from the pulmonary veins to the left heart during inspiration, and a higher gradient as the intrathoracic pressure increases on expiration. This results in increased respiratory variation of left heart filling, and because the total filling volume is fixed, right heart filling has to change in the opposite direction (48). This can be seen as respiratory shifts in the position of the ventricular and atrial septa (Fig. 23–4) (49).

The inspiratory increase in right heart filling can be seen as increase in forward flow velocity in hepatic and inferior caval veins, but often less apparent in the superior caval vein. This difference may be caused by the increase in intra-abdominal pressure on inspiration, favoring filling from the inferior caval vein, and may also help to explain the lack of decrease, or even

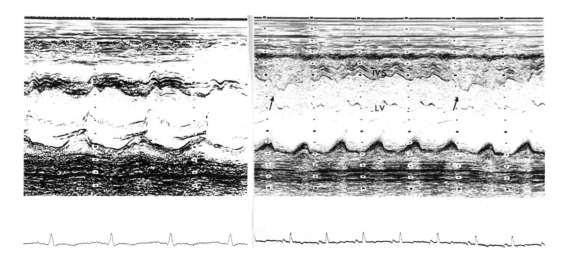

Fig. 23–4. M-mode recordings in both A and B are from patients with constrictive pericarditis. The recording in A shows thickened pericardium and a nondilated left ventricle with good systolic function. The ventricular septum shows an early diastolic notch. In B, a marked respiratory change in left ventricular (LV) diameter can be seen. Arrow points to inspiratory decrease in LV diameter (from 63 to 53 mm). IVS = intraventricular septum.

increase, in jugular venous pressure on inspiration (Kussmaul's sign).

The *degree* of respiratory variation in filling depends on the change in intrathoracic pressure, increasing with increased depth of respiration. The respiratory changes also become more prominent with increasing degree of constriction, but conversely, when filling becomes very limited, the changes may become less evident. This may result from high atrial pressure with the mitral valve opening at a time of rapid LV pressure decay; respiratory changes will then have less impact on the initial pressure gradient and peak flow velocity. Also, the more severe the constriction, the earlier the cessation of filling, and with a very short filling time, variations in this become less obvious. The degree of change may also depend on the degree of septal shift.

The degree of respiratory change in left heart filling also influences the degree of paradoxical pulse. Again, this varies with the depth of respiration, and this may explain the higher frequency of pulsus paradoxus in patients with subacute effusive/constrictive pericarditis even when there is little or no effusion present. These patients often present with more severe clinical symptoms, including more dyspnea (38). Differences between subacute and chronic constriction have been ascribed to the former being more elastic compared to a rigid shell with less transmission of intrathoracic pressure to the heart in the latter (38). A difference in the degree of septal shift in the two forms may also play a role.

The limitation to filling depends not only on the severity of the constriction, but also on ventricular size. The smaller the ventricle, the lower the possibility of an increase in stroke volume and increase in filling in the following diastole, and increase in cardiac output may only be achieved by increasing the heart rate.

Diagnosis

Signs of increased venous pressures with hepatic enlargement, ascites, and edema, in the presence of a small heart, are suggestive findings, but both clinical and hemodynamic findings may be similar to those in restrictive cardiomyopathy. The presence of a calcified pericardium on chest x ray is useful in the differential diagnosis. Pericardial thickening can be shown by echocardiography and its degree and distribution well shown by magnetic resonance imaging (MRI) and by computed tomography (CT) (50–52), but thickening or even calcified pericardium does not prove that constriction is present. Conversely, constriction may be present even if pericardial thickening cannot be shown.

At catheterization, elevated diastolic pressures with a dip and plateau pattern and pressure equalization between the chambers have been considered diagnostic. In the absence of a clear diagnosis, a fluid challenge have been suggested to confirm the presence of suspected constriction (53), but a dip-and-plateau pattern can be seen during volume loading in the absence of constriction (54, 55). Myocardial biopsy has been suggested to aid in the differentiation between constrictive pericarditis and restrictive cardiomyopathy and to avoid explorative thoracotomy (56). Atrial enlargement can be present in constrictive pericarditis (49), but is usually more marked in restriction (48), and a relative biatrial enlargement and increase in left ventricular mass have been reported to differentiate patients with restriction from those with constriction (57).

Other echocardiographic findings suggestive of constriction are the presence of an early diastolic notch on the ventricular septum (Fig. 23–4) as well as at atrial contraction (58, 59), but these have been shown to be present also in other conditions (60). A flat posterior wall (61) is seen also in restrictive cardiomyopathy, but in the latter a reduced rate of posterior wall thinning may also be present (28). It has been concluded that no single finding is diagnostic (62), but the combination of septal motion, dilated central veins, and pericardial adhesions has been reported to be helpful (63). With two-dimensional echocardiography, an increased respiratory change in the diameter of the left ventricle has been noted (49), exceeding the small inspiratory decrease seen in normal subjects (64). In Figure 23–4, recorded in a patient with constrictive pericarditis, a marked inspiratory decrease in left ventricular diameter is seen, indicating a marked decrease in left ventricular filling.

Ventricular Filling

Predominant early diastolic filling has been shown by various methods, including angiography, radionuclear methods, digitized echocardiography, and Doppler (19, 26–28, 33, 48, 65). Although this has been suggested to differentiate constriction from restriction, advanced restriction may show similar findings (8, 33, 48, 66). A slower early diastolic filling in some patients with restriction (19, 26, 28) may be caused by the presence of abnormal relaxation in addition to a decrease in passive compliance.

Doppler Echocardiography

Ventricular Filling

The recording of *mitral* flow velocity in Figure 23–5 shows the shortened duration of early diastolic filling in a patient with constrictive pericarditis as well as reduced filling at atrial contraction. These features, however, are seen also in restriction (Table 23–1). But Figure 23–5 also shows a marked change in the flow velocities with respiration, with a decrease in both peak velocity and in deceleration time on inspiration, and changes in the opposite direction on expiration. This corresponds to the increased respiratory variation in LV diameter described earlier (49) and seen in Figure 23–4. The *tricuspid* flow velocity on expiration shows a marked decrease in velocity, shortening of the deceleration time, and reduced filling at atrial contraction, indicating reciprocal filling of the two ventricles and a limitation of the total filling of the heart. The presence of both these respiratory changes and shortened deceleration times have been reported (48, 67) and with normalization after surgery as seen in Figure 23–6. Although these respiratory changes are suggestive of constriction, the degree may vary with the depth of respiration. They can be equally pronounced in subacute as in chronic constriction, but may become less obvious in severe chronic constriction. The shortening of the deceleration time is the best indicator of the severity.

The inspiratory decrease in left heart filling can also be seen in *pulmonary venous* recordings. Figure 23–7 is recorded from a

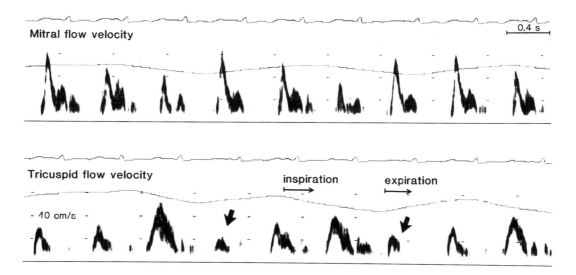

Fig. 23–5. The mitral and tricuspid flow velocity in a patient with constrictive pericarditis recorded together with respiration. Downward deflection is inspiration and upward is expiration. The mitral flow velocity shows a marked shortening of the deceleration time and, with inspiration, a decrease in velocity and further shortening of the deceleration time is seen (DT 110-70 msec). The tricuspid flow velocity changes in the opposite direction. These changes are much larger than normal. The deceleration time is markedly shortened, except during inspiration (DT 70-140 msec). The marked decrease in velocity on expiration (fourth and seventh diastole) indicates the reciprocal filling of the two ventricles caused by the limitation of total filling.

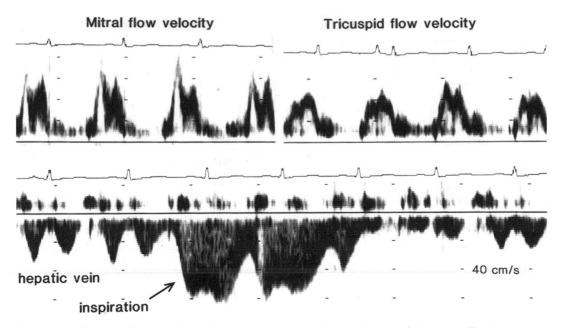

Fig. 23–6.   The recordings are from the same patient as in Figures 23–5 and 23–10. Following surgery for constriction, the velocity curves are normal. Both mitral and tricuspid flow velocities show normal deceleration times, the marked respiratory variation is no longer present, and there is more filling with atrial contraction. The hepatic vein now shows diastolic filling also on expiration and an increase in forward flow velocity throughout inspiration, indicating that the limitation to filling is no longer present. The expiratory flow reversals are also less pronounced compared to that seen in Figure 23–10.

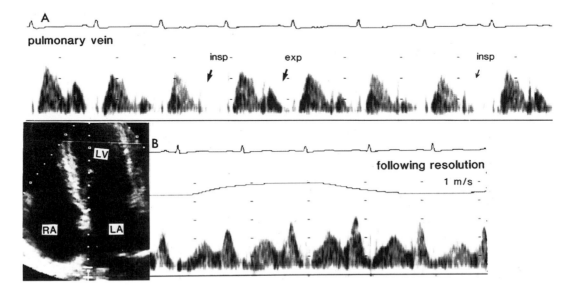

Fig. 23–7.   In *A,* the pulmonary vein recording from a patient with constriction shows both systolic and diastolic forward flow, but with marked decrease in diastolic flow on inspiration and increase on expiration. In *B,* recorded 2 months after surgery for constriction, the more prominent diastolic filling is seen, and now with only normal respiratory variation. RA = right atrium, LA = left atrium, LV = left ventricle.

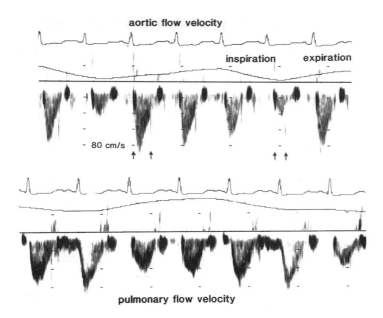

aortic flow velocity

inspiration   expiration

- 80 cm/s

pulmonary flow velocity

Fig. 23–8. The aortic flow velocity recorded from the same patient as in Figure 23–5 shows marked decrease on inspiration and increase on expiration. Small arrows point to valve opening and closure. The marked change also in the left ventricular ejection time (LVET 120-190 ms) indicates that the velocity change is caused by change in the stroke volume and not an artefact caused by change in sample volume position with respiration. The increase in pulmonary flow velocity with inspiration is normal, but the decrease seen early in expiration indicates reciprocal filling of the two ventricles.

patient with constriction and shows abnormal decrease in diastolic filling on inspiration and increase on expiration, following surgery improved diastolic filling is seen. Similar respiratory changes have also been recorded by transesophageal echocardiography, and differed from those recorded in restriction (34).

The respiratory changes in left heart filling result in marked changes also in *aortic flow velocity* as seen in Figure 23–8. The decrease in filling is followed by a decrease in stroke volume with decrease in velocity and shortening of the ejection time. The associated change in the ejection time helps to confirm that the velocity changes are caused by change in stroke volume, and not artefactual because of change in sample volume position with respiration. The respiratory changes seen in Figure 23–8 clearly exceed those seen in normal subjects or in other heart lesions except in cardiac tamponade (68). These changes correspond to the degree of pulsus alternans. The inspiratory increase in pulmonary flow velocity is also larger than usual, but it is the abnormal decrease early in expiration that indicates the limitation to filling.

Systemic Veins

The venous flow velocities usually correspond to the changes in right atrial pres-

sure with systolic and diastolic filling comparable to the X and Y descent in the pressure curves (Fig. 23–9). The flow velocity curves from the hepatic vein have been described as W-shaped with similar systolic and diastolic velocities, and both with shortened duration of forward flow reversals (69). In the majority of patients with constriction, the X-descent is reported to exceed the Y-descent (43, 45, 46), and the flow velocities recorded in the hepatic or superior caval vein in systole are often higher or similar to diastolic velocities as seen in Figure 23–10. However, in some patients diastolic velocities are higher (70), even in those with sinus rhythm as seen in Figure 23–9, but systolic filling seems to be present more often than in patients with restriction (33, 66, 71, 72). The systolic filling may be reduced because of atrial fibrillation or to impaired ventricular or atrial function (73).

The respiratory change differs from that seen in restriction. With inspiration, there is some increase in forward flow velocity in the hepatic vein, and the flow reversals may decrease or disappear, whereas expiration results in marked flow reversals and little or no diastolic filling as seen in Figure 23–10. Some increase in flow reversals on expiration is normal, but it is here more pronounced, and it is combined with short-

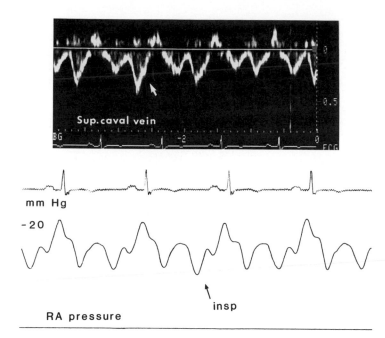

Fig. 23–9. The velocity recording from the superior caval vein shows slightly more diastolic than systolic filling with some increase in the diastolic filling on inspiration (arrow). The forward flow velocities correspond to the X and Y descents and the reversals at atrial contraction to the A-wave in the right atrial (RA) pressure tracing.

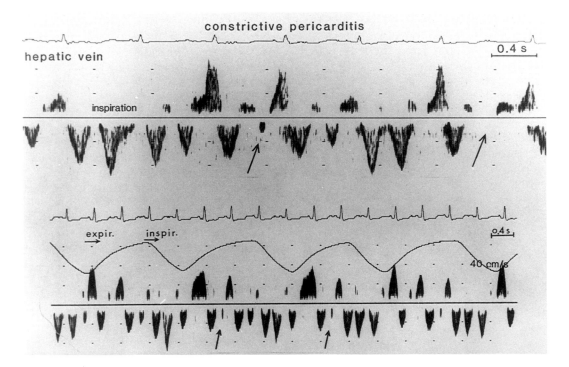

Fig. 23–10. Both panels show hepatic vein recordings, in the lower panel recorded together with respiration at 25 mm/s speed. During inspiration, the systolic and diastolic filling are approximately equal, whereas expiration results in marked flow reversals and minimal or no diastolic filling (arrows). With inspiration, there is some increase in forward flow velocity and at the same time less reversal, and the recording in the lower panel shows that this is a consistent finding.

ening of the filling periods. These respiratory changes in the hepatic veins differ from that seen in restriction (Fig. 23–3) (8, 67, 71, 72). However, in severe constriction with marked abbreviation of filling, some inspiratory increase in reversal can also be seen, but with more expiratory reversal than in restriction.

The flow velocity in the superior caval vein may show similar changes, but the respiratory changes may be less than in the hepatic veins. This could be related to the latter being more influenced by the differences between intrathoracic and intraabdominal pressures with respiration. In the superior caval vein, the opposite changes can also be seen, with decrease in forward flow velocity on inspiration. This may not, however, represent a decrease in volume flow because the diameter of the vein may increase during inspiration. An inspiratory decrease in forward flow velocity may however, be related to an inspiratory increase in right atrial pressure as seen in Figure 23–11. This suggests a preferential filling from the inferior caval vein on inspiration, possibly because of the increase in intraabdominal- and decrease in intrathoracic

pressure, that may contribute to the appearance of Kussmaul's sign in constrictive pericarditis.

With atrial fibrillation the systolic venous filling may decrease (73), resulting in a velocity curve more like that in restrictive cardiomyopathy, but the respiratory changes may still help in the differential diagnosis.

Localized Constriction

In constrictive pericarditis, the limitation of filling is usually similar for both left and right heart. In the presence of a partial constriction, the limitation to filling and the diastolic pressures and velocity curves in the left and right heart may differ, as seen in Figure 23–12.

Acute/Subacute Constriction

Constriction may develop during acute or subacute pericarditis; this may be transient (40), but may also persist with severe symptoms requiring specific treatment. When the cause is not bacterial and the duration is relatively short, rapid improvement following treatment with steroids can be seen, possibly because of reduction in

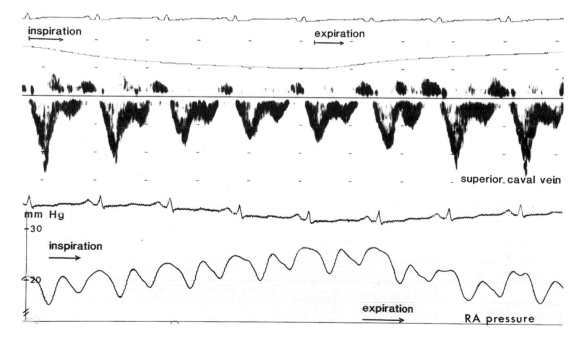

Fig. 23–11. In this patient with constrictive pericarditis, increased systolic filling is seen, corresponding to a more pronounced X than Y descent. With a prolonged inspiration, a decrease in forward flow velocity is seen, simultaneous with an increase in right atrial (RA) pressure (Kussmaul's sign).

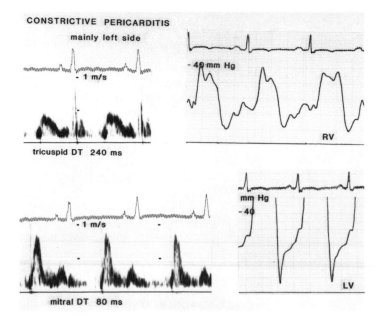

Fig. 23–12. With a localized constriction involving the left ventricle (LV) more than the right (RV), a more rapid and more marked increase in pressure on the left side is seen to correspond to a shortened mitral deceleration time, whereas the tricuspid deceleration time is normal.

edema of the pericardium. Complete resolution can be seen, but with longer duration of symptoms surgical therapy may be necessary. These patients may show marked respiratory variation, which may be partly related to more respiratory effort and more marked septal shifts than in some of the patients with chronic constriction.

Results of Treatment

Following surgery normalization of the hemodynamics and of the flow velocity pattern are seen in the majority of patients (48, 67, 74). The flow velocity curves in Figure 23–6 are from the same patient as in Figures 23–5 and 23–10 recorded 2 months after pericardectomy; they show normal filling, including marked increase in forward flow in the hepatic vein throughout inspiration showing that the earlier limitation to filling is no longer present. In patients in whom surgery does not result in relief of symptoms, shortened deceleration times and abnormal venous flow reversals may indicate the presence of additional restriction.

Respiratory Variation in Other Conditions

Increased respiratory variation in flow velocities is also seen in tamponade (68), but both atrial and ventricular filling differ

from that in constriction, with less or no diastolic venous filling and more late diastolic ventricular filling. Increased respiratory variation in mitral flow velocity is also seen in chronic obstructive lung disease (75), as well as in other conditions with increased respiratory effort, as occurs early after thoracotomy and even in obesity. However, without an abnormal limitation to filling, there is no shortening of the filling periods, and with a deeper inspiration a marked and continuous increase in venous inflow is seen (Fig. 23–6). Such respiratory variation is likely to be an exaggeration of a normal change in the relation between left atrial and left ventricular pressures during respiration. The normal decrease in left atrial pressure on inspiration can result in marked change in the mitral flow velocity in subjects with low atrial pressures, and especially if the rate of left ventricular pressure fall is reduced (Fig. 23–13). Conversely, at high left atrial pressures, when the mitral valve opens at a time with rapid ventricular pressure decay, respiratory changes may become less apparent. This is consistent with the clinical experience that the respiratory changes in left heart filling can be less well seen in the patients with the most severe constriction with very high left atrial pressures and very short filling periods.

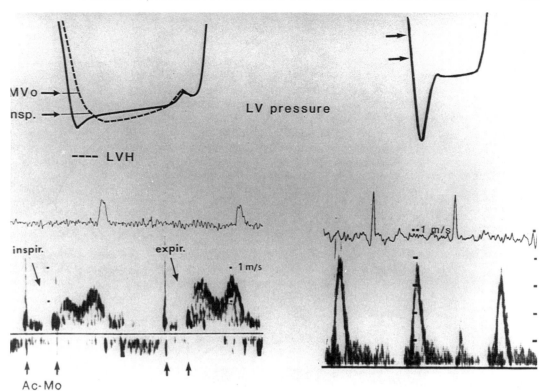

Fig. 23–13. The schematic in the upper part shows diastolic left ventricular (LV) pressures, and below corresponding mitral flow velocity curves from a patient with LV hypertrophy (LVH) to the left and to the right a patient with constriction and in atrial fibrillation. At low left atrial pressures and a slow rate of LV pressure fall in LVH. A decrease in atrial pressure on deep respiration (arrows) results in a marked delay in mitral valve opening (MVo), seen as a prolonged isovolumic relaxation time (Ac-Mo), and a reduced early diastolic flow velocity caused by a slower LV pressure fall at this time. Conversely, in the patient with constriction and elevated atrial pressure, the mitral valve opens at a time with rapid LV pressure decay, and a similar (arrows) or even larger inspiratory change in the gradient from the pulmonary veins to the left heart will result in less obvious changes in the mitral flow velocity curve. The deceleration time is 80 to 100 msec and the filling time only 160 msec. Thus, with more severe constriction and a normal LV pressure fall, high left atrial pressure, and rapid rise in LV diastolic pressure, the respiratory changes in the mitral flow velocity becomes more difficult to appreciate, especially in the presence of atrial fibrillation.

The depth of respiration also influences the findings in constriction. With very shallow respiration, only moderate changes may be seen, compared to marked changes with normal respiration as seen in Figure 23–14.

With atrial arrhythmias, respiratory changes become more difficult to assess, and in atrial flutter, the deceleration time becomes shorter, influencing the assessment in both restriction and constriction.

CONCLUSION

Reduced distensibility leads to exaggerated early diastolic filling in both restrictive cardiomyopathy and constrictive pericarditis, with shortened filling times in venous inflow and across the A-V valves. In restrictive cardiomyopathy, a reduced rate of LV pressure fall can result in less early diastolic filling in early stages. In later stages, this may no longer be evident as it is overcome by elevated atrial pressures.

The respiratory variation in constrictive pericarditis may be initiated by a change in pressure gradient from the pulmonary veins to the left heart. Its degree depends on the depth of respiration, the degree of septal shift, and the level of left atrial pressure. The degree of septal shift and the dif-

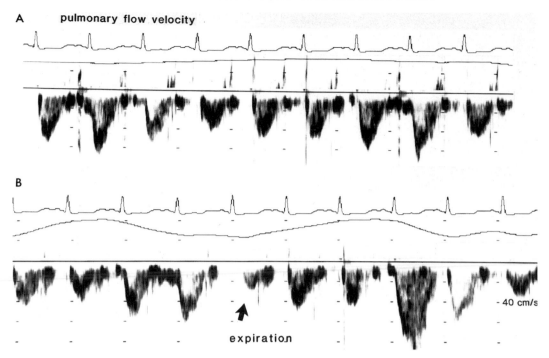

Fig. 23–14. In a patient with constriction, the recording in *A* is from a period with very superficial breathing, and the changes are not clearly more than what can be seen in a normal subject with deep respiration. With deeper respiration, the abnormal variation with marked decrease in flow velocity on expiration (arrow) is clearly seen.

ference between intrathoracic, intracardiac and intra-abdominal pressures influences the velocity pattern in hepatic veins, resulting in different respiratory changes than in restrictive cardiomyopathy. In the latter, septal involvement and possibly less difference between intrathoracic and intracardiac pressures result in similar filling of the two ventricles during respiration, compared to reciprocal filling of the ventricles in constrictive pericarditis. With increasing severity and shorter filling periods, the difference in ventricular filling may become less pronounced, and the different effect of respiration on the hepatic vein velocities can be more helpful to distinguish between the two conditions.

REFERENCES

1. Child JS, Perloff JK: The restrictive cardiomyopathies. Cardiol Clin 6:289, 1988.
2. Benotti JR, Grossman W, Cohn PF: Clinical profile of restrictive cardiomyopathy. Circulation 61:1206, 1980.
3. Hirota Y, et al: Spectrum of restrictive car-

diomyopathy: report of the national survey in Japan. Am Heart J 120:188, 1990.
4. Katritsis D, et al.: Primary restrictive cardiomyopathy: clinical and pathologic characteristics. J Am Coll Cardiol 18:1230, 1991.
5. Fitzpatrick AP, Shapiro LM, Rickards AF, Poole-Wilson PA: Familial restrictive cardiomyopathy with atrioventricular block and skeletal myopathy. Br Heart J 63:114, 1990.
6. Keren A, et al.: Mildly dilated congestive cardiomyopathy. Circulation 72:302, 1985.
7. McKenna WJ, et al.: Hypertrophic cardiomyopathy without hypertrophy: Two families with myocardial disarray in the absence of increased myocardial mass. Br Heart J 63:287, 1990.
8. Appleton CP, Hatle LK, Popp RL: Demonstration of restrictive ventricular physiology by Doppler echocardiography. J Am Coll Cardiol 11:757, 1988.
9. Valantine HA, et al.: A hemodynamic and Doppler echocardiographic study of ventricular function in long-term cardiac allograft recipients: Etiology and prognosis of restrictive/constrictive physiology. Circulation 79:66, 1989.
10. Meaney E, et al.: Cardiac amyloidosis, con-

strictive pericarditis and restrictive cardiomyopathy. Am J Cardiol 38:547, 1976.

11. Klein AL, et al.: Two-dimensional and Doppler echocardiographic assessment of infiltrative cardiomyopathy. J Am Soc Echo 1:48, 1988.

12. Roberts WC, Liegler DC, Carbone PP: Endomyocardial disease and eosinophilia. A clinical and pathologic spectrum. Am J Med 46:28, 1969.

13. Chew CYC, et al.: Primary restrictive cardiomyopathy: Non-tropical endomyocardial fibrosis and hypereosinophilic heart disease. Br Heart J 39:399, 1977.

14. Candell-Riera J, Permanyer-Miralda G, Soler-Soler J: Echocardiographic findings in endomyocardial fibrosis. Chest 82:88, 1982.

15. Fawzy ME, et al.: Endomyocardial fibrosis: Report of eight cases. J Am Coll Cardiol 5: 983, 1985.

16. Presti C, Ryan T, Armstong WF: Two-dimensional and Doppler echocardiographic findings in hypereosinophilic syndrome. Am Heart J 114:172, 1987.

17. Kennish A, Yellin E, Frater RW: Dynamic stiffness profiles in the left ventricle. J Appl Physiol 39:665, 1975.

18. Gaasch WH, et al.: Left ventricular compliance: Mechanisms and clinical implications. Am J Cardiol 38:645, 1976.

19. Hirota Y, et al.: Idiopathic restrictive cardiomyopathy: differences of left ventricular relaxation and diastolic wave forms from constrictive pericarditis. Am J Cardiol 52: 421, 1983.

20. Hirota Y: A clinical study of left ventricular relaxation. Circulation 62:756, 1980.

21. Klein AL, et al.: Doppler characterization of left ventricular diastolic function in cardiac amyloidosis. J Am Coll Cardiol 13: 1017, 1989.

22. Upton MT, Gibson DG, Brown DJ: Echocardiographic assessment of abnormal left ventricular relaxation in man. Br Heart J 38:1001, 1976.

23. Fioretti P, Brower RW, Maester GT, Serruys PW: Interaction of left ventricular relaxation and filling during early diastole in human subjects. Am J Cardiol 46:197, 1980.

24. Appleton CP, Hatle LK, Popp RL: The relationship of transmitral flow velocity patterns to left ventricular diastolic function: new insights from a combined hemodynamic and Doppler echocardiographic study. J Am Coll Cardiol 12:426, 1988.

25. Klein AL, et al.: Prognostic significance of Doppler measures of diastolic function in cardiac amyloidosis. Circulation 83:808, 1991.

26. Tyberg TI, et al.: Left ventricular filling in differentiating restrictive amyloid cardiomyopathy and constrictive pericarditis. Am J Cardiol 47:791, 1981.

27. Aroney CN, et al.: Differentiation of restrictive cardiomyopathy from pericardial constriction: assessment of diastolic function by radionuclide angiography. J Am Coll Cardiol 13:1007, 1989.

28. Janos GG, et al.: Differentiation of constrictive pericarditis and restrictive cardiomyopathy using digitized echocardiography. J Am Coll Cardiol 1:541, 1983.

29. Kitabatake A, et al.: Transmitral blood flow reflecting diastolic behavior of the left ventricle in health and disease. A study by pulsed Doppler technique. Jpn Circ J 46: 92, 1982.

30. Moreno FLL, et al.: Evaluation of size and dynamics of the inferior vena cava as an index of right-sided cardiac function. Am J Cardiol 53:579, 1984.

31. Greenberg B, et al.: The influence of left ventricular filling pressure on atrial contribution to cardiac output. Am Heart J 98: 742, 1979.

32. Rossvoll O, Hatle L: Pulmonary venous flow velocities recorded by transthoracic Doppler; relation to left ventricular diastolic pressures. Eur Heart J 13 (Abstr. Suppl):121, 1992.

33. Mancuso L, et al.: Constrictive pericarditis versus restrictive cardiomyopathy: the role of Doppler echocardiography in differential diagnosis. Int J Cardiol 31:319, 1991.

34. Schiavone WA, Calafiore PA, Salcedo EE: Transesophageal echocardiographic demonstration of pulmonary venous flow velocity in restrictive cardiomyopathy and constrictive pericarditis. Am J Cardiol 63:1286, 1989.

35. Chen C, et al.: Noninvasive estimation of the instantaneous first derivative of left ventricular pressure using continuous-wave Doppler echocardiography. Circulation 83:2101, 1991.

36. Cameron J, Oesterle SN, Baldwin JC, Hancock EW: The etiologic spectrum of constrictive pericarditis. Am Heart J 113:354, 1987.

37. Cimino JJ, Kogan AD: Constrictive pericarditis after cardiac surgery: Report of three cases and review of the literature. Am Heart J 118:1292, 1989.

38. Hancock EW: Subacute effusive-constrictive pericarditis. Circulation 43:183, 1971.

39. Robertson R, Arnold CR: Acute constrictive pericarditis. J Thorac Cardiovasc Surg 49:91, 1965.

40. Sagristà-Salueda J, et al.: Transient cardiac

constriction: an unrecognized pattern of evolution in effusive acute idiopathic pericarditis. Am J Cardiol 59:961, 1987.

41. Hefner LL, et al.: Distensibility of the dog left ventricle. Am J Physiol 201:97, 1962.

42. Santamore WP, Bartlett R, Van Buren SJ, et al.: Ventricular coupling in constrictive pericarditis. Circulation 74:597, 1986.

43. Shabetai R, Fowler NO, Guntheroth WG: The hemodynamics of cardiac tamponade and constrictive pericarditis. Am J Cardiol 26:480, 1970.

44. Svanegaard J, Thayssen P, Arendrup HK: Atrial natriuretic peptide and hemodynamic response to pericardectomy for chronic constrictive pericarditis. Am J Cardiol 66:117, 1990.

45. Reddy PS: Hemodynamics of constrictive pericarditis. *In* Pericardial Disease. Edited by P.S. Reddy et al. New York, Raven Press, 1982.

46. Lewis BS, Gotsman MS: Left ventricular function in systole and diastole in constrictive pericarditis. Am J Cardiol 34:23, 1974.

47. Hansen AT, Eskildsen P, Goetzsche H: Pressure curves from the right auricle and the right ventricle in chronic constrictive pericarditis. Circulation 3:881, 1951.

48. Hatle LK, Appleton CP, Popp RL: Differentiation of constrictive pericarditis and restrictive cardiomyopathy by Doppler echocardiography. Circulation 79:357, 1989.

49. Lewis BS: Real time two-dimensional echocardiography in constrictive pericarditis. Am J Cardiol 49:1789, 1982.

50. Schnittger I, et al.: Echocardiography: Pericardial thickening and constrictive pericarditis. Am J Cardiol 42:388, 1978.

51. Isner JM, et al.: Differentiation of constrictive pericarditis from restrictive cardiomyopathy by computed tomographic imaging. Am Heart J 105:1019, 1983.

52. Soulen RL, Stark DD, Higgins CB: Magnetic resonance imaging in constrictive pericardial disease. Am J Cardiol 55:480, 1985.

53. Bush CA, Stang JM, Wooley CF, Kilman JW: Occult constrictive pericardial disease. Diagnosis by rapid volume expansion and correction by pericardiectomy. Circulation 56:924, 1977.

54. McManus BM, et al.: Hemodynamic cardiac constriction without anatomic myocardial restriction or pericardial constriction. Am Heart J 102:134, 1981.

55. Ilia R, Weizman S, Gueron M: Effect of rapid volume expansion on the right filling pressures after prosthetic valve surgery. Cath Cardiovasc Diagn 23:169, 1991.

56. Schoenfeld MH, et al.: Restrictive cardiomyopathy versus constrictive pericarditis: Role of endomyocardial biopsy in avoiding unnecessary thoracotomy. Circulation 75:1012, 1987.

57. Francis VR, et al.: Improved echocardiographic differentiation of restrictive cardiomyopathy from constrictive pericarditis. Circulation 72:III-355 (abstr), 1985.

58. Candell-Riera J, et al.: Echocardiographic features of the interventricular septum in chronic constrictive pericarditis. Circulation 57:1154, 1978.

59. Tei C, Child JS, Tanaka H, Shah PM: Atrial systolic notch on the interventricular septal echocardiogram: an echocardiographic sign of constrictive pericarditis. J Am Coll Cardiol 1:907, 1983.

60. Candell-Riera J, del Castillo HG, Permanyer-Miralda C, Soler-Soler J: Circulation 59:847, 1979 (letter).

61. Voelkel AG, et al.: Echocardiographic features of constrictive pericarditis. Circulation 58:871, 1978.

62. Engel PJ, et al.: M-mode echocardiography in constrictive pericarditis. J Am Coll Cardiol 6:471, 1985.

63. Himelmann RB, Lee E, Schiller NB: Septal bounce, vena cava plethora, and pericardial adhesion: informative two-dimensional echocardiographic signs in the diagnosis of pericardial constriction. J Am Soc Echo 1:333, 1988.

64. Brenner JI, Waugh RA: Effect of phasic respiration on left ventricular dimension and performance in a normal population: an echocardiographic study. Circulation 57:122, 1978.

65. Agatston AS, Rao A, Price RJ, Kinney EL: Diagnosis of constrictive pericarditis by pulsed Doppler echocardiography. Am J Cardiol 54:929, 1984.

66. Izumi S, et al.: Superior vena cava and ventricular inflow in constrictive pericarditis and restrictive cardiomyopathy as measured by pulsed Doppler echocardiography. J Cardiovasc Technology 9:19, 1990.

67. Oh JK, Hatle L, Seward JB, Tajik AJ: Sensitivity of Doppler echocardiography for constrictive pericarditis. J Am Coll Cardiol 17(suppl A):49A, 1991.

68. Appleton CP, Hatle LK, Popp RL: Cardiac tamponade and pericardial effusion: respiratory variation in transvalvular flow velocities studied by Doppler echocardiography. J Am Coll Cardiol 11:1020, 1988.

69. von Bibra H, et al.: Diagnosis of constrictive pericarditis by pulsed Doppler echocardiography of the hepatic vein. Am J Cardiol 63:483, 1989.

70. Byrd BF, Linden RW: Superior vena cava

Doppler flow velocity patterns in pericardial disease. Am J Cardiol 65:1464, 1990.

71. Appleton CP, Hatle L, Popp RL: Central venous flow velocity patterns can differentiate constrictive pericarditis from restrictive cardiomyopathy. J Am Coll Cardiol 9 (suppl A):119A (abstr), 1987.

72. Appleton CP, Popp RL, Hatle LK: Differentiation of constrictive pericarditis and restrictive cardiomyopathy: new insights from two-dimensional and Doppler echocardiographic studies. *In* Pericardial disease: New insights and old dilemmas. Edited by Soler-Soler J, Permanyer-Miralda G,

Sagrista-Sauleda J. Dordrecht, Kluwer Academic Publishers, 1990.

73. Ochi H, et al.: Superior vena cava flow and tricuspid anular motion after cardioversion of atrial fibrillation, and role of right atrial relaxation on systolic venous return. Am J Cardiol 68:1335, 1991.

74. Viola AR: The influence of pericariectomy on the hemodynamics of chronic constrictive pericarditis. Circulation 48:1038, 1973.

75. Hoit B, Sahn DJ, Shabetai R: Doppler-detected paradoxus of mitral and tricuspid valve flows in chronic lung disease. J Am Coll Cardiol 8:706, 1986.

Chapter 24

DOPPLER ECHOCARDIOGRAPHIC EVALUATION OF DIASTOLIC DYSFUNCTION IN CHILDREN

A. Rebecca Snider, Jon N. Meliones, and L. LuAnn Minich

Doppler echocardiography has been used to detect abnormalities of diastolic function in children with cardiac disorders. Besides being safe, noninvasive, and useful for serial studies, the Doppler technique evaluates intracardiac blood flow, and thus is ideally suited for providing an estimate of ventricular performance that is independent of ventricular geometry. This advantage of the Doppler technique is especially important in patients with congenital heart disease in whom ventricular geometry and septal wall motion are often very distorted, making other noninvasive methods of assessing diastolic function invalid. Consequently, over the past several years, new information concerning diastolic dysfunction in children has largely been obtained using Doppler echocardiographic techniques.

In this chapter, we review (1) the normal values for right and left ventricular Doppler diastolic filling indexes throughout childhood, (2) some of the more common forms of diastolic dysfunction encountered in children, and (3) potential uses of the Doppler diastolic filling indexes in the management of pediatric heart disease.

NORMAL RIGHT AND LEFT VENTRICULAR DOPPLER DIASTOLIC FILLING INDEXES

From the mitral or tricuspid valve Doppler tracing, several different indices of ventricular diastolic function have been derived (1–7). (See Chapter 12.) For this technique, a range-gated pulsed Doppler examination of the ventricular inflow tract is performed. From the apical four-chamber view, the Doppler cursor line and sample volume are placed in the mitral or tricuspid valve orifice at an angle as nearly parallel to flow as possible. The sample volume position is adjusted to record the maximum velocity through the atrioventricular valve. This point is usually found just distal to the anulus near the tips of the valve leaflets. The position of the sample volume is critical to obtain standardized results. An adequate mitral or tricuspid valve Doppler examination consists of clear identification of the opening and closure points of the atrioventricular valve and the peak velocities at rapid ventricular filling, the peak E velocity, and during atrial contraction, the peak A velocity (Fig. 24–1).

From the Doppler tracing, several types of indexes of ventricular diastolic filling can be calculated. First, diastolic time intervals reflecting the time course of relaxation can be measured. For example, the left ventricular isovolumic relaxation time can be measured from the aortic closing component of the second heart sound to the onset of the diastolic flow velocity and usually requires a phonocardiogram to be recorded simultaneously with the mitral valve Doppler tracing (8). Likewise, the deceleration time can be measured from the peak E velocity to the time when the Doppler curve returns from peak E velocity to the baseline (8).

A second type of diastolic parameter that has been measured from the Doppler tracings is comprised of indices of velocity and acceleration. The peak velocity during rapid ventricular filling, the peak E velocity, and the peak velocity during atrial contraction, the peak A velocity, can be measured (9–12). The ratio of the peak E to peak A velocities (E/A ratio) and the ratio of the peak A to peak E velocities (A/E

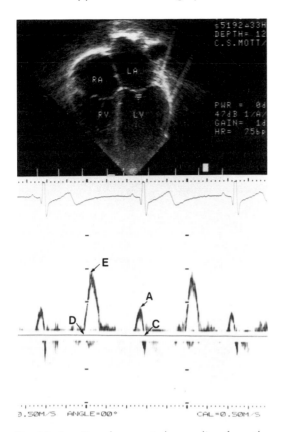

Fig. 24–1. Doppler spectral recording from the mitral valve of a normal child. The freeze-frame image (top) of the apical four-chamber view shows the position of the sample volume at the time of the Doppler recording. The Doppler spectral recording (bottom) shows normal forward flow toward the transducer and above the baseline at rapid ventricular filling (E) and during atrial contraction (A). The opening of the mitral valve leaflets occurs at the beginning of diastole (D) and the closure of the leaflets is labelled (C). Reproduced with permission from Snider AR, Serwer GA: Echocardiography in Pediatric Heart Disease. Chicago, Year Book Medical Publishers, Inc., 1990.

ing rates are calculated as the peak E velocity multiplied by the atrioventricular valve anulus cross-sectional area (calculated as $\pi\,d^2/4$ where d = the anulus diameter measured from the two-dimensional echocardiogram) (1). Normalized peak filling rate is calculated as peak filling rate divided by left ventricular end-diastolic volume (measured from the two-dimensional echocardiogram). Recent studies have shown that peak filling rate can be normalized to mitral stroke volume using the following derived equation (14):

$$\text{PFR (SV/sec)} = \frac{\text{peak E (cm/sec)}}{\text{MV VTI (cm)}}$$

where PFR (SV/sec) = peak filling rate normalized to stroke volume

MV VTI = velocity time integral of mitral valve Doppler

This index correlates well with radionuclide peak filling rate normalized for stroke volume and accounts for cardiac output without the need to calculate left ventricular end-diastolic volume. Additional filling rates have been calculated from the mitral valve Doppler examination (13). These include (1) peak atrial filling rate calculated as the product of peak A velocity and mitral anular cross-sectional area, (2) mean filling rate calculated as the product of mean diastolic velocity and mitral anular cross-sectional area, and (3) the rapid filling index calculated as the quotient of peak early diastolic filling rate divided by mean filling rate.

A fourth type of diastolic parameter that has been used to describe the patterns of ventricular filling are the Doppler area fractions or filling fractions (2). The Doppler area fractions describe the percentage of the Doppler envelope that is present in the various phases of diastole. Because the atrioventricular valve cross-sectional area changes throughout diastole, calculation of the absolute volumetric flow in the different portions of diastole would be extremely difficult. Because the volumetric flow is the product of the velocity time integral (the integrated area under the Doppler curve) and the mitral valve

ratio) have been used to describe the pattern of ventricular diastolic filling (3, 4, 9, 10, 12, 13). The deceleration of early diastolic flow can be measured as the slope of a straight line drawn from the peak E velocity to the point where peak E decreases by half on the descending limb of the early diastolic inflow (10, 12).

A third type of parameter that can be measured from the Doppler examination is comprised of indices of peak and mean ventricular filling rates. Doppler peak fill-

cross-sectional area, approximate values for the fraction of filling of the ventricle in the different phases of diastole can be obtained by measuring several areas under the Doppler curve and dividing these areas by the total area under the Doppler curve. Using this methodology, the area or filling fractions in the first third of diastole (0.33 area fraction), during early diastolic inflow (E area fraction), and during atrial contraction (A area fraction) can be calculated (Fig. 24–2). In the studies from our laboratory, the E area and A area were measured as the triangular portion under the Doppler curve formed by extrapolating a straight line down from the peak E and peak A velocities to the baseline (2, 9). Other methods have been used to define the filling fractions during early and late diastolic inflow. These include dividing the Doppler curve with a straight line in the middle of the slow filling period into early and late filling fractions (6) or drawing the triangular E area and defining all the remaining

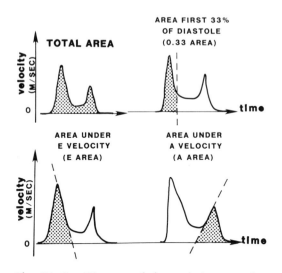

Fig. 24–2. Diagram of the technique used to measure various areas under the mitral valve Doppler tracing. The 0.33 area is measured as the area of the Doppler tracing at the completion of 1/3 of the total diastolic time. The E and A areas are measured as triangular areas under the Doppler tracing obtained by extrapolating a straight line down from the peak E and peak A velocities to the baseline. Reproduced with permission from Snider AR, Serwer GA: Echocardiography in Pediatric Heart Disease. Chicago, Year Book Medical Publishers, Inc., 1990.

area under the Doppler curve as filling caused by atrial contraction (Fig. 24–3).

For the fetus, newborn infant, and child, the Doppler patterns of right and left ventricular diastolic filling vary with age, heart rate, respiration, and ventricular loading conditions. In the evaluation of the mitral or tricuspid valve Doppler filling patterns, these normal variations must be taken into account.

Effects of Aging

Throughout gestation, the maximal flow velocity in late diastole (peak A velocity) exceeds that in early diastole (peak E velocity) for both the mitral and tricuspid valves (15–18). This probably reflects the low compliance of both fetal ventricles. In one large study of fetuses throughout gestation (15), the tricuspid valve E/A ratio increased from 0.64 ± 0.06 at 17 to 24 weeks' gestation to 0.82 ± 0.04 at 37 to 42 weeks' gestation. The increase in tricuspid valve E/A ratio was caused by an increase in the peak E velocity (from 0.26 ± 0.02 to 0.36 ± 0.02 m/sec from 17 to 42 weeks' gestation) while the peak A velocity remained relatively constant (from 0.41 ± 0.03 to 0.44 ± 0.02 m/sec from 17 to 42 weeks' gestation). For the mitral valve, the E/A ratio increased significantly from 0.64 ± 0.04 to 0.82 ± 0.06 from 17 to 42 weeks' gestation. This increase in the mitral valve E/A ratio was caused by a significant decrease in the peak A velocity (from 0.41 ± 0.03 to 0.34 ± 0.03 from 17 to 42 weeks' gestation) while peak E velocity remained unchanged (from 0.26 ± 0.02 to 0.28 ± 0.02 m/sec from 17 to 42 weeks' gestation). Thus, the human fetal ventricle fills with a pattern that suggests that ventricular compliance is lower during gestation than after birth. Previous studies in fetal lambs have also shown that the fetal ventricle is less compliant than the neonatal ventricle (19). These differences in compliance have been attributed to the distribution and relative paucity of contractile elements in the fetal myocardium compared with the adult ventricle. In the fetus, noncontractile tissue constitutes approximately 70% of the muscle mass, whereas, in the adult myocardium, noncontractile elements represent only 40% of the total mass (20). The changes in E/A ratio throughout

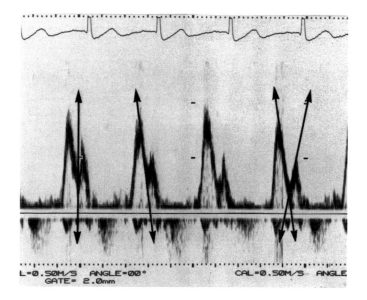

Fig. 24–3. Mitral valve Doppler tracing demonstrating the methods that have been used to calculate the filling during early and late diastole. In the first beat, the mitral valve Doppler tracing is divided in half in the middle of the slow filling period. Areas are measured in the first half and the second half of diastole. In the second beat, the triangular E area is measured and all the remaining area of the Doppler curve is defined as filling caused by atrial contraction. The fourth beat illustrates the method shown in Figure 24–2. Reproduced with permission from Snider AR, Serwer GA: Echocardiography in Pediatric Heart Disease. Chicago, Year Book Medical Publishers, Inc., 1990.

gestation are believed to reflect differences in function and maturation of the two ventricles before birth (15).

In a study of normal neonates in the first 2 days after birth, the right and left ventricular diastolic filling patterns remained abnormal compared with adult patterns and resembled those encountered in late gestation (Table 24–1) (21). All of the measurements of diastolic filling were significantly different when the right and left ventricles were compared. Compared with values in the left ventricle, the right ventricular diastolic variables indicated a shift away from early passive filling to the later period of atrial emptying. For the right compared with the left ventricle, peak E velocity, peak E/A ratio, E/total area, E/A area ratio, and 0.33 area fraction were each significantly lower, whereas peak A velocity and A/total area were significantly higher. By day two, the diastolic filling patterns of the right and

Table 24–1. Right (Tricuspid) Versus Left (Mitral) Ventricular Diastolic Filling on Days 1 and 2 in 22 Neonates

	Day 1			Day 2		
	Tricuspid	Mitral	p Value	Tricuspid	Mitral	p Value
Peak E (cm/s)	44.6 ± 10.0	53.2 + 9.30	<0.01	46.8 ± 8.50	50.2 ± 7.90	NS
E/total	0.58 ± 0.07	0.63 ± 0.05	<0.005	0.58 ± 0.05	0.61 ± 0.05	<0.05
E/A area	1.05 ± 0.23	1.63 ± 0.40	<0.0001	1.11 ± 0.21	1.36 ± 0.27	<0.001
Peak E/A	0.84 ± 0.14	1.15 ± 0.17	<0.0001	0.85 ± 0.23	1.00 ± 0.25	<0.05
⅓ area fraction	0.31 ± 0.04	0.41 ± 0.04	<0.0001	0.34 ± 0.04	0.39 ± 0.04	<0.01
Peak A (cm/s)	53.0 ± 8.40	47.6 ± 5.80	<0.05	53.4 ± 9.90	48.7 ± 8.30	<0.05
A/total	0.57 ± 0.09	0.41 ± 0.09	<0.001	0.54 ± 0.10	0.45 ± 0.12	<0.005
HR (beats/min)	121 ± 8	120 ± 7	NS	120 ± 6	118 ± 6	NS

Values are expressed as mean ± SD. A/total = ratio of atrial late active filling to total diastolic velocity-time integral; Peak A = peak flow velocity of atrial systole; E/total = ratio of early passive ventricular filling to total diastolic velocity-time integral; Peak E = peak E velocity of early passive ventricular filling; HR = heart rate; NS = not significant (that is, $p > 0.05$); Peak E/A = ratio of peak E velocity to peak A velocity; ⅓ area fraction = the proportion of diastolic filling that occurs during the first ⅓ of diastole compared with the total diastolic velocity-time integral. Reproduced with permission from Riggs TW, et al.: Doppler echocardiographic evaluation of right and left ventricular diastolic function in normal neonates. J Am Coll Cardiol 13:700, 1989.

left ventricles remained significantly different, but the difference between the mean values was less for each measured variable.

From the first to the second day of life, most of the indices of left ventricular diastolic filling did not change; however, the mitral valve E/A velocity and area ratios did decrease significantly. For the tricuspid valve, only the first third area fraction changed significantly (increasing from 0.31 ± 0.04 to 0.34 ± 0.04) from the first to the second day of life.

It is interesting that, in the first 2 days after birth, the tricuspid valve E/A velocity ratio (0.84) is nearly identical to that reported in the fetus in late gestation (0.82) (15). The mitral E/A velocity ratio in the first 2 days after birth (1.15) is significantly higher than that found in the fetus in late gestation (0.82) (15). This difference in the mitral valve peak E/A velocity ratio probably represents a shift to early passive filling from atrial emptying consistent with the increase in left ventricular preload and output that occurs during the transition from prenatal to postnatal circulation (21). In the first 2 days after birth, the diastolic filling pattern of the right ventricle shows a greater independence on atrial contraction for filling than does that of the left ventricle. This difference between the ventricular filling patterns probably indicates reduced right ventricular compliance as a result of intrauterine dominance (21).

Serial studies of normal newborn infants in the first 3 weeks of life have shown significant changes in left ventricular relaxation and compliance (22). In these studies, the E/A velocity ratio did not change significantly in the first 2 weeks of life; however, by the third week of life, this ratio increased significantly to 1.25 ± 0.1. The increase in the E/A velocity ratio was caused by an increase in peak E velocity (to 0.65 ± 0.16 m/sec by the third week of life), whereas peak A velocity remained unchanged. In addition, the mitral deceleration time (which is related to the amplitude of the rapid filling wave) increased significantly from 62 ± 14 to 87 ± 10 msec between the first day of life and age 2 weeks. This change suggests a lower early diastolic cavity pressure and muscular stiffness and, hence, improved ventricular compliance.

Likewise, the left ventricular isovolumic relaxation time increased significantly from 41 ± 12 to 51 ± 8 msec from 1 day to 3 weeks of age.

Left ventricular diastolic filling patterns have also been investigated in "normal" preterm infants (23). These infants were found to have tricuspid and mitral valve Doppler indexes identical to those of normal full-term newborn infants rather than resembling those of a fetus of corresponding age. The Doppler patterns were unrelated to gestational age and, like those of normal newborns, exhibited changes in peak E and peak A velocity after 3 weeks of age that were independent of heart rate.

In normal, healthy children and young adults, age and heart rate have been shown to account for 50% of the variation in the E/A velocity ratio, peak A velocity, and atrial filling fraction (24). Regression equations are available for determining the normal Doppler indexes at various ages and heart rates in subjects from 11 to 40 years of age (24). In general, however, the average peak E velocity in this age group is 0.73 ± 0.09 m/sec, the average peak A velocity is 0.38 ± 0.08 m/sec, and the average E/A velocity ratio is 2.0 ± 0.5 (24). In children aged 1 to 18 years old, the average first third area fraction is 0.58 ± 0.08, the average E area fraction is 0.62 ± 0.07, the average A area fraction is 0.20 ± 0.07, and the average E/A area ratio is 2.5 ± 0.69 (25). In 31 healthy subjects aged 1 day to 21 years, isovolumic relaxation time ranged from 34 to 71 msec (average 55 ± 10 msec) and deceleration time ranged from 48 to 139 msec (average 100 ± 22 msec) (26). The isovolumic relaxation time was primarily affected by age (isovolumic relaxation time = 1.31 × age + 41.4) but also correlated well with body surface area (isovolumic relaxation time = 14.3 × body surface area + 38.4). Deceleration time correlated best with body surface area (deceleration time = 27 × body surface area + 67.7) but also correlated well with age (deceleration time = 2.3 × age + 77.4). When controlled for age, neither time intervals were affected by heart rate (26).

Left ventricular diastolic function in older adults is discussed elsewhere in this text. (See Chapters 8, 11, and 25.)

Effects of Heart Rate

Several investigators have shown significant effects of heart rate on the mitral valve Doppler indexes (27–30). In a study of 20 healthy subjects aged 24 to 42 years, transesophageal atrial pacing from a baseline heart rate of 70 ± 10 beats/min to a paced rate of 88 ± 3 beats/min resulted in significant increases in peak A velocity and A area fraction, no change in peak E velocity, and consequently significant decreases in E/A velocity and area ratios. In this study, peak A velocity was related to heart rate by the regression equation: peak A velocity = 0.008 (heart rate) − 0.21. Thus, for each increase in heart rate of 10 beats/min, peak A velocity increased by 8 cm/sec (27). In another study using a dog model (30), heart rate was increased by three different methods (right atrial pacing, atropine, and isoproterenol), all of which resulted in the following similar changes on the mitral valve Doppler: (1) the peak E velocity and first third filling fraction did not change with increasing heart rate; (2) the peak A velocity increased with increasing heart rate; and (3) the "absolute" increases in peak A velocity and A area fraction were biphasic, initially decreasing as heart rate increased but then increasing when atrial contraction occurred in close proximity (< 70 msec) to mitral valve opening. Differences in the methods of increasing heart rate (related largely to their effect on PR interval and to a lesser degree on the rate of isovolumic relaxation) caused differences in the mitral velocity variables. Therefore, studies utilizing mitral flow velocity variables should probably include information on the PR interval, heart rate, and mitral flow velocity at the start of atrial contraction (30).

Effects of Respiration

The mitral and tricuspid Doppler indexes vary with the phases of respiration. In studies of adult patients, mild decreases in the mitral valve peak E velocity of 4% and 9% have been found on inspiration (31, 32). Mitral peak A velocity remains unchanged with respiration. In normal children (aged 1.5 to 11 years), the peak E velocity decreases by 8% with inspiration, whereas the peak A velocity remains unchanged (Table 24–2). As a result, the E/A velocity and area ratios for the left ventricle decrease by 14% and 12% (33). In normal children, significant large increases in both peak E and peak A velocities of the tricuspid valve occur with inspiration (Table 24–3). The tricuspid peak E velocity increases by 26%, the peak A velocity increases by 20%, and the E/A velocity and area ratios remain unchanged. Because of the changes in the Doppler velocities that occur with respiration, it is recommended that the assessment of left ventricular and especially right ventricular diastolic func-

Table 24–2. Respiratory Influence on Left Ventricular Filling (n = 20)

	Inspiration	Expiration	p Value
Peak E	85 ± 11	92 ± 14	<0.0001
E/total	0.72 ± 0.04	0.71 ± 0.03	NS
E/A area	2.72 ± 1.04	3.09 ± 1.34	<0.001
Peak E/A	1.72 ± 0.42	2.00 ± 0.64	<0.005
⅓ area fraction	0.44 ± 0.09	0.50 ± 0.09	<0.001
Peak A	52 ± 12	50 ± 13	NS
A/total	0.29 ± 0.08	0.28 ± 0.09	NS
HR	91 ± 15	86 ± 16	<0.001

Values are mean ± 1 standard deviation.
A/total = ratio of atrial late active filling to total diastolic velocity-time integral; E/total = ratio of early passive ventricular filling to total diastolic velocity-time integral; HR = heart rate in beats/min; NS = not significant (p > 0.05); ⅓ area fraction = the proportion of diastolic filling which occurs during the first ⅓ of diastole compared to the total diastolic velocity-time integral; Peak A = peak A velocity of atrial sysole in cm/s; Peak E = peak E velocity of early passive ventricular filling in cm/s; Peak E/A = ratio of peak E velocity to peak A velocity; Reproduced with permission from Riggs TW, Snider AR: Respiratory influence on right and left ventricular diastolic function in normal children. Am J Cardiol 63:858, 1989.

Table 24–3.   Respiratory Influence on Right Ventricular Filling (n = 20)

	Inspiration	Expiration	p Value
Peak E	62 ± 13	49 ± 12	<0.0001
E/total	0.72 ± 0.07	0.69 ± 0.06	NS
E/A area	2.56 ± 1.29	2.48 ± 1.34	NS
Peak E/A	1.61 ± 0.51	1.48 ± 0.46	NS
⅓ area fraction	0.40 ± 0.06	0.41 ± 0.07	NS
Peak A	42 ± 12	35 ± 9	<0.0001
A/total	0.36 ± 0.14	0.35 ± 0.13	NS
HR	90 ± 13	84 ± 15	<0.001

Values are mean ± 1 standard deviation.
Abbreviations as in Table 24-2. Reproduced with permission from Riggs, T.W. and Snider, A.R.[33]

tion in pediatric patients should include standardization for the phase of respiration (33).

ABNORMALITIES OF DIASTOLIC FILLING IN PEDIATRIC HEART DISEASE

The mitral and tricuspid valve Doppler diastolic filling indexes have been used to detect abnormalities in left and right ventricular diastolic function in a variety of pediatric cardiac disorders. In this section, some of the more common clinical settings in which diastolic dysfunction is encountered in children are reviewed.

Systemic Artery Hypertension

In children with mild systemic artery hypertension, left ventricular diastolic filling abnormalities have been detected with Doppler techniques when digitized M-mode indexes of diastolic function were still normal and before the development of systolic dysfunction or left ventricular hypertrophy on the M-mode echocardiogram (2). Children with mild systemic hypertension have a decrease in the fraction of filling in the first third of diastole, an increase in peak A velocity, and an increase in the fraction of filling under the A wave (Fig. 24–4). These findings suggest impaired left ventricular filling in early diastole accompanied by a compensatory increase in left ventricular filling in late diastole. These abnormal filling patterns could be a result of (1) increased left ventricular chamber stiffness caused by left ventricular hypertrophy with normal myocardial stiff-

ness or (2) decreased left ventricular compliance caused by myocardial dysfunction or fibrosis. (See Chapter 21.)

Hypertrophic Cardiomyopathy

In children with hypertrophic cardiomyopathy, no resting intracavitary gradient, and no mitral regurgitation, the mitral valve Doppler studies have shown prolonged isovolumic relaxation time, decreased peak E velocity in early diastole, and a decreased fraction of filling in the first third of diastole (Fig. 24–5) (34). Thus, like children with mild systemic hypertension, children with hypertrophic cardiomyopathy also had decreased filling in early diastole probably caused by impaired early left ventricular relaxation rates. Unlike the hypertensive children, the children with hypertrophic cardiomyopathy had no compensatory increase in filling in late diastole (normal peak A velocity and A area fraction) and, therefore, had a reduced left ventricular end-diastolic dimension. The lack of compensatory filling of the left ventricle during atrial contraction in children with hypertrophic cardiomyopathy as compared with hypertensive children could be caused by (1) inability of the "atrial kick" to cause thinning of the ventricular septum in hypertrophic cardiomyopathy, (2) differences in relaxation properties of left ventricular muscle in the two disease states, (3) difference in disease severity between the two groups, or (4) previous treatment with verapamil in the hypertrophic cardiomyopathy patients that may, through its negative inotropic effect,

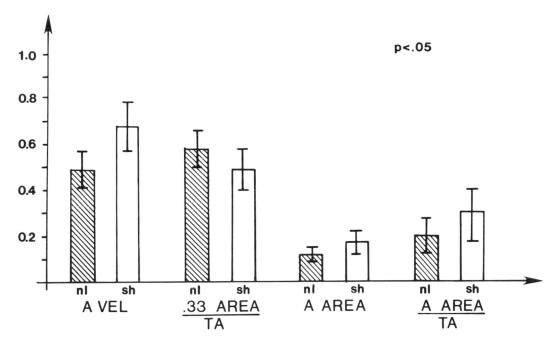

Fig. 24–4. Diagrammatic representation of the diastolic filling abnormalities found in a group of children with systemic hypertension (sh) when compared to a group of normal children (nl). The sh patients had an elevated peak A velocity. In addition, in the sh children, a decreased percentage of the total Doppler area occurred in the first 1/3 of diastole and an increased percentage of the total Doppler area occurred during atrial contraction. Thus, these children had a shift in diastolic filling toward late diastole. Reproduced with permission from Snider AR, et al.: Doppler evaluation of left ventricular diastolic filling in children with systemic hypertension. Am J Cardiol 56:921, 1985.

weaken the force of atrial contraction. (See Chapter 22.)

Left Ventricular Outflow Obstruction

Several studies have shown that children with pressure overload hypertrophy caused by left ventricular outflow obstruction have abnormalities of left ventricular diastolic filling (35, 36). In one study of children with severe aortic valve stenosis or coarctation of the aorta, the percentage of the total Doppler area occurring in the first third of diastole was significantly lower and the percentage of the total Doppler area occurring under the A wave was significantly higher than those of normal age-matched children. The percentage of the total Doppler area occurring under the E wave was the same as that of normal children; therefore, the ratio of E area to A area was significantly lower in the patient group (Figs. 24–6 to 24–8). Immediately after successful relief of the left ventricular

outflow obstruction with balloon angioplasty (gradient change from 64 ± 23 mm Hg to 33 ± 22 mm Hg), no differences were observed in any of the Doppler diastolic filling indexes.

Thus, children with severe left ventricular outflow obstruction have an abnormal pattern of left ventricular diastolic filling detectable by mitral valve Doppler examination. The decrease in the percentage of the total area in the first one-third of diastole and the increase in the percent of the total area under the A wave suggest a relative shift of left ventricular filling to late diastole probably caused by impaired early diastolic relaxation. Because diastolic filling abnormalities did not revert toward normal following removal of the high afterload and reduction of left ventricular systolic pressure to normal, it is unlikely that the filling abnormalities were caused by an afterload mismatch. In children and adults with pressure overload hypertrophy, increased wall thickness or mass has

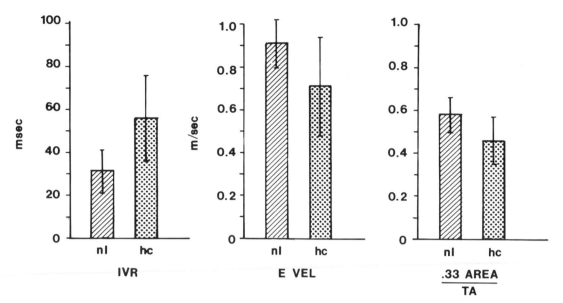

Fig. 24–5. Left ventricular diastolic filling abnormalities found in a group of children with hypertrophic cardiomyopathy (hc) and no mitral regurgitation, compared to normal (nl) age-matched children. The hc patients had a prolonged isovolumic relaxation time (IVR) and a decreased peak E velocity. In addition, in the hc patients, a decreased percentage of the total Doppler area occurred in the first 1/3 of diastole. Reproduced with permission from Gidding SS, et al.: Left ventricular diastolic filling in children with hypertrophic cardiomyopathy: Assessment with pulsed Doppler echocardiography. J Am Coll Cardiol 8:310, 1986.

been implicated as the cause of impaired left ventricular relaxation. Several studies have shown a significant correlation between the extent of hypertrophy and the severity of the diastolic filling abnormality (37–39). On the other hand, normal diastolic filling patterns have been reported in endurance-trained athletes with physiologic cardiac hypertrophy, making left ventricular hypertrophy alone an unlikely cause of impaired left ventricular relaxation (40, 41). An interaction between subendocardial ischemia and changes in cytosolic calcium transport could cause the impaired myocardial relaxation seen in patients with hypertrophy. The interaction between these two factors could explain why impaired relaxation occurs in children with pressure overload hypertrophy but not in young athletes with physiologic hypertrophy (40, 41).

If left ventricular hypertrophy alone is the cause of impaired early ventricular relaxation in children with left ventricular outflow obstruction, regression of left ventricular hypertrophy should be accompa-

nied by a return of diastolic filling patterns toward normal. This question could be addressed in long-term studies of patients who have had successful relief of left ventricular outflow obstruction and resultant decrease in left ventricular hypertrophy. Such a study was performed in children 6 years after successful repair of aortic coarctation (36). In this study, the coarctation subjects had higher peak A velocity and A area fraction, and thus showed a greater dependence on the active or atrial contraction component of left ventricular diastolic filling than the normal subjects. In addition, the coarctation patients had persistent small resting arm-leg gradients (mean 2.2 mm Hg, range −4 to 10 mm Hg) and a slightly greater indexed left ventricular mass. Diastolic filling was more impaired in older subjects with coarctation of the aorta compared to younger coarctation patients. Thus, children who have had successful repair of aortic coarctation often have persistent alterations in left ventricular diastolic function and mass that may relate to small resting arm-leg gradients. The observed

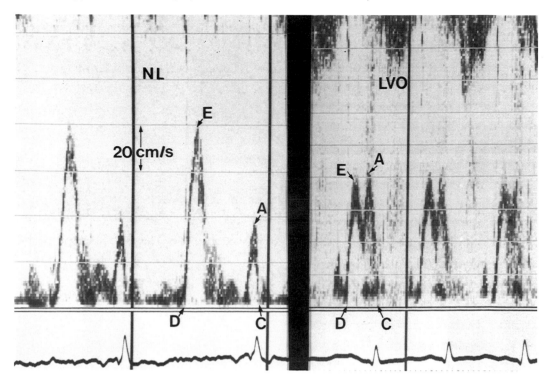

Fig. 24–6. Mitral valve Doppler recordings obtained from a normal (NL) child (left) and a child with left ventricular outflow obstruction (LVO) (right). Patients with LVO were found to have a smaller peak E velocity during rapid ventricular filling, a larger peak A velocity during atrial contraction, and a greater percentage of the Doppler area occurring during atrial contraction compared to NL children. Abbreviations: D = onset of diastole, C = mitral valve leaflet closure point.

long-term changes in left ventricular diastolic filling could be related to persistent left ventricular hypertrophy or to preoperative myocardial ischemia with resultant fibrosis (36).

Right Ventricular Outflow Obstruction

Right ventricular diastolic function can be evaluated using diastolic filling indices derived from the tricuspid valve Doppler recording. The tricuspid valve diastolic indexes are weakly affected by age and heart rate and extremely affected by the phase of respiration (42, 43). Therefore, when using the tricuspid valve Doppler indexes, care must be taken to measure complexes at a standardized time in the respiratory cycle, usually peak inspiration.

One of the first applications of the tricuspid valve Doppler indexes was the assessment of right ventricular diastolic filling in children with pressure overload hypertro-

phy of the right ventricle caused by valvular pulmonary stenosis (44). The children with pulmonary stenosis had a much higher peak A velocity than age-matched normal controls and no significant difference in peak E velocity; therefore, the ratio of peak E to peak A velocities was significantly lower in the patient group. In the patient group, the percentage of the total Doppler area occurring in the first third of diastole was significantly lower, and the percentage of the total Doppler area occurring under the A wave was significantly higher. The percentage of the total Doppler area occurring under the E wave was not significantly different between the two groups; therefore, the ratio of E area to A area was lower in the patient group (Figs. 24–9 to 24–12). Immediately after successful relief of the pulmonary stenosis with balloon valvuloplasty (gradient change from 71 ± 35 to 28 ± 15 mm Hg), no

MITRAL VALVE AREA FRACTIONS

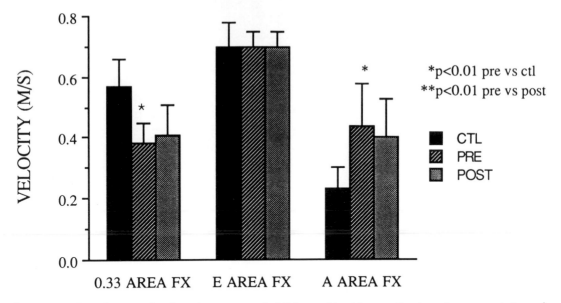

Fig. 24–7. Doppler area fractions in a group of children with either aortic stenosis or coarctation of the aorta, measured pre- and post-balloon angioplasty. Pre-angioplasty, children with left ventricular outflow tract obstruction had a decrease in the 0.33 area fraction and an increase in the A area fraction compared to normal age-matched children (CTL). Post-angioplasty, these Doppler abnormalities did not change in spite of successful relief of the left ventricular outflow tract gradient. Reproduced with permission from Meliones JN, et al.: Pulsed Doppler assessment of left ventricular diastolic filling in children with left ventricular outflow obstruction before and after balloon angioplasty. Am J Cardiol 63:231, 1989.

differences were observed in any of the Doppler velocities, area fractions, or ratios.

In children with pulmonary stenosis, the decreased percentage of the total Doppler area in the first third of diastole and the increased percentage of the total Doppler area under the A wave suggest a relative shift of right ventricular filling to late diastole. These filling abnormalities are identical to those observed for the left ventricle of children with left ventricular outflow obstruction (35). In addition, this abnormal tricuspid Doppler pattern resembles the mitral Doppler pattern I observed by Appleton et al. (8) in patients with impaired left ventricular early diastolic relaxation and normal left ventricular filling pressures. In this study, no patient had a tricuspid Doppler pattern resembling the mitral Doppler pattern II described by Appleton et al. (8) as occurring in patients with markedly elevated filling pressures, an abrupt rapid filling wave and decreased chamber compliance.

Several possible mechanisms exist to explain the impaired right ventricular early relaxation observed in children with severe pulmonary stenosis. For example, the afterload during contraction affects the extent of muscle fiber shortening and the rate of fiber lengthening. Failure to normalize right ventricular wall stress (afterload mismatch) could account for the impaired right ventricular relaxation seen in patients with pressure overload hypertrophy. Because right ventricular diastolic filling abnormalities did not return to normal after successful relief of the high afterload, it is unlikely that afterload mismatch was the cause of the observed filling abnormalities. Subendocardial ischemia has been suggested to be the cause of impaired relaxation in pressure overload hypertrophy. This may account for the occurrence of impaired relaxation with pressure overload hypertrophy, but not in young athletes with physiologic hypertrophy (41, 45).

Finally, in children and adults with pres-

DOPPLER RATIOS

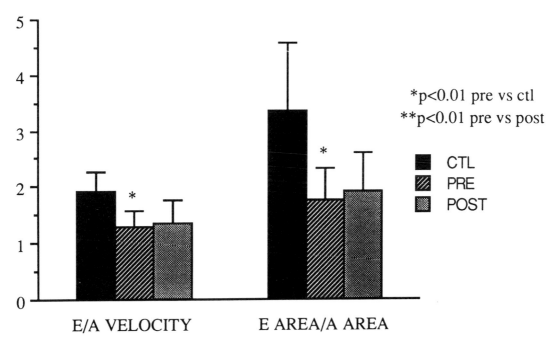

Fig. 24–8. Doppler indexes measured pre- and post-balloon angioplasty in children with either aortic stenosis or coarctation of the aorta. Pre-angioplasty (PRE), the children with left ventricular outflow tract obstruction, had a decrease in the E/A velocity and area ratios compared to control (CTL) children. Post-angioplasty (POST), these abnormal ratios did not change. Reproduced with permission from Meliones JN, et al.: Pulsed Doppler assessment of left ventricular diastolic filling in children with left ventricular outflow obstruction before and after balloon angioplasty. Am J Cardiol 63:231, 1989.

sure overload hypertrophy of the left ventricle, increased wall thickness or mass has been implicated as the cause of impaired left ventricular relaxation. Several studies have shown a significant correlation between the extent of hypertrophy and the severity of the left ventricular diastolic filling abnormality. Right ventricular mass was not assessed in these children because of the lack of an accurate means of measuring it noninvasively; however, all pulmonary stenosis patients had echocardiographic evidence of severe right ventricular hypertrophy. If right ventricular hypertrophy alone were the cause of impaired right ventricular relaxation, regression of right ventricular hypertrophy should be accompanied by a return of diastolic filling patterns toward normal. This question could be addressed in long-term studies of patients who have had successful relief of pulmonary stenosis. Such a study

was recently performed in children who were 8 ± 3 years after successful relief of pulmonary stenosis (46). In this long-term follow-up study, all right ventricular diastolic filling indexes in successfully treated pulmonary stenosis patients improved compared with untreated pulmonary stenosis patients, and approached values found in normal subjects (Table 24–4). These data suggest that right ventricular diastolic filling abnormalities in pulmonary stenosis patients are reversible and are therefore probably related to hypertrophy rather than fibrosis and scarring.

Courtois et al. (47) showed that a pattern of diastolic apex to inflow pressure gradients exists in the right ventricle during early and late diastole, similar to that reported in the left ventricle (8). (See Chapter 10.) In the right ventricle, however, the lowest early diastolic pressures are usually recorded in the outflow tract rather than

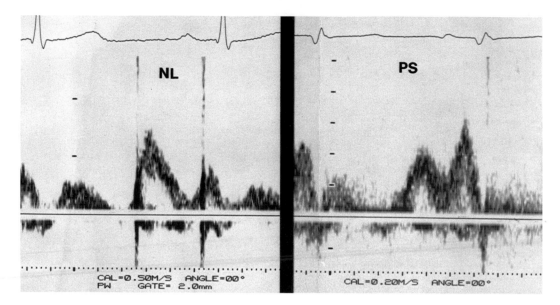

Fig. 24–9. Tricuspid valve Doppler recordings from a patient with pulmonary stenosis (PS) (right) and an age-matched normal (NL) subject (left). Note the increased velocity during atrial contraction and the larger portion of the Doppler curve occurring in late diastole in the patient with PS. Reproduced with permission from Vermilion RP, et al.: Pulsed Doppler evaluation of right ventricular diastolic filling in children with pulmonary valve stenosis before and after balloon valvuloplasty. Am J Cardiol 66:79, 1990.

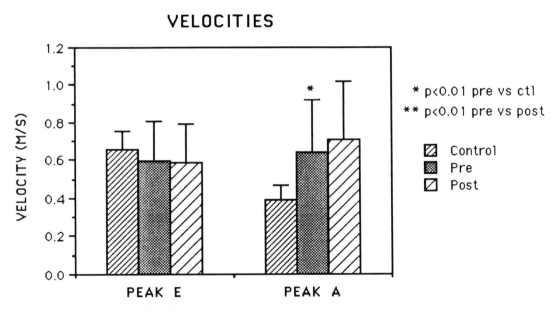

Fig. 24–10. Doppler peak velocities measured in control (ctl) subjects and patients with pulmonary stenosis (PS) before (Pre) and immediately after (Post) balloon valvuloplasty. Abbreviations: A = velocity during atrial contraction, E = velocity during rapid ventricular filling. Reproduced with permission from Vermilion RP, et al.: Pulsed Doppler evaluation of right ventricular diastolic filling in children with pulmonary valve stenosis before and after balloon valvuloplasty. Am J Cardiol 66:79, 1990.

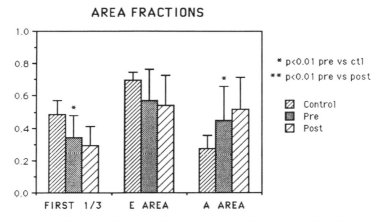

Fig. 24–11. Doppler area fractions in control (ctl) subjects and patients with pulmonary stenosis before (Pre) and immediately after (Post) balloon valvuloplasty. Other abbreviations as in Figure 24–10. Reproduced with permission from Vermilion RP, et al.: Pulsed Doppler evaluation of right ventricular diastolic filling in children with pulmonary valve stenosis before and after balloon valvuloplasty. Am J Cardiol 66:79, 1990.

in the apex. The form and timing of the regional ventricular pressure gradients found in their study suggest that mechanical suction of blood into the ventricular cavity is the primary mechanism of right ventricular filling in early diastole. Mechanisms that probably contribute to mechanical suction include downward motion of the right ventricle during systole, active contraction of muscle fibers below equilibrium and resultant storage of elastic en-

ergy, and end-systolic deformation of the walls of the right ventricular outflow tract. In the latter mechanism, blood continues to leave the ventricle after contraction has ended, thus causing the shape of the right ventricular outflow tract to be distorted, elastic energy to be stored in the myocardium, and the walls of the outflow tract to recoil in early diastole. The importance of this mechanism is supported by the finding of the lowest early diastolic pressure in the

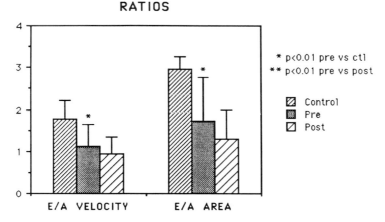

Fig. 24–12. Doppler ratios in control (ctl) subjects and patients with pulmonary stenosis (PS) before (Pre) and immediately after (Post) balloon valvuloplasty. Other abbreviations as in Figure 24–10. Reproduced with permission from Vermilion RP, et al.: Pulsed Doppler evaluation of right ventricular diastolic filling in children with pulmonary valve stenosis before and after balloon valvuloplasty. Am J Cardiol 66:79, 1990.

Table 24–4. Tricuspid Valve Doppler Measurements

Measurement	Control Subjects	PS F/U	PS Pre
Peak E (m/s)	0.63 ± 0.11	0.75 ± 0.14*†	0.59 ± 0.21
Peak A (m/s)	0.38 ± 0.09	0.47 ± 0.09*†	0.64 ± 0.28*
E/A/ vel.	1.74 ± 0.51	1.65 ± 0.33†	1.11 ± 0.52*
Total VTI (m)	0.12 ± 0.02	0.13 ± 0.03	0.12 ± 0.03
0.33 area fx	0.51 ± 0.12	0.52 ± 0.08†	0.34 ± 0.14*
E area fx	0.71 ± 0.08	0.67 ± 0.07	0.57 ± 0.19*
A area fx	0.24 ± 0.10	0.29 ± 0.06†	0.45 ± 0.21*
E/A area	3.50 ± 1.25	2.48 ± 0.82*†	1.73 ± 1.05*
Decel. time(s)	0.14 ± 0.02	0.12 ± 0.02†	0.09 ± 0.04*
PFR/SV (SV/s)	5.23 ± 0.56	5.79 ± 1.08	5.28 ± 1.96
Heart rate (beats/min)	77 ± 13	75 ± 13†	99 ± 27*

* $p < 0.03$ compared with control subjects; † < 0.03 compared with PS pre.
Values are mean ± standard deviation.
A = peak velocity at atrial contraction; E = peak velocity in early diastole; Decel. = deceleration; fx = fraction; F/U = follow-up; PFR/SV = peak filling rate normalized to stroke volume; Pre = untreated; PS = pulmonary stenosis; vel. = velocity; VTI = velocity time integral. Reproduced with permission from Vermilion RP, et al.: Long-term assessment of right ventricular diastolic filling in patients with pulmonic valve stenosis successfully treated in childhood. Am J Cardiol 68:648, 1991.

right ventricular outflow tract and the observation that significant narrowing of the outflow tract occurs at end-systole (47).

In untreated pulmonary stenosis patients, severe right ventricular hypertrophy can lead to reduced end-systolic deformation of the right ventricular outflow tract, less elastic recoil in early diastole, and a higher minimum right ventricular pressure in early diastole. With a higher minimum right ventricular diastolic pressure, the early diastolic pressure gradient and, thus, the peak E velocity are decreased, as has been observed in untreated pulmonary stenosis patients. At long-term follow-up, the return of the peak E velocity and the percentage of filling in early diastole toward normal values suggests that the end-systolic deformation of the outflow tract walls is restored as right ventricular hypertrophy regresses.

In normal subjects, the tricuspid deceleration time is longer than the mitral deceleration time, suggesting that the thin-walled right ventricle is a less effective decelerator than the thicker-walled left ventricle (47). In untreated pulmonary stenosis patients, the tricuspid deceleration time is shortened compared with age-related normal subjects. It is likely that the thick-walled right ventricle of untreated pulmonary stenosis patients quickly generates a reversed pres-

sure gradient of sufficient magnitude to decelerate flow in early diastole. As hypertrophy regresses after successful relief of pulmonary stenosis, the thin-walled right ventricle requires a longer period of time to generate a reverse pressure gradient, and thus the increase in deceleration time to normal values in follow-up pulmonary stenosis patients.

Besides abnormalities of right ventricular diastolic function, infants with isolated severe right ventricular outflow obstruction have been reported to have abnormalities of left ventricular systolic and diastolic function (48). On the mitral valve Doppler examination, these infants have a decreased early filling fraction, increased atrial filling fraction, and decreased E/A area ratio. The decrease in E/A area ratio correlated with the severity of the right ventricular obstruction and the amount of displacement of the septum toward the left ventricular free wall. In several infants evaluated after successful surgical relief of the obstruction, left ventricular geometry and function returned toward normal. These findings indicate that severe right ventricular outflow obstruction in infants can be associated with a reversible alteration in left ventricular function related to abnormal left ventricular geometry and impaired left ventricular diastolic filling.

USES OF DIASTOLIC FILLING INDEXES IN THE MANAGEMENT OF PEDIATRIC HEART DISEASE

Evaluation of Children After Cardiac Surgery

The ability to evaluate noninvasively ventricular systolic and diastolic function has led to improvements in the timing and choice of cardiac surgical procedures in children. For example, children evaluated as long as 4 years after the arterial switch operation for transposition of the great arteries with intact ventricular septum have indices of left ventricular systolic and diastolic function identical to those of age-matched normal children (49). These children were repaired in a single stage approach at a median age of 4 days. Studies performed in survivors of a two-stage approach (initial pulmonary artery banding followed by repair at ages greater than 6 months) have shown diminished left ventricular function (50); therefore, single-stage repair in the neonatal period appears to offer a measurable improvement over the results of two-stage repair, probably related to the early age of definitive surgery (49). Evaluation of ventricular diastolic function in patients long-term after the arterial switch operation has definitely contributed to improved timing and choice of the surgical approach.

Diastolic filling indexes have also been evaluated in another group of postoperative patients, children who have undergone the Fontan operation (51). Compared to age-matched control subjects, the children who had undergone the Fontan procedure had decreased peak E velocity, decreased E/A velocity ratio, decreased E area fraction, increased A area fraction, and decreased E/A area ratio. These diastolic filling abnormalities were consistent with impaired ventricular relaxation and decreased early diastolic transvalvular pressure gradient. In these children, pulmonary artery Doppler recordings showed two distinct patterns of flow. Pattern I showed biphasic forward flow with peak velocities in mid to late systole and mid-diastole. Pattern II showed decreased systolic forward flow, a late systolic to early diastolic flow reversal, and delayed onset of diastolic forward flow. Patients with pat-

tern II pulmonary artery Doppler recordings had significantly lower ejection fraction than those with pattern I pulmonary artery flow. Diastolic filling abnormalities were found in all Fontan patients; however, diastolic filling indexes did not distinguish the two different patterns of pulmonary artery blood flow velocities found in the Fontan patients. These patterns appeared to be strongly influenced by ventricular systolic function, with diminished forward systolic pulmonary flow and delayed onset of forward diastolic flow in patients with a decreased ejection fraction (pattern II). With well-preserved systolic function, biphasic forward pulmonary flow was maintained (pattern I). Several studies have described increased ventricular dimensions and diminished contractility before and after the Fontan operation in patients with a functional single ventricle (52, 53). With dilation and decreased contractility of the ventricle, systolic filling of the atrium is decreased secondary to diminished downward displacement of the atrioventricular valve during ventricular contraction. This results in reduced early diastolic atrial preload, a decreased early diastolic transvalvular pressure gradient, and decreased early ventricular filling. Increased end-systolic ventricular volume also results in decreased early diastolic flow and a shift in filling to late diastole caused by diminished ventricular relaxation and elevated early diastolic ventricular filling pressures.

Choice of Assisted Ventilation in the Intensive Care Unit

The effects of intermittent positive pressure ventilation on right and left ventricular diastolic filling patterns have been evaluated in preterm infants (54). In this study, inspiratory positive pressure varied from 16 to 24 cm H_2O, end-expiratory pressure was 4 cm H_2O, and respiratory rate varied between 21 to 71 breaths/min. Mechanical ventilation produced the opposite effects on transmitral and transtricuspid Doppler recordings to those that occur during spontaneous breathing. Across the mitral valve, peak velocities and area fractions increased during inspiration, whereas, across the tricuspid valve, peak velocities and area fractions decreased during inspiration. Intermittent positive pressure ventilation results in an increase in pleural pressure during inspiration with a resultant decrease in systemic venous return and, hence, diastolic filling of the right ventricle. With inspiration, intra-alveolar pressure increases. This leads to increased pressure in the interalveolar spaces, flushing of blood out of the capillaries into the main venous channels, and increased flow across the mitral valve. Thus, during intermittent positive pressure ventilation, inspiration decreases right ventricular filling and enhances left ventricular filling. Expiration induces opposite effects. This information is particularly useful in predicting the effects of ventilation on cardiac output and interpreting diastolic filling patterns in preterm infants requiring assisted ventilation.

The effects of positive pressure ventilation on ventricular diastolic filling have been compared to those of high-frequency jet ventilation in infants immediately after the arterial switch operation (55). Compared to the inspiratory phase of positive pressure ventilation, nonphasic high frequency jet ventilation resulted in increased tricuspid valve peak E and peak A velocities and decreased mitral valve peak E and peak A velocities. The expiratory phase of positive pressure ventilation and nonphasic high frequency jet ventilation resulted in similar effects on diastolic filling of the two ventricles. Thus, nonphasic high-frequency jet ventilation appeared to augment right heart filling, whereas the inspiratory phase of positive pressure ventilation augments left heart filling. These observations should be extremely important in the appropriate selection of the mode of postoperative ventilation.

FUTURE APPLICATIONS OF DIASTOLIC FILLING INDEXES IN PEDIATRIC HEART DISEASE

Until recently, little information has been available concerning ventricular diastolic function in pediatric heart disease. With the introduction of a noninvasive technique for the serial assessment of global ventricular diastolic function, important observations concerning ventricular diastolic dysfunction in congenital car-

diac defects have emerged. The increased awareness of the importance of diastolic function in overall ventricular performance and the ability to investigate diastolic function safely in children will undoubtedly lead to many important future investigations. For example, the Doppler indices of diastolic filling are ideally suited for assessment of the effects of drug therapy on ventricular function. This application may be important in the evaluation of the effects of cardiotoxic agents such as adriamycin or the evaluation of cardiac support agents such as nitroprusside and dobutamine. In addition, the Doppler indexes of diastolic filling should continue to be of major importance in evaluating the immediate and long term results of cardiac surgeries. For example, small residual arm-leg gradients may be unacceptable in postoperative coarctation patients if these gradients are associated with chronic alterations in left ventricular mass and function, which may predispose to ischemic heart disease in later adulthood. Longitudinal studies of these children are required to understand the impact of residual abnormalities of structure and function found in the late postoperative period (36).

Measurement of ventricular diastolic function should also be of major importance in the future determination of the "natural" and "unnatural" history of congenital heart disease. Besides structural cardiac defects, the Doppler diastolic filling indexes can be expected to be especially useful in determining the cardiac effects of systemic diseases such as diabetes mellitus, collagen vascular disease, and muscular dystrophies. These future investigations of ventricular diastolic function should provide us with information that is essential for improving the diagnostic and therapeutic approach to pediatric heart disease.

REFERENCES

1. Rokey R, et al.: Determination of parameters of left ventricular diastolic filling with pulsed Doppler echocardiography: Comparison with cineangiography. Circulation 71:543, 1985.
2. Snider AR, et al.: Doppler evaluation of left ventricular diastolic filling in children with systemic hypertension. Am J Cardiol 56: 921, 1985.

3. Spirito P, Maron BJ, Bonow RO: Noninvasive assessment of left ventricular diastolic function: Comparative analysis of Doppler echocardiographic and radionuclide angiographic techniques. J Am Coll Cardiol 7:518, 1986.

4. Fuji J, et al.: Noninvasive assessment of left and right ventricular filling in myocardial infarction with a two-dimensional Doppler echocardiographic method. J Am Coll Cardiol 5:1155, 1985.

5. Spirito P, et al.: Noninvasive assessment of left ventricular diastolic function: Comparative analysis of pulsed Doppler ultrasound and digitized M-mode echocardiography. Am J Cardiol 58:837, 1986.

6. Friedman BJ, et al.: Assessment of left ventricular diastolic function: Comparison of Doppler echocardiography and gated blood pool scintigraphy. J Am Coll Cardiol 8:1348, 1986.

7. Pearson AC, Goodgold H, Labovitz AJ: Comparison of pulsed Doppler echocardiography and radionuclide angiography in the assessment of left ventricular filling. Am J Cardiol 61:446, 1988.

8. Appleton CP, Hatle LK, Popp RL: Relation of transmitral flow velocity patterns to left ventricular diastolic function: New insights from a combined hemodynamic and Doppler echocardiographic study. J Am Coll Cardiol 12:426, 1988.

9. Wind BE, et al.: Pulsed Doppler assessment of left ventricular diastolic filling in patients with coronary artery disease before and immediately after coronary angioplasty. Am J Cardiol 59:1041, 1987.

10. Kitabatake A, et al.: Transmitral blood flow reflecting diastolic behavior of the left ventricle in health and disease: A study by pulsed Doppler technique. Jpn Circ J 46:92, 1982.

11. Miyatake K, et al.: Augmentation of atrial contribution to left ventricular inflow with aging as assessed by intracardiac Doppler flowmetry. Am J Cardiol 53:586, 1984.

12. Takenaka K, et al.: Left ventricular filling in hypertrophic cardiomyopathy: A pulsed Doppler echocardiographic study. J Am Coll Cardiol 7:1263, 1986.

13. Pearson AC, et al.: Left ventricular diastolic function in weight lifters. Am J Cardiol 58:1254, 1986.

14. Bowman LK, et al.: Peak filling rate normalized to mitral stroke volume: A new Doppler echocardiographic filling index validated by radionuclide angiographic technique. J Am Coll Cardiol 12:937, 1988.

15. Reed KL, et al.: Doppler echocardiographic studies of diastolic function in the human fetal heart: changes during gestation. J Am Coll Cardiol 8:391, 1986.

16. Kenny JF, et al.: Changes in intracardiac blood flow velocities and right and left ventricular stroke volumes with gestational age in the normal human fetus: a prospective Doppler echocardiographic study. Circulation 74:1208, 1986.

17. Reed KL, et al.: Cardiac Doppler flow velocities in human fetuses. Circulation 73:41, 1986.

18. Wladimiroff JW, Huisman TWA, Stewart PA: Fetal cardiac flow velocities in the late 1st trimester of pregnancy: A transvaginal Doppler study. J Am Coll Cardiol 17:1357, 1991.

19. Romero T, Covell J, Friedman WF: A comparison of pressure-volume relations of the fetal, newborn and adult heart. Am J Physiol 222:1285, 1972.

20. Heymann MA: Fetal and neonatal circulations. *In* Heart Diseases in Infants, Children, and Adolescents. Edited by FH Adams, GC Emmanouilides, TA Riemenschneider. Baltimore, Williams & Wilkins, 1989.

21. Riggs TW, et al.: Doppler echocardiographic evaluation of right and left ventricular diastolic function in normal neonates. J Am Coll Cardiol 13:700, 1989.

22. Areias JC, Meyer R, Scott WA, Goldberg SJ: Serial echocardiographic and Doppler evaluation of left ventricular diastolic filling in full-term neonates. Am J Cardiol 66:108, 1990.

23. Johnson GL, Moffett CB, Noonan JA: Doppler echocardiographic studies of diastolic ventricular filling patterns in premature infants. Am Heart J 116:1568, 1988.

24. Voutilainen S, et al.: Factors influencing Doppler indexes of left ventricular filling in healthy persons. Am J Cardiol 68:653, 1991.

25. Snider AR, Serwer GA: Echocardiography in Pediatric Heart Disease. Chicago, Year Book Medical Publishers, Inc., 1990.

26. Holmgren SM, Goldberg SJ, Donnerstein RL: Influence of age, body size and heart rate on left ventricular diastolic indexes in young subjects. Am J Cardiol 68:1245, 1991.

27. Harrison MR, et al.: Effect of heart rate on left ventricular diastolic transmitral flow velocity patterns assessed by Doppler echocardiography in normal subjects. Am J Cardiol 67:622, 1991.

28. Van Dam I, et al.: Normal diastolic filling patterns of the left ventricle. Eur Heart J 9:165, 1988.

29. Smith SA, et al.: Transmitral velocities mea-

sured by pulsed Doppler in healthy volunteers: effects of acute changes in blood pressure and heart rate. Br Heart J 61:344, 1989.

30. Appleton CP, Carucci MJ, Henry CP, Olajos M: Influence of incremental changes in heart rate on mitral flow velocity: Assessment in lightly sedated, conscious dogs. J Am Coll Cardiol 17:227, 1991.

31. Appleton CP, Hatle LK, Popp RL: Cardiac tamponade and pericardial effusion: Respiratory variation in transvalvular flow velocities studied by Doppler echocardiography. J Am Coll Cardiol 11:1020, 1988.

32. Dabestani A, et al.: Effects of spontaneous respiration on diastolic left ventricular filling assessed by pulsed Doppler echocardiography. Am J Cardiol 61:1356, 1988.

33. Riggs TW, Snider AR: Respiratory influence on right and left ventricular diastolic function in normal children. Am J Cardiol 63:858, 1989.

34. Gidding SS, et al.: Left ventricular diastolic filling in children with hypertrophic cardiomyopathy: Assessment with pulsed Doppler echocardiography. J Am Coll Cardiol 8:310, 1986.

35. Meliones JN, et al.: Pulsed Doppler assessment of left ventricular diastolic filling in children with left ventricular outflow obstruction before and after balloon angioplasty. Am J Cardiol 63:231, 1989.

36. Moskowitz WB, Schieken RM, Mosteller M, Bossano R: Altered systolic and diastolic function in children after "successful" repair of coarctation of the aorta. Am Heart J 120:103, 1990.

37. Fifer MA, Borow KM, Colan SD, Lorell BH: Early diastolic left ventricular function in children and adults with aortic stenosis. J Am Coll Cardiol 5:1147, 1985.

38. Eichhorn P, et al.: Left ventricular relaxation in patients with left ventricular hypertrophy secondary to aortic valve disease. Circulation 65:1395, 1982.

39. Murakami T, et al.: Diastolic filling dynamics in patients with aortic stenosis. Circulation 73:1162, 1986.

40. Lorell BH, Grossman W: Cardiac hypertrophy: the consequences for diastole. J Am Coll Cardiol 9:1189, 1987.

41. Colan SD, Sanders SP, McPherson D, Borow KM: Left ventricular diastolic function in elite athletes with physiologic cardiac hypertrophy. J Am Coll Cardiol 6:545, 1985.

42. Zoghbi WA, Habib GB, Quinones MA: Doppler assessment of right ventricular filling in a normal population. Circulation 82:1316, 1990.

43. Berman GO, Reichek N, Brownson D, Douglas PS: Effects of sample volume location, imaging view, heart rate and age on tricuspid velocimetry in normal subjects. Am J Cardiol 65:1026, 1990.

44. Vermilion RP, et al.: Pulsed Doppler evaluation of right ventricular diastolic filling in children with pulmonary valve stenosis before and after balloon valvuloplasty. Am J Cardiol 66:79, 1990.

45. Lorell BH, Grossman W: Cardiac hypertrophy: The consequences for diastole. J Am Coll Cardiol 9:1189, 1987.

46. Vermilion RP, Snider AR, Bengur AR, Meliones JN: Long-term assessment of right ventricular diastolic filling in patients with pulmonic valve stenosis successfully treated in childhood. Am J Cardiol 68:648, 1991.

47. Courtois M, Barzilai B, Gutierrez F, Ludbrook PA: Characterization of regional diastolic pressure gradients in the right ventricle. Circulation 82:1413, 1990.

48. Sholler GF, Colan SD, Sanders SP: Effect of isolated ventricular outflow obstruction on left ventricular function in infants. Am J Cardiol 62:778, 1988.

49. Colan SD, et al.: Myocardial performance after arterial switch operation for transposition of the great arteries with intact ventricular septum. Circulation 78:132, 1988.

50. Borow KM, et al.: Assessment of left ventricular contractile state after anatomic correction of transposition of the great arteries. Circulation 69:106, 1984.

51. Frommelt PC, Snider AR, Meliones JN, Vermilion RP: Doppler assessment of pulmonary artery flow patterns and ventricular function after the Fontan operation. Am J Cardiol 68:1211, 1991.

52. Gewillig MH, et al.: Impact of Fontan operation on left ventricular size and contractility in tricuspid atresia. Circulation 81:118, 1990.

53. Nakae S, et al.: Assessment of left ventricular function before and after Fontan's operation for the correction of tricuspid atresia. Heart Vessels 1:83, 1985.

54. Maroto E, et al.: Effect of intermittent positive pressure ventilation on diastolic filling patterns in premature infants. J Am Coll Cardiol 16:171, 1990.

55. Meliones JN, et al.: Effects of ventilation on diastolic filling after cardiac surgery. J Am Coll Cardiol 19:52A, 1992.

Chapter 25

CARDIAC EFFECTS OF AGING AND DIASTOLIC DYSFUNCTION IN THE ELDERLY

J. V. Nixon and Carolyn A. Burns

The principle that aging, accompanied by a more sedentary lifestyle, produces a decline in the functional capabilities of the human body is well accepted (1). From a cardiovascular perspective, changes in the structure and function of the heart and the peripheral vasculature are seen (1, 2). Left ventricular function is ultimately the most important measure of the effect of aging on myocardial tissue structure and functional capabilities, together with its responses to hormonal and other physiologic interventions (3). Furthermore, changes in other organ systems associated with aging may significantly affect cardiac performance.

In this chapter, we will review the structural and functional changes that occur in the myocardium with age, together with the altered responses to hormonal and other physiologic influences. Many changes documented in experimental studies are difficult to duplicate in humans because of the inability to obtain invasive measurements of cardiac function in a normal population. Furthermore, the rate of aging varies individually, including the aging rate of the cardiovascular system. Thus human studies, particularly of smaller numbers of subjects, may produce variable findings. Nevertheless, in reviewing the literature, it is possible to define to some degree the specific changes in cardiac structure and function that can be anticipated in a normal older population. This may provide an anatomic and physiologic baseline that can be used for the management of the older cardiovascular patient.

ALTERATIONS IN STRUCTURE

A gradual increase in cardiac weight is associated with aging (4). Histologic reports of experimental studies have identified an age-related loss of cardiac myocytes in association with an increase in fibrous tissue (5) (see Chapter 8). Both of these findings have been documented in humans in association with muscular hypertrophy. Furthermore, a series of human endomyocardial biopsies have shown an age-related increase in left ventricular mass that is principally caused by a cellular hypertrophy rather than hyperplasia (6). This latter finding is similar to findings in patients with valvular disease or hypertension.

The advent of noninvasive cardiac imaging techniques has permitted the detailed study of cardiac structure and function in humans of all ages. Echocardiography has provided further documentation of increasing left ventricular mass and wall thickness associated with age (7, 8) (Fig. 25–1). The Baltimore Longitudinal Study on Aging, in its large series of normal subjects of wide age range, has provided further details of anatomic changes associated with age (7, 9). In addition to confirming the increase in left ventricular mass and wall thickness, the study has shown evidence of aortic root dilation and left atrial enlargement. It has been suggested that these anatomic changes are adaptive responses to the alterations in cardiac function and the peripheral vasculature that are associated with the normal process of aging, including increased systolic arterial pressure, increased aortic impedance and altered left ventricular diastolic compliance. Furthermore, there are some features that remain unchanged, including cardiac volumes and ejection fraction (Table 25–1).

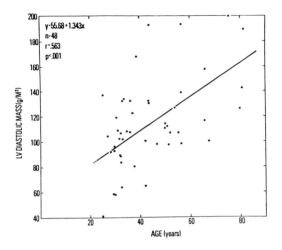

Fig. 25–1. Increasing diastolic left ventricular wall thickness associated with increasing age in the Baltimore Longitudinal Study on Aging. Reproduced with permission from Federation Proceedings from Lakatta EG: Alterations in the cardiovascular system that occur with advanced age. Fed Proc 38:163, 1979.

ALTERATIONS IN FUNCTION

Experimental Changes

Most of the cellular alterations associated with aging have been studied experimentally in rat and dog models. Several changes have been found, including a prolongation of contraction duration and relaxation, both of which are partially dependent on cellular calcium transport (5, 10, 11). In senescent rats, it has been shown that the calcium transient is prolonged, principally because of a diminished rate of calcium pumping by the sarcoplasmic reticulum (10–14). This reduction in the rate of cal-

Table 25–1.   Structural Changes in the Aging Heart

Microscopic changes
   Decreased myocytes
   Fibrous tissue proliferation
   Cellular hypertrophy
Macroscopic changes
   Increased cardiac weight
   Increased left ventricular wall mass
   Left ventricular hypertrophy
   Left atrial dilatation
   Aortic root enlargement

cium uptake by the sarcoplasmic reticulum leads to prolonged calcium-myofilament interaction, thereby contributing to the prolongation of contraction and relaxation. The prolongation of contraction with aging has also been shown in both canine and human studies (15, 16).

The prolongation of contraction duration and relaxation is associated with an increase in resting and dynamic stiffness. These findings have been reported in the isolated rat muscle as well as in intact canine hearts (13, 15). Furthermore, both the prolongation of contraction duration and the increase in dynamic stiffness in rats have been shown to be prevented by a chronic exercise program (17). Sarcoplasmic reticulum calcium transport increases with physical training, as does cellular relaxation, perhaps explaining the improvement in dynamic stiffness and normalization of contraction duration seen (18, 19). Aging is also associated with a change in myocardial ATP-ase activity, although the degree to which this alteration affects dynamic stiffness and contraction duration is difficult to ascertain because all these components of muscle function are interrelated and associated with calcium transport (17, 20). These findings suggest that the decline in the various functional parameters is not simply a function of aging per se, but may be the result of an interaction between aging and lifestyle, and therefore potentially modifiable (21).

Autonomic Changes

It has been known for some years that age alters the cardiac responses to various autonomic influences (22–25). In experimental studies, although the effects of beta-adrenergic agonists to shorten contraction duration is not age-related, it has been shown that their ability to enhance contractile force is reduced (22, 26). In human studies, plasma levels of both norepinephrine and epinephrine are higher in the elderly (27). Although alpha-adrenergic stimulation is unaffected by age, it is evident that the response to beta-adrenergic stimulation is attenuated (28). For example, a bolus infusion of isoproterenol produces a small increase in heart rate in older healthy men aged 62 and 80 years

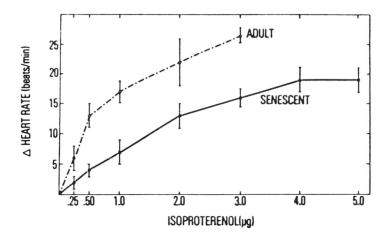

Fig. 25–2. Effects of a bolus infusion of isoproterenol on the heart rates of healthy older men and young adult controls. Reproduced with permission from Federation Proceedings from Lakatta EG: Alterations in the cardiovascular system that occur with advanced age. Fed Proc 38:163, 1979.

compared to young adult controls (Fig. 25–2) (5, 29).

Guarnieri et al. have shown that both the number of myocardial beta-adrenergic receptors and their affinity for agonists or antagonists are unaltered by age (26). Furthermore, basal levels of cyclic adenosine monophosphate and levels during peak contractile response are unaffected by age. It appears that the diminished myocardial response to beta-adrenergic stimulation is postsynaptic, and it has been suggested that the differences are in the extent or activity of protein phosphorylation (26).

Autonomic responsiveness, or lack thereof, would be exaggerated during exercise, and further detailed during adrenergic blockade. Conway et al. have shown that the difference in cardiac output between young and elderly men at comparative workloads during dynamic exercise was significantly less after beta-adrenergic blockade, suggesting that beta-stimulation is more effective in younger individuals (30). Thus, it may be concluded that autonomic nervous system function diminishes with advancing age, and this diminishing function may be compensated for by other age-related changes such as a decline in baroreceptor sensitivity.

Changes in the Intact Human Heart

It is not clear how many of the cellular changes identified in in vitro and in vivo animal models may be applied to the aged human heart. Most of the information on the aged human heart is a result of the non-invasive evaluation of a "normal" elderly population (7–9). Such information is obviously limited by indirect gross measurements and the fact that it is difficult to be certain that the population studied does not have subclinical disease or is a selected population based on survival. As previously described, simple changes in lifestyle may significantly alter microscopic cellular as well as macroscopic organ system function. Nevertheless, several unique observations can be made regarding the function of the older human heart.

Systolic function is maintained in the older human heart, both at rest and with exercise. This has been shown by studies on normal subjects enrolled in the Baltimore Longitudinal Study on Aging (7, 9). In this well-screened population, no differences in cardiac output, ejection fraction, or end-diastolic and end-systolic volumes were present at rest according to age (7). During exercise, cardiac output and ejection fraction were maintained with advancing age (9, 31) (Fig. 25–3). This was accomplished by an increase in end-systolic and end-diastolic volumes, in the presence of the well-known attenuated heart rate response to exercise that occurs with increasing age (32). In physiologic terms, this represents an enhanced dependence on the Frank-Starling mechanism, and differs from the conventional increase in both heart rate and stroke volume that occurs in younger individuals. Thus, despite different physiologic mechanisms, older subjects are able to increase their cardiac output during exercise.

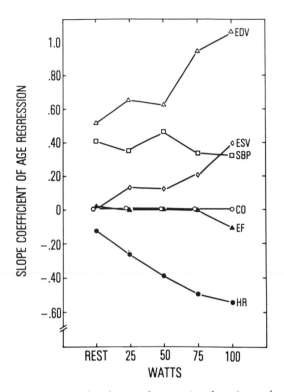

Fig. 25–3. The slopes of regression functions of age for end-diastolic volume (EDV), end-systolic volume (ESV), systolic blood pressure (SBP), cardiac output (CO), ejection fraction (EF), and heart rate (HR) at rest and at increasing incremental workloads from 25 to 100 W during dynamic exercise in the Baltimore Longitudinal Study on Aging. Reproduced with permission from Circulation from Rodeheffer RJ, et al.: Exercise cardiac output is maintained with advancing age in healthy human subjects: Cardiac dilatation and increased stroke volume compensate for diminished heart rate. Circulation 69:203, 1984.

In contrast, diastolic function as estimated by compliance has been shown to deteriorate in experimental studies (15, 16, 33, 34). Unfortunately, diastolic function or compliance is not as amenable to noninvasive measurements as systolic function. However, several indirect parameters of diastolic function have been shown to be altered with age. Table 25–2 provides a partial listing of the effects of aging on the characteristics of left ventricular filling in humans.

One indirect measure of diastolic function is left ventricular diastolic filling. The ratio of early (E) to late (A) filling velocities,

as determined by Doppler echocardiography and the ratio of the time-velocity integrals of the early and late Doppler spectral pattern have been evaluated in the elderly (35–39, 40–45). It is not clear what aspects of diastolic function these indirect measurements reflect; however, they probably represent multiple components of diastole (see Chapter 12). Bryg et al. found that the E/A ratio was significantly lower in older subjects (aged 50 to 68) compared to younger controls (35) (Fig. 25–4). In addition, they found an increase in the diameter of the late diastolic jet, by color flow analysis, with age. Taken together, their results suggest that there is an increase in the volume of blood that crosses the mitral valve in late diastole. Thus, with aging, there appears to be an exaggerated reliance on atrial systole. Other investigators have found alterations in early and late mitral inflow velocities in older normal subjects. Spirito and Maron evaluated 86 normal volunteers, aged 20 to 74 years, with regard to six Doppler indices of diastolic function (36). They found that five of the six indices, including duration of isovolumic relaxation, maximal late diastolic flow velocity, maximal early diastolic flow velocity, rate of early flow velocity deceleration, and the ratio of peak early and late

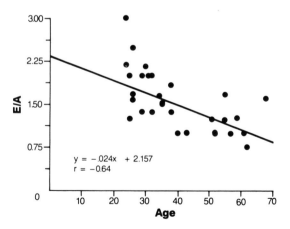

Fig. 25–4. Relationship between the Doppler echocardiographic ratio of early (E) to late (A) diastolic velocity and increasing in age. Reproduced with permission from the American Journal of Cardiology from Bryg RJ, Williams GA, Labovitz AJ: Effect of aging on left ventricular diastolic filling in normal subjects. Am J Cardiol 59:971, 1987.

Table 25–2. Left Ventricular Diastolic Filling Characteristics Related to Increasing Age, Assessed by Doppler Echocardiography and Radionuclide Ventriculography

Author	Ref.	No. of Subjects	Age	Screening	Findings
Doppler Echocardiography					
1. Bryg et al.	35	32	20–68	History, echo	↙EFD, ↙E/A
2. Spirito et al.	36	86	20–74	History, echo	↗IVRT, ↙E/A
3. Miyatake et al.	37	69	22–69	History, PE, ECG	↙E, ↙E/A
4. Swinne	38	48	45–69	History, echo	↙E/A, ↗AFF
5. Kuo et al.	39	41	20–80	History, echo	↗AFF
Radionuclide Ventriculography					
6. Arora et al.	40	13	68–86	History, PE, echo	↙PFR, ↗TPFR, ↗%AFV
7. Bonow et al.	41	66	19–77	History, PE Echo Stress Test	↙PFR, ↗TPFR ↙% early total filling
8. Iskandrian et al.	42	65	20–75	History	↙PFR
9. Miller et al.	43	30	20–80	History	↙PFR

E = early peak flow velocity rate, A = late peak flow velocity color Doppler, AFF = atrial filling fraction, E/A = ratio of early to late peak velocities, IVRT = isovolumic relaxation time, PFR = peak filling rate, TPFR = time to peak filling, EFD = early flow diameter, ECG = electrocardiogram, PE = physical examination, CATH = cardiac catheterization

flow velocities correlated significantly with age. The best index to correlate with age was the peak late diastolic flow velocity (r = 0.69) (Fig. 25–5). The correlation of these

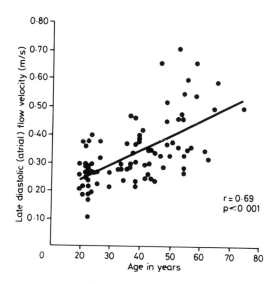

Fig. 25–5. Relationship between Doppler echocardiographic peak late diastolic (atrial) flow velocity and increasing age. Reproduced with permission from the British Heart Journal from Spirito P, Maron BJ: Influence of aging on Doppler echocardiographic indices of left ventricular function. Br Heart J 59:673, 1988.

alterations persisted after a multivariate regression analysis was done to control for the effects of left ventricular wall thickness, cavity dimension, systolic shortening, and heart rate. Kitzman and associates described an increase in atrial filling and a decrease in early filling which was independent of left ventricular mass or pulmonary capillary wedge pressure (44). Nixon et al. found a resting alteration in E/A ratio and atrial filling fraction in older subjects, and with an increase in preload by 5 degrees of head-down tilt, this alteration was reduced, mostly caused by a decrease in the atrial time-velocity integral (45). The authors suggested that such a change with augmented preload could be best explained by an intrinsic increase in left ventricular stiffness, rather than by altered relaxation.

Similarly, radionuclide gated blood pool scanning techniques have been used to evaluate the effects of age on diastolic left ventricular filling rates (40–43, 46) (See Chapter 11). Gerstenblith et al. found that the peak filling rate declined with age at rest, but this age-related decline was absent during exercise (46). The authors suggested that the effect of catecholamines on diastolic left ventricular relaxation is not affected by age. However, as pointed out by Miller and colleagues, peak filling rate reflects both the rate of relaxation and the degree of inherent stiffness of the left ventricle (43). Iskandrian and Hakki did similar studies on 65 individuals, 28 of whom had hypertension (42). As a group, the older subjects (over 50 years) had a reduced peak filling rate, both at rest and with exercise, compared to younger subjects. When the group members without hypertension were evaluated separately, the differences in peaking filling rates at rest and with exercise showed the same trend though statistical significance was not reached. Thus, the degree to which early left ventricular filling, measured by either Doppler echocardiography or radionuclide ventriculography, can discern the different altered components of diastolic function in the aging heart is not clear. Furthermore, several investigators have noted how these measurements may be altered by changes in left atrial pressure, afterload, heart rate, and contractility (24, 25, 45, 47, 48) (see Chapter 13).

An evaluation of the response of the aged heart to preload changes was done by Nixon et al. in 11 disease-free subjects, aged 61 to 73 years (49). These older hearts showed a physiologic response to increases and decreases in preload; that is, stroke volume changed in proportion to changes in end-diastolic volume. The older subjects had larger resting left ventricular volumes and the percentages of change in both end-diastolic and stroke volumes with the two preload altering maneuvers of 5 degrees of head-down tilt and graded lower body negative pressure were smaller when compared to younger controls (20 to 25 years) (Fig. 25–6). These results suggest that an alteration in diastolic performance in the older heart may not be directly related to an alteration in end-diastolic volume. Furthermore, left ventricular wall stress remained unchanged throughout the different interventions.

The observation in this study of increased end-diastolic volumes in older compared to younger subjects differs from other studies such as the evaluation by Downes et al. of 11 elderly patients determined at cardiac catheterization to be free of cardiac disease (50). Measurements of end-diastolic pressure and volume, the latter by constant ventriculography, showed that the older patients had significantly higher left ventricular end-diastolic pressures in the presence of smaller end-diastolic volumes.

Clearly, the anatomic and physiologic findings in the older human heart depend on the characteristics of the subject population. Indeed, it is conceivable that there may be no physiologically normal older population. Acknowledging the principle that each individual ages at a different rate, chronologic aging should not be directly related to anatomic physiologic aging. Nevertheless, it is reasonable to attempt to establish the constant cardiovascular changes associated with aging.

ASSOCIATED CHANGES WITH CARDIAC EFFECTS

In outlining the structural and functional changes associated with aging of the

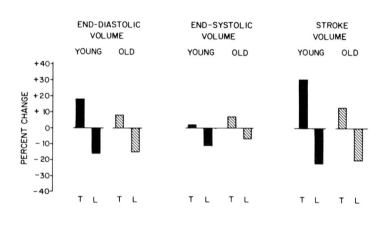

Fig. 25–6. Percentage of changes in left ventricular end-diastolic, end-systolic, and stroke volumes from control baseline values during 90 minutes of 5 degrees head-down tilt (T) and graded lower body negative pressure (L) in young (solid bars) versus old (hatched bars) normal subjects. Reproduced with permission from the American Journal of Cardiology from Nixon JV, et al.: Ventricular performance in human hearts aged 61 to 73 years. Am J Cardiol 56:932, 1985.

heart, it is critical to point out that these changes occur in the setting of an aging vascular system as well as other organ system changes. Such alterations in related systems exert a significant effect on cardiac function.

The altered cardiac responses to various anatomic influences associated with increasing age have already been discussed. In addition to altered cardiac responses, changes associated with age occur in both systemic vascular anatomy and reflex responses, including both high and low pressor baroreceptor activity. There is a significant linear decrease in peripheral vascular distensibility, attributed to a change in vascular connective tissue elasticity or an increase in the prevalence of atherosclerosis or both (51, 52). Alpha-adrenergic responsiveness appears to be unchanged with age (53, 54). However, there is abundant evidence to show that beta-adrenergic responsiveness is attentuated by age, changes that appear to be confined to the sympathetic nervous system (42, 54, 55). Thus it has been suggested that the increased peripheral vascular resistance seen in the elderly is caused partly by an imbalance of alpha and beta-adrenergic vascular tone (56).

Both renal blood flow and glomerular filtration rate diminish with age (57, 58). Plasma renin activity decreases with age (58). However, plasma nonepinephrine levels increase with increasing age (57). It has been suggested that these increases are related to the gradual reduction in beta-adrenergic responsiveness associated with aging (58). Although intravascular volume appears to be maintained in older normal individuals, the older heart appears more sensitive to relatively smaller changes in intravascular volume than younger subjects (49).

Changes in the peripheral vasculature as well as other organ systems that are related to aging affect overall cardiac structure and function in an older population. They make significant contributions to the cardiac performance of the older heart, affecting both preload and afterload characteristics.

SUMMARY

It is evident that there is a sequence of changes in cardiac structure and function with increasing age. Furthermore, there is no doubt that, in a normal aging population, left ventricular systolic function is preserved while diastolic function deteriorates. Comprehensive studies of a normal aging population have been limited by a number of factors, especially the individual variation in rates of aging and the inability of noninvasive cardiac imaging techniques to precisely measure left ventricular compliance. Nevertheless, it is clear that a series of anatomic and physiologic changes are associated with the older heart, thus providing a baseline against which the older cardiovascular patients may be compared.

Anatomic changes occur in adaptive response to the increased systolic arterial pressure, aortic impedance, and altered left ventricular diastolic compliance that is found with age. Increased cardiac weight and left ventricular hypertrophy, with dilation of the aortic root and the left atrium, have been reported.

Physiologic changes at the cellular level include prolonged contraction duration and relaxation time and diminished response to digitalis glycosides, norepinephrine, and isoproterenol. Human studies have shown that systolic function is preserved both at rest and during exercise. Ejection fraction, cardiac output, and left ventricular wall stress all remain unchanged. Furthermore, cardiac output increase is maintained during exercise, albeit by the different mechanism of an increased Frank-Starling effect in the presence of the age-related attentuated heart rate response to increasing exercise.

Diastolic function clearly deteriorates with age. The experimental documentation of altered compliance in the older heart has been difficult to duplicate in an older normal population. Nevertheless, it is clear that there are consistent changes in noninvasive parameters associated with altered left ventricular compliance both at rest and during various physiologic and pharmacologic interventions that are consistent with changes in diastolic function in older normal subjects.

It is evident that further investigation is required to more clearly document the cause and temporal sequence of changes in diastolic function with age. Questions remain regarding the effects of aging on left ventricular compliance involve genetic inheritance, rates of structural alteration, and the effects of gradual physiologic deconditioning. These are important issues for future research.

REFERENCES

1. Shock NW: Physiological aspects of aging in man. Ann Rev Physiol 23:97, 1961.
2. Befitis H, Sargent F: Human physiological adaptability through the life sequence. J Geront 32:402, 1977.
3. Weisfeldt ML: Left ventricular function. *In* the Aging Heart. Edited by ML Weisfeldt. New York, Raven Press, 1980, p. 297.
4. Linzbach AJ, Aknamoa-Boateng E: Dis alernsversanderungen des wenschlichen vcerzens. 1. Das verzgenwicht in alter. Klin Wochensk 51:156, 1973.
5. Lakatta EG: Alterations in the cardiovascular system that occur with advanced age. Fed Proc 38:163, 1979.
6. Unverforth DV, et al.: Human myocardial histologic characteristics in congestive heart failure. Circulation 68:1194, 1983.
7. Gerstenblith G, et al.: Echocardiographic assessment of a normal adult aging population. Circulation 56:273, 1977.
8. Gardin JM, et al.: Echocardiographic measurements in normal subjects: evaluation of an adult population without clinically apparent heart disease. J Clin Ultrasound 7:439, 1979.
9. Rodeheffer RJ, et al.: Exercise cardiac output is maintained with advancing age in healthy human subjects: Cardiac dilatation and increased stroke volume compensate for diminished heart rate. Circulation 69:203, 1984.
10. Lakatta EG, et al.: Prolonged contraction duration in aged myocardium. J Clin Invest 55:61, 1975.
11. Templeton GH, Willerson JT, Platt MR, Weisfeldt ML: Contraction duration and diastolic stiffness in aged canine left ventricle. *In* Recent Advances in Studies on Cardiac Structure and Metabolism, Volume II. Heart Function and Metabolism. Edited by Kobayashi T, Sano T, Dhallo T. Baltimore, University Park Press, 1978.
12. Caverto FV, Kelliher GJ, Roberts J: Electrophysiological changes in the rate atrium with age. Am J Physiol 225:1293, 1974.
13. Spurgeon HA, et al.: Increased dynamic stiffness of trabeculae carnaae from senescent rats. Am J Physiol 232:373, 1977.
14. Froelich JP, et al.: Studies of sarcoplasmic reticulum function and contraction duration in young adult and aged rat myocardiums. J Mol Cell Cardiol 10:427, 1978.
15. Templeton GH, Platt MR, Willerson JT, Weisfeldt ML: Influence of aging on left ventricular hemodynamics and stiffness in beagles. Circ Res 44:189, 1979.
16. Harrison FR, et al.: The relation of age to the duration of contraction, ejection and relaxation of the normal heart. Am Heart J 67:189, 1964.
17. Spurgeon HA, Steinbach MF, and Lakatta EG: Chronic exercise prevents characteristic age-related changed in rat cardiac contraction. Am J Physiol 244:H513, 1983.
18. Penpargkul S, Repke DI, Katz AM, Sheuer J: Effect of physical training on calcium transport by rat cardiac sarcoplasmic reticulum. Circ Res 40:134, 1977.
19. Bersolm MM, Scheuer J: Effects of physical training on end-diastolic volumes and myocardial performance of isolated rat hearts. Circ Res 40:510, 1977.
20. Alpert NR, Gale HH, and Taylor N: The effect of age on contractile protein ATPase activity and the velocity of shortening. *In* Factors Influencing Myocardial Contractility. Edited by F Kavaler, RD Tanz, J Roberts. New York, Academic Press, 1967, pp. 127–133.
21. Lakatta EG, Spurgeon HA: Effect of exercise on cardiac muscle performance in aged rats. Fed Proc 46:1844, 1987.
22. Lakatta EG, et al.: Diminished inotropic response of aged myocardium to catecholamines. Circ Res 36:262–269, 1979.
23. Gestenblith G, et al.: Diminished inotropic responsiveness to ouabain in aged rat myocardium. Circ Res 44:517, 1979.
24. Pickering TG, et al.: Effects of autonomic blockade on the baroreflex in man at rest and during exercise. Circ Res 30:177, 1972.
25. Sanchez E, Sweeney M, Nixon JV: Effects of isoproterenol and phenylephrine on cardiac function in the older normal heart. Clin Res 34:174, 1986.
26. Guarnieri T, et al.: Contractile and biochemical correlates of beta-adrenergic stimulation of the aged heart. Am J Physiol 239:H501, 1980.
27. Pfeifer MA, et al.: Differential changes of autonomic nervous system function with age in man. Am J Med 76:249, 1983.
28. Pan HY, Hoffman BB, Pershe RA, Blaschke TF: Decline in beta-adrenergic receptor mediated vascular relaxation with aging in man. J Pharmacol Exp Ther 39:802, 1986.
29. Lakatta EG: Age related alterations in the cardiovascular to adrenergic mediated stress. Fed Proc 39:P3173, 1980.

30. Conway J, Wheeler R, Hammerstedt R: Sympathetic nervous activity during exercise in relation to age. Cardiovasc Res 5: 577, 1976.

31. Fleg JL: Alterations in cardiovascular structure and function with advancing age. Am J Cardiol 57:33C, 1986.

32. Schlant RC, et al.: Guidelines for exercise testing. J Am Coll Cardiol 8:725, 1986.

33. Lee JC, Karpeles LM, Downing SE: Age-related changes in cardiac performance of male rats. Am J Physiol 222:432, 1972.

34. Yin FCP, Weisfeldt ML, Milnor WR: Role of aortic input impedance in the decreased cardiovascular response to exercise with aging in dogs. J Clin Invest 68:28, 1981.

35. Bryg RJ, Williams GA, Labovitz AJ: Effect of aging on left ventricular diastolic filling in normal subjects. Am J Cardiol 59:971, 1987.

36. Spirito P, Maron BJ: Influence of aging on Doppler echocardiographic indices of left ventricular function. Br Heart J 59:673, 1988.

37. Miyatake K, et al.: Augmentation of atrial contribution to left ventricular inflow with aging as assessed by intracardiac Doppler flowmetry. Am J Cardiol 53:586, 1984.

38. Lakatta EG: The aging heart. Ann Intern. Med 113:465, 1990.

39. Kuo LC, et al.: Quantification of atrial contribution to left ventricular filling by pulsed Doppler echocardiography and the effect of age in normal and diseased hearts. Am J Cardiol 58:1174, 1987.

40. Arora RR, et al.: Atrial kinetics and left ventricular diastolic filling in the healthy elderly. J Am Coll Cardiol 9:1255, 1987.

41. Bonow RO, et al.: Effects of aging on asynchronous left ventricular filling in normal human subjects. J Am Coll Cardiol 11:50, 1988.

42. Iskandrian AS, Haki AH: Age-related changes in left ventricular diastolic performance. Am Heart J 112:75, 1986.

43. Miller TR, et al.: Left ventricular diastolic filling and its association with age. Am J Cardiol 58:531, 1986.

44. Kitzman DW, Sheikh KH, Phillips JL, Higgenbotham MB: Normal aging is accompanied by reduced early diastolic filling independent of LV mass, heart rate, contractility and loading conditions. J Am Coll Cardiol 15:187A, 1990.

45. Nixon JV, Porter TR, Arrowood JA, and Roy V: Effects of variations in volume preload on left ventricular filling characteristics of older normal subjects. J Am Coll Cardiol 14:188A, 1990.

46. Gerstenblith G, Fleg JL, Becker LC: Maximum left ventricular filling rate in healthy individuals measured by gated blood pool scans: Effects of age. Circulation 68 (Suppl III):III-101, 1983.

47. Gribbin B, Pickering TG, Sleight P, Peto R: Effect of age and high blood pressure on baroreflex sensitivity in man. Circ Res 29: 424, 1971.

48. Porter TR, Arrowood JA, Roy V, Nixon JV: Effect of preload changes on altered left ventricular function characteristics of older normal subjects. Clin Res 38:4, 1990.

49. Nixon JV, et al.: Ventricular performance in human hearts aged 61 to 73 years. Am J Cardiol 56:932, 1985.

50. Downes T, et al.: Mechanism of altered pattern of left ventricular filling with aging in subjects without cardiac disease. Am J Cardiol 64:523, 1989.

51. Yin FCP: The aging vasculature and its effect on the heart. *In* The Aging Heart. Edited by ML Weisfeldt. New York, Raven Press, 1980, p. 137.

52. Kannel WB, et al.: Systolic blood pressure, arterial rigidity and risks of stroke: The Framingham Study. JAMA 245:1225, 1981.

53. Elliott HL, Sumner BJ, McLein K: Effect of age on vascular alpha responsiveness in man. Clin Sci 63:305A, 1982.

54. Abrass IB: Catecholamine levels and vascular responsiveness in aging. *In* Blood Pressure Regulation and Aging: An NIH Symposium. Edited by Horan MJ, Steinberg GM, Dunbar JB, Hadley EC. New York, Biomedical Information Corporation, 1986, p. 123.

55. Yin FCP, et al.: Age-associated decrease in heart rate response to isoproterenol in dogs. Mech Aging Dev 10:15, 1979.

56. Applegate WB: Hypertension in elderly patients. Ann Intern Med 110:901, 1989.

57. Masserli FJ, et al.: Essential hypertension in the elderly: hemodynamics, intervascular volume, plasma renin activity and circulating catecholamine levels. Lancet 2:983, 1983.

58. Masserli FH: Essential hypertension in the elderly. Nephron 24:35, 1985.

Part Four

MANAGEMENT OF DIASTOLIC DYSFUNCTION AND HEART FAILURE

Chapter 26

CLINICAL RECOGNITION AND TREATMENT OF DIASTOLIC DYSFUNCTION AND HEART FAILURE

Herbert J. Levine and William H. Gaasch

Basic to the recognition and treatment of congestive heart failure is an understanding of the distinction between systolic and diastolic dysfunction of the left ventricle (1, 2). Simply stated, systolic dysfunction can be considered a defect in the ability of the myofibrils to shorten against a load. Systolic dysfunction is generally detected as reduced systolic emptying caused by either impaired myocardial contractility or a heightened afterload or, as is often the case, both. Diastolic dysfunction, on the other hand, implies that the ventricle cannot accept blood at low pressures; ventricular filling is slow, delayed, or incomplete unless atrial pressure increases. Diastolic dysfunction is recognized by the major consequence of this disorder, namely venous congestion.

SYSTOLIC AND DIASTOLIC DYSFUNCTION

A graphic illustration of the hemodynamic differences between systolic and diastolic dysfunction is shown in Figure 26–1. The left panel depicts the familiar ventricular function curve relating systolic performance to an index of end diastolic fiber strain (in this instance, end-diastolic pressure). If a normal heart (Point A) were subjected to an excessive volume load (i.e., vigorous intravenous saline infusion), the coordinates of systolic performance and filling pressure would move upward along the ventricular function curve to Point B. At this point, signs and symptoms of congestive failure would be expected, yet echocardiographic or radionuclide studies would reveal perfectly normal left ventricular systolic function. Thus, this circumstance represents an example of isolated

diastolic dysfunction with its dominant clinical manifestation, venous congestion. This coordinate (Point B) can also represent the ventricle of a patient with diastolic dysfunction caused by hypertrophic heart disease. Such patients may present with congestive failure in the presence of normal systolic function (3–5).

The lower curve in this panel represents the hemodynamic characteristics of a typical patient with dilated cardiomyopathy. Systolic performance is reduced over a wide range of filling pressures; Point C indicates the coordinates of an untreated patient with evidence of both systolic and diastolic dysfunction. Were this patient to be treated vigorously with diuretic therapy, the coordinates of ventricular function would move along the depressed curve to Point D, and at this point the patient would no longer have venous congestion or evidence of diastolic dysfunction; this coordinate represents isolated systolic dysfunction. In the absence of diuretic therapy, isolated systolic dysfunction is unusual. Most patients with heart failure have combined systolic and diastolic dysfunction, but dominant or even isolated diastolic dysfunction is not uncommon.

PATHOPHYSIOLOGY OF DIASTOLIC DYSFUNCTION

The pathophysiology of diastolic dysfunction is best viewed from an analysis of the diastolic pressure-volume relationship (6). As shown in the right panel of Figure 26–1, this relationship is non-linear, and the slope of the pressure-volume relationship (dP/dV) represents left ventricular chamber stiffness. With an increase in filling pressure and volume, it is evident that

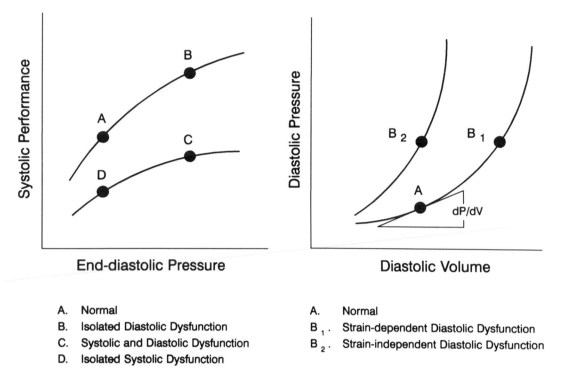

A. Normal
B. Isolated Diastolic Dysfunction
C. Systolic and Diastolic Dysfunction
D. Isolated Systolic Dysfunction

A. Normal
B_1. Strain-dependent Diastolic Dysfunction
B_2. Strain-independent Diastolic Dysfunction

Fig. 26–1. Hemodynamic differences between left ventricular systolic and diastolic dysfunction. In *A*, systolic performance is related to an index of end diastolic fiber strain (i.e., end-diastolic pressure). Point A defines the coordinate of a normal ventricle. If this heart were subjected to an excessive volume load, the coordinates of systolic performance and end-diastolic pressure would move up along the curve to point B; thus the signs and symptoms of congestive failure would exist in the presence of normal systolic performance. The lower curve represents a typical patient with dilated cardiomyopathy; point C indicates the coordinate of an untreated patient with systolic and diastolic dysfunction. Diuretic therapy might cause a transition to point B (isolated systolic dysfunction), where the patient would no longer exhibit venous congestion or diastolic dysfunction. In *B*, diastolic pressure-volume relations are shown. The slope of a tangent to this non-linear relation represents chamber stiffness (dP/dV). Point A defines the coordinate of a normal heart. A volume load causes a strain-dependent increase in chamber stiffness (a shift from point A to point B_1). In the second example (B_2), filling pressure is increased, but end-diastolic volume and muscle strain are normal; this is a typical example of increased chamber stiffness that is strain-independent.

ventricular diastolic stiffness will increase. Thus, any stretch of the diastolic ventricle will cause a *strain-dependent* increase in ventricular chamber stiffness (i.e., a shift from Point A to Point B_1) (7). This panel also illustrates the distensibility characteristics of a ventricle that is intrinsically stiffer than normal, independent of muscle strain. In the example shown, filling pressure at Point B_2 is increased (and comparable to Point B_1), although end-diastolic volume and muscle strain are normal. A classic example of *strain-independent* increased chamber stiffness is found in ventricular hypertrophy (see Chapter 9).

Although both types of diastolic dysfunction present with venous congestion, the clinical presentation and drug therapy of strain-dependent and strain-independent diastolic dysfunction may differ. Thus, there is good reason to establish an accurate etiologic diagnosis of diastolic dysfunction. Table 26–1 lists the common clinical conditions responsible for strain-dependent diastolic dysfunction. The major common denominator in this group of diseases is hypervolemia, generally as a consequence of renal retention of salt and water. The hemodynamic characteristics of this group include a normal or high cardiac

Table 26–1. Causes of Left Ventricular Diastolic Dysfunction

Strain-dependent
 1. Iatrogenic volume overload
 2. Nephrogenic congestive failure (e.g., obstructive uropathy)
 3. Anemia
 4. Cirrhosis
 5. Hyperplastic bone disease (e.g., Paget's disease)
 6. Arteriovenous fistula
 7. Heart rate mismatch
 8. Thyrotoxicosis
 9. Thiamine deficiency

Strain-independent
 1. Acute myocardial ischemia or hypoxia
 2. Chronic ischemic heart disease
 3. Concentric LV hypertrophy (e.g., aortic stenosis)
 4. Hypertrophic cardiomyopathy
 5. Endocardial fibroelastosis
 6. Infiltrative myocardial disease (e.g., amyloid)
 7. Constrictive pericardial disease

output, an increased central blood volume, and normal LV systolic function.

The major causes of strain-independent diastolic dysfunction are also listed in Table 26–1. In each instance, ventricular distensibility is reduced by virtue of a change in the passive properties of the ventricle and not by an increase in muscle strain. The prototype of this disorder is hypertrophic cardiomyopathy, in which filling pressures are high because of inappropriate hypertrophy, whereas systolic function is normal or even supernormal. Although the conditions listed in these two tables are heterogeneous, and may warrant specific therapeutic considerations, the major hemodynamic difference between strain-dependent and strain-independent types of diastolic dysfunction is that basal cardiac output is generally high in the former and normal in the latter.

CLINICAL RECOGNITION AND DIFFERENTIATION OF DIASTOLIC AND SYSTOLIC DYSFUNCTION

The signs and symptoms of heart failure are more the manifestation of a non-compliant ventricle than of a weakened, hypokinetic ventricle. That is to say, the common clinical presentation of congestive heart failure is dominated by the expression of diastolic dysfunction (venous congestion) rather than systolic dysfunction (low output). However, while signs and symptoms of reduced systolic performance may be relatively subtle, it is the consequences of systolic dysfunction that initiate the major compensatory mechanisms which drive the circulatory abnormalities of congestive heart failure. Thus, reflex arteriolar vasoconstriction, venoconstriction and chronotropy form the hemodynamic substrate for much of the modern therapy of congestive heart failure.

Systolic Dysfunction

The earliest signs of a defect in systolic ejection are apparent during stress. Thus an inadequate rise in cardiac output during exercise is manifest as fatigue and weakness. A decreased ability of the myocardial fibers to shorten reduces stroke volume and pulse pressure and, in an effort to compensate, heart rate is increased at each level of activity; this culminates in a resting sinus tachycardia. As cardiac output falls, the regional circulations best able to withstand low flow rates suffer disproportionately. Thus, skin and renal blood flow are reduced, whereas cerebral and coronary flow are maintained. The clinical expression of low skin blood flow is cool, moist skin, whereas a reduction in renal blood flow causes a defect in salt and water excretion, producing nocturia and ultimately fluid retention and edema. Fluid retention contributes to a strain-dependent diastolic dysfunction, so that the patient may now exhibit the signs of combined systolic and diastolic dysfunction. With severe reductions in cardiac output, prerenal azotemia, low-grade fever caused by defective elimination of heat, lactic acidosis, polycythemia from bone marrow hypoxia, and in agonal situations, an outpouring of reticulocytes and nucleated red blood cells may develop (8).

Some patients with chronic congestive heart failure develop a hypermetabolic state simulating thyrotoxicosis (9). The hypertrophied heart itself is largely responsible for this "oxygen trap" and thus contributes importantly to the syndrome of cardiac cachexia (10–11) which is seen in some patients with large failing hearts.

Diastolic Dysfunction

The clinical diagnosis of ventricular diastolic dysfunction depends primarily on the demonstration of elevated systemic or pulmonary venous pressures or the consequences of such elevated pressures.

Bedside Diagnosis

The combination of renal retention of salt and water and increased venous tone caused by activation of the renin-angiotensin and sympathetic nervous systems results in elevation of systemic and/or pulmonary venous pressures. Elevation of systemic venous pressure is detected clinically by examination of the internal and external jugular veins with the patient in the semirecumbent position. With chronic systemic venous congestion, dependent edema and congestive hepatomegaly develop, the latter not infrequently giving rise to abdominal fullness, ascites, anorexia, or even frank abdominal pain. The clinical manifestations of venous congestion of the abdominal viscera are extremely varied, but generally are governed by the severity and the rate at which congestion develops. In some instances, longstanding hepatic congestion may exist, with remarkably little effect on conventional liver function tests. In other cases, the clinical picture resembles that of primary hepatocellular disease. In acute right heart failure, particularly when associated with circulatory failure, extraordinary elevations of serum transaminases may be observed. Rarely, marked, chronic elevation of systemic venous pressure, as seen in constrictive pericarditis or advanced tricuspid valve disease, presents as a protein-losing enteropathy because of lymphangiectasia of intestinal villi (12) or as nephrotic syndrome (13, 14).

With left ventricular diastolic dysfunction, pulmonary venous pressure rises, initiating several disturbances of respiratory function. With an increase in pulmonary capillary pressure, interstitial and alveolar edema develop, giving rise to hypoxia and dyspnea, and increased bronchial secretions may contribute to a recumbent cough

or episodic bronchospasm. Interstitial edema by itself may initiate tachypnea even before frank alveolar transudation of fluid occurs (15). With the development of chronic pulmonary venous congestion, expansion of the pulmonary lymphatic system may enable patients to tolerate levels of pulmonary venous hypertension which acutely would evoke pulmonary edema. With a fall in lung compliance, tidal volume falls and respiratory minute volume is maintained by rapid shallow breathing. Orthopnea and particularly paroxysmal nocturnal dyspnea are characteristic of pulmonary venous congestion, but because lung volumes and vital capacity are reduced in all persons during recumbency, some patients with advanced endobronchial disease may complain of these symptoms as well.

As the diastolic pressure in the ventricle rises, chamber compliance falls and a given change in filling pressure evokes a smaller change in cardiac dimension. In this fashion, heterometric changes in systolic performance are lessened and, as a consequence, the normal sinus arrhythmia disappears and fixed or near-fixed splitting of the second heart sound may be observed. These and other consequences of diastolic dysfunction are also observed in combined systolic and diastolic dysfunction.

The third and fourth heart sounds are among the most useful and the most poorly understood signs of ventricular dysfunction. The fourth heart sound (or S_4 gallop) is perhaps the most common sign of ventricular diastolic dysfunction, but the interpretation of a third heart sound (S_3) is more complex. Without a full understanding of the hemodynamic determinants of either the S_4 or S_3 gallop, several useful correlates of these heart sounds have emerged that serve the clinician well. For example, the fourth heart sound is almost always considered an abnormal finding in children and young adults, whereas the incidence of a soft S_4 is so high among older adults as to render its detection of little or no value as a marker of ventricular dysfunction. However, an S_4 in a younger person (or a loud S_4 in an older individual) generally suggests strain-independent diastolic dysfunction (for example, LVH, coronary heart disease, etc.), or less likely acute volume overload. Atrial sounds are rarely heard in chronic volume overload (i.e., rheumatic mitral regurgitation) (16).

The older literature indicates that an S_4 gallop was essentially always present with angina pectoris and during the evolution of acute myocardial infarction. Presumably, the stiffening effect of myocardial ischemia contributed to the development of an S_4. This sound is less frequently heard nowadays, partly because of the aggressive therapeutic use of nitrates; even in the presence of a stiff ventricle, nitrates may produce a strain-dependent decrease in stiffness and a decrease in the intensity of the S_4.

Although atrial gallops suggest ventricular diastolic dysfunction (i.e., steep end-diastolic pressure-volume relationships), they are not typically a marker of venous hypertension and congestion. On the other hand, ventricular gallops in the population over 35 years of age correlate better with elevated atrial pressures and systemic or pulmonary venous congestion. Thus, although exceptions occur, the atrial gallop provides some insight into the slope of the (late diastolic) ventricular pressure volume curve, whereas the ventricular gallop reflects events in early diastole and generally indicates that mean atrial and venous pressures are high. Studies by Van der Werf et al. (17) indicate that the S_3 is invariably associated with a higher and steeper rapid filling wave on the ventricular pressure tracing, regardless of the presence or absence of systolic dysfunction. Thus, in severe mitral regurgitation with normal systolic function, a high-steep rapid filling wave with an S_3 was caused by a high filling rate, whereas in dilated cardiomyopathy, the S_3 and steep rapid wave were caused by altered diastolic properties of the ventricle.

Several bedside maneuvers may be helpful in the diagnosis of ventricular diastolic dysfunction. Simple changes in body position may bring out an elusive gallop. Elevation of the legs, prompt squatting, isometric handgrip exercise, or a few sit-ups may permit one to hear an otherwise questionable third sound. Additional information is provided by performing a Valsalva maneuver (18–20). This can be done simply with a sphygmomanometer and a stethoscope. After determining systolic blood pressure, one elevates cuff pressure approximately 30 mm Hg higher than systolic pressure as the patient executes a Valsalva maneuver. Cuff pressure is then lowered during phase 2 of the maneuver (strain phase), and if the first Korotkoff sounds are heard below the baseline systolic pressure, one is assured that the phase 2 response is normal. However, if systolic pressure during the strain phase remains above systolic levels, the observed "square wave" response is characteristic, albeit not diagnostic, of congestive heart failure. After release of the Valsalva, cuff pressure is quickly increased 30 mm Hg or so above systolic pressure once again, and the normal overshoot blood pressure response with reflex bradycardia is detected within 10 seconds of release. The mere absence of overshoot blood pressures and related reflex bradycardia during phase 4 of the maneuver is a pattern that also may be observed in patients with heart failure, but it can be produced by beta-adrenergic blocking agents in normal individuals (21). The utility of a Valsalva maneuver in distinguishing systolic from diastolic dysfunction is not well defined. However, the Valsalva maneuver has been used to unmask LV diastolic dysfunction during Doppler echocardiographic measurement of transmitral flow velocity (22). This is a potential area for future research.

The abdominojugular test, a modification of the hepatojugular reflux test, recent has been demonstrated to be useful in identifying patients with elevated pulmonary venous pressure (23). A positive test is defined as an increase in right atrial (or systemic venous) pressure during 10 seconds of firm midabdominal compression followed by an abrupt drop of at least 3 mm Hg (4 cm of blood) on pressure release. Patients with no increase in systemic venous pressure or a transient increase that returned to baseline before release of abdominal compression were generally found to have pulmonary capillary wedge pressures of 15 mm Hg or less. The extent to which the abnormal response is modulated by systolic or diastolic dysfunction is unknown. This test should be studied further in patients with isolated diastolic dysfunction.

Chest X ray

The detection of pulmonary venous congestion by physical examination is at best difficult. Indeed, except for the presence of moist rales on auscultation of the lungs, few physical signs are directly coupled to the height of the pulmonary venous pressure. The chest x ray, however, can be more useful in the diagnosis of pulmonary venous congestion. The most common radiographic signs of pulmonary venous congestion are: (1) dilation of the superior pulmonary veins (the antler appearance), (2) increased interstitial density of central lung markings (pulmonary clouding), (3) thickened septa and lymphatics (Kerley B lines), (4) alveolar edema, (5) free pleural fluid, (6) interlobar fluid (pseudotumor), and secondarily (7) dilation of the superior vena cava and azygos vein. Each of these findings may be present with or without pulmonary rales.

Exercise Testing

Hemodynamic measurements during exercise have long been used to evaluate a wide variety of cardiovascular disorders (24). Such studies have been used to differentiate constrictive pericarditis from restrictive cardiomyopathy (25), to assess the effect of pharmacologic therapy in patients with hypertrophic cardiomyopathy (26), and in patients with congestive heart failure caused by systolic dysfunction. Only recently have pulmonary artery occlusion pressures and LV volumes been measured during exercise in the evaluation of patients with the syndrome of "congestive heart failure and preserved LV systolic function" (27). Patients with this syndrome complain of symptoms (dyspnea and fatigue) that are essentially the same as those in patients with systolic dysfunction. However, LV volume measurements indicate that the LV response to exercise in isolated diastolic dysfunction differs dramatically from that seen in patients with systolic dysfunction.

Kitzman et al. (27) studied the pathophysiologic basis of symptoms of exercise intolerance in patients with heart failure and preserved systolic function. They found a reduced cardiac output during exercise that was caused by an inability to augment stroke volume by means of the Frank-Starling mechanism; this was accompanied by a substantial increase in pulmonary venous pressure, while indices of systolic function were maintained. Cuocolo et al. (28) and Clyne et al. (29) made similar observations in patients with hypertension and aortic stenosis. In distinct contrast to the expected normal increase, end-diastolic volume actually decreased during exercise (see Chapter 11). Such failure to utilize the Frank-Starling mechanism is likely to be related to the stiff ventricle seen in hypertrophic hearts (30). Another manifestation of such diastolic dysfunction may be the increased lung uptake of thallium seen during exercise testing in patients with coronary artery disease.

Measurement of pulmonary artery occlusion pressure (i.e., pulmonary capillary wedge pressure) during exercise, especially if done in conjunction with measurement of LV volume, can be useful in differentiating cardiac from pulmonary dyspnea. Such testing may also provide data that separate patients with diastolic dysfunction from those with systolic dysfunction. Recognizing the limitations of the physical examination and the potential for exercise studies, this appears to be an important area for future research.

Echocardiography and Radionuclide Ventriculography

Ultrasound and radionuclide studies provide such valuable information in patients with heart failure that it is almost mandatory to obtain at least one such study before the initiation of therapy. This is especially true if there is any question as to the diagnosis of systolic or diastolic dysfunction (see Chapters 11 and 12).

The Diagnostic-Therapeutic Trial

Occasionally, despite a careful history and physical examination and a nondiagnostic chest x-ray, the diagnosis of pulmonary venous congestion remains in doubt. In this circumstance, a reasonable next step is the diagnostic-therapeutic trial. A brief but meaningful regiment of diuretic therapy is initiated and both objective and subjective criteria for improvement are monitored. Thus, daily weights and urine volumes are measured and a frequent assessment of respiratory symptoms is made; the simple measurement of total vital capacity may demonstrate clear improvement coincident with a measurable diuresis. Thus, with utilization of a diagnostic-therapeutic trial, the clinical diagnosis of diastolic dysfunction may be confirmed without the use of invasive (right heart catheterization) diagnostic testing.

TREATMENT OF DIASTOLIC DYSFUNCTION

The treatment of diastolic dysfunction, broadly speaking, has two major objectives: (1) to reduce or eliminate the factors responsible for the diastolic dysfunction, and (2) to reverse the consequences of diastolic dysfunction, namely venous congestion. The former, for the most part, is a long-term goal. There are, however, several strain-dependent forms of diastolic dysfunction that can be reversed promptly (i.e., anemia, obstructive uropathy, thyrotoxicosis, and heart rate mismatch). On the other hand, with the exception of constrictive pericarditis, most of the reversible forms of strain-independent diastolic dysfunction require considerable time to demonstrate regression. For example, regression of hypertrophy as a consequence of antihypertensive therapy or following aortic valve replacement in the patient with aortic stenosis requires months or even years to accomplish. In some patients with diastolic dysfunction, there is no potential to reverse the cause of the altered material properties of the ventricle (i.e., amyloid disease), and one is left with the task of reducing venous congestion. A general approach to the treatment of diastolic dysfunction is presented in Table 26–2.

Diuretics

Diuretics remain the mainstay of therapy for venous congestion. Indeed, in the absence of acute renal failure, there is probably no patient who is truly refractory to vigorous diuretic therapy. For patients with mild congestion or edema, low-dose furosemide or thiazide diuretics are useful, convenient, and inexpensive. If hydrochlorothiazide is not effective, loop diuretics can be used. Correction of hypokalemia with

Table 26–2. General Approach to Treatment of Diastolic Dysfunction

Goal of Treatment	Method of Treatment

1. Reduce venous pressure	Decreased central blood volume
	  Diuretics
	  Salt restriction
	Venodilation
	  Nitrates
	  ACE inhibitors
	  Morphine
	  Tourniquets

2. Maintain atrial contraction	Cardioversion of AF Sequential A-V pacing
3. Decrease heart rate	Digitalis in atrial fibrillation Beta-adrenergic blockers Verapamil, diltiazem
4. Prevent/treat ischemia	Beta adrenergic blockers Calcium channel blockers Nitrates Coronary bypass or angioplasty
5. Improve ventricular relaxation	Systolic unloading Treat ischemia Calcium channel blockers(?)
6. Regression of hypertrophy	Antihypertensive therapy Surgery (AVR for aortic stenosis)

potassium supplements or the addition of potassium-sparing diuretics is particularly important in patients taking digitalis glycosides. Potassium-sparing diuretics should be used with caution in patients with diabetes or renal failure for fear of life-threatening hyperkalemia. Perhaps one of the major pitfalls in modern diuretic therapy relates to the use of ACE inhibitors. The addition of an ACE inhibitor to a diuretic regimen that includes potassium supplements or a potassium-sparing diuretic may place the patient at serious risk of hyperkalemia.

In patients with severe fluid overload and venous congestion, combination therapy may be necessary. The combination of furosemide and metolazone is frequently effective, and in most circumstances should be given in short courses to avoid hypovolemia and prerenal azotemia. Although aldosterone inhibitors are weak diuretics when used as monotherapy, the addition of spironolactone to a loop diuretic may be particularly gratifying in patients with conspicuous right-sided failure and substantial secondary hyperaldosteronism.

The availability of potent diuretics and combination therapy has unfortunately made today's clinicians somewhat cavalier about the need for salt restriction. Too often, the success of a well-designed diuretic regimen is thwarted by the indiscreet ingestion of dietary salt.

Venodilators

Venous congestion and its associated increase in ventricular preload is the consequence of renal retention of salt and water, and an increase in venous tone. Venodilation, therefore, provides a mechanism for reducing venous congestion in patients with diastolic dysfunction. Among vasoactive drugs, nitrates have a predominant effect on capacitance vessels and can be used with impunity in most patients with a component of strain-dependent diastolic dysfunction. In patients with strain-independent diastolic dysfunction, venodilators are also effective, but their use requires more care because abrupt preload reduction in some patients may presage a symptomatic fall in cardiac output. For example, patients with hypertrophic cardiomyopathy frequently exhibit very steep diastolic pressure-volume curves, so that a modest fall in central blood volume is accompanied by a sharp fall in ventricular filling pressure and stroke volume. This may be particularly hazardous in the patient with the obstructive variety of hypertrophic cardiomyopathy, in whom preload reduction is coupled to increased outflow obstruction and mitral regurgitation.

Nitrates effect a prompt venodilation and a reduction in systemic and pulmonary venous pressure. Although sublingual nitroglycerine is generally reserved for the management of acute coronary syndromes, its utility for treating acute pulmonary congestion should not be overlooked. Long-acting oral nitrate therapy and transcutaneous nitroglycerine preparations are also useful for chronic diastolic dysfunction, and there is reason to suspect that the benefit in mortality observed in the V-HeFT study of hydralazine-nitrate combination in chronic CHF (31) may be predominantly an effect of nitrates.

The benefit of nitrate therapy in chronic CHF is more far-reaching than a simple reduction in venous pressure (Table 26–3). The decrease in ventricular volume associated with preload reduction effects a fall in ventricular wall tension by means of the Laplace equation, which improves afterload mismatch and also decreases myocardial energy requirements. Other vasoactive properties of nitrates contribute to the benefit of these drugs in patients with congestive heart failure. Both the relief of vasospasm of extramural coronary arteries and an improvement in coronary collateral flow serve to prevent or relieve regional myocardial ischemia. Because ischemia may be responsible for both systolic and diastolic dysfunction, the value of these drugs, particularly in acute coronary syndromes, is apparent. A further benefit of preload reduction relates to perfusion of the subendocardium. When ventricular filling pressures are high, the transcoronary perfusion pressure is reduced because coronary venous pressure is elevated; as a result, the distal portion of the coronary bed (the subendocardium) suffers disproportionately. Direct coronary vascular

Table 26–3.   Beneficial Effects of Nitrates in CHF

Primary Effect	Secondary Effect
Vasodilation (venodilation)	Decrease venous congestion
Reduction in ventricular volume	Decrease wall force and MVO_2
Reduction in ventricular dimensions	Decrease dynamic mitral regurgitation
Reduction in LV diastolic pressure	Increase subendocardial perfusion
Decrease coronary vasospasm	Decrease myocardial ischemia
Improve coronary collateral blood flow	Decrease myocardial ischemia

compression by high LV diastolic pressures may also contribute to a reduced subendocardial blood flow. This circulatory dilemma can be lessened or reversed by preload reduction.

Perhaps the most dramatic effects of nitrate therapy in CHF are seen in patients with dynamic papillary muscle dysfunction. Elegant studies in a canine model have demonstrated that the major determinant of mitral regurgitant flow in this circumstance is a volume-dependent mitral systolic orifice size (32). Thus, the size of the mitral regurgitant orifice is closely coupled to left ventricular dimensions, and a reduction in preload is accompanied by an immediate decrease in regurgitant orifice size and regurgitant flow. Clinical experience with intravenous nitroglycerine in patients with dynamic papillary muscle dysfunction has confirmed this mechanism and the importance of subendocardial and papillary muscle perfusion in the genesis of the syndrome of dynamic mitral regurgitation.

ACE inhibitors reduce venous as well as arteriolar tone and thus are useful for treating diastolic dysfunction. These agents may also be useful in the prevention of LV dysfunction (see Chapter 18). However, in circumstances in which afterload reduction may have an adverse hemodynamic effect, these agents should be avoided or used with great care. Such circumstances include IHSS, critical aortic stenosis, and the condition known as hypertensive hypertrophic cardiomyopathy of the elderly (33). When using vasoactive drugs in the treatment of congestive heart failure, one must remember that preload reduction and afterload reduction are interactive. Thus, preload reduction reduces heart size and wall force by means of the Laplace equation; this can result in a secondary fall in afterload. Similarly, afterload reduction frequently effects a secondary fall in preload because relief of afterload mismatch permits more complete emptying of the ventricle and a fall in chamber volume.

Maintenance of Atrial Systole

The hemodynamic consequences of the loss of atrial systole are particularly great in the patient with advanced myocardial failure or hypertrophic cardiomyopathy. In either case, marked clinical deterioration is frequently observed with the onset of atrial fibrillation. Such deterioration may persist despite good control of the ventricular rate. In these circumstances, there is good reason to make a special effort to restore and maintain normal sinus rhythm. Similarly, among patients requiring permanent transvenous pacemakers, the importance of properly synchronized A-V sequential pacing is apparent in those with systolic dysfunction as well as in those with severe strain-independent diastolic dysfunction.

Control of Heart Rate

Congestive heart failure caused by heart rate mismatch may be a consequence of either sustained bradycardia or tachycardia. Although rarely encountered today, chronic severe bradycardia may present insidiously as congestive failure, without symptoms of cardiogenic cerebral ischemia. In this circumstance, a low cardiac output initiates renal retention of salt and water despite the presence of normal systolic function and the syndrome is promptly reversed by appropriate pacemaker therapy. Similarly, congestive heart failure, with a reversible form of both systolic and diastolic dysfunction, has also been reported in patients with prolonged supraventricular tachycardia (34).

Prolongation of diastole is one of the most important and one of the most neglected interventions in the management of diastolic dysfunction. Because the duration of diastole per beat and per minute is related inversely to heart rate, cardiac slowing provides an immediate mechanism for atrial decompression and relief of venous congestion. This effect is especially apparent in the patient with mitral stenosis. Indeed, from the orifice equation we can deduce that, in mitral stenosis, left atrial pressure varies as the square of the diastolic filling period. Thus, small increases in the latter, coincident with cardiac slowing, can exert a profound effect on pulmonary venous pressure. Not only is correction of paroxysmal rapid heart action mandatory in patients with significant mitral stenosis, but the use of beta blockers to produce chronic iatrogenic bradycardia may be extremely beneficial for the mitral stenosis patient in normal sinus rhythm.

In the absence of mitral orifice obstruction, the relationships between duration of diastole and ventricular filling are less profound, but qualitatively similar. Patients with underlying myocardial disease and diastolic dysfunction also profit from the increase in filling time associated with cardiac slowing, particularly those with substantial cardiomegaly. Biophysical principles dictate that the optimum frequency of a heart is an inverse function of its size (35). Thus, we expect the patient with long-standing hypertension and left ventricular hypertrophy to tolerate atrial fibrillation at a rate of 160/min less well than the patient with lone fibrillation and a normal left ventricle.

The inverse relation between frequency and heart size applies to systolic function as well as to diastolic function. Indeed, one of the most promising and intriguing new therapies for patients with idiopathic dilated cardiomyopathy has been the use of cardioselective beta-blocking agents introduced by Waagstein and Associates (36). The benefit reported from this chronic therapy has included not only symptomatic improvement, but increases in systolic ejection fraction and upregulation of myocardial beta receptors (37–39). Although the explanation for this response is not fully understood, cardiac slowing and a directional improvement in the frequency-heart size relationship are likely to play a role.

Although the bradycardic calcium channel blockers (verapamil and diltiazem) are useful in controlling the heart rate in patients with rapid atrial fibrillation, their utility in the treatment of patients with systolic dysfunction (i.e., dilated cardiomyopathy) has not been demonstrated. Indeed, their negative inotropic effect can have an adverse effect in such patients.

Prevention and Treatment of Myocardial Ischemia

The importance of ischemia in the genesis of both systolic and diastolic dysfunction of the ventricle cannot be overemphasized. The mechanisms involved in this phenomenon are described in detail elsewhere in this volume. In the hyperacute phase of acute myocardial infarction, the earliest

change in the diastolic properties of the ventricle is an increase in chamber compliance attributed in part to collapse of the vascular volume of the ischemic segment and a negative erectile effect of the involved myocardium (40, 41). These effects, however, are short-lived and soon replaced by impaired relaxation of the ischemic myocardium and a complex interaction between weak (ischemic) and strong (non-ischemic) regions of the ventricle. The result is a leftward and upward shift in the ventricular pressure-volume curve so that chamber stiffness increases (42). Appreciation of this fact has led clinicians to recognize that the major factor responsible for congestive heart failure in the early phases of an acute myocardial infarction is diastolic dysfunction of the ventricle. Thus, contrary to the practice of 20 years ago, clinicians have abandoned the use of digitalis glycosides for the treatment of congestive failure early in the course of a myocardial infarction and, in the absence of atrial arrhythmias, rely on diuretics and venodilators instead. In keeping with this principle is the observation that most patients with acute infarction tolerate the negative inotropic beta-blocking agents surprisingly well during the acute phase of their disease, even in the presence of congestive failure.

In this setting, the value of nitrates is preeminent. The abilities of nitrates to relieve venous congestion, decrease myocardial wall force and oxygen demands, improve collateral blood flow, and reduce subendocardial ischemia combine to establish these agents as ideal drugs for the management of diastolic dysfunction associated with acute coronary syndromes.

The role of calcium antagonists to treat myocardial ischemia in acute myocardial infarction is more controversial. Although their use in patients with normal or near-normal systolic function may be justified, an adverse effect has been reported in patients with congestive failure (43), and in this circumstance they are best avoided.

Some patients with chronic coronary heart disease may present with relatively isolated diastolic dysfunction (44). In this circumstance, optimum therapy often includes diuretics and nitrate therapy combined with antianginal agents including beta-blockers or calcium antagonists. Preload reduction and antianginal therapy are particularly important in those who have evidence of dynamic papillary muscle dysfunction.

Improvement of Ventricular Relaxation

It is well established that abnormal myocardial relaxation is common in patients with left ventricular hypertrophy. In hypertensive heart disease, some data indicate that beta-blocking agents and particularly calcium antagonists improve diastolic function, but it is not clear whether this is because of a primary effect on ventricular relaxation or a reduction in arterial pressure and/or the relief of myocardial ischemia (see Chapter 28). However, because both beta-blockers and calcium antagonists are useful in the treatment of hypertension and ischemia, their use in this setting can only be encouraged.

The evidence for improved diastolic function in hypertrophic cardiomyopathy following the use of calcium antagonists is much more compelling. In this disorder, impaired relaxation is superimposed on an increased passive stiffness; these and other factors that contribute to the hemodynamic expression of diastolic dysfunction in hypertrophic cardiomyopathy are discussed elsewhere in this text (see Chapter 22). Improved isovolumic relaxation in this disease has been demonstrated in some but not all patients during treatment with nifedipine, diltiazem, and verapamil. Because normal systolic function is a characteristic of the heart in hypertrophic cardiomyopathy, these drugs are particularly well suited for its management (see Chapter 28).

The use of calcium antagonists for the generic purpose of improving ventricular filling in the average patient with combined systolic and diastolic dysfunction warrants a word of caution. Because each of the calcium antagonists has negative inotropic properties, an adverse effect on systolic function, particularly when large doses of these drugs are used, may more than offset any anticipated benefit. Thus, it behooves the physician to restrict the use of these agents in patients with combined systolic and diastolic dysfunction to those with important myocardial ischemia or coronary

vasospastic syndromes. See subsequent text.

Regression of Hypertrophy

In the long-term therapy of diastolic dysfunction caused by left ventricular hypertrophy, regression of hypertrophy seems axiomatic. Following surgical correction of aortic stenosis, left ventricular mass declines substantially. However, such regression of hypertrophy can be associated with an increase in myocardial stiffness which seems to be caused by a relative increase in interstitial fibrosis; myocardial mass declines with little change in the absolute amount of connective tissue and as a result the relative degree of fibrosis increases and the wall stiffens (45). Recognizing the slow turnover rates of collagen (see Chapter 8), it may take months or years before a decrease in wall stiffness is seen.

The regression of hypertrophy that can be seen with the treatment of systemic arterial hypertension is much less dramatic (46). Although the associated connective tissue response is not yet defined in humans, there are data that support the notion that regression of hypertrophy may be associated with improved diastolic function in some such patients (see Chapter 21). Successful antihypertensive therapy is known to reduce the mortality and morbidity of stroke and, to a lesser extent, the manifestations of coronary disease. Based on such observations, it is reasonable to expect that successful antihypertensive therapy and the regression of hypertrophy would have a beneficial effect on left ventricular diastolic function. This is an important area for future research.

COMBINED SYSTOLIC AND DIASTOLIC DYSFUNCTION

The cardinal features of isolated systolic dysfunction, isolated diastolic dysfunction, and combined dysfunction are shown in Table 26–4. Instances of chronic, pure systolic dysfunction in clinical medicine are not common, but occasionally one encounters a patient with a dilated hypokinetic left ventricle who has normal systemic and pulmonary pressures and little or no need for diuretic therapy. Their clinical syndrome is generally characterized by symptoms of a

Table 26–4. Features of LV Systolic and Diastolic Dysfunction

	Pure Systolic Dysfunction	Pure Diastolic Dysfunction	Combined Dysfunction
Pulmonary congestion	No	Yes	Yes
Cardiac output	Low	Normal or increased	Normal or decreased
Ejection fraction	Depressed	Normal	Depressed
LV dilation	Yes	No*	Yes
Inotropic agents	Yes	No	Yes
Afterload reduction	Yes	No	Yes
Venodilators	No	Yes	Yes
Diuretics	No	Yes	Yes
Calcium antagonists	No	Yes	Questionable†

* In strain-dependent diastolic dysfunction, the LV size may be normal or slightly increased; by contrast, LV chamber dimensions are normal or small in the strain-independent forms of diastolic dysfunction.
† In combined systolic and diastolic dysfunction, the calcium channel blockers may be useful in the treatment of hypertension or angina.

low output state with fatigue and weakness, but signs and symptoms of congestive failure are absent. In some instances, surprisingly, a normal or near-normal resting cardiac output is found despite the presence of a markedly depressed systolic ejection fraction. This apparent paradox can be explained by the fact that a greatly enlarged ventricle need shorten little to eject a normal stroke volume. In this circumstance, there is little rationale for the use of diuretics and venodilators; in fact, preload reduction may prove counterproductive by evoking a negative heterometric response and a further fall in stroke volume. Appropriate therapy in this condition includes inotropic support and afterload reduction to augment forward flow and relieve afterload mismatch. Contrariwise, patients with pure diastolic dysfunction have little to gain from the use of inotropic agents, and in the absence of arterial hypertension or valvular regurgitation, there is little rationale for the use of (arterial) vasodilators.

Most patients with congestive heart failure exhibit combined systolic and diastolic dysfunction; effective therapy should be targeted to deal with both of these abnormalities. Large clinical trials indicate that vasodilator therapy prolongs life in patients with congestive heart failure (31, 47, 48); asymptomatic patients with LV dysfunction may also benefit from this therapy. ACE inhibitors, in particular, have been found to be extremely well tolerated and effective and have emerged as first-line therapy for patients with combined ventricular dysfunction (see Chapter 18). Their success in this setting likely is caused, at least partly, by their ability to effect both preload and afterload reduction. Although qualitative similar hemodynamic and clinical response can be expected from the combination of hydralazine and oral nitrate therapy (31), a high incidence of side effects suggests that this combination therapy is best reserved for patients who are unable to tolerate ACE inhibitors.

Although there is a general consensus concerning the utility of digitalis in heart failure patients who have atrial arrhythmias, there has been considerable skepticism as to whether digitalis glycosides are of real benefit in those with normal sinus rhythm. In a thorough review of this subject, Kimmelstiel and Benotti (49) conclude that digitalis exerts "a moderate salutary effect in patients with congestive heart failure who are in sinus rhythm." A similar conclusion was expressed in recent reviews by Kelly (50) and others (51).

In patients with functional class 3 or 4 CHF and combined ventricular dysfunction, there is good reason to use both ACE inhibitors and digitalis glycosides as well as diuretic therapy. In those with conspicuous venous congestion, especially when associated with ischemic heart syndromes, the addition of nitrate therapy is recommended. In heart failure, calcium antagonists are best reserved for those with hypertension.

The time course of response to therapeutic agents in CHF varies substantially. Some agents evoke potent responses with initial use, but benefit is not sustained with chronic use (i.e. beta agonists). The utility of chronic diuretic therapy is well sustained without evidence of tachyphylaxis. Among the inotropic agents, the same can be said for digitalis glycosides, the bypyridines, and perhaps the imidolazines, whereas downregulation of the myocardial beta receptors limits the effectiveness of continuous administration of beta agonists (52). Responses to vasodilator therapy, too, differ with the choice of drug. ACE inhibitors and combination therapy with hydralazine and oral nitrates retain their effectiveness with chronic use, whereas prolonged use of prazosin is characterized by the appearance of tachyphylaxis. Quite the opposite has been observed with the use of beta-blocker therapy in idiopathic dilated cardiomyopathy. Examination of the short-term responses to these drugs has failed to demonstrate clinical or hemodynamic improvement (53, 54). Indeed, the immediate responses to intravenous metoprolol in these patients, not infrequently, are adverse (36, 37). With chronic drug administration (6 to 12 months), however, salutary effects have been demonstrated (37–39).

TREATMENT OF DIASTOLIC DYSFUNCTION ASSOCIATED WITH VALVULAR REGURGITATION

The treatment of strain-dependent diastolic dysfunction and heart failure associated with valvular regurgitation is aided by consideration of the specific hemodynamic determinants of regurgitant flow. For example, in aortic regurgitation, the hydraulic variables that determine the size of the regurgitant volume are the aortic regurgitant orifice area during diastole, the duration of diastole, and the gradient across the aortic valve in diastole. The first of these is a relatively constant value that can only be reduced surgically. The duration of diastole, however, is a function of heart rate, and it should be apparent that profound bradycardia increases the magnitude of aortic regurgitant flow, and this may increase the severity of strain dependent diastolic dysfunction. In addition, consideration of aortic valve orifice dynamics provides some rationale for treating arterial hypertension in patients with aortic regurgitation. The benefit reported in patients with aortic regurgitation treated with hydralazine (55) remains unexplained. Indeed, the observation that the reported decrease in LV volume can not be explained simply on the basis of a lower regurgitant volume indicates that other factors contribute to the beneficial effects of vasodilators (56).

The effect of vasoactive drugs on the magnitude of regurgitant flow in mitral regurgitation is more complex. This is partly because the causes of mitral regurgitation are diverse. In some instances, the mitral orifice during systole is fixed (i.e., rheumatic disease, mitral annular calcification, or ruptured chordae tendineae), whereas in other diseases the regurgitant mitral orifice is dynamic (hypertrophic cardiomyopathy, mitral valve prolapse and papillary muscle dysfunction). In fixed orifice forms of mitral regurgitation, the major determinants of regurgitant flow are the mitral regurgitant orifice size during systole, the duration of systole, and the systolic gradient across the mitral valve. In this circumstance, drugs that reduce systolic blood pressure can be expected to reduce regurgitant mitral flow, whereas venodilators could reduce venous congestion without a reduction in the magnitude of regurgitation.

In patients with dynamic forms of mitral regurgitation, the response to vasoactive agents is determined by the specific cause of the regurgitation. For example, preload reduction (as with venodilators) can aggravate mitral regurgitation in patients with IHSS or mitral valve prolapse, whereas the same intervention in patients with papillary muscle dysfunction caused by coronary disease generally effects a gratifying reduction in mitral regurgitation and pulmonary venous congestion.

REFRACTORY DIASTOLIC DYSFUNCTION

In some cases of severe diastolic dysfunction, extraordinary measures are required to relieve symptoms of systemic and/or pulmonary venous congestion. In acute renal failure or extreme volume overload, dialysis or hemofiltration may be required to relieve hypervolemia and life-threatening elevations of central venous pressure. If these measures are impractical or unavailable, phlebotomy or plasmapheresis may be helpful. Direct removal of pleural or ascitic fluid can produce symptomatic improvement, and occasionally such an approach may initiate a diuresis. In rare instances of inferior vena caval obstruction with massive anasarca, the use of Southey-Leech tubes to relieve dependent edema has proved useful; this ancient therapy may also be useful for symptomatic relief in some patients with refractory heart failure.

In the treatment of all forms of congestive heart failure, the role of surgery to correct valvular stenosis, regurgitation, or myocardial ischemia should always be considered. When all else fails, the ultimate therapeutic measure is cardiac transplantation.

REFERENCES

1. Stauffer JC, Gaasch WH: Recognition and treatment of left ventricular diastolic dysfunction. Prog Cardiovasc Dis 32:319, 1990.
2. Grossman W: Diastolic dysfunction in congestive heart failure. N Engl J Med 325:1557, 1991.
3. Echeverria HH, Bilsker MS, Myerburg RJ, et al.: Congestive heart failure: Echocardiographic insights. Am J Med 75:750, 1983.
4. Dougherty AH, et al.: Congestive heart failure with normal systolic function. Am J Cardiol 54:778, 1984.
5. Soufer R, et al.: Intact systolic left ventricular function in clinical congestive heart failure. Am J Cardiol 55:1032, 1985.
6. Gaasch WH, Apstein CS, Levine HJ: Diastolic properties of the left ventricle. *In* The Ventricle. Edited by HJ Levine and WH Gaasch. Boston, Martinus Nijhoff Publishers, 1985.
7. Levine HJ: Diastolic dysfunction in patients with congestive heart failure. *In* Echocardiography 1990. Edited by A Dagianti and H Feigenbaum. Amsterdam, Elsevier Science Publishers, 1990.
8. Frumin AM, et al.: Nucleated red blood cells in congestive heart failure. Circulation 20:367, 1959.
9. Smith JA, Levine SA: Aortic stenosis with elevated metabolic rate simulating hyperthyroidism. Arch Intern Med 80:265, 1947.
10. Levine HJ, Wagman RJ: Energetics of the human heart. Am J Cardiol 9:372, 1962.
11. Estes NAM III, Levine HJ: Cardiac cachexia. Med Grand Rounds 1:188, 200, 1982.
12. Davidson JD, Waldman TA, Goodman DS, Gordon RS Jr.: Protein-losing gastroenteropathy in congestive heart failure. Lancet 1:899, 1961.
13. Burack WR, Pryce J, Goodwyn JF: A reversible nephrotic syndrome associated with congestive heart failure. Circulation 18:562, 1958.
14. Pastor BH, Cahn M: Reversible nephrotic syndrome resulting from constrictive pericarditis. N Engl J Med 262:872, 1960.
15. Fishman AP: Pulmonary edema: The water exchanging function of the lung. Circulation 46:390, 1972.
16. Criscitiello MG: Pathophysiology of heart sounds and murmurs. *In* Clinical Cardiovascular Physiology. Edited by HJ Levine. New York, Grune and Stratton, 1976.
17. Van de Werf F, et al.: Diastolic properties of the left ventricle in normal adults and in patients with third heart sounds. Circulation 69:1070, 1984.
18. Gorlin R, Knowles JH, Storey CF: Valvular maneuver as test of cardiac function: Pathologic physiology and clinical significance. Circ 23:197, 1957.
19. Nishimma RA, Tajik AJ: The Valsalva maneuver and response revisited. Mayo Clin Proc 61:211, 1986.
20. McInytre KM, Vita JA, Lambrew CT, Freeman J, Loscalzo J: A non-invasive method of predicting pulmonary capillary wedge pressure. N Engl J Med 327:1715, 1992.
21. Hoshino PK, Blaustein AS, Gaasch WH: Effect of propranolol on the left ventricular response to the Valsalva maneuver in normal subjects. Am J Cardiol 61:400, 1988.
22. Dumesnil JG, Gaudreault G, Honos GN, Kingma JG: Use of Valsalva maneuver to unmask left ventricular diastolic function abnormalities by Doppler echocardiography in patients with coronary artery disease or systemic hypertension. Am J Cardiol 68:515, 1991.
23. Ewy G: The abdominojugular test: technique and hemodynamic correlates. Ann Intern Med 109:456, 1988.
24. Lorell BH, Grossman W: Dynamic and isometric exercise during cardiac catheterization. *In* Cardiac Catheterization and Angiography. Edited by W Grossman. Philadelphia, Lea & Febiger, 1986.
25. Meaney E, Shabetai R, Bhargava V: Cardiac amyloidosis constrictive pericarditis and restrictive cardiomyopathy. Am J Cardiol 38:547, 1976.

26. Bonow RO, et al.: Verapamil induced improvement in left ventricular diastolic filling and increased exercise tolerance in patients with hypertrophic cardiomyopathy: short and long term effects. Circulation 72: 853, 1985.

27. Kitzman DW, et al.: Exercise intolerance in patients with heart failure and preserved left ventricular systolic function: failure of the Frank-Starling mechanism. J Am Coll Cardiol 17:1065, 1991.

28. Cuocolo A, et al.: Left ventricular hypertrophy and impaired diastolic filling in essential hypertension: Diastolic mechanisms for systolic dysfunction during exercise. Circulation 81:978, 1990.

29. Clyne CA, et al.: Systemic and left ventricular response to exercise stress in asymptomatic patients with valvular aortic stenosis. Am J Cardiol 68:1469, 1991.

30. Gaasch WH, et al.: Left ventricular stress and compliance in man: with special reference to normalized ventricular function curves. Circulation 45:746, 1972.

31. Cohn JN, et al.: Effect of vasodilator therapy on mortality in chronic congestive heart failure: Results of a Veterans Administration Cooperative Study. N Engl J Med 314: 1547, 1986.

32. Borgenhagen DM, et al.: The effects of left ventricular load and contractility on mitral regurgitation orifice size and flow in the dog. Circulation 56:106, 1977.

33. Topol EJ, Traill TA, Fortuin NJ: Hypertensive hypertrophic cardiomyopathy of the elderly. N Engl J Med 312:277, 1985.

34. Packer DL, et al.: Tachycardia-induced cardiomyopathy: A reversible form of left ventricular dysfunction. Am J Cardiol 57:563, 1986.

35. Levine HJ: Optimum heart rate of large failing hearts. Am J Cardiol 61:633, 1988.

36. Waagstein F, Hjalmmarson A, Varnauskas E, Wallentin I: Effect of chronic beta adrenergic receptor blockade in congestive cardiomyopathy. Br Heart J 37:1022, 1975.

37. Waagstein F, et al.: Long-term beta blockade in dilated cardiomyopathy. Circulation 80:551, 1989.

38. Anderson JL, et al.: A randomized trail of low-dose beta blockade therapy for idiopathic dilated cardiomyopathy. Am J Cardiol 55:471, 1985.

39. Engelmeier RS, et al.: Improvement in symptoms and exercise tolerance by metoprolol in patients with dilated cardiomyopathy: a double-blind, randomized, placebo-controlled trial. Circulation 72:536, 1985.

40. Forrester JS, Diamond G, Parmley WW, Swan HJC: Early increase in left ventricular compliance after myocardial infarction. J Clin Invest 51:598, 1972.

41. Vogel WM, Apstein CS, Briggs LL, Gaasch WH: Acute alterations in left ventricular diastolic chamber stiffness: Role of the "erectile" effect of coronary arterial pressure and flow in normal and damaged hearts. Circ Res 51:465, 1982.

42. Hood WB Jr, Bianco JA, Kumar R, Whiting RB: Experimental myocardial infarction IV: Reduction of left ventricular compliance in the healing phase. J Clin Invest 49: 1316, 1970.

43. The Multicenter diltiazem Post-infarction Trial Research Group: The effect of diltiazem on mortality and reinfarction after myocardial infarction. N Engl J Med 319: 385, 1988.

44. Dodek A, Kassebaum DG, Brislow JD: Pulmonary edema in coronary artery disease without cardiomegaly: Paradox of the stiff heart. N Engl J Med 286:1347, 1972.

45. Hess OM, et al.: Diastolic stiffness and myocardial structure in aortic valve disease before and after valve replacement. Circulation 69:855, 1984.

46. Georgiou D, Brundage BH: Regression of left ventricular mass in systemic hypertension. Clin Cardiol 15:5, 1992.

47. The CONSENSUS trial study group: Effects of enalapril on mortality in severe congestive heart failure. N Engl J Med 316: 1429, 1987.

48. The SOLVD Investigators: Effect of enalapril on survival in patients with reduced left ventricular ejection fractions and congestive heart failure. N Engl J Med 325:293, 1991.

49. Kimmelstiel C, Benotti Jr: How effective is digitalis in the treatment of congestive heart failure? Am Heart J 116:1063, 1070, 1988.

50. Kelly RA: Cardiac glycosides and congestive heart failure. Am J Cardiol 65:10E, 1990.

51. Kulick DL, Rahimtoola SH: Current role of digitalis therapy in patients with congestive heart failure. JAMA 265:2995, 1991.

52. Colucci WS, et al.: Decreased lymphocyte beta-adrenergic-receptor density in patients with heart failure and tolerance to the beta-adrenergic agonist pirbuterol. N Engl J Med 305:185, 1981.

53. Ikram H, Fitzpatrick D: Double blind trial of chronic oral beta blockade in congestive cardiomyopathy. Lancet 2:490, 1981.

54. Currie PJ, et al.: Oral beta adrenergic blockade with metoprolol in chronic severe dilated cardiomyopathy. J Am Coll Card 3: 203, 1984.

55. Greenberg B, et al.: Long term vasodilator therapy of chronic aortic insufficiency: A randomized double-blinded placebo-controlled clinical trial. Circulation 78:92, 1988.

56. Gaasch WH, Levine HJ: Prediction of the left ventricular response to surgical correction of chronic aortic regurgitation: The ratio of regurgitant volume to end-diastolic volume. *In* Chronic Aortic Regurgitation. Edited by WH Gaasch and HJ Levine. Boston, Kluwer Academic Publishers, 1988.

Chapter 27

BETA-ADRENERGIC RECEPTOR BLOCKERS AND CALCIUM CHANNEL BLOCKERS IN LEFT VENTRICULAR HYPERTROPHY

Otto M. Hess and Hans P. Krayenbuehl

Myocardial hypertrophy represents a fundamental compensatory mechanism of the heart to compete with an increased load imposed upon the ventricle (1–4). Chronic pressure or volume overload are, after a period of compensation, associated with a reduction and, finally, exhaustion of myocardial function with development of cardiac failure. To prevent myocardial failure, several therapeutic approaches have been used to normalize either the abnormal load or to improve the reduced contractile performance (5, 6). Medical therapy with beta-blocking agents, calcium antagonists, and ACE inhibitors became popular in the past, because hypertrophy was found to be an independent risk factor for cardiovascular morbidity and mortality (7). The purpose of this chapter is to discuss the effect of beta-blockers and calcium antagonists on diastolic dysfunction in patients with left ventricular hypertrophy.

PHARMACOLOGIC ACTION OF BETA-BLOCKING AGENTS AND CALCIUM ANTAGONISTS

Left ventricular hypertrophy is associated with a series of changes in regard to contractile function, myocardial metabolism, morphology, myocardial architecture, and neurohormonal control. Not only myocytes but also the interstitial tissue undergoes alterations when cardiac muscle has to produce chronically an increased force (see Chapters 20 and 21). The myocytes show hypertrophy with increased muscle fiber diameter, whereas the interstitium elicits architectural changes with rearrangement of collagen structure and cross-hatching of orthogonally oriented fibers

(8–10). These structural alterations represent an adaptive mechanism, but might become irreversible in the presence of long-standing pressure or volume overload. Structural alterations are associated with functional changes in systolic and/or diastolic function; however, a reduced systolic ejection performance may be reversible after correction of the abnormal loading conditions (3). The cardiac interstitium and the renin-angiotensin system have gained a lot of interest in the past few years, and medical therapies to reduce collagen formation or to increase collagen degradation have been discussed widely (8–10). Beta-blocking agents and calcium antagonists have been used for many years to control blood pressure and thus to reduce myocardial hypertrophy and to improve systolic and diastolic function in patients with left ventricular hypertrophy. Besides the antihypertensive action of these drugs, the negative chrono- and inotropic action of the beta-blockers as well as the negative inotropic and positive lusitropic effect of the calcium antagonists have been studied extensively in patients with primary or secondary myocardial hypertrophy. Beta blockers have been found to reduce heart rate, blood pressure, and the inotropic state of the myocardium but to induce vasoconstriction of the coronary arteries (11). Different beta blockers may show differences in the pharmacologic action, and newly developed beta blockers with vasodilating properties (carvedilol) are associated with coronary vasodilation, which might be especially important in patients with severe myocardial hypertrophy and subendocardial ischemia. The lusitropic effect of the

Table 27–1.   Cumulative Survival Rates in Patients with Hypertrophic, Obstructive Cardiomyopathy*

	n	5-year Cumulative Survival Rate	10-year Cumulative Survival Rate
Control patients	22	72%	65%
Propranolol-treated patients	20	81% *	67% *
Verapamil-treated patients	18	88%	80%

* Reproduced with permission from Seiler CH, et al.: Long-term follow-up of medical versus surgical therapy for hypertrophic cardiomyopathy: A retrospective study. J Am Coll Cardiol 17:634, 1991.
5- and 10-year cumulative survival rates in patients with hypertrophic cardiomyopathy. No significant difference in survival rates was observed between propranolol-treated and control patients. However, 10-year survival rate was significantly better under verapamil than in untreated controls or propranolol-treated patients. n = number of patients. Mean follow-up was 8–9 years.

ment after beta blocker treatment in patients with dilated cardiomyopathy. More recently, the same authors reported an upregulation of myocardial betareceptor density after long-term treatment with metoprolol (25), suggesting that a higher number of beta-receptors may exert a stronger response to sympathetic stimulation. Possible other mechanisms include a reduction of heart rate resulting in a better myocardial perfusion and possibly a reduced oxygen consumption as well as prevention of a toxic effect of the increased catecholamines levels (see Chapter 26).

Parallel to the improvement in systolic function, an improvement in diastolic dysfunction, with a decrease in diastolic filling pressure and an increase in diastolic

filling rates, was observed in patients with dilated cardiomyopathy after beta blocker treatment.

A beneficial effect of calcium antagonists on diastolic heart failure has been reported in patients with dilated cardiomyopathy after long-term treatment with diltiazem (26). The exact mechanism of action is not clear, but was thought to be the afterload-reducing and/or the negative chronotropic effect of the calcium blocker. However, other data in patients with congestive heart failure (27) have indicated that calcium antagonists may exert an adverse effect on outcome and survival rate, probably because of its negative inotropic effect and/or its activation of the neurohormonal system, especially the renin-angiotensin system.

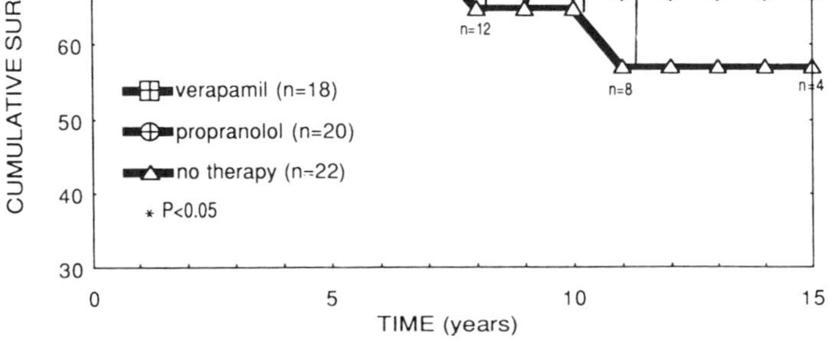

Fig. 27–3. Cumulative survival rates in 60 patients with hypertrophic cardiomyopathy. The best survival rates can be observed in patients treated with verapamil, whereas no difference was found in propranolol-treated and untreated patients. Thus, the best long-term results were obtained in patients with chronic verapamil therapy. Reproduced with permission from Seiler CH, et al.: Long-term follow-up of medical versus surgical therapy for hypertrophic cardiomyopathy: A retrospective study. J Am Coll Cardiol 17:634, 1991.

Valvular Heart Disease

Chronic pressure overload, as in aortic stenosis, is associated with increased systolic wall stress and increased wall thickness. Whereas hypertrophy restores wall stress toward normal and improves systolic contraction, the increase in mass predisposes the heart to subendocardial ischemia. In advanced forms of hypertrophy, systolic performance becomes depressed with slowing of myocardial relaxation and increased myocardial stiffness (28). On the other hand, long-term volume overload, as in mitral or aortic regurgitation, is associated with enlargement of cardiac chambers and increased diastolic wall stress. Both forms lead to diastolic dysfunction, which reflects qualitative and quantitative changes in myocardial collagen structure. Primary diastolic dysfunction has been observed (4) in a large proportion of patients with aortic valve disease and normal systolic ejection performance (Fig. 27–4). However, in the presence of systolic dysfunction, all patients have also diastolic dysfunction. Thus, either diastolic function parameters are more sensitive for detection of left ventricular dysfunction or diastolic functional abnormalities precede systolic dysfunction.

Beta blockers have been used rarely in patients with valvular lesions, mainly because of the negative inotropic effect of these drugs. Antihypertensive treatment in patients with valvular heart disease is usually done with ACE inhibitors because these drugs have, besides their antihypertensive effect, a direct action on the cardiac muscle by way of the local renin-angiotensin system. The effect of calcium antagonists on left ventricular diastolic function has been evaluated in patients with chronic pressure overload (29); in contrast to hypertrophic cardiomyopathy (16, 18–22, 29), the speed of relaxation is prolonged and diastolic filling remains abnormal after intravenous administration of verapamil (Fig. 27–5). Thus, worsening of diastolic function after verapamil in patients with secondary myocardial hypertrophy is probably related to the negative inotropic action of the drug (29).

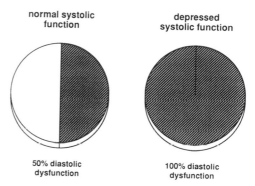

Diastolic dysfunction in aortic valve disease

Fig. 27–4. Occurrence of diastolic dysfunction in 58 patients with severe aortic valve disease in the presence of normal (left hand) or depressed systolic function (right hand). Fifty percent of all patients (n = 40) with normal systolic function already had an abnormal diastolic function (either prolonged time constant of relaxation, reduced peak filling rate, or increased constant of myocardial stiffness). However, all patients with depressed systolic function (n = 18) also had abnormal diastolic function. Thus, systolic and diastolic dysfunction occur at the same time in most patients with aortic valve disease, but 50% of all patients with normal systolic function already have diastolic dysfunction. Diastolic function parameters seem either to be more sensitive for detection of a functional derangement of the left ventricle or to precede systolic dysfunction.

Hypertension

Left ventricular hypertrophy is a compensatory mechanism to maintain a normal wall stress and, thus, a normal ventricular ejection performance in patients with hypertension. However, hypertrophy per se is a risk factor for acute myocardial infarction, congestive heart failure, sudden death, and other cardiovascular events (7) (see Chapter 21). The awareness of the increased risk of cardiovascular diseases with systemic hypertension has led to attempts to identify and utilize drugs that would be useful not only in lowering blood pressure but also in reversing left ventricular hypertrophy, and thus in improving its functional characteristics. Some of the most commonly used antihypertensive drugs are beta blockers, calcium antagonists, and

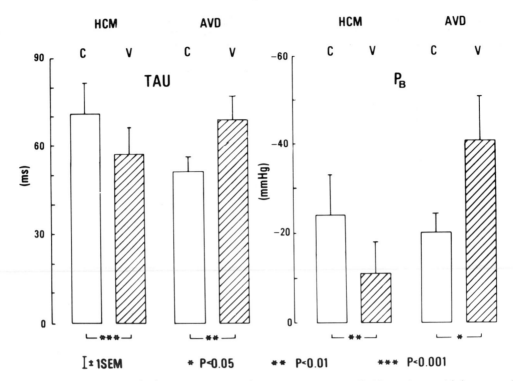

Fig. 27–5.   Time constant of relaxation (TAU) and pressure asymptote (P_B) in patients with hypertrophic cardiomyopathy (HCM) and in patients with aortic valve disease (AVD) before (open bars) and after 0.1 mg/kg verapamil I.V. (hatched bars). Relaxation is improved after intravenous administration of verapamil in patients with HCM (decrease in TAU and P_B) but deteriorates in patients with AVD (increase in TAU and P_B). Thus, verapamil has a beneficial effect on relaxation in the primary form of hypertrophy but a negative effect on diastolic function in secondary hypertrophy. Reproduced with permission from Hess OM, et al.: Does verapamil improve left ventricular relaxation in patients with myocardial hypertrophy? Circulation 74:530, 1986.

ACE inhibitors, which have been shown to be especially useful in reducing blood pressure and causing regression of myocardial hypertrophy. However, vasodilators, such as alpha-adrenergic blockers or diuretics, appear less effective and have been shown not to induce regression of left ventricular hypertrophy (30). The effect of beta blockers and calcium antagonists on the reversal of left ventricular muscle mass has been evaluated by several authors and is summarized in Tables 27–2 and 27–3. With a short-term antihypertensive treatment, a 10 to 20% decrease in mass can be expected.

Coronary Artery Disease

In patients with myocardial infarction, ventricular hypertrophy serves as a compensatory mechanism, e.g., the nonin-

farcted regions of the left ventricle undergoes regional hypertrophy and thus compensates for the reduced pump function of the infarcted segment (31). The changes in regional wall stress associated with myocardial infarction result in extensive remodeling of the ventricle (see Chapter 18). Because of the abnormal LV shape, wall stress becomes elevated in the normal myocardium and regional hypertrophy ensues. Both scar formation in the infarcted region and compensatory hypertrophy are important for the decrease in diastolic distensibility of the left ventricle and, thus, diastolic dysfunction. Whether diastolic dysfunction can be influenced beneficially with a reduction in regional hypertrophy by lowering afterload with medical therapy is unknown. A decrease in left ventricular muscle mass has been reported (32) after

Table 27–2. **Effects of Calcium Entry Blocking Agents on LV Mass, Evaluated by Echo, in Patients with Arterial Hypertension**

Drug	Study		Patients (no.)	Dose (mg/d)	Follow-up (Months)	LVM Before	LVM After	Change in %
Nitrendipine	Ferrara[33]	1985	20	20	2	195	188 g	− 3.4
	Drayer[35]	1986	30	10–80	12	243	236 g	− 2.9
	Grossman[34]	1988	14	10–30	3	133	116 g/m²	− 12.7
Nifedipine	Strauer[38]	1984	12	120	3.9	171	153 g	− 10.5
	Mace[37]	1985	9	3 × 10	4	126	117 g/m²	− 7.1
	Muiesan[36]	1986	7	2 × 20	3	224	194 g	− 13.4
	Kleine[39]	1987	11	30	6	400	297 g	− 25.7
Verapamil	Mulesan[36]	1986	7	2 × 120	3	207	172 g	− 16.9
	Schmieder[10]	1987	7	240 SR	3	190	179 g	− 6.1
Diltiazem	Amodeo[41]	1986	9	300	1	242	217 g	− 10.3
	10 studies		126		4.1	234 g	205 g	− 10.9

└P < 0.05┘
(n = 8)

successful aortocoronary bypass surgery when full revascularization has been achieved.

CLINICAL IMPLICATIONS

Beta-adrenergic blockers and calcium antagonists play an important role in the treatment of hypertrophic cardiomyopathy, hypertension, and coronary heart disease. These drugs have been shown to be efficient in the reduction of left ventricular mass in the presence of long-standing pressure overload caused by hypertension. A beneficial effect of calcium antagonists was also reported in patients with hypertrophic cardiomyopathy. This effect was not directly related to the reduction in myocardial muscle mass, but more to an improvement in myocardial relaxation and diastolic chamber filling. Calcium blockers reduce the calcium influx into the myocardial cell and thus improve relaxation by removing the calcium from the cytosol (28). However, relaxation is improved only in patients with hypertrophic cardiomyopathy, not in patients with secondary hypertrophy

Table 27–3. **Effects of Beta-Blocking Agents on LV Mass, Evaluated by Echo, in Patients with Arterial Hypertension**

Drug	Study		Patients (no.)	Dose (mg/d)	Follow-up (Months)	LVM Before	LVM After	Change in %
Metoprolol	Franz[42]	1986	25	200	6.1	147	126 g/m²	− 14.0
			25	200	12.7	147	114 g/m²	− 22.5
	Corea[43]	1984	8	200	16–18	134	112 g/m²	− 16.1
Labetalol	Kaul[44]	1984	10	580	3	241	160 g	− 33.6
Atenolol	Sau[45]	1982	15	100	12	157	126 g/m²	− 19.7
	Dunn[46]	1987	12	100	12	144	127 g/m²	− 11.8
	6 studies		95		10.4	146	121 g/m²	− 19.6

└P < 0.01┘
(n = 5)

from aortic stenosis. This different behavior could be explained by differences in the type of hypertrophy (primary versus secondary form). Beside the effect on relaxation, calcium antagonists are associated with an improvement in the cumulative survival rate of patients with hypertrophic cardiomyopathy which was not observed with beta-blocking agents, suggesting that the reduction in intracellular calcium has a potentially beneficial effect on diastolic dysfunction (17).

SUMMARY

Hypertrophy represents an adaptive process of the myocardium to compete with an increased mechanical load. Several adaptations of the myocardium, the peripheral circulation, and the neurohormonal system are involved and lead ultimately to architectural changes of the myocardium with alterations in the collagen network. Beta-blockers and calcium antagonists have been associated with different myocardial effects in patients with primary and secondary forms of hypertrophy. In patients with hypertrophic cardiomyopathy, calcium antagonists elicit a beneficial effect on relaxation and diastolic filling, but beta blockers do not; in patients with dilated cardiomyopathy, beta blockers may show a beneficial effect on ventricular function and survival but calcium antagonists do not; in patients with hypertension, both drugs have a beneficial effect on the regression of myocardial hypertrophy. Thus, the effect of beta blockers and calcium antagonists on diastolic function may vary according to the type and severity of disease and may be beneficial or detrimental depending on the origin of the hypertrophic process.

REFERENCES

1. Wikman-Coffelt J, Parmley WW, Mason DT: The cardiac hypertrophy process. Analyses of factors determining pathological vs. physiological development. Circ Res 45:697, 1979.
2. Grossman W: Cardiac hypertrophy: Useful adaptation or pathologic process? Am J Med 69:576, 1980.
3. Krayenbuehl HP, Hess OM, Schneider J, Turina M: Physiologic or pathologic hypertrophy. Eur Heart J 4(Suppl. A): 29, 1983.
4. Villari B, Hess OM, Kaufmann PH, et al.: Effects of aortic valve stenosis (pressure overload) and regurgitation (volume overload) on left ventricular systolic and diastolic function. Am J Cardiol 69:927–34, 1992.
5. Tarazi RC, Frohlich ED: Is reversal of cardiac hypertrophy a desirable goal of antihypertensive therapy? Circulation 75(Suppl. I):114, 1987.
6. Pearson AC, Pasierski T, Labovitz AJ: Left ventricular hypertrophy: diagnosis, prognosis, and management. Am Heart J 121: 148, 1991.
7. Messerli FH, Ketelhut R: Left ventricular hypertrophy: an independent risk factor. J Cardiovasc Pharm 17(Suppl. 4):S59, 1991.
8. Rodbard S: Negative feedback mechanisms in the architecture and function of the connective and cardiovascular tissues. Perspect Biol Med 13:507–527, 1970.
9. Jalil JE, Doering CW, Janicki JS, Pick R, Schroff SG, Weber KT: Fibrillar collagen and myocardial stiffness in the intact hypertrophied rat left ventricle. Circ Res 64: 1041, 1989.
10. Weber KT: Cardiac interstitium in health and disease: The fibrillar collagen network. J Am Coll Cardiol 13:1637, 1989.
11. Bortone AS, Hess OM, Suter T, et al.: Effect of intravenous propranolol on coronary vasomotion at rest and during dynamic exercise in patients with coronary artery disease. Circulation 81:1225, 1990.
12. Hanrath P, Mathey DG, Kremer P, et al.: Effect of verapamil on left ventricular isovolumic relaxation time and regional left ventricular filling in hypertrophic cardiomyopathy. Am J Cardiol 45:1258, 1980.
13. Stewart S, Mason DT, Braunwald E: Impaired rate of left ventricular filling in idiopathic hypertrophic subaortic stenosis and valvular aortic stenosis. Circulation 37:8, 1968.
14. Wigle ED, Sasson Z, Henderson MA, et al.: Hypertrophic cardiomyopathy. The importance of the site and the extent of hypertrophy. A review. Prog Cardiovasc Dis 28: 1, 1985.
15. Speiser K, Krayenbuehl HP: Reappraisal of the effect of acute betablockade on left ventricular filling dynamics in hypertrophic obstructive cardiomyopathy. Eur Heart J 2: 21, 1981.
16. Hess OM, Grimm J, Krayenbuehl HP: Diastolic function in hypertrophic cardiomyopathy: effects of propranolol and verapamil on diastolic stiffness. Eur Heart J 4(Suppl. F):47, 1983.
17. Seiler CH, Hess OM, Schoenbeck M, et al.:

Long-term follow-up of medical versus surgical therapy for hypertrophic cardiomyopathy: A retrospective study. J Am Coll Cardiol 17:634, 1991.

18. Betocchi S, Bonow RO, Bacharach SL, et al.: Isovolumic relaxation period in hypertrophic cardiomyopathy: assessment by radionuclide angiography. J Am Coll Cardiol 7:74, 1986.

19. Bonow RO, Vitale DF, Maron BJ, et al.: Regional left ventricular asynchrony and impaired global left ventricular filling in hypertrophic cardiomyopathy: Effect of verapamil. J Am Coll Cardiol 9:1108, 1987.

20. Suwa M, Hirota Y, Kawamura K: Improvement in left ventricular diastolic function during intravenous and oral diltiazem therapy in patients with hypertrophic cardiomyopathy: an echocardiographic study. Am J Cardiol 54:1047, 1984.

21. Lorell BH, Paulus WJ, Grossman W, et al.: Modification of abnormal left ventricular diastolic properties by nifedipine in patients with hypertrophic cardiomyopathy. Circulation 65:499, 1982.

22. Toshima H, Koga Y, Nagatam H, et al.: Comparable effects of oral diltiazem and verapamil in the treatment of hypertrophic cardiomyopathy. Jpn Heart J 27:701, 1986.

23. Cohn JN, Johnson G: Veterans Administration Cooperative Study Group: Heart failure with normal ejection fraction: The V-Heft study. Circulation 81(Suppl. III):48, 1990.

24. Waagstein F, Hjalmarson A, Varnauskas E, Wallentin I: Effect of chronic beta-adrenergic receptor blockade in congestive cardiomyopathy. Br Heart J 37:1022, 1975.

25. Waagstein F, Caidahl K, Wallentin I, et al.: Long-term beta-blockade in dilated cardiomyopathy. Circulation 80:551, 1989.

26. Figulla HR, Rechenberg JV, Wiegand V, et al.: Beneficial effects of long-term diltiazem treatment in dilated cardiomyopathy. J Am Coll Cardiol 13:653, 1989.

27. Packer M: Pathophysiological mechanisms underlying the adverse effects of calcium channel-blocking drugs in patients with chronic heart failure. Circulation 80(Suppl. IV):IV59, 1989.

28. Grossman W: Diastolic dysfunction in congestive heart failure. N Engl J Med 325:1557, 1991.

29. Hess OM, Murakami T, Krayenbuehl HP: Does verapamil improve left ventricular relaxation in patients with myocardial hypertrophy? Circulation 74:530, 1986.

30. Fouad-Tarazi M: Structural cardiac and vascular changes in hypertension: Response to treatment. Curr Opin Cardiol 2:782, 1987.

31. Hess OM, Schneider J, Nonogi H, et al.: Myocardial structure in patients with exercise-induced ischemia. Circulation 77:967, 1988.

32. Meester GT, Brower RW, Hugenholtz PG: Regression of left ventricular wall mass index after coronary artery bypass surgery in a group of patients with stable angina pectoris. Eur Heart J 3(Suppl. A):155, 1982.

33. Ferrera LA, Fasano ML, de Simone G, et al.: Antihypertensive and cardiovascular effects of nitrendipine: A controlled study vs. placebo. Clin Pharmacol Ther 38:434, 1985.

34. Grossman E, Oren S, Garavaglia GE, et al.: Systemic and regional hemodynamic and humoral effects of nitrendipine in essential hypertension. Circulation 78:1394, 1988.

35. Drayer JIM, Hall WD, Smith VE, et al.: Effect of calcium channel blocker nitrendipine on left ventricular mass in patients with hypertension. Clin Pharmacol Ther 40:679, 1986.

36. Muiesan G, Agabiti-Rosei E, Romanelli G, et al.: Adrenergic activity and left ventricular function during treatment of essential hypertension with calcium antagonists. Am J Cardiol 57:44D, 1986.

37. Mace PJ, Littler WA, Glover DR, et al.: Regression of left ventricular hypertrophy in hypertension: Comparative effects of three different drugs. J Cardiovasc Pharmacol 7(Suppl. 2):52, 1985.

38. Strauer BE, Mahmoud MA, Bayer F, et al.: Reversal of left ventricular hypertrophy and improvement of cardiac function in man by nifedipine. Eur Heart J 5(Suppl. F):53, 1984.

39. Kleine P, Meissner E, von Bruchhausen V, Bruckner S: Effects of clonidine and nifedipine on left ventricular hypertrophy and muscle mass in hypertensive patients. J Cardiovasc Pharmacol 10(Suppl. 12):180, 1987.

40. Schmieder RE, Messerli FH, Garavagli GE, Nunez BD: Cardiovascular effects of verapamil in patients with essential hypertension. Circulation 75:1030, 1987.

41. Amodeo C, Kobrin I, Ventura HO, et al.: Immediate and short-term hemodynamic effects of diltiazem in patients with hypertension. Circulation 73:108, 1986.

42. Franz IW, Wiewel D, Behr M, Ketelhut R: Rückbildung der Myokardhypertrophie Hochdruckkranker unter chronischer Beta-Rezeptorenblockade. Deutsch Med Wschr 111:530, 1986.

43. Corea L, Bentivoglio M, Verdecchia P, et al.: Left ventricular hypertrophy regression

in hypertensive patients treated with metoprolol. Int J Clin Pharmacol 22:365, 1984.

44. Kaul U, Mohan JC, Bhatia ML: Effects of labetalol on left ventricular mass and function in hypertension—an assessment by serial echocardiography. Int J Cardiol 5:461, 1984.

45. Sau F, Cherchi A, Seguo C: Reversal of left ventricular hypertrophy after treatment of hypertension by atenolol for one year. Clin Sci 63:367s, 1982.

46. Dunn FG, Ventura HO, Messerli FH, et al.: Time course of regression of left ventricular hypertrophy in hypertensive patients treated with atenolol. Circulation 76:254, 1987.

Chapter 28

LEFT VENTRICULAR DIASTOLIC FUNCTION AND CALCIUM CHANNEL BLOCKERS IN HYPERTROPHIC CARDIOMYOPATHY

James E. Udelson and Robert O. Bonow

Hypertrophic cardiomyopathy (HCM) is a primary disorder of cardiac muscle of unknown origin. In most patients, the disease appears to be genetically determined in an autosomal-dominant fashion with a variable penetrance (1), and studies have identified several genetic loci that appear to be associated with the presence of disease in certain families (2–4). In some patients, the disease appears to be sporadic and unrelated to genetic mechanisms.

The presence of HCM is defined by the echocardiographic demonstration of a hypertrophied, nondilated ventricle in the absence of a cardiac or systemic stimulus that could be responsible for causing hypertrophy (5). Although early studies of patients with HCM emphasized the asymmetric nature of the septal hypertrophy and the presence of left ventricular outflow tract obstruction, the advent of more sophisticated echocardiographic techniques to investigate ventricular morphology in patients with HCM has revealed wide variation in the site and extent of hypertrophy that may be present (5). Hypertrophy may be mild and localized, not necessarily involving the basal septum, or extensive, severe, and diffuse, involving all aspects of the left ventricle. The morphologic site and extent of hypertrophy may differ even among first-degree relatives who have the disease (6). Histologically, the regions of hypertrophy are characterized by areas of myocyte hypertrophy and cellular disorganization, with the hypertrophied myocytes arranged in such a way that they may form a loop or perpendicular angles to one another (7–10). Although such cellular disorganization is not unique to HCM, it tends

to be extensive in such patients, and when this histopathologic abnormality is found in myocardium of patients with other types of cardiac disease, it tends to be of much smaller magnitude (10). Other histologic features seen in patients with HCM include variable degrees of myocardial scarring with fibrous tissue formation ranging from patchy interstitial fibrosis to large confluent scars that may be transmural, findings that may occur in the absence of epicardial coronary artery disease (11). Finally, in approximately 80% of patients with HCM studied at autopsy, the small intramural coronary arteries are histologically abnormal, with an increase in the width of the intima or media, with apparent compromise of the lumen (12). These abnormal intramural arteries are found in increased numbers within or at the margins of areas of fibrosis (12). Such small vessel abnormalities are likely to contribute in an important manner to myocardial ischemia and myocardial infarction in such patients.

PATHOPHYSIOLOGIC ABNORMALITIES IN HCM

Left Ventricular Diastolic Dysfunction

Elevation of left ventricular end-diastolic pressure in patients with HCM, in the presence of normal or reduced end-diastolic volume, led early investigators to suggest that impaired filling of the hypertrophied ventricle may contribute importantly to the clinical manifestations of the disease (13–15). The concept of an impairment in early, rapid diastolic filling resulting from a hypertrophied and "stiff" left ventricle was supported by the hemodynamic obser-

465

vation that the magnitude and rate of decrease in left atrial pressure during early diastole are diminished in HCM (15), as well as by the echocardiographic observation that the mitral valve EF slope is decreased (16). Subsequent invasive and noninvasive studies of left ventricular diastolic function have identified abnormalities in relaxation, distensibility (compliance), and filling in most patients with the nonobstructive and obstructive forms of HCM (17–22): the early filling phase is prolonged, and the rate and volume of rapid filling are decreased. Consequently, there is a compensatory increase in the contribution of atrial systole to overall left ventricular filling. Although diastolic dysfunction sufficient to produce symptoms is usually associated with considerable left ventricular hypertrophy, diastolic abnormalities may also be identified in patients with only mild and localized wall thickening (23). (See Chap. 22.)

Left Ventricular Distensibility

Two factors contribute to impaired diastolic filling of the hypertrophied left ventricle in HCM: decreased distensibility (or compliance) and prolonged (and/or incomplete) relaxation. Decreased distensibility results from increases in stiffness of both the left ventricular chamber and the muscle (17, 18). The increase in muscle stiffness reflects abnormalities in the intrinsic elastic properties of the myocardium that may be caused by areas of interstitial and, in some cases, transmural fibrosis (11, 12, 24), or possibly to cell disorganization (9). The increase in chamber stiffness results from the combination of increased muscle stiffness, increased ventricular mass, and dynamic abnormalities caused by incomplete relaxation. Diminished distensibility is manifested by an abnormally steep slope of the late diastolic pressure-volume curve, so that a given increase in diastolic volume results in a disproportionately greater augmentation in diastolic pressure.

Left Ventricular Relaxation

Abnormal left ventricular relaxation in HCM, as manifested by a prolonged isovolumic relaxation period and a reduced rate of decline in left ventricular pressure

(17–20, 23, 25, 26), is evident in most patients. An association between prolonged relaxation and subsequent reduction in the rate and magnitude of the rapid filling phase has also been demonstrated (17, 20, 26).

Myocardial relaxation is a complex, energy-requiring process that may be altered by several mechanisms. The primary mechanism influencing relaxation is the inactivation process, by which calcium ions are sequestered in the sarcoplasmic reticulum, thereby lowering intracellular calcium concentration in the region of the myofibrillar contractile proteins (27). Because the energy-dependent systems responsible for this process are sensitive to even mild degrees of ischemia or hypoxia (27, 28), the myocardial ischemia that occurs in HCM could alone diminish the rate and completeness of left ventricular relaxation. Relaxation may also be influenced by several load-dependent mechanisms (29, 30), including left ventricular end-systolic pressure and volume, afterload, wall stress, coronary blood flow, and regional asynchrony (29). Any or all of these factors may be altered to variable degrees in HCM, and could contribute to prolonged or incomplete relaxation.

The interrelated abnormalities in relaxation, distensibility, and filling in HCM affect global left ventricular diastolic function. For example, prolonged (or incomplete) relaxation, in which increased myocardial wall tension persists into the rapid filling phase of the cardiac cycle, impairs both the rate and the degree of left ventricular filling, and also increases the diastolic intracavitary pressure as volume increases. The diastolic pressure-volume relations that determine distensibility are therefore influenced not only by the myocardial mass and stiffness (which may be considerable in HCM) but also by the dynamic relation between left ventricular relaxation and filling (18, 28, 29).

The concepts that impaired ventricular relaxation is a dynamic process that may be modified, and that abnormal relaxation influences diastolic pressure-volume relations in patients with HCM, are supported by data involving beta-adrenergic stimulation (31). Instantaneous relations between LV pressure and volume throughout the cardiac cycle were compared in patients with obstructive HCM during rapid atrial pacing to induce ischemia and during isoproterenol infusion to a matched heart rate. During pacing, the diastolic pressure-volume relation shifted upward, indicating diminished distensibility, and in many patients LV pressure continued to decline throughout much of the filling period, evidence of incomplete relaxation. During beta-adrenergic stimulation with isoproterenol, there was an increase in outflow gradient and evidence of more severe myocardial ischemia with worsening chest pain and more abnormal lactate metabolism by coronary sinus sampling. Nonetheless,

there was an increase in both the rate and the extent of LV pressure decline, indicating an enhanced relaxation process. This was associated with a downward and rightward shift of the diastolic pressure-volume relation toward its baseline position before pacing (Fig. 28–1), as well as a more complete decline of pressure before the onset of filling. Regional nonuniformity also improved during beta-adrenergic stimulation, consistent with a favorable effect of isoproterenol on the synchrony of regional LV performance. Thus, beta-adrenergic stimulation resulted in favorable effects on LV relaxation and global diastolic function in patients with HCM, despite potential de-

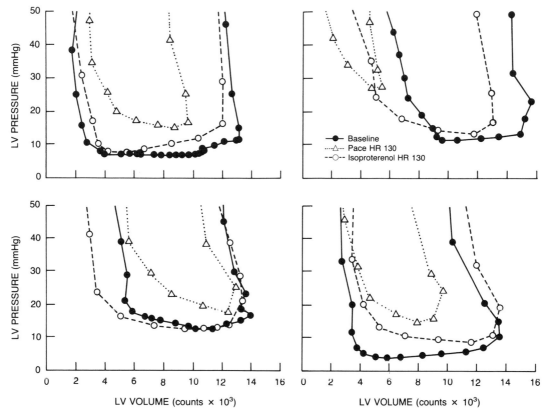

Fig. 28–1. Plots of diastolic pressure-volume relation in four patients with hypertrophic cardiomyopathy. Instantaneous diastolic pressure-volume relations are shown during baseline control conditions, atrial pacing (pace) to a heart rate (HR) of 130, and isoproterenol infusion. During atrial pacing, the curves shift upward and leftward and left ventricular (LV) pressure continues to decline through the filling period. During isoproterenol, the curves shift downward and rightward toward the baseline despite evidence of more severe myocardial ischemia (by symptoms and metabolic parameters) in all cases, and there is less evidence of impaired relaxation. Reproduced with permission from Udelson JE, et al.: β-adrenergic stimulation with isoproterenol enhances left ventricular diastolic performance in hypertrophic cardiomyopathy despite potentiation of myocardial ischemia: Comparison to rapid atrial pacing. Circulation 79:371, 1989.

leterious effects on the LV outflow gradient and on myocardial ischemia (31).

The mechanism for improved diastolic function during beta stimulation may relate to beneficial loading effects on the left ventricle. Systolic shortening increased, which in the normal ventricle leads to enhanced elastic recoil and restoring forces to augment the rate and extent of LV pressure decline during diastole (32–34). However, because myocardial ischemia would be expected to impair the inactivation process and result in relative insensitivity to changes in load (29), additional effects of isoproterenol must also play a role. We hypothesize that beta-adrenergic stimulation directly enhances the myocardial inactivation process (31, 35), thereby restoring load sensitivity. This is suggested by data in animal models, in which beta-adrenergic stimulation enhances myocardial relaxation related to its ability to speed the calcium sequestration process (36). In addition, the improvement in regional asynchrony is another possible mechanism with which to explain the improvement in diastolic hemodynamics.

It is clear that isoproterenol is not a clinically useful drug for the treatment of HCM (especially in patients with outflow obstruction). However, these findings provide further evidence that the disturbances of LV diastolic function in this disease state are not merely related to the abnormal passive myocardial properties that develop in response to hypertrophy, fibrosis, and cellular disarray. Rather, diastolic dysfunction in HCM also involves dynamic disorders of LV relaxation stemming from the complex interrelationships of hypertrophy, ischemia, and asynchrony. (See Chap. 4.)

Myocardial Ischemia

There is growing awareness that, in the absence of coronary artery disease, myocardial ischemia occurs commonly in patients with HCM. Several lines of evidence support this concept. Angina pectoris is a common symptom; although angina may occur at rest, it characteristically develops with increases in myocardial oxygen demand [such as with exercise or with atrial pacing (37, 38)]. The increased demands of exercise are often associated with reversible regional thallium-201 perfusion defects, compatible with transient ischemia (39–41).

Abnormalities of both coronary blood supply and myocardial oxygen demand may underlie myocardial ischemia in HCM (Fig. 28–2) (42). Coronary vasodilator capacity is reduced, so that incremental increases in myocardial demand are not balanced by appropriate increases in coronary flow; this imbalance is associated with disproportionate increases in left ventricular filling pressures and reduction in myocardial lactate consumption (37, 38, 43). Reduced coronary flow reserve may result from left ventricular diastolic dysfunction alone because increases in myocardial wall tension arising from prolonged or incomplete relaxation restrict early diastolic coronary flow, and elevated left ventricular cavity pressures in late diastole have a

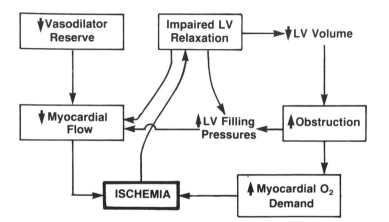

Fig. 28–2. Influence of reduced coronary vasodilator reserve, impaired left ventricular (LV) relaxation, and the presence of subaortic obstruction on myocardial ischemia in hypertrophic cardiomyopathy. Reproduced with permission from Bonow RO, et al.: Medical and surgical therapy of hypertrophic cardiomyopathy. *In* Cardiomyopathies: Clinical Presentation, Differential Diagnosis, and Management. Philadelphia, FA Davis, 1988, pp. 221–239.

compressive effect on the intramyocardial coronary arteries, which further limits blood supply (38), especially in the subendocardial regions. Reduction in vasodilator capacity could also develop in HCM because of abnormalities of the small intramural coronary arteries (12, 44), which are only rarely present in other forms of hypertrophy. The intramyocardial coronary arteries in HCM are characterized by thickening of the intima or media (or both) of the arterial walls, often with apparent luminal compromise (12). Myocardial oxygen demand is increased in HCM as the result of excessive oxygen requirements of the hypertrophied ventricular myocardium and, in many patients, of the added demands of greatly elevated systolic pressures resulting from outflow tract obstruction. Once ischemia develops, it may be self-perpetuating, inasmuch as ischemia results in further impairment of left ventricular relaxation (27–29) and further increase in end-diastolic pressure, resulting in a greater compromise of myocardial blood flow (Fig. 28–2).

Left Ventricular Systolic Function

Indexes of LV systolic performance in patients with HCM usually demonstrate normal or supernormal values (13, 45). Although this may reflect augmentation in the primary state of contractility per se, it may also reflect reduced afterload because the hypertrophied and nondilated ventricle would demonstrate reduced wall stress throughout the ejection period (46). Some studies have suggested that primary contractile performance in HCM is normal or may even be depressed despite supernormal ejection fractions (46). In patients with hypertrophy of the basal anterior ventricular septum, the hyperdynamic left ventricular systolic function is often associated with a pressure gradient across the left ventricular outflow tract, which can be demonstrated at cardiac catheterization or by Doppler echocardiography.

The presence of LV outflow obstruction and hyperdynamic systolic performance has important implications for diastolic function in HCM. To the extent that the greatly increased systolic chamber pressure in the presence of a pressure gradient acts as a "contraction load" (29, 47), both the onset and rate of isovolumic pressure decline may be subsequently impaired by means of load-dependent mechanisms (29). (See Chaps. 13 and 22.) However, although contraction and relaxation loading are determinants of myocardial relaxation in isolated myocardial preparations (29) and experimental models (48), their influence on relaxation in the intact normal and diseased human heart is undefined. Enhanced oxygen demand resulting from high LV chamber pressures in the presence of outflow obstruction may aggravate myocardial ischemia, resulting in detrimental effects on diastolic performance (27–29). This concept is supported by studies following surgical relief of outflow tract obstruction. After septal myectomy or mitral valve replacement, thallium perfusion abnormalities are improved or normalized (49), in association with both lower LV filling pressures and diminished metabolic evidence of inducible ischemia (50). These data suggest that outflow obstruction is associated with clinically relevant myocardial ischemia, and operative relief of obstruction has favorable effects of inducible ischemia as well as on diastolic performance.

THEORETIC RATIONALE FOR THE USE OF CALCIUM CHANNEL BLOCKERS IN HCM

Although no unifying hypothesis regarding the microscopic or cellular events responsible for the morphologic and clinical expression of HCM has been forthcoming to this point, speculation has focused on two hypotheses, which are not, in and of themselves, mutually exclusive. The "catecholamine hypothesis" postulates that the morphology and physiology of HCM are the end result of abnormalities in adrenergic stimulation caused by excessive production of circulating catecholamines or an abnormal response to the presence of catecholamines at the level of the membrane adrenergic receptor (51, 52). Experimentally, subhypertensive chronic infusions of norepinephrine in dogs may cause a hypertrophic response, histologic evidence of cellular disarray and a hemodynamic picture similar to that seen in HCM (53). Furthermore, diseases such as pheochromocytoma (52), Freidreich's ataxia (54), and Von Recklinghausen's disease

(55), which are associated with abnormalities of the adrenergic nervous system, have been reported in some patients with HCM. Although these studies and associations suggest a possible link of the adrenergic system to the pathogenesis of HCM, studies of myocardial norepinephrine concentration and density of beta-adrenergic receptors have not revealed important differences from controls (56–58). More recent data, however, examining cardiac norepinephrine kinetics in HCM, have identified significant differences from controls in norepinephrine release and uptake, supporting a role for altered sympathetic nerve function in the genesis of morphologic and pathophysiologic abnormalities in HCM (59).

The coexistence of normal to hyperdynamic systolic performance and impaired diastolic characteristics appear to implicate abnormal regulation of calcium fluxes as a potentially important pathogenetic mechanism in HCM. (See Chap. 1.) Increased intramyocellular calcium content is associated with an increase in the inotropic state of the ventricle (60). Deactivation of myocardial actin-myosin crossbridges requires the rapid and extensive re-uptake of calcium into the sarcoplasmic reticulum from the myocellular cytosol (27), and this energy-dependent process is extremely sensitive to low levels of myocardial ischemia or hypoxia (27, 28). Thus, cytosolic calcium overload during systole, alone or in combination with diminished ability to remove calcium, is expected to impair myocardial relaxation and allow an increase in diastolic tone throughout the left ventricular filling period.

The most compelling evidence to support an abnormality in transmembrane calcium regulation as an important underlying mechanism in HCM comes from studies of calcium channel antagonist receptors in cardiac tissue of patients with HCM as well as studies of calcium membrane transients in ventricular tissue of patients with HCM (61–63). Wagner et al. demonstrated an increase in the number of calcium channel antagonist receptors in atrial tissue of patients with HCM compared to atrial tissue from patients with other cardiac disorders, and a strong correlation was observed between the levels of

receptors in the right atrium and levels of calcium channel receptors in the ventricular septum of HCM patients undergoing myotomy/myectomy, suggesting that the abnormal receptor density is a diffuse phenomenon in HCM (61). Morgan and Morgan demonstrated prolonged calcium transients in ventricular tissue of patients with HCM, further supporting the concept that disordered calcium regulation is an important phenomenon in this disease (62). Moreover, Gwathmey et al. have demonstrated that intracellular calcium overload in excised operative HCM tissue specimens is associated with prolonged and incomplete relaxation and resulting impairment in active tension development during systole (63); these abnormalities were potentiated at increasing stimulation frequencies (63). These data are the first to directly link abnormal calcium regulation with the pathophysiologic abnormalities in HCM.

In the Syrian hamster model of cardiomyopathy, elevated myocyte calcium concentrations are found, microvascular abnormalities are common (64, 65), the numbers of calcium channel antagonist receptors are increased (66–68), and treatment with the calcium channel blocker verapamil prevents or delays the development of cardiomyopathy (64, 65). Although it is tempting to speculate a common pathophysiologic pathway involving disordered calcium regulation based on the common membrane abnormalities and response to calcium antagonists, the morphologic and clinical expression of Syrian hamster cardiomyopathy and human HCM are distinct, and whether the data from this animal model further support a role for abnormal calcium fluxes as an etiologic mechanism in human HCM is unclear.

Taken together, these observations and data provide a theoretic framework for the use of calcium channel blockers in the treatment of HCM, although it is important to note that definitive data describing exact mechanisms of the effect of calcium channel blockers on calcium homeostasis in HCM are lacking at present.

INFLUENCE OF CALCIUM-CHANNEL BLOCKING AGENTS ON DIASTOLIC FUNCTION

A large body of clinical data has demonstrated that abnormal LV diastolic function in HCM may be favorably modified by calcium channel blocking agents. Investigations have been performed, examining the acute hemodynamic effects as well as the short- and long-term effects of oral therapy on indexes of systolic and diastolic LV performance, exercise tolerance, and symptoms.

Acute Effects

Verapamil

Several groups of investigators have examined the acute hemodynamic effects of calcium channel blocking agents to assess the mechanisms by which these agents may have their salutary influence on symptoms in patients with HCM. Hanrath et al. examined echocardiographic indexes of left ventricular relaxation and filling following acute treatment with intravenous verapamil (69). Isovolumic relaxation time decreased significantly, associated with an increase in the peak rate posterior wall thinning, an increase in the duration of the rapid filling period, and an increase in the LV dimension during the LV filling period accompanied by a small but significant increase in end-diastolic dimension. There was no change in end-systolic dimension, fractional shortening, cycle length, or systolic blood pressure (69).

Using a combined radionuclide and hemodynamic technique to measure instantaneous pressure-volume relations throughout the cardiac cycle, the hemodynamic effects of serial infusions of low, medium, and high dose intravenous verapamil were examined in HCM (70). Verapamil produced a dose-related increase in end-diastolic counts (directly reflecting end-diastolic volume) as well as increases in end-systolic counts and stroke counts. Associated with these changes were a decrease in ejection fraction as well as a reduction in the outflow tract gradient in those patients with resting gradients under control conditions. A negative inotropic effect was evident in all patients, in that the end-systolic pressure volume relation was shifted downward and rightward in all patients. Of the 10 patients in whom instantaneous LV pressure-volume loops were constructed from simultaneous micromanometer pressure recordings and radionuclide time-activity curves, a downward and

rightward shift of the diastolic pressure volume limb of the curve was evident in five patients, reflecting improved pressure-volume relations despite the negative inotropic effect (Fig. 28–3). In these five patients, the time constant of isovolumic relaxation was favorably modified by verapamil, and these changes were associated with an increase in the peak rate of rapid diastolic filling. The improvement in these indexes of LV diastolic function after acute intravenous administration of verapamil suggests that verapamil directly modified left ventricular relaxation and compliance properties to more than offset the negative inotropic effect, which by itself would be expected to cause deterioration in LV diastolic performance. In the patients in whom diastolic pressure-volume relations were unaltered by verapamil, increased end-diastolic volumes occurred at higher end-diastolic pressures, suggesting no change in intrinsic late diastolic properties. Peak rate of left ventricular diastolic filling was unaltered by verapamil in these patients. Although the negative inotropic effects of intravenous verapamil may be potentially beneficial in patients with HCM by decreasing left ventricular contractile function, reducing oxygen demand, and increasing left ventricular volume, these data also demonstrate that in a subset of patients with HCM, acute treatment with verapamil enhances left ventricular relaxation and diastolic filling and improves diastolic pressure-volume relations (70).

Using a combined hemodynamic-M-mode echocardiographic technique, Ten-Cate et al. studied 10 patients with HCM following completion of a 5-minute infusion of 10 mg of intravenous verapamil (71). In contrast to previous studies, no apparent salutary change in indexes of relaxation, filling, or distensibility was demonstrated. Time constants derived by three different methods reflected a slower rate of pressure fall or were unchanged after verapamil. LV end-diastolic pressure rose slightly but significantly, and echocardiographic measurements reflecting left ventricular filling either did not change or were diminished, reflecting slower filling, associated with no change in end-diastolic dimension. Pressure-dimension loops did not show any change compatible with im-

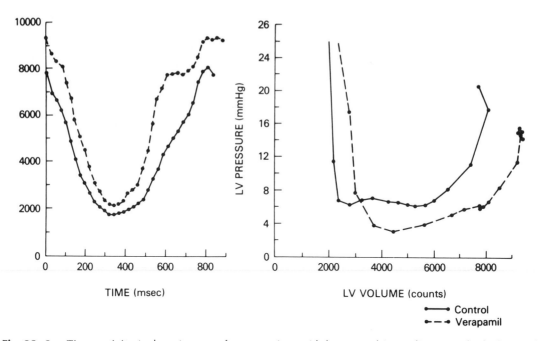

Fig. 28–3. Time-activity (volume) curves from a patient with hypertrophic cardiomyopathy before and after acute intravenous verapamil (left panel). Verapamil results in an increase in left ventricular (LV) end-systolic and end-diastolic counts, stroke counts, and peak filling rate, and a decrease in ejection fraction. These changes were associated with a downward and rightward shift in the instantaneous diastolic pressure-volume relation (right panel), obtained with simultaneous micromanometry and radionuclide angiography. Reproduced with permission from Bonow RO, et al.: Effects of verapamil on left ventricular systolic and diastolic function in patients with hypertrophic cardiomyopathy: Pressure-volume analysis with a nonimaging scintillation probe. Circulation 68:1062, 1983.

proved distensibility. It is important to note that individual patient data were not presented in this study, only mean data for the entire group. As earlier data demonstrate that only a subset of patients with HCM demonstrated favorable modification of abnormal diastolic properties after acute administration of verapamil (70), such changes may not have been apparent by examining only the effects on group data.

Using similar techniques, Hess et al. studied the acute effects of verapamil on left ventricular relaxation and late diastolic pressure-dimension relations in HCM and compared the findings to patients with aortic stenosis (72). (See Chap. 27.) The time constant of isovolumic pressure decay decreased in all patients with HCM, associated with improvement in echocardiographic indexes of diastolic filling. End-diastolic pressure remained unchanged, as did peak systolic LV pressure and heart rate; LV end-diastolic volume or dimen-

sions were not reported. Combined data representing late diastolic properties demonstrated no important changes following verapamil in pressure-dimension relationships during late diastole (Fig. 28–4). Left ventricular cycle efficiency (the ratio of the area of the pressure-volume loop to that area of the rectangle enclosing the pressure-volume loop, considered a measure of the effective synchrony of LV systolic and diastolic performance) increased in the HCM patients following verapamil, suggesting diminished nonuniformity. In contrast, intravenous verapamil had no important effect on echocardiographic indexes of LV filling in patients with aortic stenosis, time constants increased, associated with no change in cycle efficiency, and a slight but significant increase in end-diastolic pressure was observed (72). These data suggest that the effects of verapamil on diastolic properties depend partly on the etiology of left ventricular hypertrophy.

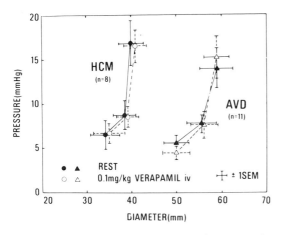

Fig. 28–4. Late diastolic pressure-diameter relations in patients with hypertrophic cardiomyopathy (HCM) and aortic stenosis (AVD) obtained before (solid line) and after (dashed line) verapamil. Data are averaged at minimum diastolic pressure, mid-diastole, and end-diastole from 8 patients with HCM and 11-patients with aortic stenosis. There is no apparent effect of verapamil on late diastolic pressure volume relations. Reproduced with permission from Hess OM, Murakami T, Krayenbuehl HP: Does verapamil improve left ventricular relaxation in patients with myocardial hypertrophy? Circulation 74:530, 1986.

In studying 16 HCM patients, Tendera et al. found that end-diastolic pressure decreased slightly but significantly in association with a 10% increase in end-diastolic volume, suggesting improved distensibility following intravenous verapamil (73). Wilmshurst et al. studied 12 patients with HCM at incremental pacing levels under control conditions and again after infusion of intravenous verapamil (74). There was no change in end-diastolic volume or end-diastolic pressure, no change in cardiac output, and a trend toward diminished outflow tract gradients following verapamil in patients with gradients under control conditions. Left ventricular systolic pressure and aortic systolic pressure decreased, and end-systolic volume increased, suggesting a predominant negative inotropic effect on the ventricle; cardiac output was unchanged because of significantly diminished systemic vascular resistance (74).

Thus, the effects of acute intravenous verapamil on ventricular performance in HCM are variable: a negative inotropic effect is often seen, and in a subset of patients, a favorable effect on myocardial relaxation and chamber distensibility is evident, associated with enhanced LV filling.

Nifedipine

The acute effects of nifedipine on diastolic properties in HCM has been studied by several groups of investigators. Lorell et al. studied 15 HCM patients 20 minutes after the sublingual administration of 10 mg of nifedipine (75). Echocardiographic data demonstrated a shortening of isovolumic relaxation time, and improved echocardiographic indexes of left ventricular filling. There was no change in end-diastolic diameter in this study, possibly related to the shortened diastolic filling time associated with the observed increase in heart rate. A subset of 10 patients underwent simultaneous invasive hemodynamic assessment: end-diastolic pressure diminished slightly but significantly, and in all patients, a favorable effect on the time constant of isovolumic pressure decay was noted. Simultaneous left ventricular pressure and chamber dimension data demonstrated a downward and sometimes rightward shift in most patients (75), suggesting improved left ventricular distensibility.

In an attempt to delineate the mechanism of the acute effects of nifedipine, Paulus et al. studied 10 patients with nonobstructive HCM using a similar nifedipine protocol, as well as during intravenous infusion of sodium nitroprusside in equihypotensive doses, to separate loading effects from direct myocardial effects on hemodynamic and echocardiographic indexes (76). Heart rate increased significantly from control during both drugs, and peak systolic LV pressure diminished similarly, by design. The time constant of isovolumic relaxation diminished significantly during both nitroprusside and nifedipine, whereas isovolumic relaxation time improved to a greater extent during nifedipine compared to nitroprusside. Peak rates of posterior wall thinning and LV internal dimension change were more favorably enhanced by nifedipine compared to nitroprusside; end-diastolic dimension was unchanged during nifedipine compared to control but diminished with nitroprusside. These data suggest that, although both agents have a similar effect on the rate of isovolumic relaxation in nonobstructive HCM patients, nifedipine more consistently improved indexes of left ventricular filling and diminished left ventricular end-diastolic pressure without changing end-diastolic dimension, consistent with a favorable effect on late diastolic chamber properties (76). Pressure-dimension loops supported this contention (Fig. 28–5). The data suggest that the beneficial effects of nifedipine on diastolic performance in these patients with HCM were related to direct effects on myocardial properties rather than systemic loading conditions; whether such direct effects involve primary alterations in myocardial inactivation, changes in regional non-

uniformity, improvement in subclinical ischemia, or a change in the extent of relaxation could not be discerned from the data.

In contrast to these findings, Betocchi et al., using higher doses of sublingual nifedipine in 11 HCM patients (77), found no important change in time constants of isovolumic relaxation, an increase in left ventricular end-diastolic pressure and pulmonary arterial wedge pressure (primarily because of an increase in patients with normal baseline wedge pressures), and no change in radionuclide indexes of the rate or timing of left ventricular filling. There was also no consistent change in diastolic pressure-volume relations: three patients demonstrated improved pressure-volume relations; three patients showed no change; and there was a deleterious left-

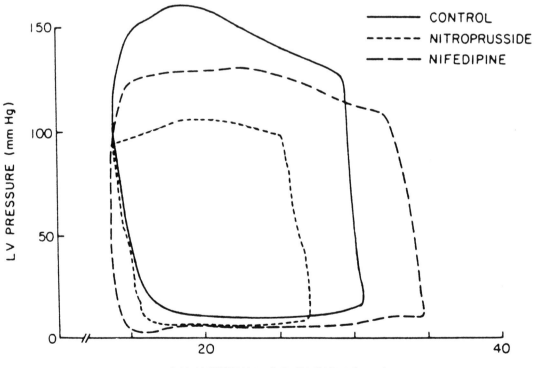

Fig. 28–5. Instantaneous left ventricular (LV) pressure-dimension relations in a patient with HCM under control conditions, during the infusion of nitroprusside, and after the administration of sublingual nifedipine. There is a downward shift in the diastolic pressure-dimension relation during both nitroprusside and nifedipine; however, end-diastolic dimension is significantly greater during nifedipine at an unchanged end-diastolic pressure, suggesting a favorable effect of nifedipine on diastolic distensibility. Reproduced with permission from Paulus WJ, et al.: Comparison of the effects of nitroprusside and nifedipine on diastolic properties in patients with hypertrophic cardiomyopathy: Altered left ventricular loading or impaired muscle inactivation? J Am Coll Cardiol 2:879, 1983.

ward and upward shift in four patients (77). In this study, the invasive radionuclide-hemodynamic measurements were made with heart rate controlled by atrial pacing. An analysis of the relation between serum levels of nifedipine following acute sublingual dosing and hemodynamic effects in a subgroup of nonobstructive HCM patients showed that, at lower nifedipine concentrations (≤ 120 ng/mL), vasodilator effects were most evident, whereas negative inotropic effects predominated at higher serum levels (78).

Similar findings suggesting little direct effect of acute nifedipine therapy on diastolic performance were reported by Yamkado et al. (79), in a study of asymptomatic or minimally symptomatic HCM patients with no evidence of outflow obstruction. LV end-diastolic pressure increased, with no change in end-diastolic volume. Isovolumic relaxation time decreased with nifedipine, as in the studies of Lorell (75) and Paulus (76); however, this appeared to be entirely a result of diminished LV end-systolic pressure and an increase in mitral valve opening pressure as there were no changes in pressure-derived indexes of relaxation rate (79). Diastolic pressure-volume relations demonstrated a favorable shift in only one patient (79).

Diltiazem

Few studies have addressed the acute effect of diltiazem on diastolic properties in HCM. Nagao et al. studied HCM patients with pulmonary artery catheterization at rest and during exercise under control conditions and again after intravenous diltiazem (80). There was no change during exercise in peak values of heart rate, systolic or diastolic blood pressure, pulmonary artery systolic pressure, or cardiac output. There was, however, a diminished exercise pulmonary artery diastolic pressure, suggesting improved diastolic properties during exercise. These investigators subsequently reported significantly diminished isovolumic relaxation time as measured by M-mode echocardiography and phonocardiography following intravenous diltiazem (81). Suwa et al. also examined M-mode echocardiographic indexes before and after intravenous diltiazem in HCM and

found both diminished isovolumic relaxation time and time to peak rate of LV dimension change, with no significant changes in LV dimensions or fractional shortening, again suggesting that diltiazem may improve LV relaxation properties in HCM (82).

Interpretive Difficulties with Acute Studies

It is clear from this review of acute hemodynamic effects of the various calcium channel blockers in patients with HCM that in a subset of patients, acute administration of calcium channel blockers has a beneficial effect on diastolic properties. This is most notable in studies reporting individual patient data. When these agents favorably modify indexes of relaxation, LV filling is augmented, associated with improved diastolic pressure-volume or pressure-dimension relations. The reasons for the disparate results seen in various studies (Table 28–1) undoubtedly lie in the complex and interrelated pathophysiologic abnormalities in patients with HCM. There may be a differing effect in patients with or without outflow obstruction, as well as in patients with or without underlying myocardial ischemia as an important contributor to abnormal diastolic properties. There may also be a potential detrimental effect when peripheral vasodilation lowers systemic pressure, possibly aggravating outflow tract gradients or lowering coronary perfusion pressure to the hypertrophied myocardium and inducing myocardial ischemia. In addition to the heterogeneous nature of the disease itself, studies from different laboratories have used different drug protocols, as well as varying methods of data acquisition and analysis. For example, the analysis of isovolumic relaxation using pressure-derived indexes, controversial in the normal heart, is more complex in HCM. We (31, 70) and others (75, 76) have found that the exponential fits of isovolumic pressure data in HCM generally have unsatisfactory correlation coefficients, as the concepts of exponential pressure fall derived in the isolated and normal intact heart (32) may not apply to HCM because of regional LV nonuniformity. Finally, although acute studies highlight he-

Table 28–1. **Influence of Acute Calcium Channel Blockade on Indexes of Myocardial Relaxation in HCM**

Author (Ref)	Index	Method	Agent	Dose	Result	%HOCM
Hanrath (69)	IVRT	M-mode echo	V	0.15 mg/kg IV	↓	55
Bonow (70)	T	Micromanometry	V	Incremental IV	↓, ↑	71
Ten Cate (71)	T	Micromanometry	V	10 mg IV	↑,—	60
Hess (72)	T	Micromanometry	V	0.1 mg/kg IV	↓	80
Lorell (75)	IVRT	M-mode echo	N	10 mg sl	↓	
	T	Micromanometry	N	10 mg sl	↓	47
Paulus (76)	T	Micromanometry	N	10 mg sl	↓	0
Betocchi (77)	T	Micromanometry	N	10–20 mg sl	—	78
Yamakado (79)	T	Micromanometry	N	20 mg sl	—	0
Suwa (82)	IVRT	M-mode echo	D	10 mg IV	↓	66
Nagao (81)	IVRT	M-mode echo	D	0.2 mg/kg IV	↓	45

Abbreviations: D = diltiazem, IV = intravenously, IVRT = isovolumic relaxation time, N = nifedipine, sl = sublingually, T = time constant of isovolumic pressure decline, V = verapamil, ↓ ↑ — = decrease, increase or no change of index, %HOCM = percent of study patients with resting or provocable outflow gradients.

modynamic and physiologic effects of these agents on LV performance, the relation between these acute changes and chronic drug effects on hemodynamic and clinical parameters is complex.

Short and Long-Term Oral Therapy

Verapamil

The acute intravenous effects of calcium channel blockers on left ventricular function in HCM can be compared and contrasted to short- and long-term effects of oral administration of these agents. In 40 HCM patients studied at the NIH, the effect of short-term oral therapy with verapamil (320 to 640 mg a day) was evaluated by radionuclide angiography (22). Quantitative indices of left ventricular systolic function and diastolic filling were computed from the left ventricular time-activity curve, which represents a relative measure of the left ventricular volume changes throughout an average cardiac cycle. Before verapamil, each patient manifested normal or supernormal left ventricular systolic performance, as assessed by ejection phase indexes. Impaired diastolic filling was demonstrated in 28 patients (70%), manifested by a subnormal peak filling rate, prolonged time to peak filling rate, or both. Follow-up radionuclide angiograms after 5 to 7 days of oral verapamil therapy demonstrated that, unlike the acute intravenous studies, oral verapamil did not alter

left ventricular systolic function because there was no change in the mean ejection fraction for the group, although several individual patients manifested a decrease in ejection fraction. The predominant effect of oral verapamil was on indices of left ventricular diastolic filling: peak filling increased significantly (by 21%), and time to peak filling rate decreased (by 15%) (Fig. 28–6) (22). Improvement in both variables was seen in 75% of patients, and improvement in either variable was seen in the 39 of the 40 patients. Overall, abnormal diastolic filling, which had been present in 70% of the patients, was present in only 30% of patients after short-term oral verapamil therapy. The extent of left ventricular filling during the rapid diastolic filling period was also improved following oral verapamil, as the contribution of atrial systole to total LV filling volume, and thus to LV stroke volume, was diminished following verapamil therapy (83). Further radionuclide angiographic analysis demonstrated that the improvement in the time to peak filling rate during verapamil was entirely caused by favorable effects of the drug on the prolonged isovolumic relaxation time (26).

These results with verapamil are in contrast to those obtained in a subset of the same group of HCM patients who were also studied during short-term oral propranolol therapy (22). Propranolol did not alter any of the diastolic indexes, consistent with

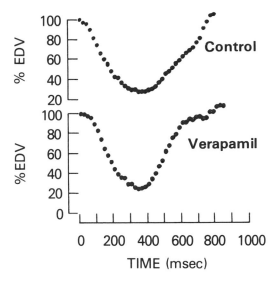

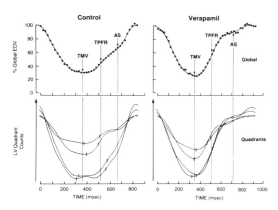

Fig. 28–6. Raw time-activity curve data obtained by radionuclide angiography from a patient with hypertrophic cardiomyopathy before (control) and during oral verapamil therapy. Verapamil results in an increase in peak filling rate and reduced time-to-peak filling rate. EDV = end-diastolic volume. Reproduced with permission from Bonow RO, et al.: Effects of verapamil on left ventricular systolic function and diastolic filling in patients with hypertrophic cardiomyopathy. Circulation 64:787, 1981.

Fig. 28–7. Assessment of regional left ventricular (LV) asynchrony in a patient with hypertrophic cardiomyopathy studied at rest by radionuclide angiography before (control) and during oral verapamil therapy. Global left ventricular time-activity (volume) curves are presented in the top panels, with points indicating time-to-minimum volume (TMV), time-to-peak filling rate (TPFR), and the onset of atrial systole (AS). Regional quadrant curves are shown in the bottom panels. The variation among quadrants in TMV and TPFR before verapamil indicates a considerable degree of systolic and diastolic asynchrony. Reduction in diastolic asynchrony after verapamil, with greater homogeneity in the relative contributions of rapid filling and atrial systole to regional filling, is associated with an improvement in global rapid diastolic filling, an increase in the global peak filling rate, and a decrease in the percent atrial contribution to total filling volume. EDV = end-diastolic volume. Reproduced with permission from Bonow RO, et al.: Regional left ventricular asynchrony and impaired global left ventricular filling in hypertrophy cardiomyopathy: Effect of verapamil. J Am Coll Cardiol 9:1108, 1987.

subsequent data of Speiser et al. (84), who found no change in left ventricular filling dynamics or diastolic pressure-volume relations after acute propranolol administration.

Short-term therapy with oral verapamil also has an important effect on diminishing the extent of regional nonuniformity in patients with HCM (85). The concept of ventricular diastolic asynchrony as contributing to impaired diastolic performance in patients with HCM (86) is supported by the correlation seen under control conditions of the regional variation in time-to-peak filling rate (an index of diastolic asynchrony) and global peak filling rate, as well as the correlation observed between regional variation in stress dissipation during isovolumic relaxation and global indexes of relaxation (87). Following short-term therapy with oral verapamil, the regional variation in timing and magnitude of rapid filling is reduced, associated with enhanced global left ventricular filling (Fig. 28–7).

Radionuclide angiographic studies performed during exercise also demonstrate enhanced LV diastolic filling after verapamil (Fig. 28–8) (88, 89). (See Chap. 11.) These findings are consistent with the hemodynamic data reported in a study by Hanrath et al. (90), in which 18 patients with HCM were studied before and after 7 weeks of treatment with oral verapamil at doses up to 720 mg a day. Both resting and peak exercise stroke-volume index increased significantly, in association with a significant decrease in pulmonary artery diastolic pressure during exercise. To the extent that pulmonary artery diastolic pressure reflects pulmonary capillary

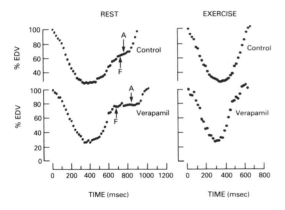

Fig. 28–8. Left ventricular time-activity (volume) curves obtained by radionuclide angiography at rest and during exercise in a patient with hypertrophic cardiomyopathy. Oral verapamil results in enhanced diastolic filling at rest: there is a shortened isovolumic phase, an increased rate and extent of rapid diastolic filling, and reduced contribution of atrial systole to total filling volume. An increased rate of filling is also evident during exercise following verapamil. EDV = end diastolic volume. Reproduced with permission from Bonow RO: Impaired left ventricular diastolic function in hypertrophic cardiomyopathy and coronary artery disease: Effect of calcium channel blocking agents. Am J Cardiol 55:172B, 1985.

wedge pressure and left atrial pressure, these data suggest that verapamil therapy was associated with enhanced transmitral flow (and thus stroke volume) during exercise; the enhanced transmitral pressure gradient must have resulted from lower left ventricular diastolic pressures during exercise, suggesting improved diastolic pressure-volume relations, as a result of verapamil therapy. These salutary changes in exercise hemodynamics following verapamil therapy were associated with an improvement in exercise capacity. Hence, enhanced LV diastolic performance may account, at least in part, for the objective improvement in exercise tolerance seen in this (90) and other studies (91). This concept is supported by the results of treadmill exercise testing in patients following 1 to 4 weeks of oral verapamil therapy (89). Among patients in whom peak filling rate increased, exercise capacity improved significantly. Among those patients with an unchanged or decreased peak filling rate

after verapamil, exercise capacity was not altered (Fig. 28–9) (89).

Longer-term effects of treatment with oral verapamil were studied in patients with HCM before and again 1 to 2 years after chronic therapy (89). Peak filling rate remained increased above baseline values at the late study, but to a lesser degree than that seen during short-term therapy; time-to-peak filling rate was not changed compared to control values after long-term

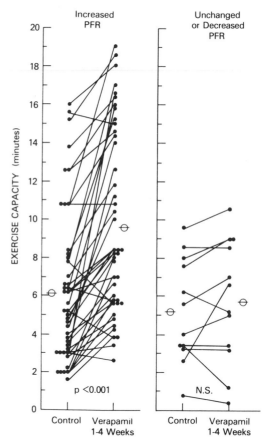

Fig. 28–9. Effects of short-term therapy with verapamil on exercise capacity in hypertrophic cardiomyopathy. Among patients whose peak filling rate (PFR) increased on verapamil, there was a significantly increased exercise capacity (left panel). There was no significant change in exercise capacity among patients with an unchanged or decreased PFR (right panel). Reproduced with permission from Bonow RO, et al.: Verapamil-induced improvement in left ventricular diastolic filling and increased exercise tolerance in patients with hypertrophic cardiomyopathy: Short- and long-term effects. Circulation 72:853, 1985.

therapy. Nonetheless, over 50% of patients had a persistent increase in peak filling rate greater than the reproducibility of that index, and exercise capacity over long-term drug administration remained significantly longer than control values. Furthermore, the association of salutary changes in diastolic filling with improved exercise capacity continued to hold over the long term: the 16 patients with a persistent increase in resting peak filling rate after 1 to 2 years of therapy manifested a significant increase in exercise tolerance over this period. In contrast, of the 9 patients with no change or decrease in peak filling rate compared with initial control values, exercise tolerance at 1 to 2 years was unchanged compared to control. Furthermore, the magnitude of change in exercise capacity during treatment with verapamil was related to the magnitude of change in peak filling rate over both short- and long-term studies, suggesting that both short- and long-term changes in exercise capacity are importantly related to improvement in left ventricular diastolic filling in HCM (Fig. 28–10) (89). Withdrawal of verapamil after long-term therapy and repeat study of diastolic filling parameters by radionuclide angiography indicated a significant deterioration in LV filling variables following verapamil withdrawal (89), supporting the presence of a persistent drug effect of verapamil on left ventricular filling during long-term therapy.

Kaltenbach et al. were the first investigators to study the long-term effect of oral verapamil therapy (92); serial cardiac catheterizations were performed in 10 patients before and again an average of 15 months after treatment. In these patients, end-diastolic volume increased by 10% in association with no change in ejection fraction, suggesting that the improved stroke volume observed at rest was a result of the favorable increase in end-diastolic volume.

In a study of 11 patients who underwent repeat catheterization 6 months after treatment with oral verapamil (average dose 690 mg per day), Anderson et al. (93) observed a 28% increase in end-diastolic volume index without a significant change in end-diastolic pressure. There was no change in either ejection fraction or outflow tract gradient; stroke volume in-

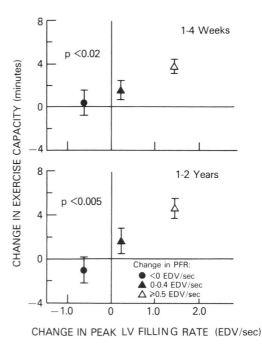

Fig. 28–10. Change in exercise capacity with verapamil therapy in hypertrophic cardiomyopathy plotted as a function of the change in resting left ventricular (LV) peak filling rate (PFR). Top panel—changes with short-term therapy; bottom panel—changes with long-term therapy. Over both the short and long term, there is a significant correlation between change in PFR and change in exercise capacity following verapamil therapy. EDV = end-diastolic volume. Reproduced with permission from Bonow RO, et al.: Verapamil-induced improvement in left ventricular diastolic filling and increased exercise tolerance in patients with hypertrophic cardiomyopathy: Short- and long-term effects. Circulation 72:853, 1985.

creased by 15%. No evidence for a significant negative inotropic effect was seen during chronic oral therapy, as the ratio of end-systolic pressure to end-systolic volume was unchanged. In four patients, the diastolic pressure-volume curve shifted to the right or downward and to the right, in one patient there was no change; and in two there was a shift upward and to the left. These data suggest that chronic oral verapamil therapy was associated with an improvement in diastolic distensibility in a subset of patients, similar to that seen with acute therapy (70), translating to increased resting stroke volume in the absence of changes in systolic function or in the outflow tract gradient.

Nifedipine

Few studies have examined short- or long-term effects of oral nifedipine therapy on indexes of LV filling in HCM. In one report, improvement in diastolic indexes of LV function similar to those seen with verapamil were observed during exercise following short-term oral nifedipine therapy (94), although resting parameters were not significantly changed.

Diltiazem

The influence of therapy with diltiazem on left ventricular filling in HCM has been studied by Suwa et al. (82), examining echocardiographic indexes following 180 mg of diltiazem daily for 2 weeks. The peak rate of LV dimensional lengthening increased, associated with a reduction in isovolumic relaxation time and the time-to-peak rate of LV dimensional lengthening, indicating an improvement in the rate and timing of early diastolic filling. In contrast, the treatment of the same group of patients with 60 mg to 120 mg a day of propranolol for 2 weeks caused no significant changes, consistent with earlier radionuclide angiographic findings (22). These data with diltiazem were extended by Iwase and colleagues (95) who found, using similar techniques, that treatment with diltiazem improved exercise LV filling indexes in HCM patients to a degree at which they did not differ from controls.

The data on acute intravenous effects as well as short- and long-term effects of oral therapy with calcium channel blockers indicate that these agents favorably modify diastolic performance in patients with HCM, although the effects are not manifest in all patients. The exact mechanism for the salutary effect of these agents on diastolic performance has not been clearly elucidated, but is likely to involve effects on the inactivation process itself (either directly or indirectly), improvement in regional nonuniformity, or favorable alterations in loading of the left ventricle. Many of these effects may be mediated by influence of calcium channel blockers on regional myocardial ischemia. The correlations between changes in indexes of left ventricular filling and changes in exercise performance during both short- and long-term therapy (89) supports the concept that the enhanced diastolic performance mediated by calcium channel blockers is an important factor in the improvement in exercise tolerance and symptoms in these patients, particularly as changes in the magnitude of other pathophysiologic abnormalities during treatment with verapamil, such as the outflow tract gradient, do not have clear-cut associations with changes in symptoms or exercise performance (94).

EFFECT OF CALCIUM CHANNEL BLOCKERS ON MYOCARDIAL ISCHEMIA IN HCM

As noted previously, myocardial ischemia plays an important role in the pathophysiology and the natural history of patients with HCM. Studies using exercise thallium scanning provide a noninvasive means of identifying myocardial perfusion abnormalities in HCM (39–41), and studies from our laboratory involving a large, heterogeneous group of patients with HCM demonstrated that thallium perfusion defects occur in most patients (96), including over 50% of those without symptoms (97).

The morphologic findings of structurally abnormal intramural coronary arteries with thickened media and apparent luminal compromise in previously asymptomatic HCM patients who died suddenly (12) as well as the noninvasive evidence of exercise induced reversible perfusion abnormalities in such patients (39–41) raised the possibility that some asymptomatic patients may experience recurrent episodes of silent myocardial ischemia. We tested the hypothesis that this might be a dynamic abnormality that could be favorably modified by therapy by studying the effects of verapamil on myocardial perfusion and function in a group of 29 asymptomatic or minimally symptomatic patients with HCM (97). Eleven patients (38%) of this group had evidence of resting left ventricular outflow obstruction by echocardiography or cardiac catheterization. Patients were studied by exercise thallium tomographic imaging and by radionuclide angiographic before and after 1 week of treatment with oral verapamil in doses ranging from 240 mg to 480 mg a day (mean 453 mg). During verapamil therapy, exercise treadmill time increased slightly but significantly, whereas the rate-pressure product did not change significantly.

Under control conditions, 15 of the 29 patients (52%) developed regional thallium perfusion defects during exercise, with an average of 3.7 abnormal regions per patient. Most of these perfusion abnormalities occurred in the interventricular septum. In the 14 patients with reversible perfusion abnormalities under control conditions, 10 (71%) demonstrated improved regional perfusion at peak exercise during verapamil therapy (Fig. 28–11) (97), including 8 patients whose exercise scans returned completely to normal. The perfusion pattern improved in approximately 70% of all initially abnormal regions.

That these perfusion defects represent myocardial ischemia is supported by their relation to LV morphologic and functional data. In patients developing perfusion defects during exercise under control conditions, the LV peak filling rate at rest was significantly lower than in patients with a normal perfusion pattern. Those with improved perfusion defects during verapamil had a greater increase in peak filling rate than those with persistently inducible perfusion defects during verapamil (97). Moreover, there was a significant correlation between the number of improved regions in these patients and the increase in global peak filling rate (98). Finally, patients with more extensive LV hypertrophy by echocardiography were more likely to have reversible thallium perfusion defects during exercise than those with less severe hypertrophy, and the improvement in exercise perfusion defects during verapamil was most pronounced in patients with the greatest degree of myocardial hypertrophy. These findings indicate that the reversible perfusion defects induced by exercise are caused by some process that is associated with (rather than caused by) hypertrophy, and that process may be modified favorably by verapamil therapy.

It is possible that the regional heterogeneity of thallium uptake in patients with HCM may merely represent abnormal local transmembrane cation transport rather than true myocardial ischemia. However, the perfusion defects are associ-

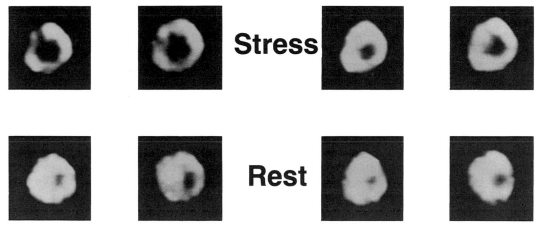

Fig. 28–11. Short-axis thallium-201 tomograms obtained immediately after maximal treadmill exercise (top) and 3 hours of rest (bottom) in an 18-year-old asymptomatic man with hypertrophic cardiomyopathy. Under control conditions, severe septal and inferoposterior perfusion defects develop during exercise, and are reversible at rest. There is also apparent reversible cavity dilation induced by exercise. During oral verapamil (right), myocardial perfusion and apparent cavity dilation are improved during exercise to a similar workload. Reproduced with permission from Udelson JE, et al.: Verapamil prevents silent myocardial perfusion abnormalities during exercise in asymptomatic patients with hypertrophic cardiomyopathy. Circulation 79:1052, 1989.

ated with functional abnormalities of left ventricular filling (97, 98), previous studies demonstrate the common occurrence of myocardial ischemia in HCM (37, 38, 43), and there is necropsy evidence of small vessel pathology in asymptomatic HCM patients who die suddenly (12). In addition, the thallium defects noted in HCM are reproducible using the perfusion agent technetium-99m sestamibi (which does not rely on an energy-requiring transmembrane cation transport mechanism to enter the myocardial cell) (99). Thus, the available data overwhelmingly support the contention that even asymptomatic patients are subject to inducible, silent myocardial ischemia, and that verapamil can ameliorate this process. The mechanism responsible for reduction in inducible ischemia by verapamil in HCM is likely to involve either a direct effect on the small coronary vessels or an improvement in regional myocardial relaxation allowing greater regional coronary flow during diastole (97).

Because regional myocardial ischemia profoundly affects LV relaxation, diminished myocardial ischemia in patients with HCM appears to be a critically important mechanism by which verapamil enhances ventricular diastolic function. This concept is supported by the correlation between the improvement in regional perfusion and improvement in indexes of LV filling during verapamil therapy (97, 98).

EFFECT OF CALCIUM CHANNEL BLOCKERS ON SYMPTOMS AND EXERCISE CAPACITY IN HCM

Verapamil

In a study of 19 patients with HCM, most of whom were in New York Heart Association Functional Class III despite what was considered optimal medical therapy, a placebo-controlled, double-blind trial compared the effects of verapamil and propranolol on exercise tolerance (91). Compared to placebo values, the average exercise time increased significantly during both verapamil (by $26 \pm 35\%$) and propranolol (by $21 \pm 35\%$) administration. There was no difference between the increases seen with verapamil and propranolol. In a preliminary comparison of a short-term oral course of verapamil to a similar

duration of nifedipine treatment in 27 patients with HCM, verapamil improved exercise time over control values by $38 \pm 58\%$, a statistically significant increase, whereas there was a tendency for improved exercise time with nifedipine, by $20 \pm 47\%$, although this increase did not reach statistical significance (94). For verapamil therapy, there was no relationship between changes in either exercise time or symptomatic response and the acute intravenous effects of verapamil on left ventricular outflow tract gradients measured at catheterization in the same patients (100).

In a follow-up study of a larger group of patients studied during long-term treatment with oral verapamil, the initial in-hospital improvement in exercise time was maintained at 12 months, and continued at 24 months. Over 70% of patients had a persistent or continuing improvement in exercise time during long-term oral verapamil therapy (101).

In a subset of 24 patients who had been taking verapamil for at least 1 year, exercise duration was evaluated after withdrawal of verapamil (101). Although the exercise time during the withdrawal treadmill test was higher than at the initial baseline, the difference did not achieve statistical significance. Of the individual patients, 12 of 24 who were studied following verapamil withdrawal had an increase of greater than 30% in their treadmill time compared to controls, suggesting the possibility that verapamil therapy may have altered the course of their disease, although this change may have also been the result of a training effect, because the functional capacity of most patients improved during therapy. The statistically insignificant difference between treadmill time following withdrawal of long-term verapamil compared to initial baseline suggests that the long-term improvement in exercise time seen during verapamil therapy is most likely caused by persistently favorable drug effect.

In a multicenter randomized study, Kober et al. compared long-term oral therapy with verapamil to propranolol (each at maximally tolerated dosage) in 137 patients with HCM (102). Symptoms improved significantly only during verapamil therapy, and deterioration in clinical status was seen only during propranolol therapy. At the conclusion of the 2-year study, cardiac catheterization was repeated, and although the maximum provocable outflow gradient had diminished more with propranolol, no other hemodynamic index differed between the groups, and no baseline index predicted the improvement seen with verapamil.

Nifedipine

Preliminary data involve long-term administration of nifedipine in HCM. In an unblinded study, Koide et al. studied 11 HCM patients and compared the long-term effects of nifedipine with that of propranolol (103). More effective symptomatic relief was attained with beta blockers compared with nifedipine, although anginal chest pain was more commonly alleviated with nifedipine therapy. A similar number of HCM patients, all of whom had no outflow obstruction, were studied in a randomized, double-blind, placebo-controlled, two month trial by Ruddy et al. (104). There was effective symptomatic relief during nifedipine therapy compared to placebo.

Diltiazem

Although several studies have addressed the short-term effect of oral diltiazem on the echocardiographic indexes of diastolic performance, only one report has investigated the effect of this agent on exercise tolerance or symptoms. In a double-blind, cross-over study of 32 HCM patients, Toshima et al. (105) compared short-term oral therapy with diltiazem (180 mg/day) to verapamil (240 mg/day). Although verapamil improved peak oxygen consumption to a greater degree, there was no difference between the agents in treadmill time increment or symptom relief.

ADVERSE EFFECTS OF CALCIUM CHANNEL BLOCKERS IN HCM

The adverse effects of calcium channel blockers in HCM relate primarily to their electrophysiologic effects, peripheral vasodilating effects, potential interaction with other drugs, and in some patients, the potential for negative inotropic effects.

Among a large group of patients treated with verapamil at the NIH, most adverse events occurred early during treatment, and importantly, this was particularly true of the significant and potentially life-threatening adverse events (106). Approximately 10% of patients in this group had evidence of AV dissociation, a result of verapamil effects on AV nodal conduction. These effects generally disappeared with a decrease in dosage, and most patients were able to continue to take verapamil. Continuation of verapamil required the use of a pacemaker in only two patients. Rare instances of sudden death from heart block and asystole in HCM temporally related to oral verapamil therapy have been reported (107).

Approximately 5% of patients in the NIH series had significant and symptomatic hypotension, which often responded to a decrease in dose. Worsening pulmonary congestion was seen in approximately 8% of patients, with most of these having resting or provocable LV outflow tract gradients greater than 50 mm (106).

Excessive peripheral vasodilation may lead to hypotension with augmentation of the outflow tract gradient either directly or by an increase in inotropic state mediated by means of a reflex increase in sympathetic activity. Increased left ventricular chamber pressures developing simultaneously with systemic hypotension may diminish coronary flow substantially. The aggravation of myocardial ischemia by this mechanism may result in potentially severe hemodynamic consequences. This mechanism may also precipitate acute pulmonary edema, as was observed in several patients during early studies with verapamil (106). Similar reports of systemic hypotension with an increase in outflow tract gradient and elevated diastolic pressures have also been reported after acute administration of nifedipine (108). Severe congestive symptoms may also result from an excessive negative inotropic effect. These observations form the basis for the cautious use of these agents in patients with HCM in the presence of a large outflow gradient and symptoms of pulmonary congestion (106).

Potentially important drug interactions include the increase in digoxin levels seen following initiation of verapamil therapy as well as a potential interaction with quinidine in the development of postural hypotension.

EFFECTS OF CALCIUM CHANNEL BLOCKERS ON ARRHYTHMIA AND PROGNOSIS

The efficacy of calcium channel blockers, particularly verapamil, on the long-term clinical course and outcome in HCM is unknown. There have been no long-term, randomized trials comparing verapamil or other calcium channel blockers with other forms of medical therapy or with surgical therapy. Although the electrophysiologic actions of verapamil may lead to control of ventricular response in atrial fibrillation because of its actions on the AV node, verapamil appears to have no consistent effect on ventricular arrhythmias in HCM, an important determinant of prognosis. McKenna et al. compared verapamil to amiodarone in 19 patients with HCM complicated by supraventricular and ventricular arrhythmias (109). Amiodarone reduced the number of patients who had complex ventricular arrhythmias and ventricular tachycardia, whereas there was no change in arrhythmia density during verapamil therapy. Similarly, there was no change in the incidence of supraventricular arrhythmias during verapamil, whereas amiodarone significantly reduced supraventricular tachycardia and converted several patients from atrial fibrillation to sinus rhythm (109). Although oral verapamil did not affect ambient arrhythmias in this study, reports have suggested that acute administration of verapamil may in some cases prevent the induction of monomorphic ventricular tachycardia, which had been inducible under control conditions (110).

A recent retrospective analysis of a large group of HCM patients followed for almost 9 years compared long-term outcome in groups treated medically and surgically (111). Although this study was retrospective and without randomization, the 10-year cumulative survival among medically treated patients was significantly greater in those treated with verapamil than in those treated with propranolol or those receiving no therapy. Among those treated with verapamil after undergoing surgery, there were no deaths over a 10-year period. Although these data reflect an obvious patient selection bias in the various therapeutic groups, there is the suggestion that long-term treatment with verapamil may have favorable effects on natural history and prognosis compared to other therapies, or in combination with septal myectomy. Theoretically, the combination of surgical treatment to abolish the outflow obstruction, when present, and subsequent medical treatment with verapamil to address diastolic abnormalities is physiologically sound, and would eliminate or reduce the potential untoward effects seen with verapamil therapy in patients with outflow tract obstruction. Similar long-term survival data during verapamil therapy were reported by Hopf and Kaltenbach in a large group of HCM patients in a non-randomized uncontrolled study (112).

Insofar as myocardial ischemia may contribute to a milieu for malignant ventricular arrhythmias, the ability of verapamil to diminish inducible myocardial ischemia in HCM (97) may have important implications for long-term prognosis. In this regard, a recent study by Dilsizian et al. found that, among young HCM patients, the presence of inducible perfusion abnormalities on thallium scintigraphy was more importantly related to syncope or cardiac arrest than were the results of Holter monitoring or electrophysiologic study (113).

Moreover, in a subset of patients with HCM, the clinical course is characterized by recurrent transmural or nontransmural fibrosis with wall thinning, cavity dilation, and progressive reduction in systolic function leading ultimately to congestive heart failure (11, 114, 115). This process may involve repetitive episodes of myocardial ischemia because histologic abnormalities of small intramural vessels are observed in autopsy studies in the vicinity of large areas of myocardial necrosis (12), suggesting (but not proving) a causal relation between myocardial ischemia and this unfavorable clinical course. Prevention of episodes of myocardial ischemia, as has been demonstrated with verapamil (97), may alter this untoward outcome.

The diversity of clinical expression of patients with HCM, as well as the heterogeneous natural history of the various subsets of patients, including the likelihood that a large subset has a rather benign prognosis (116), makes a definitive, long-term, randomized clinical study of therapies a difficult objective. More likely, in the future, better recognition and definition of clinical subsets and their probable outcomes, such as those with inducible myocardial ischemia and those at highest risk for malignant ventricular arrhythmias, will lead to more directed therapies with more favorable short-term and long-term clinical outcomes.

REFERENCES

1. Maron BJ, Mulvihill JJ: The genetics of hypertrophic cardiomyopathy. Ann Intern Med 105:610, 1986.
2. Jarcho JA, McKenna W, Pare JAP, et al. Mapping a gene for familial hypertrophic cardiomyopathy to chromosome 14q1. N Engl J Med 321:1372, 1989.
3. Epstein N, Fananapazir L, Lin H, et al.: Genetic heterogeneity in hypertrophic cardiomyopathy: Evidence that HCM maps to chromosome 2p. Circulation 82:III-399, 1990 (Abstr).
4. Hejtmancik JF, Brink PA, Towbin J, et al.: Localization of the gene for familial hypertrophic cardiomyopathy to chromosome 14q1 in a diverse American population. J Am Coll Cardiol 17:165A, 1991 (Abstract).
5. Maron BJ, Gottdiener JS, Epstein SE: Patterns and significance of distribution of left ventricular hypertrophy in hypertrophic cardiomyopathy: A wide angle, two-dimensional echocardiographic study of 125 patients. Am J Cardiol 48:418, 1981.
6. Maron BJ, Nichols PF, Pickle LW, et al.: Patterns of inheritance in hypertrophic cardiomyopathy: Assessment by M-mode and two-dimensional echocardiography. Am J Cardiol 53:1087, 1984.
7. Maron BJ, Epstein SE: Hypertrophic cardiomyopathy: Recent observations regarding the specificity of three hallmarks of the disease: Asymmetric septal hypertrophy, septal disorganization and systolic anterior motion of the anterior mitral leaflet. Am J Cardiol 45:141, 1980.
8. VanNoorden S, Olsen EGJ, Pearse AGE: Hypertrophic obstructive cardiomyopathy, a histological, histochemical, and ultrastructural study of biopsy material. Cardiovasc Res 5:118, 1971.
9. Ferrans VJ, Morrow AG, Roberts WC: Myocardial ultrastructure in idiopathic hypertrophic subaortic stenosis: a study of operative excised left ventricular outflow tract muscle in 14 patients. Circulation 45:769, 1972.
10. Maron BJ, Roberts WC: Quantitative analysis of cardiac muscle cell disorganization in the ventricular septum of patients with hypertrophic cardiomyopathy. Circulation 59:689, 1979.
11. Maron BJ, Epstein SE, Roberts WC: Hypertrophic cardiomyopathy and transmural myocardial infarction without significant atherosclerosis of the extramural coronary arteries. Am J Cardiol 43:1086, 1979.
12. Maron BJ, Wolfson JK, Epstein SE, Roberts WC: Intramural ("small vessel") coronary artery disease in hypertrophic cardiomyopathy. J Am Coll Cardiol 8:545, 1986.
13. Wigle ED, Heimbecker RO, Gunton RW: Idiopathic ventricular septal hypertrophy causing muscular subaortic stenosis. Circulation 26:325, 1962.
14. Goodwin JF: Congestive and hypertrophic cardiomyopathies: A decade of study. Lancet 1:731, 1970.
15. Stewart S, Mason DT, Braunwald E: Impaired rate of left ventricular filling in idiopathic hypertrophic subaortic stenosis and valvular aortic stenosis. Circulation 37:8, 1968.
16. Moreyra E, Klein JJ, Shimada H, Segal BL: Idiopathic hypertrophic subaortic stenosis diagnosed by reflected ultrasound. Am J Cardiol 23:32, 1969.
17. Gaasch WH, Levine HJ, Quinones MA, Alexander JK: Left ventricular compliance: Mechanisms and clinical implications. Am J Cardiol 38:645, 1976.
18. Grossman W, McLaurin LP: Diastolic properties of the left ventricle. Ann Intern Med 84:316, 1976.
19. Sanderson JE, Gibson DG, Brown DJ, Goodwin JF: Left ventricular filling in hypertrophic cardiomyopathy: an angiographic study. Br Heart J 39:661, 1977.
20. St. John Sutton MG, Tajik AJ, Gibson DG, et al.: Echocardiographic assessment of left ventricular filling and septal and posterior wall dynamics in idiopathic hypertrophic subaortic stenosis. Circulation 57:512, 1978.
21. Hanrath P, Mathey DG, Siegert R, Bleifeld W: Left ventricular relaxation and filling pattern in different forms of left ventricular hypertrophy: An echocardiographic study. Am J Cardiol 45:15, 1980.

22. Bonow RO, Rosing DR, Bacharach SL, et al.: Effects of verapamil on left ventricular systolic function and diastolic filling in patients with hypertrophic cardiomyopathy. Circulation 64:787, 1981.

23. Spirito P, Maron BJ, Chiarella F, et al.: Diastolic abnormalities in patients with hypertrophic cardiomyopathy: relation to magnitude of left ventricular hypertrophy. Circulation 72:310, 1985.

24. Tanaka M, Fujiwara H, Onodera T, et al.: Quantitative analysis of myocardial fibrosis in normals, hypertensive hearts, and hypertrophic cardiomyopathy. Br Heart J 55:575, 1986.

25. Alvares RF, Shaver JA, Gamble WH, Goodwin JF: Isovolumic relaxation period in hypertrophic cardiomyopathy. J Am Coll Cardiol 3:71, 1984.

26. Betocchi S, Bonow RO, Bacharach, et al.: Isovolumic relaxation period in hypertrophic cardiomyopathy: assessment by radionuclide angiography. J Am Coll Cardiol 7:74, 1986.

27. Nayler WC, Williams A: Relaxation in heart muscle: Some morphological and biochemical considerations. Eur J Cardiol 7(Suppl):35, 1978.

28. Mann T, Goldberg S, Mudge GH, Grossman W: Factors contributing to altered left ventricular diastolic properties during angina pectoris. Circulation 59:14, 1979.

29. Brutsaert DL, Rademakers FE, Sys SU: Triple control of relaxation: implications in cardiac disease. Circulation 69:190, 1984.

30. Hess OM, Grimm J, Krayenbuehl HP: Diastolic function in hypertrophic cardiomyopathy: Effects of propranolol and verapamil on diastolic stiffness. Eur Heart J 4(Suppl F):47, 1983.

31. Udelson JE, Cannon RO, Bacharach SL, et al.: β-adrenergic stimulation with isoproterenol enhances left ventricular diastolic performance in hypertrophic cardiomyopathy despite potentiation of myocardial ischemia: Comparison to rapid atrial pacing. Circulation 79:371, 1989.

32. Weiss JL, Frederiksen JW, Weisfeldt ML: Hemodynamic determinants of the time course of fall in canine left ventricular pressure. J Clin Invest 58:751, 1976.

33. Karliner JS, LeWinter M, Mahler F, et al.: Pharmacologic and hemodynamic influence on the rate of isovolumic left ventricular relaxation in the normal conscious dog. J Clin Invest 60:511, 1977.

34. Udelson JE, Bacharach SL, Cannon RO, Bonow RO: Minimum left ventricular pressure during β-adrenergic stimulation in human subjects: Evidence for elastic recoil and diastolic "suction" in the normal heart. Circulation 82:1174, 1990.

35. Blaustein AS, Gaasch WH: Myocardial relaxation: IV. Effects of β-adrenergic tone and synchrony on LV relaxation rate. Am J Physiol 244:H417, 1983.

36. Morad M: Ionic mechanisms mediating the inotropic and relaxant effects of adrenaline on the heart muscle. *In* Catecholamines in the Nonischaemic and Ischaemic Myocardium. Edited by Riemersma RA, Oliver MF. New York, Elsevier Biomedical, 1981.

37. Pasternac A, Noble J, Streulens Y, et al.: Pathophysiology of chest pain in patients with cardiomyopathies and normal coronary arteries. Circulation 65:778, 1982.

38. Cannon RO, Rosing DR, Maron BJ, et al.: Myocardial ischemia in patients with hypertrophic cardiomyopathy: Contribution of inadequate vasodilator reserve and elevated left ventricular filling pressures. Circulation 71:234, 1985.

39. Rubin KA, Morrison J, Padnick MB, et al.: Idiopathic hypertrophic subaortic stenosis: Evaluation of anginal symptoms with thallium-201 myocardial imaging. Am J Cardiol 44:1040, 1979.

40. Pitcher D, Wainwright R, Maisey M, et al.: Assessment of chest pain in·hypertrophic cardiomyopathy using exercise thallium-201 myocardial scintigrapy. Br Heart J 44:650, 1980.

41. Hanrath P, Mathey D, Montz R, et al.: Myocardial thallium-201 imaging in hypertrophic obstructive cardiomyopathy. Eur Heart J 2:177, 1981.

42. Bonow RO, Maron BJ, Leon MB, et al.: Medical and surgical therapy of hypertrophic cardiomyopathy. *In* Cardiomyopathies: Clinical Presentation, Differential Diagnosis, and Management. Edited by Davis FA, Shaver JA. Philadelphia, 221, 1988.

43. Thompson DS, Naqvi N, Juul SM, et al.: Effects of propranolol on myocardial oxygen consumption, substrate extraction, and haemodynamics in hypertrophic obstructive cardiomyopathy. Br Heart J 44:488, 1980.

44. James TH, Marshall TK: De subitaneis mortibus. XII. Asymmetrical hypertrophy of the heart. Circulation 51:1149, 1975.

45. Braunwald E, Lambrew CT, Rockoff SD, et al.: Idiopathic hypertrophic subaortic stenosis. I. A description of the disease based upon an analysis of 54 patients. Circulation 30(Supp IV):IV-3, 1964.

46. Pouleur H, Rousseau MF, van Eyll C, et al.: Force-velocity-length relations in hypertrophic cardiomyopathy: evidence of normal or depressed myocardial contractility. Am J Cardiol 52:813, 1983.

47. Wigle ED, Sasson Z, Henderson MA, et al.: Hypertrophic cardiomyopathy: the importance of the site and the extent of hypertrophy: A review. Prog Cardiovasc Dis 28:1, 1985.

48. Ariel Y, Gaasch WH, Bogen DK, McMahon TA: Load-dependent relaxation with late systolic volume steps; servo-pump studies in the intact canine heart. Circulation 75:1287, 1987.

49. Cannon RO, Dilsizian V, O'Gara PT, et al.: Impact of operative relief of outflow obstruction on thallium perfusion abnormalities in hypertrophic cardiomyopathy. Circulation, in press. Circulation 85:1039, 1992.

50. Cannon RO, McIntosh CL, Schenke WH, et al.: Effect of surgical reduction of left ventricular outflow obstruction on hemodynamics, coronary flow, and myocardial metabolism in hypertrophic cardiomyopathy. Circulation 79:766, 1989.

51. Perloff JK: Pathogenesis of hypertrophic cardiomyopathy: hypothesis and speculations. Am Heart J 101:219, 1981.

52. Goodwin JF: Prospects and predictions for the cardiomyopathies. Circulation 50:210, 1974.

53. Lake MM, Morady F, Swan HJC: Myocardial hypertrophy produced by chronic infusion of subhypertensive doses of norepinephrine in the dog. Chest 64:75, 1973.

54. Smith ER, Sangalang VE, Helterman LP, et al.: Hypertrophic cardiomyopathy: The heart disease of Freidreich's ataxia. Am Heart J 94:428, 1977.

55. Elliot CM, Tajik AJ, Giuliani ER, et al.: Idiopathic hypertrophic subaortic stenosis associated with cutaneous neurofibromatosis. Am Heart J 92:368, 1976.

56. Van Noorden S, Olsen EGJ, Pearse AGE: Hypertrophic obstructive cardiomyopathy, a histological, histochemical and ultrastructural study of biopsy material. Cardiovasc Res 5:118, 1971.

57. Kawai C, Yui Y, Hishino T, et al.: Myocardial catecholamines in hypertrophic and dilated (congestive) cardiomyopathy: A biopsy study. J Am Coll Cardiol 2:834, 1983.

58. Golf S, Myhre E, Abdelnoor M, et al.: Hypertrophic cardiomyopathy characterized by β-adrenoceptor density, relative amount of β-adrenoceptor subtypes and adenylate cyclase activity. Cardiovasc Res 19:693, 1985.

59. Brush JE, Eisenhofer G, Garty M, et al.: Cardiac norepinephrine kinetics in hypertrophic cardiomyopathy. Circulation 79:836, 1989.

60. Nayler WG: Calcium exchange in cardiac muscle. A basic mechanism of drug action. Am Heart J 73:379, 1967.

61. Wagner JA, Sax FL, Weisman HF, et al.: Calcium-antagonist receptors in the atrial tissue of patients with hypertrophic cardiomyopathy. N Engl J Med 320:755, 1989.

62. Morgan JP, Morgan KG: Calcium and cardiovascular function: Intracellular calcium levels during contraction and relaxation of mammalian cardiac and vascular smooth muscle as detected with aequorin. Am J Med 77(Suppl 5A):33, 1984.

63. Gwathmey JK, Warren SE, Briggs GM, et al.: Diastolic dysfunction in hypertrophic cardiomyopathy. Effect on active force generation during systole. J Clin Invest 87:1023, 1991.

64. Lossnitzer K, Janke J, Hein B, et al.: Disturbed myocardial calcium metabolism: a possible pathogenetic factor in the hereditary cardiomyopathy of the Syrian hamster. *In* Recent Advances in Studies on Cardiac Structure and Metabolism. Vol. 6. Edited by A. Fleckenstein and G. Rona. Pathophysiology and Morphology of Myocardial Cell Alteration. Baltimore, University Park Press, 1975.

65. Rouleau JL, Chuck HSC, Hollosi G, et al.: Verapamil preserves myocardial contractility in the hereditary cardiomyopathy of the Syrian hamster. Circ Res 50:405, 1982.

66. Wagner JA, Reynolds IJ, Weisman HF, et al.: Calcium antagonist receptors in cardiomyopathic hamsters: Selective increase in heart, muscle, brain. Science 232:515, 1986.

67. Finkel MS, Marks ES, Patterson RE, et al.: Increased cardiac calcium channels in hamster cardiomyopathy. Am J Cardiol 57:1205, 1986.

68. Kobayashi A, Yamashita T, Kaneko M, et al.: Effects of verapamil on experimental cardiomyopathy in the Bio 14.6 Syrian hamster. J Am Coll Cardiol 10:1128, 1987.

69. Hanrath P, Mathey DG, Kremer P, et al.: Effect of verapamil on left ventricular isovolumic relaxation time and regional left ventricular filling in hypertrophic cardiomyopathy. Am J Cardiol 45:1258, 1980.

70. Bonow RO, Ostrow HG, Rosing DR, et al.: Effects of verapamil on left ventricular systolic and diastolic function in patients with hypertrophic cardiomyopathy: Pressure-volume analysis with a nonimaging scintillation probe. Circulation 68:1062, 1983.

71. TenCate FJ, Serruys PW, Mey S, Roelandt J: Effects of short-term administration of verapamil on left ventricular relaxation and filling dynamics measured by a combined hemodynamic-ultrasonic technique in patients with hypertrophic cardiomyopathy. Circulation 68:1274, 1983.

72. Hess OM, Murakami T, Krayenbuehl HP: Does verapamil improve left ventricular relaxation in patients with myocardial hypertrophy? Circulation 74:530, 1986.

73. Tendera M, Polonski L, Kozielska E: Left ventricular end-diastolic pressure-volume relationships in hypertrophic cardiomyopathy: Changes induced by verapamil. Chest 84:54, 1983.

74. Wilmshurst PT, Thompson DS, Juul SM, et al.: Effects of verapamil on haemodynamic function and myocardial metabolism in patients with hypertrophic cardiomyopathy. Br Heart J 56:544, 1986.

75. Lorell BH, Paulus WJ, Grossman W, et al.: Modification of abnormal left ventricular diastolic properties by nifedipine in patients with hypertrophic cardiomyopathy. Circulation 65:499, 1982.

76. Paulus WJ, Lorell BH, Craig WE, et al.: Comparison of the effects of nitroprusside and nifedipine on diastolic properties in patients with hypertrophic cardiomyopathy: altered left ventricular loading or impaired muscle inactivation? J Am Coll Cardiol 2:879, 1983.

77. Betocchi S, Cannon RO, Watson RM, et al.: Effects of sublingual nifedipine on hemodynamics and systolic and diastolic function in patients with hypertrophic cardiomyopathy. Circulation 72:1001, 1985.

78. Betocchi S, Bonow RO, Cannon RO, et al.: Relation between serum nifedipine concentration and hemodynamic effects in nonobstructive hypertrophic cardiomyopathy. Am J Cardiol 61:830, 1988.

79. Yamakado T, Okano H, Higashiyama S, et al.: Effects of nifedipine on left ventricular diastolic function in patients with asymptomatic or minimally symptomatic hypertrophic cardiomyopathy. Circulation 81:593, 1990.

80. Nagao M, Yasue H, Omote S, et al.: Diltiazem-induced decrease of exercise-elevated pulmonary arterial diastolic pressure in hypertrophic cardiomyopathy patients. Am Heart J 102:789, 1981.

81. Nagao M, Omote S, Takizawa A, Yasue H: Effect of diltiazem on left ventricular isovolumic relaxation time in patients with hypertrophic cardiomyopathy. Jpn Circ J 47:54, 1983.

82. Suwa M, Hirota Y, Kawamura K: Improvement in left ventricular diastolic function during intravenous and oral diltiazem therapy in patients with hypertrophic cardiomyopathy: an echocardiographic study. Am J Cardiol 54:1047, 1984.

83. Bonow RO, Frederick TM, Bacharach, et al.: Atrial systole and left ventricular filling hypertrophic cardiomyopathy: Effect of verapamil. Am J Cardiol 51:1386, 1983.

84. Speiser KW, Krayenbuehl HP: Reappraisal of the effect of acute beta blockade on left ventricular filling dynamics in hypertrophic obstructive cardiomyopathy. Eur Heart J 2:21, 1981.

85. Bonow RO, Vitale DF, Maron BJ, et al.: Regional left ventricular asynchrony and impaired global left ventricular filling in hypertrophic cardiomyopathy: Effect of verapamil. J Am Coll Cardiol 9:1108, 1987.

86. Pagani M, Pizzinelli P, Gussoni M, et al.: Diastolic abnormalities of hypertrophic cardiomyopathy reproduced by asynchrony of the left ventricle in conscious dogs (Abstract). J Am Coll Cardiol 1(2):641, 1983.

87. Hayashida W, Kumada T, Kohno F, et al.: Left ventricular regional relaxation and its nonuniformity in hypertrophic nonobstructive cardiomyopathy. Circulation 84:1496, 1991.

88. Bonow RO: Impaired left ventricular diastolic function in hypertrophic cardiomyopathy and coronary artery disease: Effect of calcium channel blocking agents. Am J Cardiol 55:172B, 1985.

89. Bonow RO, Dilsizian V, Rosing DR, et al.: Verapamil-induced improvement in left ventricular diastolic filling and increased exercise tolerance in patients with hypertrophic cardiomyopathy: Short- and long-term effects. Circulation 72:853, 1985.

90. Hanrath P, Schluter M, Sonntag F, et al.: Influence of verapamil therapy on left ventricular performance at rest and during exercise in hypertrophic cardiomyopathy. Am J Cardiol 52:544, 1983.

91. Rosing DR, Kent KM, Maron BM, Epstein SE: Verapamil therapy: A new approach to the pharmacologic treatment of hypertrophic cardiomyopathy. II. Effects on exercise capacity and symptomatic status. Circulation 60:1208, 1979.

92. Kaltenbach M, Hopf R, Kober G, et al.: Treatment of hypertrophic obstructive cardiomyopathy with verapamil. Br Heart J 42:35, 1979.

93. Anderson DM, Raff GL, Ports TA, et al.: Hypertrophic obstructive cardiomyopathy: effects of acute and chronic verapamil treatment on left ventricular systolic and diastolic function. Br Heart J 51:523, 1984.

94. Rosing DR, Idanpaan-Heikkila U, Maron BJ, et al.: Use of calcium-channel blocking drugs in hypertrophic cardiomyopathy. Am J Cardiol 55(Suppl):185B, 1985.

95. Iwase M, Sotobata I, Takagi S, et al.: Effects of diltiazem on left ventricular diastolic behavior in patients with hypertrophic cardiomyopathy: evaluation with exercise pulsed Doppler echocardiography. J Am Coll Cardiol 9:1099, 1987.

96. O'Gara PT, Bonow RO, Maron BJ, et al.: Myocardial perfusion abnormalities in patients with hypertrophic cardiomyopathy: Assessment with thallium-201 emission computed tomography. Circulation 76:1214, 1987.

97. Udelson JE, Bonow RO, O'Gara PT, et al.: Verapamil prevents silent myocardial perfusion abnormalities during exercise in asymptomatic patients with hypertrophic cardiomyopathy. Circulation 79:1052, 1989.

98. Udelson JE, Maron BJ, O'Gara PT, Bonow RO: Relation between left ventricular hypertrophy, filling, and perfusion in asymptomatic hypertrophic cardiomyopathy (Abstract). J Am Coll Cardiol 13:80A, 1989.

99. Dilsizian V, Smeltzer WR, Dextras R, et al.: Regional thallium abnormalities in hypertrophic cardiomyopathy: myocardial ischemia or disturbed cellular activation uptake? (Abstract). Circulation 82:III-9, 1990.

100. Rosing DR, Kent KM, Borer JS, et al.: Verapamil therapy: A new approach to the pharmacologic treatment of hypertrophic cardiomyopathy. I. Hemodynamic effects. Circulation 60:1201, 1979.

101. Rosing DR, Condit JR, Maron BJ, et al.: Verapamil therapy: A new approach to the pharmacologic treatment of hypertrophic cardiomyopathy. III. Effects of long-term administration. Am J Cardiol 48:545, 1981.

102. Kober G, Hopf R, Biamino G, et al.: Long-term treatment of hypertrophic cardiomyopathy with verapamil or propranolol in matched pairs of patients: results of a multicenter study. Z Kardiol 76(Suppl 3):113, 1987.

103. Koide T, Kakihana M, Takabatake Y, et al.: Long-term clinical effect of calcium inhibitors in hypertrophic cardiomyopathy compared to the effect of beta-blocking agents: A preliminary report with special reference to the beneficial effect of nifedipine on angina pectoris. Jpn Heart J 22:87, 1981.

104. Ruddy TD, Koilpillai C, Liu PP, et al.: Evaluation of chronic nifedipine therapy in nonobstructive hypertrophic cardiomyopathy. Circulation 66:II-24, 1982.

105. Toshima H, Koga Y, Nagata H, et al.: Comparable effects of oral diltiazem and verapamil in the treatment of hypertrophic cardiomyopathy. Double-blind crossover study. Jpn Heart J 27:701, 1986.

106. Epstein SE, Rosing DR: Verapamil: Its potential for causing serious complications in patients with hypertrophic cardiomyopathy. Circulation 64:437, 1981.

107. Perrot B, Danchin N, Terrier-de-la-Chaise A: Verapamil: A cause of sudden death in a patient with hypertrophic cardiomyopathy. Br Heart J 51:352, 1984.

108. Fedor JM, Stack RS, Pryor DB, Phillips HR: Adverse effects of nifedipine therapy on hypertrophic obstructive cardiomyopathy. Chest 83:704, 1983.

109. McKenna WJ, Harris L, Perez G, et al.: Arrhythmia in hypertrophic cardiomyopathy-II: Comparison of amiodarone and verapamil in treatment. Br Heart J 46:173, 1981.

110. Miyajima S, Aizawa Y, Suzuki K, et al.: Sustained ventricular tachycardia responsive to verapamil in patients with hypertrophic cardiomyopathy. Clinical and electrophysiological assessment of drug efficacy. Jpn Heart J 30:241, 1989.

111. Seiler C, Hess OM, Schoenbeck M, et al.: Long-term follow-up of medical versus surgical therapy for hypertrophic cardiomyopathy: A retrospective study. J Am Coll Cardiol 17:634, 1991.

112. Hopf R, Kaltenbach M: 10-year results and survival of patients with hypertrophic cardiomyopathy treated with calcium antagonists. Z Kardiol 76(Suppl 3):137, 1987.

113. Dilsizian V, Bonow RO, Epstein SE, Fananapazir L: Myocardial ischemia is a frequent cause of cardiac arrest and syncope in young patients with hypertrophic cardiomyopathy (Abstract). Circulation 82:III-9, 1990.

114. TenCate FJ, Roeland J: Progression to left ventricular dilatation in patients with hypertrophic obstructive cardiomyopathy. Am Heart J 97:762, 1979.

115. Spirito P, Maron BJ, Bonow RO: Occurrence and significance of progressive wall thinning and relative cavity dilatation in patients with hypertrophic cardiomyopathy. Am J Cardiol 60:123, 1987.

116. Spirito P, Chiarella F, Carratino L, et al.: Clinical course and prognosis of hypertrophic cardiomyopathy in an outpatient population. N Engl J Med 320:749, 1989.

Index

Note: Page numbers in italics indicate figures; page numbers followed by t indicate tables.